Cardiac Arrhythmias 2001

Springer-Verlag Italia Srl.

Cardiac Arrhythmias 2001

Edited by
Antonio Raviele

Proceedings of the
7th International Workshop
on Cardiac Arrhythmias

(Venice, 7-10 October 2001)

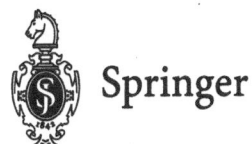 Springer

Antonio Raviele, MD
Divisione di Cardiologia
Ospedale Umberto I
Via Circonvallazione 50
I-30174 Venezia Mestre

The Editor and Authors wish to thank KNOLL FARMACEUTICI S.p.A. for the support and help in the realization of this volume

© Springer-Verlag Italia 2002
Originally published by Springer-Verlag Italia, Milan in 2002.
Softcover reprint of the hardcover 1st edition 2002

ISBN 978-88-470-2165-5   ISBN 978-88-470-2103-7 (eBook)
DOI 10.1007/978-88-470-2103-7

Library of Congress Cataloging-in-Publication Data: Applied for

Cover design: Simona Colombo, Milan
Typesetting: Graphostudio, Milan

SPIN: 10847894

Preface

The field of cardiac arrhythmias has been evolving so fast during the last years that scientific meetings are frequently necessary to present technological advances, to communicate results of relevant and innovative researches, to assess the impact of recently developed diagnostic and therapeutical tools, to discuss controversial aspects, and to reach a consensus on the most appropriate evaluation and management of specific problems. This is the main reason why in 1988 we started to organize a biannual International Workshop on Cardiac Arrhythmias. Since then many editions of the workshop have taken place and over the years the fame and popularity of the event have increased continuously.

This book contains the Proceedings of the Seventh Edition of the Workshop held in Venice at the Fondazione Giorgio Cini from the 7th to the 10th of October 2001. During the meeting all the principal aspects of the different arrhythmias, from epidemiology to physiopathology, electrogenetic mechanisms, diagnosis, prognosis, treatment, pshycological implications and economic costs have been discussed among the numerous experts and participants.

The book is divided in seven sections, each dedicated to a different topic: evaluation and management of syncope; rationale, indications and results of cardiac resynchronization therapy; risk stratification and prevention of ventricular arrhythmias and sudden death; diagnosis and therapy of atrial flutter and other supraventricular tachyarrhythmias; electrogenetic, clinical and therapeutical aspects of atrial fibrillation; non-pharmacological therapy of atrial fibrillation; technological and practical issues of pacemaker therapy. In my opinion, the book represents a comprehensive and modern overview of all pertinent aspects of cardiac arrhythmias and should be of interest not only to electrophysiologists and experts of the sector but also to general cardiologists, internists and medical students. I hope it will contribute to a better diffusion of current knowledge on cardiac arrhythmias and motivate researches in this field.

Many recognized authors have contributed to this volume. I am deeply indebted to all of them. Without their dedicated efforts and talents this book would not have been completed. I also wish to express my appreciation to Springer-Verlag and its staff, in particular Donatella Rizza, Executive Editor, for the great professionalism and meticulous attention to all the details of the editorial process. I am especially grateful to Rita Reggiani, Project Manager of

Adria Congrex, for the exceptional skill and enthusiasm in preparing the work-shop. Moreover, I would like to thank my colleagues at Umberto I Hospital, Drs. De Piccoli, Di Pede, Bonso, Gasparini, Giada, Themistoclakis, Zuin, Rigo for their support in the organization of the meeting and their scientific collabora-tion over the years.

Also the personal involvement and help of Gloria Leandro, Susanna Orbolato, Stefania Damiani and other members of the secretarial and nurse staff at my institution is sincerely appreciated. A special word of gratitude to my mentor, professor Piccolo, whose example and advices continue to represent an inestimable guidance and stimulus. Finally, my sincere thanks to my wife Carmen and my children, Francesca and Michele. Their continuous encourage-ment, assistance and patience helped me during the long hours of preparing the meeting and editing the book.

Antonio Raviele

Table of Contents

CARDIAC RESYNCHRONIZATION THERAPY: WHEN, HOW AND WHY

ATRIAL FIBRILLATION: ELECTROGENETIC, CLINICAL AND
THERAPEUTICAL ASPECTS

PACEMAKER THERAPHY: TECHNOLOGICAL AND PRACTICAL ASPECTS

List of Contributors

LECTURE

Progress in Arrhythmia and Sudden Cardiac Death Research Support

P. M. SPOONER

"It was the best of times, it was the worst of times, it was a season of darkness, it was a season of light...". This schismatic opening of Dickens's *A Tale of Two Cities*, published the same year Einthoven was born, provides perspective on the sometimes extraordinary consequences of social and political change on a range of activities spanning from law to the pursuit of science in medicine. Although Dickens had in mind contrasts between what was occurring in England and in France in the eighteenth century, his depiction of the ways progress is affected in "times of plenty" versus "times of hardship" is also one that helps in understanding how biomedical research has changed over recent decades. Dickens's view of events in his time are also instructive in understanding the impact of the various "evolutionary" and "revolutionary" changes that have occurred in how research is financed and managed, and how changes in the public's perception and willingness to participate in this process have such an enormous impact on its success. In the relatively brief period since Dickens's *Tale* was published, we have evolved from a system of relatively modest public funding of individual investigators in local or regional academic and university laboratories, to today's more richly endowed, broad-based programs that may embrace many different aspects of a problem simultaneously in both academic and large corporate research centers. Today, both nontargeted basic research and all manner of applied and clinical investigations frequently involve studies undertaken on an international scale, using tens of different disciplines and engaging the efforts of thousands of scientists and the investment of billions of private and public dollars, euros, and yen each year! Clearly the scale, medical impact, and public health implications of biomedical research have increased to the extent where it has become a very important economic aspect of today's world agenda.

Division of Heart and Vascular Diseases, National Heart, Lung, & Blood Institute, National Institutes of Health, Bethesda, Maryland, USA

*The views expressed in this discussion summary represent the personal opinions of the author and do not in any way reflect those of the National Institutes of Health or National Heart, Lung, and Blood Institute, nor do these organizations necessarily agree or disagree with positions expressed. Data cited in this article are taken exclusively from those available in the public domain

Progress in the ways biomedical science is pursued and directed has not occurred linearly over time and we have indeed gone through periods of "darkness" and of "light," rises and declines in public popularity, support, and funding. Like the political progress depicted by Dickens, however, enormous strides have in fact been achieved and new developments are occurring with unprecedented speed and efficiency. In cardiovascular medicine in particular, results have been remarkable. In the United States and other developed nations, death rates from heart disease have declined by almost 50% since just the late 1970s. Similar advances have occurred in the treatment of many forms of vascular disease and of stroke. Achievements in the basic sciences underlying these clinical developments have been even more productive, resulting for instance, in investigative technologies sufficiently powerful to allow molecular delineation of the three-billion-byte DNA sequence of now at least a half-dozen different individuals and structural determinations on amounts of protein too small to see. Impressive, and likely also impossible, without equivalent developmental changes in the ways and means by which medical research is directed, organized, and financed. This then leads to the first topic to be considered in this discussion: that is, what are these developments in project support and administration, and how, over the last few decades, have they contributed to institutional processes to facilitate and manage these activities on such a very large scale?

The federally sponsored National Institutes of Health (NIH) is the primary publicly funded means by which biomedical research is administered in the US. The NIH today is essentially a confederation of 27 separate institutes, each with its own director, staff, and scientific, medical, and political constituencies, and each has a congressionally directed mission and reporting responsibilities. Although revisions of this current structure are often discussed, major NIH operating units (Institutes and Centers) have, for much of their history, been organized on the basis of either disease issues addressed, (e.g., National Cancer Institute; National Institute of Neurological Diseases and Stroke; National Heart, Lung, and Blood Institute, etc.), or categorical resources provided, such as those developed by the National Human Genome Institute, the National Library of Medicine, or the recently constituted National Institute of Biomedical Imaging and Engineering. The activities of each of these semi-independent entities are coordinated through a "Central NIH" authority which establishes guidelines for the NIH's grant and contract program, and for the scientific evaluation of both solicited and unsolicited research proposals. NIH Central also ensures that operations of each of the different divisions are consistent and in compliance with operating policies and programmatic directives established by the Office of the President and the Department of Health and Human Services. Jointly and individually, NIH, the Institutes, and Centers also report regularly and directly to specific House and Senate Congressional Oversight and Budget committees. Although the several lines of authority and review involved might appear somewhat cumbersome, it is this participation of multiple levels of government and public involvement that helps ensure that the system remains responsive to the country's health research needs. Another factor is that, despite pressures to become involved in other health issues, NIH has remained tightly focused on its research mission, leaving regulatory, and other public health issues to other branches of the federal establishment.

The history of how the NIH evolved into its present position reflects to a considerable extent the ways the institution has responded to the US public's awareness of which health research issues are most critical, and as a result, the development of new Institutes and Centers often has followed changes in this perception. As specific problems increase in public awareness, the structure and organization of the NIH has been frequently altered to accommodate these new interests. For example, the establishment of the National Human Genome Institute and of a Center for Women's Health Studies within the office of the NIH Director were relatively recent developments that followed this pattern. Originally however, NIH began as a single "Laboratory of Hygiene" dealing with issues of infectious disease, only a half dozen years after Dickens's death (from, interestingly, cardiovascular complications of stroke) in 1870. The original NIH building continues today at the center of a burgeoning campus of more than 75 buildings employing more than 16 000 scientists, administrators, and technical specialists in Bethesda, Maryland, just outside Washington. The on-campus laboratories here, as most are aware, have garnered multiple Nobel prizes for their work in basic science. At any one time the Bethesda labs and clinics typically provide facilities for scientists from every continent, and through collaborative arrangements, now support close to a hundred different international programs. NIH's clinical research hospital, once current construction is complete, is expected to provide one of the largest facilities in the world for comprehensive, hands-on, patient-oriented investigations. Here hundreds of individuals who enroll each year assist in studies on underlying causes of disease and are treated at no personal cost. In addition to the various on-campus "intramural" research programs, each of the individual NIH institutes provides research funds for an "extramural" grants and contract program that supports research in every major research and academic center across the country. Through the "extramural" programs of each of the institutes, NIH provides most of the support for a majority of biomedical investigators working in the US today. In addition, working with the US Public Health Service, NIH provides support for comprehensive biomedical training programs that guide professional development at virtually every career stage, from predoctoral student, to lifetime clinical career investigator.

The financial assistance provided by the taxpaying US public for this enormous level of activity is, not surprisingly, considerable. NIH's present annual budget (US$ 20 300 000 000) is likely among the world's largest, although, as was indicated in a recent study, a number of nations, including several within the EU, actually devote a higher percentage of their net Gross Domestic Product to health research. Nevertheless, growth rates over the last decade are up and on the rise, and there is much enthusiasm for increasing future appropriations even further. In fact, NIH as a whole is presently 3 years into a congressionally mandated effort to *double* its annual appropriation over the 5-year period between 1999 and 2003; this following a *tripling* since 1985! Table 1 summarizes recent information on

Table 1. National Institutes of Health: actual obligations FY 1993–FY 2002 (US$ 000's)

	1993	1994	1994	1996	1997	1998	1999	2000	2001	Est. 2002
Extramural grants	8 152 984	8 611 809	8 876 764	9 366 589	10 032 594	10 800 971	12 543 618	14 366 082	16 524 329	18 678 018
% of total	79%	79%	78%	79%	79%	79%	80%	81%	81%	81%
Intramural labs	1 160 950	1 201 091	1 222 646	1 294 777	1 346 127	1 434 635	1 564 547	1 746 220	1 959 249	2 159 230
% of total	11%	11%	11%	11%	11%	11%	10%	10%	10%	9%
Research management and support	493 200	497 886	506 415	479 746	479 297	487 229	542 188	600 203	692 736	779 173
% of total	5%	5%	5%	4%	4%	4%	4%	3%	3%	3%
Other research costs	520 983	600 183	735 016	739 535	912 753	964 024	992 922	1 101 234	1 121 955	1 425 481
% of total	5%	6%	7%	6%	7%	7%	6%	6%	6%	6%
Total NIH	10 328 118	10 910 970	11 340 842	11 880 648	12 770 772	13 686 860	15 643 276	17 813 740	20 298 270	23 041 903
Annual % change	3.2%	5.6%	3.9%	4.8%	7.5%	7.2%	14.3%	13.9%	12.2%	13.5%
% of applications awared	25.0%	25%	27%	28%	31%	31%	32%	32%	31%	33%

Table 2. National Heart, Lung, and Blood Institute: actual obligations FY 1993–FY 2002 (US$ 000's)

	1993	1994	1995	1996	1997	1998	1999	2000	2001	Est. 2002
Extramural grants	1 057 100	1 117 800	1 156 500	1 194 800	1 272 800	1 357 100	1 604 600	1 837 100	2 091 338	2 339 833
% Total	87%	88%	88%	88%	89%	89%	93%	91%	91%	91%
Intramural labs	98 200	101 700	98 900	101 800	104 400	111 600	119 500	122 300	133 986	145 705
% Total	8%	8%	8%	8%	7%	7%	7%	6%	6%	6%
Research management and other support	59 400	58 400	59 500	54 800	54 600	57 600	63 900	67 900	73 776	81 891
% Total	5%	5%	5%	4%	4%	4%	4%	4%	3%	3%
Total NHLBI	1 214 600	1 277 799	1 314 799	1 351 300	1 431 700	1 526 200	1 787 896	2 027 199	2 299 000	2 567 329
Annual % change	2.1%	5.2%	2.9%	2.8%	5.9%	6.6%	17.1%	13.4%	13.4%	11.7%
% of applications awared	22%	23%	27%	25%	26%	30%	36%	35%	35%	

federal obligations for NIH since 1993 and includes information on how these sums are being used. As illustrated in the table, funding for the "off-campus" extramural research program accounts for about 80% of the total allocation. The data also show that this figure has increased by a factor of 2.3 between 1993 and the budget presently estimated for fiscal year (FY) 2002. Also reflected in the table is the fact that funding for extramural studies dwarfs expenditures on all other activities combined. Thus, funding percentages in support of research infrastructure (e.g., "other research costs") and for its administration (e.g., "research management and support") can be seen to have remained relatively constant or decreased to comparatively smaller levels during this 10-year period. Table 2 provides similar data on expenditures of the National Heart, Lung, and Blood Institute (NHLBI), and it is from this appropriation that most research on cardiovascular issues is derived. Note that in 2001 the data indicate that NHLBI received about 13% of the total dollars allocated to the NIH. Here funding between 1993 and the figure estimated for 2002 increased by a factor of 2.2, while support for extramural activities accounts for 91% of the budget. Management and infrastructure again account for relatively small percentages, with changes over recent years that reflect improvements in efficiency unexpected from an agency of this size.

There are the two principal factors that have been most powerful in justifying recent and earlier NIH budgetary expansions. These are: scientific opportunity and public health need. In the assessment of scientific opportunity, all NIH institutes have traditionally relied on the principle that it is the investigators themselves who are most knowledgeable as to where progress can be made. This is one of the chief reasons why a majority of extramural support is allocated to so-called "investigator-initiated" research proposals. In this funding category, awards are made largely on the basis of how well an investigator's peers rate his or her proposal on the basis of scientific merit. Applications are prioritized during an assessment of the following factors: (1) significance of the work; (2) the approach and its feasibility; (3) scientific innovation; (4) abilities of the investigative staff; and (5) the research environment where the project will be performed. Evaluations are conducted by multidisciplinary "study sections" of independent scientists expert in the subject being investigated. These groups thus perform the "triage" function asked of Dickens's "people's tribunals," but since revisions for proposals that are not funded are permitted, less than stellar outcomes are of considerably less dire consequence!

Public health needs are assessed through a similarly complex process with political and societal as well as scientific dimensions. These evaluations are typically directed at obtaining input from a wide range of groups and individuals within the scientific and medical communities at large, from panels of community and professional lay advisors who function much like corporate boards of directors, from various patient and disease advocacy groups, and other divisions of the federal health establishment. Another very important source governing program directions resides with the various Congressional leaders, committees, and staff who represent interests of their special constituencies. It is at this level of input that fiscal realities eventually are aligned with intellectual opportunities and competing societal interests. It is also at this level that intense "educational" or lobbying activities may occur, in which the various stake holders in the process attempt to affect outcome allocations. In the arena of cardiovascular and arrhythmia research, this most usually includes participants such as the American College of Cardiology, and North American Society of Pacing and Electrophysiology, and others acting on behalf of their memberships, as well as voluntary organizations like the American Heart or Diabetes Associations. Cross-cutting patient disease groups and broad scientific coalition leaders like Research! America often act as advocates in supporting the entire research establishment and, as in the case of the latter, play an important role in forging coalitions among competing special interests. Non-science influences also play a role. For example, the philosophical agendas of the different political parties, which may change from one administration to another, can have major effects on programs that deal with controversial issues such as the use of animals and embryonic tissues and the acceptability of new approaches like human gene therapy or cloning.

How well do such complex processes work in stimulating new medical discoveries and state-of-the-art therapies? So far the record is good, but as was also true in Dickens's contrast between an unfinished democracy and an autocratic oligarchy, answers usually depend on the state of the administering system's evolution and the scarcity of available resources. Obviously, as management improves and budgets increase, the process becomes much easier, whereas the converse is true when support levels decline – as may in fact be not too far on the horizon.

The very recent surge in NIH and NHLBI funding is a phenomenon that has occurred only since 1999 (see Tables 1 and 2), and the attendant increases in project and grant funding rates occurring as a result of this effort have in fact been extraordinary. Overall grant paylines are currently sufficient to allow funding of approximately a third of all funding requests in the NHLBI and most of the NIH Institutes. Since about two-thirds of the NHLBI budget is allocated to support studies on cardiovascular problems, the current budget represents the highest levels of expenditure ever committed to further progress in this field. The magnitude of this change can be appreciated by recalling that funding paylines have now more than doubled since just the 1980s. Certainly these early years of the new millennium are likely to be considered by future researchers as "the good old days" in cardiovascular support! And this leads us to the second topic to consider: How was this indeed "revolutionary" acceleration in progress achieved, what contributed to such increases in support, and what happens when these extraordinary increases decline?

In an era of increasing communications concerning health advances, clearly one important factor has been an increase in public and political interest in improved health. As the realist, Citizen Doctor Manette noted in Dickens's *Tale*, such profound expressions of public endorsement (and in this case expenditures) are, however, seldom associated solely with a nonspecific zeal for humanitarian causes in general, but more frequently involve expectations of increased longevity, freedom from fear and pain, as well as significant economic expectations. The question then is: How can these goals best be delivered? Another is: How will progress be maintained if and when the targeted budget doubling is achieved in 2003, and then growth rates return to "normal" levels? Once this goal of doubling is complete, previous escalating commitments will likely impose an increasing burden on the percentage of available funds to support new grants and paylines will again decrease to even below "normal" levels. The problem is similar to what Dickens saw in Paris, that is: How we can manage a "soft landing," at the back end of the revolution without threatening a "meltdown"? These impending reductions in growth rates will be especially important for new investigators just entering the system, and programs for their accommodation will require special attention during this transition.

What does this imply for programs in the cardiovascular sciences and for research on sudden cardiac death and arrhythmias in particular? Are there implications for basic and clinical research that could have a differential impact on resource-intense studies (e.g., new clinical trials) versus cell- or animal-based laboratory studies? Will recent insights in the areas of new antiarrhythmic drug and device design continue as productively as in the recent past? Although much has been achieved in developing effective therapies for both atrial and ventricular arrhythmias, these disorders are still responsible for close to half of all deaths due to cardiovascular disease. Major research challenges clearly remain: improvements in risk stratification for individual patients are clearly needed, and we are only beginning to explore the first genetic dimensions of susceptibility. While today's implantable electrical devices are surely lifesavers, they have major limitations, and it seems certain that new generations of drugs will be required to help prevent arrhythmic deaths that occur in close to half the patients receiving these technologies. Biventricular pacing appears to be a fresh start to help resolve unique deficiencies in heart failure patients, but we have much to learn regarding in whom it is most effective. SCD-HeFT will soon provide other important new answers for this population, but an important issue here will then be whether we can afford whatever that answer may be? The goal for the concluding part of this discussion will then be to raise some questions about the highest priorities in this research area and where future progress is most required. To reverse the very last words ascribed to Citizen Evrémonde at the end of Dickens's *Tale*, the problem here is *not* to focus on whether "...it is far, far better, thing we do today, than we have ever done before..." but rather to ask where it is we need to be to maintain progress in the future.

SYNCOPE: DIAGNOSTIC, PROGNOSTIC AND THERAPEUTICAL ISSUES

Syncope or Drop Attack?

R.A. KENNY

Definitions

Syncope (derived from the Greek words, *syn* meaning with and the verb *koptein* meaning "to cut", or, more appropriately in this case, "to interrupt") is a symptom, defined as a transient, self-limited loss of consciousness, usually leading to falling. The onset of syncope is relatively rapid, and the subsequent recovery is spontaneous, complete: and usually prompt [1, 3].

A drop attack is traditionally defined as a sudden fall to the ground or other lower level, without loss of consciousness, and frequently associated with difficulty in standing up after the event [4].

A fall is an event whereby a person lands on the ground or another lower level without loss of consciousness.

Reasons for Overlap

One of the reasons for overlap of these symptoms is amnesia for loss of consciousness. Up to 20% of older adults have amnesia for loss of consciousness during syncope; if episodes are unwitnessed (which is the case in 40%-60% of over-70-year-olds [5, 6]) then it may be impossible to determine from the history alone whether a fall or syncopal episode has occurred. Amnesia for loss of consciousness is a well-described phenomenon in epilepsy, and has been observed even in fit young adults during physiologically-induced situational syncope [3, 7]. It is not uncommon for older adults with locomotor problems to have difficulty standing unaided after falling. Thus, older patients with sudden non-accidental falls or with amnesia for syncope may present with symptoms consistent with "drop attacks". Gait and balance instability are well-described risk factors for falls. Falls may be more likely to occur during hypotensive

Cardiovascular Investigation Unit, University of Newcastle and Royal Victoria Infirmary, Newcastle upon Tyne, UK

episodes in older adults who have gait and balance disorders. Up to 20% of adults over 80 years have mild cognitive impairment. Falls and syncope are more common in persons with cognitive impairment and dementia, thus rendering an accurate recall of events unlikely [8-12]. In older adults the margins of these definitions are frequently blurred and symptoms of unwitnessed drop attacks or falls and syncope may be difficult to differentiate.

A number of studies have described this overlap for symptoms of falls, syncope and drop attacks. In one study of older patients with carotid sinus hypersensitivity (CSH) who only complained of recurrent falls and denied syncope, two-thirds lost consciousness during asystole induced during upright carotid sinus massage. Over 80% denied loss of consciousness on recovery, thus demonstrating amnesia for loss of consciousness [13]. Orthostatic hypotension (OH) is a well-recognized risk factor for falls and fractures. In patients who benefited from targeted treatment of OH, 30% of pre-treatment episodes were falls and 50% were falls and syncope [14]. Fall rates were also reduced after pacing in a pilot study of elderly patients who were paced for sinus node disease or atrioventricular conduction disturbances [15]. In another retrospective series of older patients who were paced for carotid sinus syndrome (CSS), two-thirds had complained of falls before pacing and a majority had not experienced falls after pacing [16].

In a small pilot study, the prevalence of CSH was significantly higher in older adults who experienced non-accidental falls (i.e., self-reported falls with no recall for events such as a slip or trip which caused the fall) compared with accidental falls, suggesting a causal association [17]. In a series of older patients (over 65 years) who attended a syncope and falls facility for the investigation of symptoms consistent with the classical description of drop attacks, cardiovascular causes were present in the majority. A diagnosis was attributed to symptoms if the symptoms were reproduced during a specific procedure or if a targeted intervention abolished the symptoms (Table 1). CSH was the attributable cause in 50% and possible attributable cause in a further 20% [18].

Syncopal episodes not only present as falls or drop attacks, but there is emerging evidence of misdiagnosis of syncope as epilepsy. This has particularly been reported for vasovagal syncope and CSS [19-21].

In a large prospective series of older adults screened in the accident and emergency department, falls were the single commonest reason for attendance – 37% over age 50 and 45% over age 65.

In order to determine, in a prospective study, whether cardiac pacing reduces the frequency of falls, fallers with cardio-inhibitory CSH were recruited to a ran-

Table 1. Diagnosis in 35 cases of drop attacks (aged > 65 years) [18]

	Associated diagnosis	Attributable diagnosis
Carotid sinus syndrome	24	18
Orthostatic hypotension	10	5
Vasovagal syncope	4	1
Gait and visual defect	1	1
Unexplained	3	10

domized controlled trial. Consecutive older patients (> 50 years) attending an accident and emergency facility because of a non-accidental fall were randomized to dual-chamber pacemaker implant (paced patients) or standard treatment (controls). The primary outcome was the number of falls during 1 year of follow-up.

We screened 71 299 adult attendees over age 50. Thirty-seven per cent attended because of a fall. Fourteen per cent (3384) had non-accidental falls, of whom 1630 agreed to further cardiovascular assessment; of these, 262 (16%) had cardio-inhibitory CSH, 175 eligible patients (mean age 73 ± 10 years, 60% female) were randomized to the trial: pacemaker 87, controls 88 (see Table 2). Falls (without loss of consciousness) were reduced by two-thirds: the controls reported 669 falls (mean 9.3, range 0-89) and paced patients 216 falls (mean 4.1, range 0-29). Thus, paced patients were significantly less likely to fall (OR, 0.42; 95% CI, 0.23-0.75) than controls. Injurious events were also reduced by 70% (202 in controls compared to 61 in paced patients). Syncopal events were also reduced during the follow-up period but there were much fewer syncopal events than falls – 28 episodes in paced patients and 47 in controls.

The results of this trial suggest a strong association between non-accidental falls and cardio-inhibitory CSS. Pacing is already recommended for recurrent syncope in these patients. In the present study, pacing also significantly reduced falls during 1 year of follow-up in patients who had single or recurrent falls as the presenting symptom. These patients would not usually be referred for cardiovascular assessment. Assessment of CSH should be considered in all older adults who have non-accidental falls.

In summary, falls and syncope are the commonest reasons for adults to attend the accident and emergency department. Of these, one-third are non-accidental falls or "drop attacks", one-sixth of these fallers have cardio-inhibitory CSS which, if paced, will reduce subsequent falls by 70% – more than any other single intervention for falls to date. The prevalence of CSS in fallers with "drop attacks" or unexplained falls also increased with advancing years – one in 10 of over-50-year-olds to one in six of over-65-year-olds and one in four of over-75-year-olds. Screening and appropriate interventions for falls will have enormous health care and cost implications.

Another recent series [22] (Table 3) compared the clinical characteristics of 34 patients with CSS who had presented with syncope with 34 patients who had presented with non-accidental falls or "drop attacks". The mean age of patients was 75 years, and symptoms had been present for on average 20 months. Over one-third had sustained an injury during events. However, a number of charac-

Table 2. Outcome in randomized controlled trial of pacing in cardio-inhibitory CSS

Variable	Control	Pacemaker
All events	746	238
Falls	699	216
Syncope	47	22
Injury	198	58
Fracture	4	3

(OR, 0.42; CI, 0.23-0.75)

Table 3. Results

	Drop attacks (n = 34)	Syncope (n = 34)	p
Mean age (SD)	76.8 (9)	74.7 (9)	0.26
Sex	27 (79%) F	16 (47%) F	0.006
Soft tissue injury	9 (26%)	19 (56%)	0.02
Mean no. of episodes in 6 months	7 (median 6)	3 (median 3)	0.03
Mean symptom duration	13 months	28 months	0.009
Initial CSM +ve upright	20 (59%)	9 (26%)	0.009
Loss of consciousness during carotid sinus massage	22 (55%)	15 (44%)	0.09
Amnesia for loss of consciousness	21 (95% of LOC)	4 (27% of LOC)	0.0006

teristics were different for the two groups. Patients presenting with drop attacks were more likely to be female, and have more frequent symptoms over a shorter period of time before presentation.

Both groups exhibited similar rates of loss of consciousness during carotid sinus massage-induced asystole, but almost all of the "drop attack" group had amnesia for loss of consciousness compared with a small minority of the syncopal group. There was no overt difference in the cognitive status of the groups.

Causes

The commonest causes of syncope and cardiovascular causes of falls or "drop attacks" in older adults are orthostatic hypotension, carotid sinus hypersensitivity, vasovagal syncope and cardiac arrhythmias. The prevalence of orthostatic hypotension in older adults varies from 6% in the community-dwelling elderly to 33% in elderly hospital inpatients. Orthostatic hypotension is an attributable cause of syncope in 20%-30% of older patients. In symptomatic patients, up to 25% have "age-related" orthostatic hypotension. In the remainder, orthostatic hypotension is predominantly due to culprit medications, primary autonomic failure, secondary autonomic failure (diabetes), Parkinson's disease and multisystemic atrophy [23-27]. Carotid sinus hypersensitivity is an age-related diagnosis. Rare before the age of 40, the prevalence increases with advancing years and with cardiovascular, cerebrovascular and neurodegenerative comorbidity [28-30]. Cardio-inhibitory CSS has been considered in recent reports to be an attributable cause of symptoms in up to 20% of older adults who have syncope; further study is ongoing to better assess the true frequency, but it is fair to point out that it is likely to be more common than previously thought. CSS of predominantly the vasodepressor form is equally prevalent, but its potential role in causing syncope in this population is much less certain [5, 17].

Up to 15% of syncope in older adults is vasovagal [6]. In over half, episodes are related to the prescription of cardiovascular medications. The pattern of blood pressure and heart rate responses during testing is similar to that described in younger patients, although patterns reflecting dysautonomia are more common in drug-related episodes [31]. Up to 20% of syncope in older patients is due to cardiac arrhythmia [32, 33]. Assessment and management of brady-and tachyarrhythmias is as for younger adults.

Conclusions

The symptoms of syncope/falls/drop attack are not necessarily distinct entities in older patients. At present, the majority of patients with cardiovascular causes of falls and drop attacks are rarely captured by cardiology practice. Yet there is evidence that targeted cardiovascular interventions are of great benefit to these patients. The challenge is to develop care pathways within European cultures that screen and treat those older patients currently not receiving cardiac assessment and intervention.

References

1. Rossen R, Kabat H, Anderson JP (1943) Acute arrest of cerebral circulation in man. Arch Neurol Psychiatr 50:510-528
2. Fenton AM, Hammill SC, Rea RF et al (2000) Vasovagal syncope. Ann Intern Med 133:714-725
3. Hoefnagels WAJ, Padberg GW, Overweg J et al (1991) Transient loss of consciousness: the value of the history for distinguishing seizure from syncope. J Neurol 238:39-43
4. Dey AB, Kenny RA (1997) Drop attacks in the elderly revisited. Qu J Med 90:1-3
5. McIntosh SJ, Lawson J, Kenny RA (1993) Clinical characteristics of vasodepressor, cardioinhibitory, and mixed carotid sinus syndrome in the elderly. Am J Med 95:203-208
6. McIntosh SJ, Lawson J, Kenny RA (1994) Heart rate and blood pressure responses to carotid sinus massage in healthy elderly subjects. Age Ageing 23:57-61
7. Lempert T, Bauer M, Schmidt D (1994) Syncope: a videometric analysis of 56 episodes of transient cerebral hypoxia. Ann Neurol 36:233-237
8. Cummings SR, Nevitt MC, Kidd S (1988) Forgetting falls: the limited accuracy of recall of falls in the elderly. J Am Geriatr Soc 36:613-616
9. Nevitt MC, Cummings SR, Kidd S (1989) Risk factors for recurrent non syncopal falls. A prospective study. J Am Med Assoc 261:2663-2667
10. Robbins AS, Rubenstein LZ, Josephson KT (1989) Predictors of falls among elderly people. Results of two population-based studies. Arch Intern Med 149:1628-1631
11. Tinnetti ME, Williams TF, Mayewski R (1986) Fall risk index for elderly patients based on number of chronic disabilities. Am J Med 80:429-451
12. Shaw FE, Kenny RA (1997) The overlap between syncope and falls in the elderly. Postgrad Med J 73:635-639

13. Kenny RA, Traynor G (1991) Carotid sinus syndrome - clinical characteristics in elderly patients. Age Ageing 91:669-675
14. Ward C, Kenny RA (1996) Reproducibility of orthostatic hypotension in the elderly. Am J Med 100:418-422
15. Seifer C, Cox J, Bexton RS, Kenny RA (2001) Falls and bradyarrhythmic disorders. J Amer Geriatr Soc (in press)
16. Crilley JG, Herd B, Khurana CS et al (1997) Permanent cardiac pacing in elderly patients with recurrent falls, dizziness and syncope, and a hypersensitive cardioinhibitory reflex. Postgrad Med J 73:415-418
17. Richardson DA, Bexton RS, Shaw FE, Kenny RA (1997) Prevalence of cardioinhibitory carotid sinus hypersensitivity in patients 50 years or over presenting to the accident and emergency department with "unexplained" or "recurrent" falls. Pacing Clin Electrophysiol 20:820-823
18. Dey AB, Stout NR, Kenny RA (1996) Cardiovascular syncope is the commonest cause of drop attacks in the older patient. Eur Card Pacing Elect 2:84-88
19. Zaidi A, Cotter L, Fitzpatrick A (1997) Head-up tilt testing has a place in distinguishing certain conditions from epilepsy. Br Med J 314:1048
20. Zaidi A, Clough P, Scheepers B, Fitzpatrick A (1998) Treatment resistant epilepsy or convulsive syncope? Br Med J 317:869-870
21. Parry SW, Kenny RA (2001) Vasovagal syncope masquerading as unexplained falls in an older patient. Can J Cardiol (in press)
22. Parry SW, Baptist M, Kenny RA (2000) Clinical characteristics in carotid sinus syndrome presenting with drop attacks versus syncope: implications for investigation and management of older subjects with atypical presentations of cardiovascular syncope. Heart 83(Suppl 1):18, A47
23. Palmer KT (1983) Studies into postural hypotension in elderly patients. N Z Med J 96:43-45
24. Masaki KH, Schatz IJ, Burchfiel CM et al (1998) Orthostatic hypotension predicts mortality in elderly men: the Honolulu Heart program. Circulation 98:2290-2295
25. Tonkin A, Wing L (1994) Effects of age and isolated systolic hypertension on cardiovascular reflexes. Hypertension 12:1083-1088
26. Tonkin A, Wing LMH, Morris MJ, Kapoor V (1991) Afferent baroreflex dysfunction and age-related orthostatic hypotension. Clin Sci 81:531-538
27. Strangaard S (1976) Autoregulation of cerebral blood flow in hypertensive patients: the modifying influence of prolonged antihypertensive treatment on the tolerance of acute drug induced hypotension. Circulation 53:720-729
28. Brignole M, Gigli G, Altomonte F et al (1985) The cardioinhibitory reflex evoked by carotid sinus stimulation in normal and in patients with cardiovascular disorders. G Ital Cardiol 15:514- 519
29. Brown KA, Maloney JA, Smith HC et al (1980) Carotid sinus reflex in patients undergoing coronary angiography: relationship of degree and location of coronary artery disease to response to carotid sinus massage. Circulation 62:697-703
30. Brignole M, Menozzi C, Gianfranchi L et al (1991) Carotid sinus massage, eyeball compression and head-up tilt test in patients with syncope of uncertain origin and in healthy control subjects. Am Heart J 122:1644-1651
31. Brignole M, Menozzi C, Del Rosso A et al (2000) New classification of haemodynamics of vasovagal syncope: beyond the VASIS classification. Analysis of the pre-syncopal phase of the tilt test without and with nitroglycerin challenge. Europace 2:66-76
32. Kapoor WN (1991) Diagnostic evaluation of syncope. Am J Med 90:91-106
33. Lipsitz LA, Wei JY, Rowe JW (1985) Syncope in an elderly, institutionalised population: prevalence, incidence and associated risk. Qu J Med 55:45-54

Syncope or Seizures: What Have We Learned from Electrocardiographic Monitoring?

L. Bergfeldt

Syncope is a symptom defined as "a transient, self-limited loss of consciousness, usually leading to falling" [1]. The onset of syncope is relatively rapid, and the subsequent recovery is spontaneous, complete and usually prompt. The underlying mechanism is a transient global cerebral hypoperfusion. *Seizure* is, according to the same document, synonymous with *an epileptic fit*, and "...whatever its immediate or remote cause, an epileptic attack is the manifestation of a paroxysmal discharge of abnormal rhythms in some part of the brain" [2]. In order to differentiate between the two, simultaneous electroencephalographic (EEG) and electrocardiographic (ECG) recording with multiple scalp and chest electrodes is required, a situation that is rarely fulfilled.

Involuntary movements (myoclonic jerks) might accompany syncope [3], and (wrongly) lead to a suspicion of a seizure disorder. In contrast to seizure disorders, myoclonic jerks in syncope, however, follow upon the initial phase with loss of muscular tone, leading to a fall, when cerebral hypoperfusion occurs with the patient in the upright position. During the initial evaluation of a patient with a transient loss of consciousness, it is important to consider this sequence of events in order to avoid a misdiagnosis of syncope as an epileptic fit. This is important for several reasons, discussed more in detail below: 1) syncope with a cardiac cause, which generally has a severe prognosis [1] if not correctly attended to, may be overlooked; 2) treatment with anti-epileptic drugs might not only fail to relieve symptoms but might also be harmful in the presence of overt or latent cardiac conduction system abnormalities; 3) the psychological and socio-economic consequences of a wrong diagnosis might be severe.

In one article the authors reported on 12 patients in whom an initial diagnosis of seizure disorder proved wrong 0.5-20 years after the initial evaluation [4]. The correct diagnosis was obtained from Holter monitoring ($n = 2$), loop recorder ($n = 1$), loop recorder plus exercise testing ($n = 1$), tilt table test ($n = 4$), ECG ($n = 2$), ECG plus invasive electrophysiologic study ($n = 1$) and ECG plus tilt testing ($n = 1$). Five patients were diagnosed as having neurally-medi-

Electrophysiology and Arrhythmia Service, Department of Cardiology, Karolinska Hospital, Stockholm, Sweden

ated reflex syncope (two with asystole), four of whom received pharmacological therapy, while the fifth patient received drugs plus a pacemaker. Four patients had torsade de pointes polymorphic ventricular tachycardia, and all received pharmacological therapy, in one supplemented by an implantable cardioverter defibrillator (ICD). Two patients received a pacemaker because of asystole and sinus arrests, respectively, and the remaining patient underwent a successful radiofrequency ablation because of a paroxysmal supraventricular tachycardia. Reference was also made to other reports on patients with the long QT syndrome, presenting with symptoms interpreted as caused by a seizure disorder. The authors concluded their report by suggesting that both tilt testing and prolonged ambulatory ECG recording (with Holter or loop recorders) should be "...considered in patients with presumed seizures and negative or nonspecific EEGs, especially when accompanied by atypical seizure-like symptoms (such as nausea, warmth, lightheadedness, palpitations, diaphoresis, or pallor) and a failure to respond to anticonvulsive therapy".

Some antiepileptic drugs have significant ion channel effects, including effects on sodium, potassium and calcium channels. Typical examples are phenytoin and carbamazepine, which have negative dromotropic and chronotropic effects via sodium and potassium channel-blocking properties. Similar properties in procainamide, disopyramide and ajmaline are utilized for provocation of latent His-Purkinje system defects (transient or impending high-degree AV block) [5]. However, and especially documented for carbamazepine [6, 7], if used inadequately in patients with overt or latent cardiac conduction system disorders, such therapy might not only lead to bradycardia/asystole and syncope, misinterpreted as inefficient seizure therapy, but also put patients at a risk for sudden cardiac death. The effects on the normal conduction system is, however, minimal [7, 8].

It was also pointed out that cardiac syncope and seizure disorders co-exist [6], which raises a question as to whether the central nervous system activities during seizure might lead to severe arrhythmias. This question was pursued also in one study in attempt to shed light on the increased risk for sudden death in "young" patients with epilepsy. Thus, simultaneous 20-24 h ECG and EEG recording was performed in 338 consecutive patients with epilepsy [9]. In 17 patients there were 56 episodes of electrographic seizures (both focal and generalized) lasting at least 10 s. First, there was sinus tachycardia during seizures, but no ventricular arrhythmias or conduction defects. Second, although 18 patients were classified as having "high-risk cardiac arrhythmias", the occurrence of arrhythmias was not increased compared to what has been reported in a "general" population with the same age structure. In addition, and according to this author's personal opinion, the listed arrhythmias in those 18 patients were not of a malignant character.

So, what we have learned from electrocardiographic monitoring in syncope or seizure?

1. That torsade de pointes ventricular tachycardia as part of the long QT syndrome, and asystole (whether or not part of a neurally-mediated reflex syncope) might cause syncope with myoclonic jerks, which should not immediately raise the suspicion of a seizure disorder.

2. That spontaneously resolving seizures rarely, if ever, cause arrhythmias other than sinus tachycardia.
3. That antiepileptic drug therapy with ion channel-active substances might provoke clinically significant bradycardia and syncope in susceptible patients (i.e. those with latent or overt cardiac conduction system abnormalities), with or without concomitant seizure disorders.

References

1. Brignole M, Alboni P, Benditt D et al (2001) Task Force report. Guidelines on management (diagnosis and treatment) of syncope. Eur Heart J 22:1256-1306
2. Bannister R (1973) Brain's clinical neurology. Oxford Medical, London, New York, Delhi, p 142
3. Lempert T, Bauer M, Schmidt D (1994) Syncope: a videometric analysis of 56 episodes of transient cerebral hypoxia. Ann Neurol 36:233-237
4. Linzer M, Grubb BP, Ho S et al (1994) Cardiovascular causes of loss of consciousness in patients with presumed epilepsy: a cause of the increased sudden death rate in people with epilepsy? Am J Med 96:146-154
5. Englund A, Bergfeldt L, Rosenqvist M (1998) Pharmacological stress-testing of the His-Purkinje system in patients with bifascicular block. Pacing Clin Electrophysiol 21:1979-1987
6. Kennebäck G, Bergfeldt L, Vallin H et al (1991) Electrophysiologic effects and clinical hazards of carbamazepine treatment for neurologic disorders in patients with abnormalities of the cardiac conduction system. Am Heart J 121:1421-1429
7. Kennebäck G, Bergfeldt L, Tomson T et al (1992) Carbamazepine-induced bradycardia - a problem in general or only in susceptible patients? A 24 h long-term electrocardiogram study. Epilepsy Res 13:141-145
8. Kennebäck G, Bergfeldt L, Tomson T (1995) Electrophysiological evaluation of the sodium-channel blocker carbamazepine in healthy human subjects. Cardiovasc Drugs Ther 9:709-714
9. Keilson MJ, Hauser A, Magrill JP, Goldman M (1987) ECG abnormalities in patients with epilepsy. Neurology 37:1624-1626

Postprandial Hypotension: Pathophysiology and Management

L.A. LIPSITZ

Over the past two decades, postprandial hypotension (PPH) has become recognized as a common problem among elderly people and patients with autonomic insufficiency, Parkinson's Disease, diabetes mellitus, and renal failure [1]. Defined as a 20 mmHg or greater decline in systolic blood pressure within 2 h of the start of a meal, PPH has been reported to occur in 24% [2] to 36% [3] of nursing-home residents, and in 23% of elderly persons admitted to a geriatric hospital with syncope or falls [4]. Meal-related hypotension is particularly common among elderly people with hypertension and is more prevalent than orthostatic hypotension in the elderly population.

Clinical Consequences

Although PPH is usually asymptomatic, it may have serious clinical consequences. Meal-related declines in blood pressure of sufficient magnitude to reduce cerebral perfusion have been found in 8% of nursing-home residents presenting with syncope [5], and 50% of elderly patients recruited for a study of unexplained syncope [6]. In a large long-term care facility, the decrease in systolic blood pressure after a meal was associated with falls, syncope, new coronary events, new stroke, and total mortality [2]. Large postprandial blood pressure declines have been reported in elderly patients with angina pectoris or transient ischemic attacks that resolved when pressure returned to normal [3, 7]. In a recent study of hospitalized hypertensive patients, the prevalence of asymptomatic lacunar infarctions and leukoaraiosis on magnetic resonance imaging of the brain was significantly correlated with the mean reduction of systolic blood pressure within 2 h after a meal [8]. It is currently not clear whether postprandial hypotension is a cause or effect of cerebrovascular disease. However, the observation by transcranial Doppler ultrasonography that middle cerebral artery cerebral vascular resistance appears to increase following a meal in elderly patients with PPH suggests that these patients may develop cerebral ischemia during periods of marked blood pressure decline [9].

Hebrew Rehabilitation Center for Aged, Boston, Massachusetts, USA

Pathophysiologic Mechanisms

The mechanisms of PPH are not fully understood and may differ depending on whether meal-associated blood pressure reduction is associated with aging, hypertension, or frank autonomic failure. Our current understanding of the pathophysiology of this phenomenon is summarized in Fig. 1.

After eating in healthy humans of all ages, there is a decline in splanchnic vascular resistance, an increase in superior mesenteric artery blood flow [10, 11], and approximately a 20% increase in bowel blood volume [12]. The consequent reduction in venous return to the heart activates cardiopulmonary, aortic, and carotid baroreceptors, resulting in an increase in central sympathetic outflow and reduction in cardiovagal activity [13]. This is manifested by an increase in plasma norepinephrine levels [14-16] and muscle sympathetic nerve activity [17] and a reduction in high frequency heart rate variability [13]. As a result, heart rate and cardiac output increase, and systemic vascular resistance is returned to baseline, thus maintaining a relatively stable arterial pressure.

Elderly subjects and autonomic failure patients with PPH have been shown to have blunted cardioacceleratory and vascular responses to meal ingestion [12]. As a result, they fail to maintain arterial pressure. It appears as though the stimulus for these hemodynamic adjustments is unaltered, since splanchnic blood volume is unaffected by aging or autonomic failure [11, 12]. However,

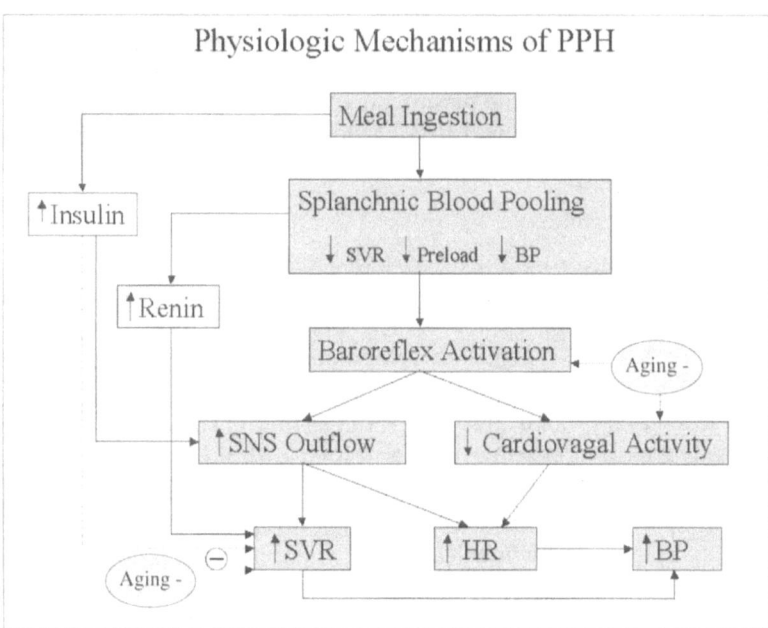

Fig. 1. Physiologic mechanisms of postprandial hypotension

cardioacceleratory and vasoconstrictor responses may be attenuated in these patients as a result of inadequate sympathetic outflow from the central nervous system [12, 18, 19]. Furthermore, aging has been shown to impair cardiac β-adrenergic and vascular α-adrenergic responses to sympathetic activity [20]. Finally, age-related impairments in ventricular diastolic filling may diminish stroke volume when preload is reduced by meal digestion [21].

A variety of hormones and vasoactive peptides released following meal ingestion have been investigated as potential mediators of PPH [1]. Measurements of pre- and postprandial levels of vasoactive intestinal polypeptide, neurotensin, substance P, cholecystokinin, gastrin, and motilin in subjects with and without PPH, have failed to demonstrate an etiologic role for these peptides. In healthy subjects, plasma renin levels and renin activity also increase after a high carbohydrate meal [13], possibly preventing hypotension by increasing vascular resistance and intravascular volume. However, renin responses to meal ingestion in subjects with PPH has not been adequately studied.

In contrast to the vasoactive peptides discussed above, the hormone insulin has been the subject of numerous studies [1]. The observation that blood pressure falls after the ingestion of glucose or a high carbohydrate meal, but not after fructose or a high fat meal, suggests that insulin may play an important role in PPH [11, 15, 16, 22, 23]. Insulin is known to have vasodilatory and sympathoexcitatory effects [1]. When a high-fat meal was given with insulin infusion to reproduce the plasma insulin concentration associated with isocaloric carbohydrate ingestion, blood pressure fell to the same extent as it did with carbohydrate [11]. Also, after the high-carbohydrate or high-fat plus insulin meals, calf vascular resistance failed to increase as it did after the high-fat meal alone. There was no difference in the plasma norepinephrine response to these three meals. These data lend support to a vasodepressor action of insulin in the pathogenesis of PPH.

Diagnostic Evaluation

Any patient with a fall, syncope, or symptoms of dizziness or lightedheadedness within 2 h of eating a meal should be evaluated for PPH. Although it is advisable to measure blood pressure in the sitting position before, and at 15 min intervals after a standardized 400 kcal high-carbohydrate meal (70-80% of calories from carbohydrate) [1], this is not always practical in the clinical setting. Instead, patients can be asked to bring a meal, similar to that associated with their symptoms, to the medical office, where blood pressure can be measured before and at least 30 and 60 min after they eat it. Alternatively, blood pressure can be measured by patients in their homes using a portable automated device, or throughout the day using ambulatory blood pressure monitoring.

If PPH is detected in an elderly patient, it is not appropriate to attribute it to age. Healthy, ambulatory elders without hypertension or cardiovascular disease do not develop PPH [13]. On the other hand, frail, sedentary, hypertensive elderly people with multiple diseases and medications are most vulnerable. Therefore, a careful history of diseases and medications is essential. Alcohol ingestion with the meal should also be considered. The history should inquire about autonomic symptoms, such as poor night vision, orthostatic intolerance, diarrhea, constipation, urinary incontinence, impotence, and abnormal sweating, which are clues to the presence of autonomic insufficiency. The physical examination should look for evidence of cerebrovascular disease, structural heart disease, Parkinson's disease, peripheral neuropathy, and diseases associated with autonomic failure. Formal autonomic testing may be required to confirm the presence of autonomic dysfunction.

Since the patient with PPH may be experiencing cardiac ischemia as a cause or result of blood pressure reduction, an electrocardiogram should be obtained, preferably after a meal. If autonomic failure is suspected, blood tests to detect anemia, diabetes, and dysproteinemias such as amyloidosis should be obtained, and imaging studies to look for multiple cerebral infarctions or occult malignancies should be considered. Dumping syndrome, which may also cause PPH, can be diagnosed by the presence of rapid gastric emptying on scintigraphy.

Management

Nonpharmacologic

Often, meal-related declines in blood pressure can be prevented by discontinuing hypotensive medications or avoiding their administration before meals. In patients with heart failure and preserved systolic function, the withdrawal of furosemide ameliorates PPH, possibly by improving diastolic ventricular filling [21].

Adjustments in the composition or size of meals may also help, although this has not been rigorously studied. Large carbohydrate meals and alcohol ingestion with meals should be avoided. Instead, multiple small meals, composed primarily of fat and protein, can be given throughout the day. Food temperature might also influence postprandial blood pressure. One study found that a warm glucose solution reduced blood pressure in elderly subjects, while a cold glucose solution increased it [24].

In frail elderly nursing home residents with PPH, there is evidence that walking exercise 35 min after the start of a meal can restore blood pressure to its pre-meal value. Curiously, these patients do not develop orthostatic hypotension when they stand up after a meal. However, when they stop walking and resume sitting, pressure falls to the same level that it would be without exercise [25]. Therefore, patients should avoid prolonged sitting after meals. They should be encouraged to walk if they can do so without hypotension, or lie semi-recumbent for 90 min after a meal.

In patients with end-stage renal failure who have PPH, meals should not be given during dialysis. All patients with meal-related hypotension should take adequate fluids to maintain intravascular volume, and avoid diuretics if possible.

Pharmacologic

If the above measures are ineffective, pharmacologic therapy should be considered. However, this can be quite challenging. Currently accepted pharmacologic approaches are summarized in Table 1.

Table 1. Pharmacologic Approaches to the Treatment of PPH

Caffeine	250 mg (two cups of brewed coffee) before breakfast
Octreotide	50 μg subcutaneously, 30 min before each meal
Indomethacin	25-50 mg orally, three times a day (may cause confusion)
Fludrocortisone	0.1-1.0 mg orally once daily (watch for heart failure, supine hypertension, and hypokalemia)
Midodrine	2.5-10 mg orally, three times a day (watch for supine hypertension)

The role of caffeine is controversial, but it is useful in some patients. Unfortunately, many patients develop tolerance, especially if it is given more than once a day. In four patients with multiple systems atrophy, vasopressin was shown to prevent hypotension when infused intravenously for 60 min following oral glucose [18]. In a randomized, double-blind, placebo-controlled study of 11 patients with autonomic failure, oral 3,4-DL-threo-dihydroxyphenylserine, a norepinephrine precursor, attenuated the postprandial fall in blood pressure [26]. In a recent study, guar gum was shown to reduce PPH in 10 elderly subjects, possibly by slowing gastric emptying and glucose absorption [27]. Although these treatments are promising, they are not approved for general use.

The widely observed relationship between hypertension and PPH, and known association between hypertension and impaired blood pressure regulation, raises the question of whether antihypertensive therapy will improve or worsen PPH. In two previous studies of elderly patients with and without cardiovascular disease, blood pressure lowering with either isosorbide dinitrate, nicardipine, nitrendipine, or hydrochlorothiazide all ameliorated PPH [28, 29]. Therefore, the judicious treatment of hypertension may actually improve cardiovascular adaptation to a meal.

Acknowledgments. Supported in part by Grant No. AG04390 from the National Institute on Aging, US Public Health Service, Bethesda, MD, USA. Dr Lipsitz holds the Irving and Edyth S. Usen and Family Chair in Geriatric Medicine at the Hebrew Rehabilitation Center for the Aged.

References

1. Jansen RWMM, Lipsitz LA (1995) Postprandial hypotension: epidemiology, pathophysiology, and clinical management. Ann Intern Med 122:286-295
2. Aronow WS, Ahn C (1994) Postprandial hypotension in 499 elderly persons in a long-term health care facility. J Amer Geriatr Soc 42:930
3. Vaitkevicius PV, Esserwein DM, Maynard AK et al (1991) Frequency and importance of postprandial blood pressure reduction in elderly nursing-home patients. Ann Intern Med 115:865
4. Puisieux F, Bulckaen, Fauchais AL et al (2000) Ambulatory blood pressure monitoring and postprandial hypotension in elderly persons with falls or syncope. J Gerontol 55A:M535
5. Lipsitz LA, Pluchino FC, Wei JY, Rowe JW (1986) Syncope in institutionalized elderly: the impact of multiple pathological conditions and situational stress. J Chron Dis 39:619
6. Jansen RWMM, Connelly CM, Kelley-Gagnon MM et al (1995) Postprandial hypotension in elderly patients with unexplained syncope. Arch Int Med 155:945-952
7. Kamata T, Yokota T, Jurukawa T, Tsukagoshi H (1994) Cerebral ischemic attack caused by postprandial hypotension. Stroke 25:511-513
8. Kohara K, Jiang Y, Igase M et al (1999) Postprandial hypotension is associated with asymptomatic cerebrovascular damage in essential hypertensive patients. Hypertension 33:565-568
9. Krajewski A, Freeman R, Ruthazer R et al (1993) Transcranial Doppler assessment of the cerebral circulation during postprandial hypotension in the elderly. J Amer Geriatr Soc 41:19-24
10. Kooner JS, Raimbach S, Watson L et al (1989) Relationship between splanchnic vasodilation and postprandial hypotension in patients with primary autonomic failure. J Hypertension 7[Suppl 6]:S40
11. Kearney MT, Cowley AJ, Stubbs TA et al (1988) Depressor action of insulin on skeletal muscle vasculature: a novel mechanism for postprandial hypotension in the elderly. J Am Coll Cardiol 31:209
12. Lipsitz LA, Ryan SM, Parker JA et al (1993) Hemodynamic and autonomic nervous system responses to mixed meal ingestion in healthy young and old subjects and dysautonomic patients with postprandial hypotension. Circulation 87:391
13. Oberman AS, Gagnon MM, Kiely DK et al (2000) Autonomic and neurohumoral control of postprandial blood pressure in healthy aging. J Gerontol 55A:M477-M483
14. Lipsitz LA, Pluchino FC, Wei JW et al (1986) Cardiovascular and norepinephrine responses after meal consumption in elderly (older than 75 years) persons with postprandial hypotension and syncope. Am J Cardiol 58:810
15. Jansen RWMM, Penterman JM, van Lier HJJ, Hoefnagels WHL (1987) Blood pressure reduction after oral glucose loading and its relation to age, blood pressure and insulin. Am J Cardiol 60:1087
16. Sidery MB, Cowley AJ, MacDonald IA (1993) Cardiovascular responses to a high-fat and a high-carbohydrate meal in healthy elderly subjects. Clin Sci 84:263
17. Fagius J, Berne C (1994) Increase in muscle nerve sympathetic activity in humans after food intake. Clin Sci 86:159
18. Hakusui S, Sugiyama Y, Iwase S et al (1991) Postprandial hypotension: microneurographic analysis and treatment with vasopressin. Neurology 41:712
19. Fagius J, Ellerfelt K, Lithell H, Berne C (1996) Increase in muscle nerve sympathetic activity after glucose intake is blunted in the elderly. Clin Autonom Res 6:195

20. Hogikyan RV, Supiano MA (1994) Arterial α-adrenergic responsiveness is decreased and SNS activity is increased in older humans. Am J Physiol 266:E717-E724

21. Van Kraaij DJW, Jansen RWMM, Bouwels LHR, Hoefnagels WHL (1999) Furosemide withdrawal improves postprandial hypotension in elderly patients with heart failure and preserved left ventricular systolic function. Arch Int Med 159:1599

22. Potter JF, Heseltine D, Hartley G (1989) Effects of meal composition on the postprandial blood pressure, catecholamine and insulin changes in elderly subjects. Clin Sci 77:265-272

23. Jansen RWMM, Peeters TL, van Lier HJJ, Hoefnagels WHL (1990) The effect of oral glucose, protein, fat and water loading on blood pressure and the gastrointestinal peptides VIPO and somatostatin in hypertensive elderly subjects. Eur J Clin Invest 20:192

24. Kuipers HMM, Jansen RWMM, Peeters TL, Hoefnagels WHL (1991) The influence of food temperature on postprandial blood pressure reduction and its relation to substance-P in healthy elderly subjects. JAGS 38:181

25. Oberman AS, Harada RK, Gagnon MM et al (1999) Effects of postprandial walking exercise on meal-related hypotension in frail elderly patients. Am J Cardiol 84:1130-1132

26. Freeman R, Young J, Landsberg L, Lipsitz L (1996) The treatment of postprandial hypotension in autonomic failure with 3,4-DL-threo-dihydroxyphenylserine. Neurology 47:1414-1417

27. Jones KL, MacIntosh C, Su Y-C et al (2001) Guar gum reduces postprandial hypotension in older people. JAGS 49:162-167

28. Jansen RWMM, van Lier HJJ, Hoefnagels WHL (1988) Effects of nitrendipine and hydrochlorothiazide on postprandial blood pressure reduction and carbohydrate metabolism in hypertensive patients over 70 years of age. J Cardiol Pharmacol 12[Suppl 4]:S59-S63

29. Connelly CM, Waksmonski C, Gagnon MM, Lipsitz LA (1995) Effects of isosorbide dinitrate and nicardipine hydrochloride on postprandial blood pressure in elderly patients with stable angina pectoris or healed myocardial infarction. Am J Cardiol 75:291-293

Psychogenic Syncope: How Frequent Is It?

F. Giada[1], A. Raviele[1], I. Silvestri[2], P. G. Nicotera[2], A. Rossillo[1], G. Leandro[1] and C. Ravenna[2]

Introduction

A high prevalence of psychiatric disorders such as anxiety, depression, and somatization disorders has been reported in patients with syncope of unknown origin [1-3]. Psychiatric disturbances are most frequently encountered in young female patients with a history of numerous syncopal episodes. Although it is well known that vasovagal syncope may be triggered by mental and emotional stress, data on the prevalence of psychiatric disorders in patients with vasovagal syncope, and on their quality of life, are somewhat scant and incomplete [4, 5].

The aim of the present study was to evaluate the prevalence of psychiatric disorders and quality of life (QOL) in female patients with documented recurrent vasovagal syncope, and to compare these data with those of a control group made up of healthy sex- and age-matched subjects without syncope.

Materials and Methods

Patients

Twenty-seven consecutive female patients referred to the Syncope Unit of the Cardiology Department of Umberto I Hospital in Mestre-Venice for recurrent syncope of unknown origin were enrolled in the study (Table 1). Inclusion criteria were: age over 18 years (since the method used for psychological evaluation is valid only for adult subjects); at least three syncopal episodes in the patient's lifetime; head-up tilt testing positive for vasovagal syncope; complete diagnostic work-up negative for other causes of syncope. The presence of other concomitant pathological conditions or declared psychiatric disorders were taken as exclusion criteria.

[1]Cardiovasculary Department, Division of Cardiology; [2]Division of Neurology, Umberto I Hospital, Mestre-Venice, Italy

Table 1. Patients' clinical characteristics

	Patients (N = 27)	Controls (N = 27)	p value
Age (years)	40 ± 19	39 ± 11	ns
Number of syncope	23 ± 27 (10)	-	-
Duration of symptoms (years)	9 ± 14 (4)	-	-
Number of pre-syncopal	14 ± 23 (6)	-	-
Associated injuries	10 (37%)	-	-

Values are expressed as mean ± SD

Controls

The control group consisted of 27 healthy, age-matched female subjects with no history of syncope or presyncope and with negative head-up tilt testing (Table 1). Control subjects with concomitant diseases or declared psychiatric disorders were excluded from the study.

All subjects taking part in the study underwent complete anamnesis including collection of some demographic data, thorough objective examination, head-up tilt testing, and all other tests deemed necessary in order to exclude other causes of syncope .

Head-Up Tilt Testing

The protocol used in head-up tilt testing involved a first phase of tilting at 60° for 20 min without drug challenge; if this proved negative, it was followed by a second phase of tilting at the same angle for 15 min, after sublingual administration of 400 µg nitroglycerin spray [6]. Head-up tilt testing was considered positive if it elicited syncope with reproduction of the patient's spontaneous symptoms, associated with a sudden and significant fall in blood pressure (systolic blood pressure < 60 mmHg).

Psychiatric Evaluation

At least 3 days after head-up tilt testing, all subjects taking part in the study underwent a structured interview with a psychologist, and were asked to complete the Minnesota Multiphasic Personality Inventory-2 (MMPI-2) questionnaire for psychological assessment. The MMPI-2 is a widely recognized instrument for assessing the psychological profile of adult subjects [7, 8]. Made up of over 500 items, the questionnaire uses specific scales to explore various aspects of the individual's personality. The higher the score assigned on each scale, the greater the personality disorder. The score is considered pathological when higher than 65 points. Subjects were asked to complete the MMPI-2 questionnaire alone at home and to return it to the Syncope Unit. Subsequently, the questionnaires were evaluated by two expert psychologists, working "blind", by means of special software (MMPI-2 Psy-System, OS, Florence, Italy). Clinical diagnoses were formulated on the basis of the interview and the questionnaire results, in accordance with the criteria of the Diagnostic and Statistical Manual of Mental Disorders IV (DSM-IV) [9].

Assessment of QOL

Assessment of Quality of life (QOL) was performed by means of the Short-Form Health Survey (SF-36) questionnaire, which was distributed to patients at least 3 days after head-up tilt testing. The SF-36 is an international standardized instrument for assessing the general state of health, which measures physical and psychological functions on eight specific scales [10, 11]. The lower the score assigned on each scale, the higher the degree of impairment of that particular aspect of QOL. The SF-36 questionnaire was analyzed "blind" by two expert psychologists.

Statistical Analysis

Statistical analysis was carried out using the Systat software. Continuous variables were expressed as means ± standard deviation; comparison between groups was made by Student's t-test for unpaired data in the case of variables with normal distribution, and by the Mann-Whitney nonparametric test in the case of variables with nonlinear distribution. Discrete variables were expressed as percentages; comparison between groups was made by using the χ^2 test. Correlation among different variables was assessed by means of Pearson correlation matrix. The criterion of statistical significance was taken as $p < 0.05$.

Results

Clinical Characteristics

All of the patients participating in the study proved to be affected by recurrent vasovagal syncope, with serious injuries resulting from loss of consciousness being recorded in a large number of cases (Table 1). There were no differences between patients and control subjects in terms of age, marital status, number of children or level of education, while a higher percentage of control subjects held steady jobs (74% vs 37%, $p < 0.05$).

Psychiatric Evaluation

In comparison with control subjects, patients had significantly higher scores on the scales assessing hypochondria (60 ± 13 vs 49 ± 8, $p < 0.005$), depression (54 ± 10 vs 47 ± 5, $p < 0.01$), hysteria (58 ± 14 vs 44 ± 7, $p < 0.001$), fear (56 ± 10 vs 51 ± 9, $p < 0.05$), and worry over health (61 ± 12 vs 52 ± 10, $p < 0.01$). The number of scales with pathological scores was higher in the patient group than in the control group (1.5 ± 1.8 vs 0.6 ± 1.1, $p < 0.05$).

The number of subjects with at least one psychiatric disorder according to the criteria of the DSM-IV was statistically higher among patients than among controls (Table 2), with a prevalence of somatization disorders and mood disorders. By contrast, there were no statistical differences between the two groups with regard to anxiety disorders or personality disorders. In neither group were any psychiatric disorders such as a tendency to alcohol or drug abuse recorded. In one control group subject, two simultaneous psychiatric disorders were detected, while in the syncope group two patients had two simultaneous psychiatric disorders and one patient had three.

Table 2. Psychiatric diagnoses

	Patients (N = 27)	Controls (N = 27)	p Value
Any disorders	20 (74%)	6 (22%)	0.01
Somatoform disorders	9 (33%)	0 (0%)	0.01
Mood disorders	6 (22%)	1 (4%)	0.04
Anxiety disorders	3 (11%)	1 (4%)	ns
Personality disorders	7 (26%)	5 (18%)	ns

There was no significant difference between patients with psychiatric disorders and those without in terms of age, number of syncopal episodes, duration of syncopal symptoms, or occurrence of syncope-related injury (Table 3). No significant differences were observed in the scores of the personality scales between patients with more than six syncopal episodes and those with fewer than six, between patients with and without syncope-related injury, or between patients over 40 years of age and those under 40. Finally, no significant correlation was seen between the various MMPI-2 scales and the syncopal burden, that is the number of syncopal episodes during the patient's lifetime and the duration of syncopal symptoms.

Table 3. Clinical characteristics of patients with and without psychiatric diagnoses

	With (N = 20)	Without (N = 7)	p Value
Age (years)	39 ± 19	43 ± 20	ns
Number of syncope episodes	23 ± 30	22 ± 21	ns
Duration of symptoms (years)	10 ± 15 (5)	8 ± 10 (2)	ns
Number of presyncope episodes	14 ± 23	13 ± 20	ns
Associated injuries	8 (40%)	2 (29%)	ns

Values are expressed as mean $\pm$ SD

QOL Evaluation

The scores on all of the SF-36 scales, in both the physical (Table 4) and psychosocial domains (Table 5), proved to be statistically lower in patients than in controls. No significant differences were observed in the scores of the various scales between patients with more than six syncopal episodes and those with fewer than six episodes, though only the former showed a significant reduction on the scales of physical functioning ($p < 0.005$) and general health ($p < 0.005$) in comparison with the control group. Finally, inverse correlations were seen between the number of syncopal episodes during the patient's lifetime and the scales of physical functioning (r = - 0.612, $p < 0.001$) and role-physical function (r = - 0.501, $p < 0.01$), and between the severity of syncope-related injury and the scale of vitality (r = - 0.548, $p < 0.01$).

Table 4. QOL measurements: "physical domain"

	Patients (N = 27)	Controls (N = 27)	p value
Physical functioning	75 ± 23	90 ± 13	0.01
Role-physical	41 ± 36	83 ± 31	0.01
Bodily pain	54 ± 31	80 ± 26	0.04
General health	53 ± 21	70 ± 15	0.01

Values are expressed as mean ± SD

Table 5. QOL measurements: "psychosocial domain"

	Patients (N = 27)	Controls (N = 27)	p value
Vitality	44 ± 18	68 ± 15	0.001
Social functioning	57 ± 26	82 ± 17	0.001
Role-emotional	50 ± 41	90 ± 20	0.001
Mental health	56 ± 23	77 ± 14	0.001

Values are expressed as mean ± SD

Discussion

The relationship between syncope and disorders within the mental sphere, though not thoroughly explored, has long been known. Indeed, syncope is such a frequent symptom in some psychiatric illnesses that, according to the DSM-IV, it constitutes one of the criteria on which the diagnosis of somatization disorders, depression disorders, and anxiety disorders is based [9].

A few clinical studies conducted at the beginning of the 1990s in the United States reported a high prevalence of psychiatric disorders such as anxiety, depression, somatization disorders, and alcoholism in patients with unexplained syncope [1-3]. Moreover, studies conducted during the same period [4, 5] found that patients with recurrent syncope of various etiologies also suffered a significant reduction in their QOL in both the physical and the psychosocial domains. However, the above-mentioned studies present some confounding factors which deserve to be highlighted. The first is the poor homogeneity of the study population. As these studies were carried out before the days of head-up tilt testing, patients with syncope of various origins, including vasovagal origin, were probably classified as suffering from unexplained syncope. Moreover, the patients studied were very often affected by other diseases in addition to syncope. We cannot, therefore, rule out the possibility that these concomitant illnesses may have affected the psychological profile and QOL of the patients examined. Finally, these studies lack a suitable control group that is representative of the general population. This last point is of fundamental importance, in that recent epidemiological studies have revealed that the prevalence of psychiatric disorders in the general population is somewhat high, and is steadily rising [12]. Thus, the lack of comparison with a control group made up of healthy subjects without syncope may lead to overestimation of the results recorded on syncope patients.

In the international literature, data on the prevalence of psychiatric disorders and on QOL in patients suffering from vasovagal syncope are rather scanty and incomplete [13-16]. Nevertheless, various factors seem to suggest the presence of an association between vasovagal syncope and psychological disturbances. In patients with vasovagal syncope, mental stress and particular emotional states can facilitate and/or trigger the neurally mediated reaction that underlies the syncopal episode [17, 18]. Furthermore, it is well known that, when patients are reassured of the substantially benign nature of their problem, they have significantly fewer syncopal recurrences [19]. Finally, it should be pointed out that the only drug shown to be efficacious in preventing vasovagal syncope in placebo-controlled studies [20] is paroxetine, an inhibitor of serotonin re-uptake commonly used as an antidepressant.

To our knowledge, the present study is the first to analyze psychological profile and QOL systematically in patients with documented vasovagal syncope and no concomitant associated diseases, and to compare these data with those obtained in a control group of healthy sex- and age-matched subjects without syncope. We observed a higher frequency of pathological scores on the various MMPI-2 scales among patients than among control subjects, with the highest scores being recorded on the scales for hypochondria, depression, hysteria, fear, and worry over health. The number of individuals with psychiatric diagnoses was also higher among patients than among controls, especially with regard to somatization and mood disorders. Obtained in patients with vasovagal syncope, the present results are in agreement with those reported in subjects with unexplained syncope in the era before tilt testing [1-3], and appear to suggest that these two populations partially overlap. However, we did not find disorders linked to drug or alcohol abuse in our patients, as has been reported in patients with unexplained syncope. Such disorders would therefore appear to be peculiar to patients with unexplained syncope. Indeed, the mechanisms through which alcohol or drug abuse can elicit syncope do not seem to be linked to neurally mediated reflexes [21].

Anxiety disorders were more frequent in our patients than in controls, though not significantly so from the statistical point of view. This finding is in line with that of two recent studies which examined the degree of anxiety in patients with unexplained syncope who underwent head-up tilt testing [13, 14].

In the present study, no significant differences in the various MMPI-2 scales were seen between patients with more than six syncopal episodes and those with fewer than six, nor between patients with and without syncope-related injury. Moreover, there were no differences in syncopal burden between patients with and without psychiatric disorders. These findings, together with the absence of significant correlations among the MMPI-2 scales, the number of syncopal episodes and the duration of syncopal symptoms, would seem to exclude a direct relationship between the presence and severity of psychiatric disorders and the syncopal burden. By contrast, studies conducted on patients with unexplained syncope have reported a higher number of syncopal episodes, and a higher risk of syncopal recurrence in patients with psychiatric syncope than in those with other causes of syncope [1, 2]. Moreover, in the study by Linzer et al. [2] patients with psychiatric syncope treated by psychotherapy or drug therapy are reported as having fewer syncopal recurrences during follow-up, supporting the hypothesis of an etiopathogenetic link between syncope and psychiatric disorders. The explanation for the discrepancy between the results of the present study and those of the studies quoted above is unclear. It may, however, lie in the small size of our patient population, which was made up almost exclusively of extremely symptomatic patients.

In patients with syncope of various etiologies and other concomitant diseases, a significant impairment of QOL has been described, relating to the psychosocial domain more than the physical domain. This QOL impairment seems to be of similar magnitude to that observed in some chronic illnesses such as rheumatoid arthritis and chronic low back pain [4, 5]. In our patients with recurrent vasovagal syncope and without other associated diseases, we also observed a marked reduction in all of the QOL indexes in comparison with control subjects; this reduction was more significant with regard to the psychosocial indexes. Moreover, in the present study, we observed a significant inverse correlation between syncopal burden and the scales of physical functioning and role-physical function, and between the severity of syncope-related injury and the scale of vitality. Our data, in agreement with those recently published by Rose et al. [15], seem to suggest a direct association between the syncopal burden and the state of well-being of patients with recurrent vasovagal syncope. Furthermore, these results are supported by data from Sheldon et al. [16] about the effects of pacemakers in patients with recurrent vasovagal syncope. These authors found a significant improvement in QOL in subjects who experienced a reduction in syncopal recurrences following pacemaker implantation.

Conclusions

Although our study population was small, selected, and restricted to female patients, the following conclusions are suggested:
1. Patients with recurrent vasovagal syncope, like patients with syncope of unknown origin, frequently display psychiatric disorders, especially somatization disorders and depression. However, unlike in patients with syncope of unknown origin, there seems to be no correlation between syncopal burden and the presence and severity of the psychiatric disorders.
2. Patients with recurrent vasovagal syncope suffer a significant impairment of QOL, especially in the psychosocial domain, even in the absence of other concomitant pathologies. QOL seems to be inversely correlated with the patients' syncopal burden.
3. Thorough psychiatric evaluation should be included in the diagnostic work-up, not only in patients with syncope of unknown origin, but also in patients with recurrent vasovagal syncope, especially if refractory to therapy.
4. The present study might lead to important future developments in the therapeutic management of patients with vasovagal syncope, in terms both of the selection of patients to treat and the kind of treatment to undertake.

References

1. Kapoor WN, Fortunato M, Hanusa BH, Shulberg HC (1995) Psychiatric illnesses in patients with syncope. Am J Med 99:505-512
2. Linzer M, Felder A, Hackel A et al (1990) Psychiatric syncope: a new look at on old disease. Psychosomatics 31:181-188
3. Koenig D, Linzer M, Pontinen M, Divine GW (1992) Syncope in young adults: evidence for combined medical and psychiatric approach. J Intern Med 232:169-176
4. Linzer M, Pontinen M, Gold DT et al (1991) Impairment of physical and psychosocial function in recurrent syncope. J Clin Epidemiol 44:1037-1043
5. Linzer M, Gold DT, Pontinen M et al (1994) Recurrent syncope as a chronic disease: preliminary validation of a disease-specific measure of functional impairment. J Gen Intern Med 9:181-185
6. Bartoletti A, Alboni P, Ammirati F et al (2000) Tilt test potenziato con nitroglicerina orale nei pazienti con sincope inspiegata: "Il protocollo italiano". Ital Heart J 1:226-231
7. Hathaway SR, McKinley JC (1995) MMPI-2 Minnesota Multiphasic Personality Inventory – 2 Manual. Italian adaptation by Pancheri P, Sirigatti S. OS, Organizzazioni Speciali, Florence

8. Butcher JN, Williams CL (1996) Fondamenti per l'interpretazione del MMPI-2 e del MMPI-A. OS, Organizzazioni Speciali, Florence

9. American Psychiatric Association (1994) Diagnostic and Statistical Manual of Mental Disorders, 4th edn (DSM-IV). American Psychiatric Association, Washington, DC

10. Ware JE, Sherbourne CD (1992) The RAND 36 Short-Form Health Survey: I. Conceptual framework and item selection. Med Care 30:473-481

11. McHorney CA, Ware JE, Raczek AE (1993) The MOS 36-Item Short-Form Health Survey (SF-36): II. Psychometric and clinical tests of validity in measuring physical and mental health constructs. Med Care 31:247-263

12. Kessler RC (1994) Lifetime and 12-month prevalence of DSM-III-R psychiatric disorders in the United States: results from the National Comorbidity Survey. Arch Gen Psychiatry 51:8-19

13. Kouakam C, Lacroix D, Baux P et al (1996) Anxiety neurosis and unexplained syncope of presumed vaso-vagal origin. Arch Mal Coeur 89:1247-1254

14. Cohen TJ, Thayapran N, Ibrahim B et al (2000) An association between anxiety and neurocardiogenic syncope during head-up tilt table testing. Pacing Clin Electrophysiol 23:837-841

15. Rose MS, Koshman ML, Spreng S, Sheldon R (2000) The relationship between health-related quality of life and frequency of spells in patients with syncope. J Clin Epidemiol 53:1209-1216

16. Sheldon R, Koshman ML, Wilson W et al (1998) Effect of dual-chamber pacing with automatic rate-drop sensing on recurrent neurally mediated syncope. Am J Cardiol 81:158-162

17. Schmidt RT (1975) Personality and fainting. J Psychosom Res 19:21-25

18. Sledge WH (1978) Antecedent psychological factors in the onset of vasovagal syncope. Psychosom Med 40:568-579

19. Sheldon R, Rose S, Flanagan P et al (1996) Risk factors for syncope recurrence after a positive tilt-table test in patients with syncope. Circulation 93:973-981

20. Di Girolamo E, Di Iorio C, Sabatini P et al (1999) Effects of paroxetine hydrochloride, a selective serotonin reuptake inhibitor, on refractory vasovagal syncope: a randomized, double-blind, placebo-controlled study. J Am Coll Cardiol 33:1227-1230

21. Kapoor WN, Fortunato M, Hanusa B, Schulberg HC (1998) Psychiatric disorders in patients with syncope. In: Grubb BP, and Olshansky B (eds): Syncope: mechanisms and management. Futura, Armonk, NY, pp 253-263

Syncope with Exercise: Mechanisms and Management

D.G. BENDITT

Introduction

Syncope associated with exercise is infrequent but warrants special considera-tion, both because of the adverse prognostic implications in certain situations, and because of the community concern that often arises when these events occur in otherwise healthy active individuals such as student athletes or prominent professionals.

Exercise-related syncope may occur during or immediately after exercise. The former should immediately raise concern regarding a possible structural or arrhythmic cardiac origin, even though in many cases it may ultimately prove to be due to inappropriate reflex vasodilatation. By contrast, postexer-tional syncope is most often due to neurally mediated hypotension-bradycar-dia [1-11], autonomic failure [12, 13], or on rare occasion inappropriate sinus slowing as a manifestation of chronotropic incompetence (or inadequate rate response settings in patients with rate-adaptive pacemakers) [14].

For the purposes of this discussion, exercise-related syncope is classified in terms of three generally distinct settings in which it occurs: (1) underlying structural heart disease (e.g., myocardial ischemia), (2) primary electrophysio-logical disorders (e.g., long QT syndromes), and (3) apparently healthy indi-viduals (e.g., exercise variant of neurally mediated syncope).

Structural Heart Disease

Exercise-induced syncopal episodes resulting directly from structural abnor-malities of the heart or blood vessels (excluding arrhythmias) are uncommon. Probably the most common are those that occur in conjunction with acute myocardial ischemia or infarction [15-20].

Cardiac Arrhythmia Center, University of Minnesota Medical School, Minneapolis, Minnesota, USA

Either congenital or acquired coronary artery disease may be responsible for exercise-induced syncope. The former tends to be more often recognized in younger individuals, in whom any of a variety of anatomic disturbances may be present. These include abnormal take-off of the coronary vessels, entrapment of coronary arteries between the great vessels, or even hypoplastic coronararteries. Intramyocardial tunneling of coronary arteries also occurs, although the relationship of this finding to myocardial ischemia is difficult to establish. The pathophysiologic basis for syncope in congenital or acquired coronary artery disease is complex, incorporating transient reduction of cardiac output, important neural reflex effects, and ischemia-related cardiac arrhythmias (usually ventricular tachycardia).

Syncope associated with left ventricular outflow tract obstruction [especially hypertrophic obstructive cardiomyopathy (HOCM)] is relatively rare [21-25], but nevertheless receives considerable attention since it tends to occur most often in younger athletic individuals. The basis for the faint is multifactorial. Ventricular mechanoreceptor-mediated bradycardia and hypotension (i.e., a form of neurally mediated syncope) is thought to play an important role [26], but syncope may also be the result of diminished cardiac output in conjunction with abrupt onset of atrial tachyarrhythmias (particularly atrial fibrillation) or ventricular tachycardia. McKenna et al. [22] reported syncope to be an important predictor of sudden death in these patients, a finding yet to be confirmed by others.

Finally, syncope during exercise can be due to aggravation of structural atrioventricular conduction system disease. Tachycardia-related second-degree and high-grade atrioventricular block is invariably located distal to the atrioventricular node, and the baseline electrocardiogram frequently shows an intraventricular conduction abnormality [27-31]. Further, this clinical scenario is associated with subsequent progression to complete atrioventricular block. Consequently, cardiac pacemaker therapy is warranted.

Primary Electrophysiologic Disturbances

In general, supraventricular tachyarrhythmias (SVT) are less often implicated as causes of syncope than are ventricular tachycardias [32-36], and are particularly infrequent causes of exercise-related syncope. Among the exercise-induced ventricular tachycardias associated with syncope, those accompanying myocardial ischemia (see above) and those associated with certain forms of long QT syndrome are the most important.

Long QT syndrome (LQTS) presents a special form of ventricular tachycardia risk known for its presentation as syncope. LQTS may not be among the most common causes of syncope, but must always be kept in mind [37-39]. Syncope is primarily due to "torsades de pointes" ventricular tachycardia, a form of polymorphous ventricular tachycardia. The acquired form of LQTS is by far the more common, and is most frequently the result of drugs which prolong the QT interval. Torsades in this setting is most often seen during periods of bradycardia (e.g., sleep) or following pauses in the cardiac rhythm (e.g., post PVC) which accentuate the QT interval. Congenital, idiopathic, or familial LQTS is caused by mutations in cardiac ion channels that contribute to the action potential repolarization process. Congenital LQTS is a very infrequent cause of syncope, but its identification can be life saving. Syncope and sudden death in this setting is frequently associated with emotional arousal such as may be triggered by fear or loud noises, or physical activity accompanying exertion. LQTS1 has been particularly associated with exercise. Heterogeneity in clinical presentation exists, however, so that in other individuals torsades de pointes occurs due to bradycardia or during sleep in conjunction with rate-dependent QT interval prolongation.

Neurally Mediated Post-Exertional Syncope

Neurally mediated reflex syncope may manifest as postexertional syncope [1-3, 5-11, 40]. Usually the affected individual has no evidence of underlying structural heart or cardiovascular disease. A failure of reflex vasoconstriction during exercise in the splanchnic capacitance bed and in forearm resistance vessels may play a role. As a rule, the syncopal event occurs after termination of exercise, and this historical feature is crucial to establishing the diagnosis. On rare occasions, however, reflex syncope occurs during exercise. In this case it is caused by marked hypotension without bradycardia [3, 4, 8, 41]. However, in the case of syncope during exercise, it is imperative that all other potentially more dangerous causes be excluded before the syncope is attributed to a neurally mediated origin.

Exercise testing is not particularly cost-effective when used in a general population with syncope. Its diagnostic yield was less than 1% in a population study [42]. However, when its use is limited to selected patients with exertional syncope, it may represent an important diagnostic test. Exercise testing should be performed in patients who experienced episodes of syncope during or shortly after exertion. Exercise testing should be symptom-limited, and close electrocardiographic monitoring should be performed during both the test and the recovery phase.

References

1. Yerg JE II, Seals DR, Hagberg JM, Ehsani AA (1986) Syncope secondary to ventricular asystole in an endurance athlete. Clin Cardiol 9:220-222
2. Huycke EC, Card HG, Sobol SM et al (1987) Postexertional cardiac asystole in a young man without organic heart disease. Ann Intern Med 106:844-845
3. Greci ED, Ramsdale DR (1991) Exertional syncope in aortic stenosis: evidence to support inappropriate left ventricular baroreceptor response. Am Heart J 121:603-606

4. Arad M, Solomon A, Roth A et al (1993) Postexercise syncope: evidence for increased activity of the sympathetic nervous system. Cardiology 83:121-123

5. Osswald S, Brooks R, O'Nunain SS et al (1994) Asystole after exercise in healthy persons. Ann Intern Med 120:1008-1011

6. O'Connor FG, Oriscello RG, Levine BD (1999) Exercise-related syncope in the young athlete: Reassurance, restriction or referral? Am Fam Phys 60:2001-2008

7. Sneddon JF, Scalia G, Ward DE et al (1994) Exercise induced vasodepressor syncope. Br Heart J 71:554-557

8. Sakaguchi S, Shultz JJ, Remole SC et al (1995) Syncope associated with exercise, a manifestation of neurally mediated syncope. Am J Cardiol 75:476-481

9. Calkins H, Seifert M, Morady F (1995) Clinical presentation and long-term follow-up of athletes with exercise-induced vasodepressor syncope. Am Heart J 129:1159-1164

10. Tse HF, Lau P (1995) Exercise-associated cardiac asystole in persons without structural heart disease. Chest 107:572-576

11. Abe H, Nakashima Y, Kohshi K, Kuroiwa A (1997) Exercise-induced neurally mediated syncope. Jpn Heart J 38:535-539

12. Smith GPD, Mathias CJ (1995) Postural hypotension enhanced by exercise in patients with chronic autonomic failure. Q J Med 88:251-256

13. Hainsworth R (1999) Syncope and fainting: classification and pathophysiological basis. In: Mathias CJ, Bannister R (eds) Autonomic failure: a textbook of clinical disorders of the autonomic nervous system, 4th edn. Oxford University Press, Oxford, pp 428-436

14. Benditt DG, Milstein S, Goldstein MA et al (1990) Sinus node dysfunction: pathophysiology, clinical features, evaluation and treatment. In: Zipes DP, Jalife J (eds) Cardiac electrophysiology: from cell to bedside. Saunders, Philadelphia, pp 708-734

15. Pathy MS (1967) Clinical presentation of myocardial infarction in the elderly. Br Heart J 29:190-199

16. Kovac JD, Murgatroyd FD, Skehan JD (1997) Recurrent syncope due to complete atrioventricular block, a rare presenting symptom of otherwise silent coronary artery disease: successful treatment by PTCA. Cathet Cardiovasc Diagn 42:216-218

17. Ascheim DD, Markowitz SM, Lai H et al (1997) Vasodepressor syncope due to subclinical myocardial ischemia. J Cardiovasc Electrophysiol 8:215-221

18. Havranek EP, Dunbar DN (1992) Exertional syncope caused by left main coronary artery spasm. Am Heart J 123:792-794

19. Hattori R, Murohara Y, Yui Y et al (1987) Diffuse triple-vessel coronary artery spasm complicated by idioventricular rhythm and syncope. Chest 92:183-185

20. Watanabe K, Inomata T, Miyakita Y et al (1993) Electrophysiologic study and ergonovine provocation of coronary spasm in unexplained syncope. Jpn Heart J 34:171-182

21. Romeo F, Cianfrocca C, Pelliccia F et al (1990) Long-term prognosis in children with hypertrophic cardiomyopathy: an analysis of 37 patients aged $\leq$ 14 years at diagnosis. Clin Cardiol 13:101

22. McKenna WJ, Deanfield J, Faruqui A et al (1981) Prognosis in hypertrophic cardiomyopathy: role of age and clinical electrocardiographic and hemodynamic features. Am J Cardiol 47:532-538

23. Shapira Y, Kusniec J, Birnbaum Y, Strasberg B (1996) Exercise-induced syncope and Holter-documented asystole in an endurance runner with moderate aortic stenosis. Clin Cardiol 19:71-73

24. Chamarthi B, Dubrey SW, Cha K et al (1997) Features and prognosis of exertional syncope in light-chain associated AL cardiac amyloidosis. Am J Cardiol 80:1242-1245

25. Atwood JE, Kawanishi S, Myers J, Froelicher VF (1988) Exercise testing in patients with aortic stenosis. Chest 93:1083-1087

26. Sneddon JF, Slade A, Seo H et al (1997) Assessment of the diagnostic value of head-up tilt testing in the evaluation of syncope in hypertrophic cardiomyopathy. Am J Cardiol 80:1242-1245

27. Dhingra RC, Amat-y-Leon F et al (1976) Infranodal block: diagnosis, clinical significance and management. Med Clin North Am 60:175-192

28. Byrne JM, Marais HJ, Cheek GA (1994) Exercise-induced complete heart block in a patient with chronic bifascicular block. J Electrocardiol 27:339-342

29. Woeifel AK, Simpson RJ, Gettes LS, Foster JR (1983) Exercise-induced distal atrio-ventricular block. J Am Coll Cardiol 2:578-582

30. Barra M, Brignole M, Menozzi CA et al (1985) An exercise induced intermittent atrio-ventricular block. Report of three cases report (*in Italian*). G Ital Cardiol 15:1051-1055

31. Yuzuki Y, Horie M, Makita T et al (1997) Exercise-induced second-degree atrioventricular block. Jpn Circ J 61:268-271

32. Leitch JW, Klein GJ, Yee R et al (1992) Syncope associated with supraventricular tachycardia: an expression of tachycardia or vasomotor response. Circulation 85:1064-1071

33. Camm AJ, Lau CP (1988) Syncope of undetermined origin: diagnosis and management. Prog Cardiol 1:139-156

34. Dhingra RC, Denes P, Wu D et al (1974) Syncope in patients with chronic bifascicular block. Significance, causative mechanisms, and clinical implications. Ann Int Med 81:302-306

35. Middelkauff HR, Stevenson WG, Stevenson LW, Saxon LA (1993) Syncope in advanced heart failure: high risk of sudden death regardless of origin of syncope. J Am Coll Cardiol 21:110-116

36. Morady F, Shen E, Schwartz A et al (1983) Long-term follow-up of patients with recurrent unexplained syncope evaluated by electrophysiologic testing. J Am Coll Cardiol 2:1053-1059

37. Jackman WM, Friday KJ, Anderson JL et al (1988) The long QT syndromes: a critical review, new clinical observations and a unifying hypothesis. Prog Cardiovasc Dis 31:115-172

38. Moss AJ, Schwartz PJ, Crampton RS et al (1991) The long QT syndrome: prospective longitudinal study of 328 families. Circulation 84:1136-1144

39. Schwartz PJ, Zaza A, Locati E, Moss AJ (1991) Stress and sudden death. The case of the long QT syndrome. Circulation 83(Suppl II):71-80

40. Kosinski D, Grubb BP, Kip K, Hahn H (1996) Exercise-induced neurocardiogenic syncope. Am Heart J 132:451-452

41. Thomson HL, Atherton JJ, Khafagi FA, Frenneaux MP (1996) Failure to reflex venoconstriction during exercise in patients with vasovagal syncope. Circulation 93:953-959

42. Kapoor W (1990) Evaluation and outcome of patients with syncope. Medicine 69:160-175

The Postural Tachycardia Syndrome: Etiology, Diagnosis and Treatment

B.P. Grubb

Syncope, the transient loss of consciousness and postural tone, has long been recognized by medical science. Only relatively recently, however, was it established that many episodes of syncope were due to transient periods of autonomically-mediated hypotension and bradycardia. During the last 15 years, tilt-table testing has been employed as a useful modality for the diagnosis of these conditions, while simultaneously providing a controlled setting where precise observations and measurements of these phenomena could be made [1]. Thus, during this period there was a very rapid increase in our knowledge of these disorders. One such observation was that these transient disturbances in autonomic nervous system tone could produce varying degrees of hypotension, while not enough to result in loss of consciousness, could nonetheless be great enough to produce symptoms such as vertigo, dizziness, near-syncope and focal neurologic deficits that appeared remarkably similar to transient ischemic attacks. At the same time, several groups of investigators noted that there was a group of patients who exhibited a less severe form of autonomic disturbance, resulting in a form of orthostatic intolerance manifested by postural tachycardia, severe fatigue, blurred vision, exercise intolerance, dizziness and near-syncope. Detailed analysis of these patients uncovered the fact that their clinical histories, physical examinations, and responses to upright posture and head upright tilt were essentially similar. Taken together, these observations, made by multiple different groups, determined that these patients suffer from a common disorder that is now most commonly referred to as the postural orthostatic tachycardia syndrome (POTS) [2]. This paper will try to review the unique characteristics of this disorder as well as recent advances in our knowledge of its pathophysiology and treatment.

Division of Cardiology, Department of Medicine, Medical College of Ohio, Toledo, Ohio, USA

Physiologic Aspects

A full description of all the physiologic changes that occur during upright posture is beyond the scope of this review. However, briefly, approximately 25% of the body's blood is in the thorax while supine [1]. Almost immediately after assuming upright posture, gravity causes a downward displacement of about 500 ml of blood to the lower extremities and inferior mesenteric area. One-half of the amount is redistributed within seconds after standing and up to 25% of the total blood volume may be involved in the process. This causes a decrease in venous return to heart and stroke volume may fall by 40%. In the normal subject, orthostatic stabilization after standing is achieved in 1 min or less. Immediately after standing there is a slow progressive decline in arterial pressure and cardiac filling, which results in an activation of the high-pressure receptors of the aortic arch and the carotid sinus (as well as low-pressure cardiac and pulmonary receptors). The cardiac mechanoreceptors are joined by unmyelinated vagal effects from both the atria and ventricles. These cause continuous inhibitory actions on the cardiovascular areas of the brain stem (especially the nucleus tractus solitarii) [3]. The reduced venous return caused by upright posture produces less stretch on these receptors, decreasing their discharge rates. This alteration in input to the medulla results in an increase in sympathetic outflow and there is an increase in systemic vasoconstriction. Simultaneously, the decline in arterial pressure while upright activates the high-pressure receptors in the carotid sinus, which then increase heart rate. Therefore, steady-state adaptation to upright posture causes a 10-15 beats/min increase in heart rate, an increase in diastolic blood pressure of approximately 10 mmHg, with little or no change in systolic blood pressure. More detailed descriptions of the process are available elsewhere [4]. The inability of this complex process to respond adequately (or in a coordinated fashion) can result in a failure to respond normally to sudden changes in posture (and to maintain adequate responses). Failure in this system may manifest itself as hypotension, which, if severe, may cause cerebral hypoperfusion, hypoxia and loss of consciousness.

Etiology

In the early nineteenth century, physicians described patients who suffered from severe fatigue, exercise intolerance and tachycardia that occurred without an obvious cause. One of the earliest reports was made by DeCosta during the American Civil War, who used the term "inevitable heart syndrome" to describe the condition [5]. Further reports of a similar condition were made during the First and Second World Wars, when terms such as "neurocirculatory asthenia" or "vasoregulatory asthenia" were often used [6]. In 1944 MacLean et al. described patients with orthostatic tachycardia associated with mild hypotension who complained of palpitations, dizziness, weakness, and exercise intolerance [7]. Similar reports were made by a number of investigators over the next half century. By the late 1980s, Streeten had employed γ camera counting of sodium pertechnetate ^{99}Tc-labeled erythrocytes in similar patients and demonstrated evidence of extensive gravity-dependent venous pooling in the lower extremities [8]. By the mid-1990s, both Low et al. and Schondorf et al. reported on 16 patients who suffered from postural tachycardia, severe fatigue, exercise intolerance, lightheadedness, and bowel hypomotility. During tilt-table testing, these patients demonstrated abnormal cardiovascular responses, with heart rates that would accelerate to as high as 120-170 beats/min (often in the first few minutes of upright tilt) [9, 10]. Although few patients had a mild fall in blood pressure, the majority remained normotensive, while some actually developed hypertension.

These investigators dubbed this condition the postural orthostatic tachycardia syndrome (POTS) and postulated that it represented a mild form of autonomic dysfunction. Grubb et al. then reported on a group of 28 patients with postural tachycardia, fatigue, exercise intolerance, cognitive impairment, and near-syncope [2]. At tilt-table testing, each patient demonstrated a heart rate increase of at least 30 beats/min (after exceeding rates of 110 beats/min) during the first 10 min of the test. Systolic blood pressure only fell about 20 mmHg. A similar report from Karas et al. [11] demonstrated identical findings in a group of 35 adolescent patients, suggesting that there is a large age range affected by the disorder.

Investigators quickly noted that in some patients there was a marked familial predisposition to these disorders, raising suspicions that there was a possible genetic basis to them. This suspicion was recently confirmed by investigators at Vanderbilt, where the exact genetic basis for this disorder was determined in one severely affected family [12]. The defective gene causes a dysfunction in a norepinephrine transporter protein, producing excessive serum norepinephrine levels. Many investigators have postulated that there are multiple genetic forms of the disorder and more detailed investigations are currently in progress.

At the same time, a large number of patients report that symptoms appear after a severe viral infection, suggesting that an immune-mediated mechanism may be involved. This concept was recently confirmed by investigators at the Mayo Clinic, who found that many patients had high serum levels of auto-antibodies to peripheral acetylcholine receptors [13]. The levels of these antibodies seemed to vary with the severity of the illness. There may be a considerable degree of overlap between POTS and "inappropriate" sinus tachycardia. Support for this concept has also come from the Mayo Clinic, who reported that radiofrequency ablation had little effect in these disorders, and sometimes made people worse [14].

Definitions

Taken together, these observations begin to present a fairly consistent picture of this disorder. While a number of different terms have been coined to describe this phenomenon, we prefer "postural orthostatic tachycardia syndrome"

(POTS) because it is a fairly descriptive term and easy to remember. These patients manifest an orthostatic intolerance, in that they develop symptoms while standing that are relieved by recumbency. POTS patients frequently present with complaints of fatigue, exercise intolerance, lightheadedness, nausea, loss of concentration and memory, tremulousness, and recurrent near-syncope (and sometimes syncope). These patients may frequently be misdiagnosed as having panic attacks or chronic anxiety. Relatively simple activities, such as modest exercise, showering (or sometimes even eating), may intensify these symptoms and profoundly limit even the most basic activities of daily life. Because severe autonomic failure is not present, the general physical examination is often unrevealing and patients are told that "nothing is wrong".

At present we define POTS as the development of orthostatic symptoms that are associated with at least a 30 beats/min increase in heart rate or a heart rate of $\geq$ 120 beats/min that occurs within the first 10 min of standing or upright tilt. With respect to the age range of patients with POTS (aged 10-60 years), this increase in heart rate exceeds the 99th percentile for control subjects (aged 10-83 years) [15].

Classification

While the etiology of POTS is still unclear, it most likely represents a heterogenous group of disorders with similar clinical characteristics. The largest group of patients appear to have a mild form of idiopathic peripheral autonomic neuropathy (a "partial dysautonomia"), in which an inability to increase peripheral vascular resistance during upright posture results in an excessive compensatory postural tachycardia. Venous pooling appears to be present, which results in a reduction in ventricular preload, which in turn leads to baroreceptor unloading while upright, with a resultant increase in sympathetic outflow. Interestingly, many of these patients will be noted to develop a bluish discoloration of the lower extremities on prolonged standing.

A second group of patients may have a component of β-receptor supersensitivity. Some investigators have used the term "hyperadrenergic orthostatic intolerance" to describe the subset. Many of these patients complain of extreme tremulousness and anxiety, in addition to palpitations and tachycardia while standing. They also demonstrate exaggerated responses to low-dose isoproterenol infusions while supine (it is not uncommon to see heart rate increases of 30 beats/min or more in response to a 1 µg/min isoproterenol infusion). Serum catecholamine levels are quite high (serum norepinephrine levels are often > 600 ng/ml). It is unclear whether this supersensitivity is primary in nature or due to a secondary denervation supersensitivity. Indeed, some of these patients appear to display excessive sympathetic activation in some distributions almost all the time. This excessively sympathetic activation is not appropriately attenuated by baroreflex mechanisms. Indeed, recent genetic studies alluded to previously have demonstrated a mutation that results in a deficiency of the norepinephrine transporter that clears it from the synaptic cleft. Impairment of synaptic norepinephrine clearance could potentially result in a state of excessive sympathetic activation in response to physiologic stimuli.

While these patients share a number of characteristics with those who suffer from the partial dysautonomic form of POTS, they more often complain of tremor, migraine headache and cold sweaty extremities. Furthermore, detailed studies are presently under way to better understand the differences present in these two groups, and whether other subtypes may also exist.

The term "secondary POTS" is applied to those patients with a known autonomic disorder with preserved cardiac innervation despite peripheral autonomic denervation. This can be due to diseases such as diabetes, amyloidosis, Sjögren's syndrome or lupus. In occasional patients it may be the presenting sign of more severe disorders, such as pure autonomic failure or multiple systems atrophy [16].

Evaluation and Management

The first step is a detailed history and physical examination that includes a careful neurologic examination. Patients should also be evaluated for recognizable causes of orthostatic intolerance, such as anemia, dehydration, or any chronic debilitating illness. Any drug that the patient may be taking that could cause or aggravate the problem (such as vasodilators, tricyclic antidepressants, MAO inhibitors, or alcohol) should be identified. Heart rate and blood pressure should be measured in the supine, sitting, and standing positions. The standing pressures and heart rates should be checked immediately upon standing, and after 2 min and 5 min upright. If cardiac causes are suspected, these should be appropriately evaluated. Sinus tachycardia that is abrupt in onset and termination, unrelated to posture, suggests possible sinus node re-entry and may require electrophysiologic studies.

Tilt-table testing is often useful as a standardized measure of response to postural change [1].

The treatment of these patients can be somewhat of a challenge, as no single approach is uniformly successful. The first step in management of these patients is to rule out any correctable cause that might need special treatment. Conditions such as diabetes, significant weight loss, chronic debilitating disease, or prolonged immobilization are usually self-evident. One should also determine if any medications the patient may be taking could be contributing to the problem (and in some individuals one must consider whether illicit drug use could potentially play a role). An extremely important part of therapy is educating the patient and his/her family as to the nature of the disorder and to avoid aggravating factors such as extreme heat, dehydration, and excess alcohol consumption. Next, we try to increase salt and fluid intake. Patients are encouraged to sleep with the heads of their beds elevated. Mild aerobic exercise is strongly encouraged, with an eventual goal of performing 20 min activity three times a week. Resistance training to build up the lower extremities can be particularly helpful. Elastic support hose are useful in some patients. The hose should be waist high and provide 30 mmHg ankle counterpressure. Pharmacologic therapy must be tailored to meet the needs of each individual patient, and it should be remembered that those needs will change over time. Fludrocortisone is useful in many patients, with the usual dose around 0.2 mg/day. Midodrine is quite useful, due to its peripheral vasoconstrictive action, and is usually given in 5-10 mg doses three times a day. Patients with the β-receptor hypersensitivity form may respond to either β-blocking agents or to clonidine. In patients refractory to other forms of therapy, erythropoietin may be useful [16]. Some groups have reported that phenobarbital may be useful in selected patients. We have found the selective serotonin reuptake inhibitors useful in many patients, the most effective one being venlafaxine [17]. Frequently patients will require a combination of various therapies to be effective. A comprehensive review of potential treatments is beyond the scope of this review and more in-depth discussions of therapy can be found elsewhere [15].

Conclusions

POTS is a potentially recognizable and treatable disorder, in which patients present with a marked orthostatic intolerance manifested by postural tachycardia, palpitations, weakness, fatigue, and exercise intolerance. The importance of this disorder goes beyond the number of people it affects, as it may cause substantial disability among young, otherwise healthy individuals. During passive upright tilt, these patients demonstrate a heart rate increase of > 30 beats/min or a peak rate of > 120 beats/min within the first 10 min, reproducing the patients' symptoms. Some patients may exhibit an exaggerated response to isoproterenol. Therapies directed at correcting autonomic balance can often relieve the severity of the symptoms. Greater efforts will be necessary to better understand this syndrome and its various subtypes and provide therapies that will help this group of highly symptomatic patients return to normal life. Continuing research will help provide greater insight into this and other autonomic disturbances associated with chronic orthostatic intolerance.

Acknowledgements. The author gratefully acknowledges the unending encouragement and support of Barbara Straus, MD as well as the support of The Sheller-Globe Foundation. This study has been supported in part by a grant from The Sheller-Globe Foundation.

References

1. Grubb BP (1998) Neurocardiogenic syncope. In: Grubb BP, Olshansky B (eds) Syncope: mechanisms and management. Futura, Armonk, NY, pp 73-106

2. Grubb BP, Kosinski D, Boehm K, Kip K (1997) The postural orthostatic tachycardia syndrome: a neurocardiogenic variant identified during tilt table testing. Pacing Clin Electrophysiol 20:2205-2212
3. Benarroch E (1993) The central autonomic network: functional organization, dysfunction and perspective. Mayo Clinic Proc 68:988-1001
4. Wieling W, Lieshout J (1993) Maintenance of postural normotension in humans. In: Low P (ed) Clinical autonomic disorders. Little, Brown, Boston, MA, pp 69-73
5. DaCosta JM (1871) An irritable heart. Am J Med Sci 27:145-163
6. Holmgren A et al (1957) Low physical work capacity in suspected heart cases due to inadequate adjustment of peripheral blood flow (vasoregulatory asthenia). Acta Med Scand 158:413-415
7. MacLean AR, Allen EV, Magath TB (1944) Orthostatic tachycardia and orthostatic hypotension: defect in the return of venous blood to the heart. Am Heart J 27:145-163
8. Streeten DHP, Anderson GH Jr, Richardson R et al (1988) Abnormal orthostatic changes in blood pressure and heart rate in subjects with intact sympathetic nervous system function: evidence for excessive venous pooling. J Lab Clin Med 111:326-335
9. Schondorf R, Low P (1993) Idiopathic postural orthostatic tachycardia syndrome: an attenuated form of acute pandysautonomia? Neurology 43:132-137
10. Low P, Opfer-Gehrking T, Textor S et al (1995) Postural tachycardia syndrome. Neurology 45:519-525
11. Karas B, Grubb BP, Boehm K, Kip K (2000) The postural orthostatic tachycardia syndrome: a potentially treatable cause of chronic fatigue, exercise intolerance and cognitive impairment in adolescents. Pacing Clin Electrophysiol 23:344-351
12. Shannon JR, Flattem NL, Jordan J et al (2000) Orthostatic intolerance and tachycardia associated with norepinephrine-transporter deficiency. N Engl J Med 342:541-549
13. Vernino S, Low P, Fealey R et al (2000) Auto-antibodies to ganglionic acetylcholine receptors in auto-immune autonomic neuropathies. N Engl J Med 343:847-855
14. Shen WK, Low P, Tahangir A et al (2001) Is sinus node modification appropriate for inappropriate sinus tachycardia with features of postural orthostatic tachycardia syndrome? Pacing Clin Electrophysiol 24:217-230
15. Grubb BP, Kanjwal MY, Kosinski DJ (2001) The postural orthostatic tachycardia syndrome: current concepts in pathophysiology, diagnosis and management. J Intervent Cardiac Electrophysiol 5:9-16
16. Grubb BP (1998) Dysautonomic syncope. In: Grubb BP, Olshansky B (eds) Syncope: mechanisms and management. Futura, Armonk, NY, pp 107-126
17. Grubb BP, Karas BJ (1998) The potential role of serotonin in the pathogenesis of neurocardiogenic syncope and related autonomic disturbances. J Intervent Cardiac Electrophysiol 2:325-332

Syncope in Hypertrophic Cardiomyopathy: What are the Potential Mechanisms and Therapeutic Implications?

S. Betocchi and F. Manganelli

Incidence

Syncope is a common occurrence in hypertrophic cardiomyopathy. About one symptomatic patient out of three has already experienced or will experience one or more syncopal episodes [1]. Although an exhaustive epidemiological assessment of syncope in hypertrophic cardiomyopathy has never been performed, some clinical characteristics are widely recognized.

Syncope is somewhat more common in youth; this finding is also found in vasovagal syncope, and suggests that the two forms of syncope have some mechanisms in common. The clinical presentation of patients with hypertrophic cardiomyopathy and syncope is rather bizarre: some patients have one or two episodes in a lifetime, while others experience numerous spells that are quite debilitating. A somewhat typical pattern is that syncopal episodes are clustered in a short time frame, followed by a "free" period. As we will see later, syncope may be an ominous sign and should not be overlooked. Syncope can occur while the patient is resting, or during exercise, or it may be related to postural changes (such as suddenly rising from bed). The modality of occurrence of syncope may be related to the pathophysiological mechanisms, but this link remains sometimes elusive.

Pathophysiology

Left Ventricular Outflow Tract Obstruction

The presence of a left ventricular outflow tract gradient (observed in about 25% of patients with hypertrophic cardiomyopathy [1]) has classically been related to the occurrence of syncope. The mechanism for syncope (especially

Department of Clinical Medicine, Cardiovascular and Immunological Sciences, Federico II University of Naples, Italy

exercise-related syncope) was thought to be similar to that in severe valvular aortic stenosis: that exercise-induced vasodilation not associated with a parallel increase in cardiac output, owing to a "fixed" outflow tract area.

Recently, the relevance of left ventricular outflow tract gradient to syncope has been questioned: first, because the incidence of syncope is the same in patients with and without obstruction [2]; secondly, because obstruction does not explain syncope at rest or postural syncope; and thirdly, because the relief of obstruction is not always associated with a decrease in the occurrence of syncope. Only treatment of obstruction by dual-chamber pacing has been shown, in one study [3], to reduce the occurrence of syncope; but pacing could prevent syncope through other mechanisms than a decreased left ventricular outflow tract gradient. It is noteworthy that surgical myotomymyectomy or septal ablation obtained by injecting alcohol into septal branch(es), as well as DDD pacing in other studies [4, 5] have no impact on syncope.

The link between left ventricular outflow tract gradient and syncope remains elusive, and obstruction is not presently considered an important determinant of syncope.

Arrhythmias

Short-lasting, spontaneously recovering ventricular tachyarrhythmias, namely ventricular tachycardia and fibrillation, have the potential to induce syncope, although the complex pathophysiology of hypertrophic cardiomyopathy may lead to hemodynamic syncope through several different mechanisms. Probably some, but not most syncopal episodes have these arrhythmias as a background.

ECG Holter monitoring has proved of dubious help in identifying an arrhythmic substrate for syncope in hypertrophic cardiomyopathy. While the relationship between ventricular tachycardia and sudden death has been elucidated in sufficient detail [6], the association with syncope is less clear. In electrophysiological studies, sustained monomorphic ventricular tachycardia can be induced in virtually all patients with hypertrophic cardiomyopathy and a history of resuscitation from sudden death, and in many patients with a history of syncope. Fananapazir and coworkers have shown that inducible sustained ventricular tachycardia has a good positive predictive power for major arrhythmic events in patients with history of syncope [7]: this finding suggests that this approach can single out those patients in whom previous syncope was due to arrhythmias, while those in whom ventricular tachycardia could not be induced might be the ones with hemodynamic syncope. Clearly, an electrophysiological study could not be proposed as a screening method to identify patients at risk, because of ethical and practical considerations, but also because in the general population of patients with hypertrophic cardiomyopathy its diagnostic power is much less than in subgroups of patients with symptoms of impaired consciousness (aborted sudden death or syncope) [7].

It has been demonstrated that supraventricular tachycardia (as induced by rapid atrial pacing) can evoke hypotension and presyncope in 25% of patients with hypertrophic cardiomyopathy; of note is that this acute hemodynamic deterioration was more marked in patients with than in those without a history of syncope [8]. Another study reports a higher prevalence of induced sustained supraventricular tachycardia in patients with previous dizziness or syncope (73%) than in those without (16%); this finding supports a potential role of atrial tachyarrhythmias in syncope of patients with hypertrophic cardiomyopathy [9]. Moreover, Lopez Gil et al. showed recently that short runs of atrial pacing induce a QRS widening and then a ventricular fibrillation in three patients with hypertrophic cardiomyopathy, two of whom had a history of previous ventricular fibrillation [10]. Therefore, in some clinical instances, rapid atrial rates may per se lead to hemodynamic collapse, by critically impairing left ventricular filling, or may trigger major ventricular arrhythmias responsible for syncope.

Complete atrioventricular block is very unusual in patients with hypertrophic cardiomyopathy and it has been demonstrated as a cause of syncope only in anecdotal case reports [11, 13].

Myocardial Ischemia

Angina pectoris and myocardial ischemia are prominent features of hypertrophic cardiomyopathy and several mechanisms (intramural small vessels abnormalities, abnormal myocellular architecture, massive hypertrophy) may account for impaired coronary reserve, even in the absence of epicardial coronary artery stenosis. Recurrent myocardial ischemia may cause myocardial injury and scarring, which can reduce the threshold for ventricular arrhythmias.

Dilsizian et al. demonstrated that, in young patients with a history of cardiac arrest, exercise-induced myocardial ischemia is invariably present, whereas a primary arrhythmogenic ventricular substrate could be found in a minority of them [14]. All 15 patients with history of cardiac arrest or syncope had reversible thallium abnormalities, whereas ventricular tachycardia was induced by electrophysiological study in only 4 (27%); these findings suggest that myocardial ischemia plays a role in cardiac arrest and, possibly, syncope that is more relevant than the presence of arrhythmogenic substrates. Lazzeroni et al. reported that ECG signs of myocardial ischemia elicited by dipyridamole infusion may identify patients with hypertrophic cardiomyopathy at higher risk of cardiac events (among them syncope), supporting a potential role of myocardial ischemia in causing frank collapse [15]. Conversely, in another study assessing myocardial blood flow by positron emission tomography, coronary reserve was found to be similar in patients with and in those without syncope [16]. These conflicting data are the consequence of the inherent difficulties in assessing ischemia in hypertrophic cardiomyopathy.

Peripheral Nervous System Activation

In patients with vasovagal (also called neurally mediated) syncope, loss of consciousness is generally attributed to the activation of left ventricular mechanoreceptors that mediate the Bezold-Jarisch reflex. Since a small left ventricular cavity with vigorous systolic function is deemed an ideal substrate to elicite this reflex, Gilligan et al. suggested that reflex hypotension and bradycardia could be a mechanism of syncope in some patients with hypertrophic cardiomyopathy [17]. According to this view, exercise-induced hypotension, due to a fall in systemic vascular resistance despite a rise in cardiac index, could be responsible for symptoms of impaired consciousness (including frank syncope) during effort [18].

Conversely, little is known about the role of sympathovagal balance in the pathogenesis of syncope. Although patients with hypertrophic cardiomyopathy have a selective impairment of vagal modulation of heart rate compared to controls, a relation between autonomic dysfunction and syncope has not been clearly proved [19, 20].

Diastolic Dysfunction

Impairment of diastolic function is common in patients with hypertrophic cardiomyopathy and pieces of evidence support the hypothesis that diastolic dysfunction could be implicated in some clinical circumstances. Nienaber and coworkers showed that small left ventricular end-diastolic volume, nonsustained ventricular tachycardia, and young age may identify patients at risk for syncope [21]. Accordingly, in a large population of outpatients with hypertrophic cardiomyopathy, we found left ventricular end-diastolic diameter to be the only independent predictor of syncopal events among several clinical, echocardiographic and radionuclide variables [22]. Since left ventricular end-diastolic diameter is directly correlated to peak filling rate, a small cavity size may be considered as a morphological marker of inadequate filling characteristics in patients with hypertrophic cardiomyopathy. Our preliminary results during head-up tilt extend these findings: while the hemodynamic adaptation of patients without a history of syncope is similar to that of normal subjects, in patients with a history of syncope, volume unloading resulted in an abnormal reduction in cardiac output, causing significant hypotension and sometimes frank syncope [23]. In other words, in some patients, higher left ventricular filling pressures, due to a more severe diastolic dysfunction, might involve a major susceptibility to sudden unloading.

Therapeutic Implications

Hypertrophic cardiomyopathy is the most common cause of sudden death in otherwise healthy individuals and, over the past decade, progress has been made in identifying patients at higher risk of sudden death. Syncope is a well-known risk factor, and patients who have experienced recurrent syncope deserve an aggressive therapeutic strategy, particularly if they have a family history of sudden death, nonsustained ventricular tachycardia, marked hypertrophy, and abnormal blood pressure response during exercise [24]. A very recent study by Elliot et al. showed a significant interaction between syncope and a family history of sudden death, and found a risk ratio for sudden death of 5.3:1 when these features were taken together [25]. Patients with two or more risk factors have a substantially increased risk of sudden death and warrant consideration for prophylactic therapy. In a study investigating patients' outcome after resuscitated ventricular fibrillation or sustained ventricular tachycardia with syncope, only implantable cardioverter-defibrillators seem to improve survival [26]. Recently, a multicenter study enrolling 128 high-risk patients demonstrated that implantable defibrillators are an effective therapeutic option in both primary and secondary prevention of sudden death in hypertrophic cardiomyopathy by effectively terminating ventricular tachycardia or fibrillation [27]. Interestingly, two-thirds of patients underwent implantation prophylactically for primary prevention of sudden death, and in almost half of these patients syncope, alone or in combination with other markers, was the clinical reason for implantation. Despite the nonrandomized design of the study, the protection provided by an implantable defibrillator does indeed appear to be considerably superior to that with conventional antiarrhythmic therapy. However, during follow-up in patients with hypertrophic cardiomyopathy after cardioverter-defibrillator implantation, a low incidence of recurrence of ventricular tachycardia/fibrillation was observed [28].

There is evidence that ventricular tachyarrhythmias are not the only mechanism of syncope in patients with hypertrophic cardiomyopathy. Although in selected patients (i.e. patients with two or more risk factors) implantable defibrillators must be regarded as the therapy of choice against a devastating feature of hypertrophic cardiomyopathy, it cannot be the solution for all patients with syncope. Consequently, physicians involved in the management of patients with syncope must take into account the different potential mechanisms which could be involved in the individual case.

References

1. Maron BJ, Bonow RO, Cannon RO III et al (1987) Hypertrophic cardiomyopathy. Interrelations of clinical manifestation, pathophysiology, and therapy. N Engl J Med 316:844-852
2. Wigle ED, Sasson Z, Henderson MA et al (1989) Hypertrophic cardiomyopathy: the importance of the site and the extent of hypertrophy: a review. Prog Cardiovasc Dis 28:1-83
3. Fananapazir L, Cannon RO III, Tripodi D, Panza JA (1992) Impact of dual-chamber permanent pacing in patients with obstructive hypertrophic cardiomyopathy with symptoms refractory to verapamil and β-adrenergic blocker therapy. Circulation 85:2149-2161
4. Jeanrenaud X, Goy JJ, Kappenberger L (1992) Effects of dual-chamber pacing in hypertrophic obstructive cardiomyopathy. Lancet 339:1318-1323

5. Slade AKB, Sadoul N, Shapiro L et al (1996) DDD pacing in hypertrophic cardiomyopathy: a multicentre clinical experience. Heart 75:44-49

6. Spirito P, Rapezzi C, Autore C et al (1994) Prognosis of asymptomatic patients with hypertrophic cardiomyopathy and nonsustained ventricular tachycardia. Circulation 90:2743-2747

7. Fananapazir L, Chang AC, Epstein E, McArevey D (1992) Prognostic determinants in hypertrophic cardiomyopathy. Prospective evaluation of a therapeutic strategy based on clinical-Holter, hemodynamic, and electrophysiological findings. Circulation 86:730-740

8. Nakatani M, Yokota Y, Yokoyama M (1996) Acute hemodynamic deterioration during rapid atrial pacing in patients with HCM. Clin Cardiol 19:385-392

9. Brembilla-Perrot B, Jacquot A, Beurrier D, Jacquemin L (1997) Hypertrophic cardiomyopathy: value of atrial programmed electrical stimulation in patients with or without syncope with special reference to the role of atrial arrhythmias. Int J Cardiol 59:47-56

10. Lopez Gil M, Arribas F, Cosio FG (2000) Ventricular fibrillation induced by rapid atrial rates in patients with hypertrophic cardiomyopathy. Europace 2:327-332

11. Chmielewski CA, Riley RS, Mahendran A, Most AS (1977) Complete heart block as a cause of syncope in asymmetric septal hypertrophy. Am Heart J 93:91-93

12. Khair GZ, Bamrah VS (1985) Syncope in hypertrophic cardiomyopathy. Association with atrioventricular block. Am Heart J 110:1081-1083

13. Yes LM, Bayata S, Susam I et al (1999) Rare association of hypertrophic cardiomyopathy and complete atrioventricular block with prompt disappearance of outflow gradient after DDD pacing. Europace 1:280-282

14. Dilsizian V, Bonow RO, Epstein SE, Fananapazir L (1993) Myocardial ischemia detected by thallium scintigraphy is frequently related to cardiac arrest and syncope in young patients with hypertrophic cardiomyopathy. J Am Coll Cardiol 22:796-804

15. Lazzeroni E, Picano E, Morozzi L et al (1997) Dipyridamole-induced ischemia as a prognostic marker of future adverse cardiac events in adult patients with hypertrophic cardiomyopathy. Echo Persantine Italian Cooperative (EPIC) Study Group, Subproject Hypertrophic Cardiomyopathy. Circulation 96:4268-4272

16. Lorenzoni R, Gistri R, Cecchi F et al (1997) Syncope and ventricular arrhythmias in hypertrophic cardiomyopathy are not related to derangement of coronary microvascular function. Eur Heart J 18:1946:1950

17. Gilligan DM, Nihoyannopoulos P, Chan WL, Oakley CM (1992) Investigation of a hemodynamic basis for syncope in hypertrophic cardiomyopathy. Use of a head-up tilt test. Circulation 85:2140-2148

18. Frenneaux MP, Counihan PJ, Caforio ALP et al (1990) Abnormal blood pressure response during exercise in hypertrophic cardiomyopathy. Circulation 82:1995-2000

19. Gilligan DM, Chan WL, Sbauroni E et al (1993) Autonomic function in hypertrophic cardiomyopathy. Br Heart J 69:525-529

20. Bonaduce D, Petretta M, Betocchi S et al (1997) Heart rate variability in patients with hypertrophic cardiomyopathy: association with clinical and echocardiographic features. Am Heart J 134:165-172

21. Nienaber CA, Hiller S, Spielmann RP et al (1990) Syncope in hypertrophic cardiomyopathy: multivariate analysis of prognostic determinants. J Am Coll Cardiol 15:948-955

22. Manganelli F, Betocchi S, Losi MA et al (1999) Influence of left ventricular cavity size on clinical presentation in hypertrophic cardiomyopathy. Am J Cardiol 83:547-552

23. Manganelli F, Betocchi S, Ciampi Q et al (1999) Hemodynamic determinants of syncope in hypertrophic cardiomyopathy. Eur Heart J 20:622 (abstr)

24. Spirito P, Seidman CE, McKenna WJ, Maron BJ (1997) The management of hypertrophic cardiomyopathy. N Engl J Med 336:775-785
25. Elliott PM, Poloniecki J, Dickie S et al (2000) Sudden death in hypertrophic cardiomyopathy. Identification of high risk patients. J Am Coll Cardiol 36:2212-2218
26. Elliott PM, Sharma S, Varnava A et al (1999) Survival after cardiac arrest or sustained ventricular tachycardia in patients with hypertrophic cardiomyopathy. J Am Coll Cardiol 33:1596-1601
27. Maron BJ, Shen W-K, Link MS et al (2000) Efficacy of implantable cardioverter-defibrillators for the prevention of sudden death in patients with hypertrophic cardiomyopathy. N Engl J Med 342:365-373
28. Primo J, Geelen P, Brugada J et al (1998) Hypertrophic cardiomyopathy: role of the implantable cardioverter-defibrillator. J Am Coll Cardiol 31:1086-1088

Intraventricular Conduction Disturbances and Negative Electrophysiologic Study in Patients with Syncope: What Should One Do?

C. MENOZZI[1], N. BOTTONI[1] AND M. BRIGNOLE[2]

Patients with bundle branch block (BBB), right bundle branch block plus left anterior or left posterior fascicular block or left bundle branch block are at higher risk of developing high-degree atrioventricular (AV) block. A significant problem in the evaluation of syncope and BBB is the transient nature of high-degree AV block and, therefore, the long periods required to document it by ECG.

Data from two syncope units (Lavagna and Reggio Emilia) showed that in 15% of the patients referred for syncope and BBB the diagnosis had remained unexplained at the end of the conventional work-up [1]. Even if the finding of BBB in patients with syncope suggests that paroxysmal AV block may be the cause of syncope, we observed that several causes of syncope were found during conventional investigations in an unselected population of 55 consecutive patients with BBB. *Cardiac* syncope was found in 25 patients (45%): AV block in 20 patients, sick sinus syndrome in 2, sustained ventricular tachycardia in 1, and aortic stenosis in 2. *Neuromediated* syncope was found in 22 (40%): carotid sinus syndrome in 5, tilt-induced syncope in 15, and adenosine-sensitive syncope in 2. Syncope remained *unexplained* in 8 (15%).

Is the Diagnostic Value of the Electrophysiological Study High Enough to be Acceptable?

In studies conducted by Gronda et al. [2] and Bergfeldt et al. [3], complete electrophysiologic investigation, including drug stress, was able to predict the development of stable AV block in 87% and 80% of patients, respectively. In patients with negative electrophysiologic studies, Link et al. [4] observed development of stable AV block in 18% (after 30 months) and Gaggioli et al. [5] in

[1]Department of Interventional Cardiology and Arrhythmologic Center, Ospedale S. Maria Nuova, Reggio Emilia; [2]Department of Cardiology and Arrhythmologic Center, Ospedali Riuniti, Lavagna, Italy

19% (after 62 months), suggesting that some results are false negatives; the syncope recurrence rate was 19% after 2.2 years in one study [6] and about 40% after 3 years in another [4]; mortality was generally low [4, 6, 7]. Thus, even if electrophysiologic study remains an obligatory step in the evaluation of patients with syncope and BBB, there nevertheless exist a substantial number of patients with false negative results that require further investigation.

So far, little is known about the mechanism of syncope in patients with a negative electrophysiologic investigation. An implantable event monitor has recently become available and has been validated in patients with unexplained syncope [8]. Its use seems promising in patients with BBB and negative electrophysiologic study as well, to evaluate the natural history of these patients and obtain further information on the mechanism of syncope.

Mechanism of Syncope in Patients with BBB and Negative Electrophysiologic Result

The International Study of Syncope of Uncertain Etiology (ISSUE) is a multicenter international prospective study aimed at analyzing the diagnostic contribution of implantable loop recorders (ILR) in four predefined groups of patients with syncope of uncertain origin: (1) the isolated syncope group, i.e., patients without structural heart disease or with minor cardiac abnormalities considered to be without clinical relevance and not suggestive of a cardiac cause of syncope, and with absence of intraventricular conduction defects and negative complete work-up including tilt testing; (2) the tilt-positive group, i.e, patients as above but who had a positive response to tilt testing; (3) the suspected bradycardia group, i.e., patients with BBB and negative electrophysiologic test; and (4) the suspected tachycardia group, i.e, patients with overt heart disease at risk of ventricular arrhythmia, as these were patients with previous myocardial infarction or cardiomyopathy with depressed ejection fraction or nonsustained ventricular tachycardia in whom an electrophysiologic study did not induce sustained ventricular arrhythmias. The patients in the present study belong to subgroup 3 with BBB and negative electrophysiologic test result [9].

Findings

An ILR was applied in 52 patients. During a follow-up of 3-15 months, syncope recurred in 22 patients (42%) and the event was documented in 19 patients after a median of 48 days. The most frequent finding – which occurred in 17 patients – was one or multiple prolonged asystolic pauses, mainly due to AV block (Fig. 1). The remaining two patients had normal sinus rhythm or sinus tachycardia. The onset of the bradycardic episodes was always sudden, but sometimes it was preceded by ventricular premature beats. The median duration of the arrhythmic event was 47 s. Three other patients developed nonsyn-

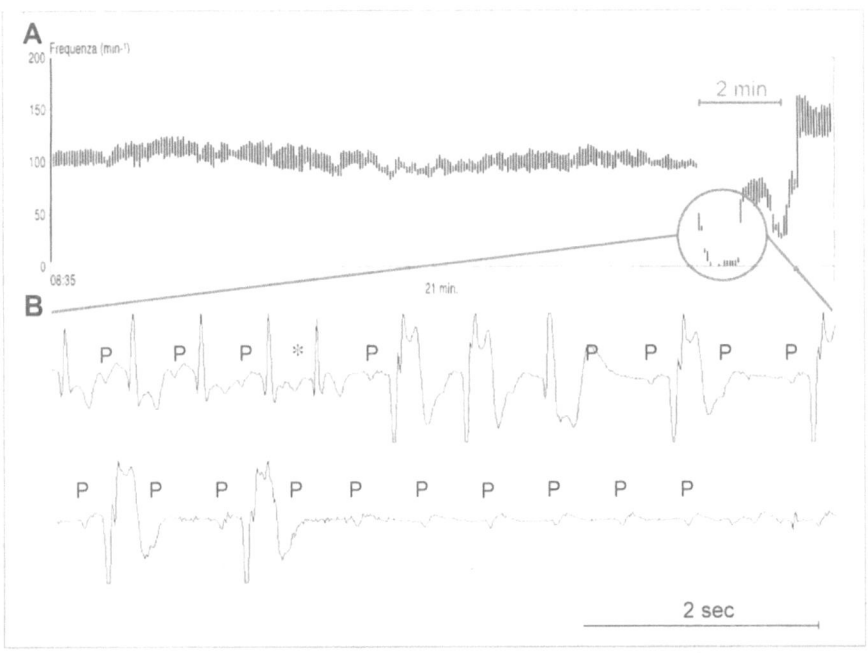

Fig. 1. Syncopal event observed in a patient. *Panel A:* Heart rate trend during the whole 21-min loop recording. Initially, the heart rate is stable at approximately 100 bpm, but it suddenly falls at the time of the syncope. *Panel B:* The expanded ECG shows a premature atrial beat (*) that seems to trigger the AV block. Initially during the block there are seven idioventricular beats, then prolonged asystole occurs

copal persistent third degree AV block and two patients had presyncope due to AV block with asystole. Overall, an intermittent or stable AV block was observed in 17 patients (33%), with actuarial estimates of 24%, 34%, and 34% at 3, 9, and 15 months. No clinical variable at baseline was able to predict the development of AV block. No patients had injury due to syncopal relapse.

Conclusions

In patients with BBB and negative electrophysiologic study, most syncopal recurrences have a homogeneous mechanism characterized by prolonged asystolic pauses mainly due to sudden-onset paroxysmal AV block. However, the majority of the patients remain free of events for more than 1 year.

Using the results of the present study as a reference standard for arrhythmic causes of syncope, we can shed new light on the diagnostic value of electrophysiologic investigation. In particular, this study shows that electrophysiologic investigation has a low sensitivity in detecting paroxysmal AV block as the cause of syncope, yielding at least a 33% rate of false negative results. Until now, this figure could be calculated only indirectly from the rate of development of stable AV block, which was roughly 5% per year in the literature [3, 4], a figure confirmed in this study.

Practical Implications: Pacemaker or Not ?

In patients with BBB and negative electrophysiologic study, an ILR-guided strategy seems reasonable, with pacemaker implantation safely delayed until symptomatic bradycardia is documented. In accordance with this approach, 44% of our patients received a pacemaker after their first documented syncope. Other patients would probably have had a documented syncopal recurrence if the monitoring phase had been prolonged further. The usefulness of a very prolonged monitoring phase and the efficacy of therapy in suppressing further syncopal recurrences remain to be proved. Owing to the high rate of AV block observed, the only acceptable alternative strategy is to implant a pacemaker in all patients with BBB and unexplained syncope. Which of these two strategies is more cost-effective remains to be shown. The present study forms the background for programming research in this direction.

References

1. Donateo P, Alboni P, Brignole M et al (2000) The mechanism of syncope in patients with bundle branch block (abstract). Europace (Suppl)2:A43
2. Gronda M, Magnani A, Occhetta E et al (1984) Electrophysiologic study of atrio-ventricular block and ventricular conduction defects. G Ital Cardiol 14:768-773
3. Bergfeldt L, Edvardsson N, Rosenqvist M et al (1994) Atrioventricular block progression in patients with bifascicular block assessed by repeated electrocardiography and a bradycardia-detecting pacemaker. Am J Cardiol 74:1129-1132
4. Link M, Kim KM, Homoud M et al (1999) Long-term outcome of patients with syncope associated with coronary artery disease and a non-diagnostic electrophysiological evaluation. Am J Cardiol 83:1334-1337
5. Gaggioli G, Bottoni N, Brignole M et al (1994) Progression to second- or third-degree atrioventricular block in patients electrostimulated for bundle branch block: a long-term study. G Ital Cardiol 24:409-416
6. Click R, Gersh B, Sugrue D et al (1987) Role of invasive electrophysiologic testing in patients with symptomatic bundle branch block. Am J Cardiol 59:817-823
7. Englund A, Bergfeldt L, Rehnquist N et al (1995) Diagnostic value of programmed ventricular stimulation in patients with bifascicular block: a prospective study in patients with and without syncope. J Am Coll Cardiol 26:1508-1515
8. Krahn AD, Klein GJ, Yee R et al (1999) Use of an extended monitoring strategy in patients with problematic syncope. Reveal Investigators. Circulation 99:406-410
9. Brignole M, Menozzi C, Moya A et al (2001) The mechanism of syncope in patients with bundle branch block and negative electrophysiologic test. Circulation (in press)

Unexplained Syncope with Inducible Sustained Ventricular Arrhythmias: to Implant or Not to Implant an ICD?

A. Raviele

Introduction

The induction of a sustained ventricular arrhythmia in patients with otherwise unexplained syncope is generally regarded as an important finding with an unfavorable prognosis that deserves aggressive treatment with an implantable cardioverter-defibrillator (ICD). However, the real significance of an induced arrhythmia in patients with syncope of unknown origin varies greatly according to different factors, especially the programmed stimulation protocol used, the type of arrhythmia induced, and the patient characteristics, in particular the presence, type, and severity of underlying heart disease.

As general rule, the proportion of patients who are inducible at programmed ventricular stimulation – that is the sensitivity of the test – is higher and the specificity is lower when an aggressive protocol (≥ 3 extrastimuli, very short coupling intervals, 2 stimulation sites) is used [1, 2]. Moreover, it is universally accepted that the induction of a monomorphic ventricular tachycardia is a specific event that should guide therapy, whereas the induction of a polymorphic ventricular tachycardia or ventricular fibrillation is a less specific feature, especially when obtained with an aggressive protocol [3, 4]. Finally, the meaning of an inducible sustained ventricular arrhythmia in cases of syncope of undetermined nature is strictly dependent on the particular clinical context of the patient. It is better known for patients with cardiac disease, especially those with ischemic cardiomyopathy, but is less clear for patients with an apparently normal heart [2].

In this paper, the role of programmed ventricular stimulation as a diagnostic tool to unmask a potentially lethal arrhythmia as a cause of syncope in different clinical settings, and the usefulness of ICD implantation in inducible patients, will be reviewed.

Cardiovascular Department, Division of Cardiology, Umberto I Hospital, Mestre-Venice, Italy

Value of Programmed Ventricular Stimulation

In patients with organic heart disease and otherwise unexplained syncope, a sustained ventricular arrhythmia is frequently induced during an electrophysiologic study (20%-26% of the cases) [5-9]. Patients who are more prone to this event are men with ischemic heart disease (in particular with previous myocardial infarction), left ventricular ejection fraction (EF) ≤ 40%, bundle branch block, ventricular late potentials, nonsustained ventricular tachycardia by Holter monitoring, and injury related to loss of consciousness [7-13]. The prognosis of these patients is usually poor, similar to that of patients with documented spontaneous ventricular tachyarrhythmia [7] and (at least for patients with ischemic heart disease) significantly worse of that of noninducible patients [9, 14]. For example, in the ESVEM trial (pre-ICD era), the reported arrhythmic and all-cause mortality rates of patients with syncope of unknown origin and positive electrophysiologic study were 21% and 24%, respectively, at 1 year and 37% and 42%, respectively, at 4 years [9].

However, not in all clinical circumstances does programmed ventricular stimulation have good predictive value. This is particularly true for patients with idiopathic dilated cardiomyopathy or severe heart failure and undetermined syncope, who have a substantially increased risk of sudden death regardless of the outcome of electrophysiologic study [15-18]. In patients with hypertrophic cardiomyopathy and syncope or presyncope, the inducibility of polymorphic ventricular tachycardia or ventricular fibrillation is a common finding [19, 20], but its clinical and prognostic significance is still uncertain [19, 21, 22]. A sustained ventricular arrhythmia is inducible in 43% of patients with valvular heart disease and unexplained syncope (monomorphic ventricular tachycardia in 14% and ventricular fibrillation in 29%); however, only the induction of ventricular tachycardia seems to be predictive of future arrhythmic events [23]. In patients with mitral valve prolapse the percentage of induction is similar (23%), but to date it is unclear in which patients this feature is really important and in which it is by contrast a nonspecific response to programmed ventricular stimulation [24]. The inducibility of life-threatening ventricular arrhythmias in patients with bifascicular block and undocumented syncope is particularly high (20%-34%); however, on the basis of literature data, it seems that the occurrence of clinical events during follow-up is not accurately predicted by the results of programmed ventricular stimulation in this condition [25, 26].

The usefulness of electrophysiologic study to stratify the arrhythmic risk in patients with arrhythmogenic right ventricular cardiomyopathy and undetermined syncope has not yet been established [27]. Programmed ventricular stimulation, by contrast, has proven to be of limited value in the diagnosis and treatment of patients with long QT syndrome with syncope or cardiac arrest [28]. In patients with Brugada syndrome, ventricular fibrillation or sustained polymorphic ventricular tachycardia is often induced at programmed ventricular stimulation (67%-80% of cases), with similar proportions in patients who are symptomatic and in those who are asymptomatic for syncope or cardiac arrest [29, 30]. The inducibility of sustained ventricular arrhythmia in these patients, however, is apparently not correlated to the clinical outcome during follow-up [29, 30].

Finally, in patients with apparently normal heart and syncope of unknown origin, an electrophysiologic study rarely yields positive results (< 5% of cases) [5, 31, 32]. Moreover, when an arrhythmia is induced, only the occurrence of monomorphic sustained ventricular tachycardia seems to have clinical relevance, whereas the induction of polymorphic ventricular tachycardia and ventricular fibrillation is generally considered a nonspecific response to aggressive stimulation protocols [3, 4], a concept that probably needs to be modified.

Value of ICD Therapy

The advent of the ICD and its use in patients with unexplained syncope and inducible sustained ventricular tachyarrhythmias allows accurate documentation of the arrhythmic events during the follow-up and, consequently, verification of the real diagnostic and prognostic accuracy of programmed ventricular stimulation in different categories of patients. The majority of currently available data refer to patients with ischemic heart disease and idiopathic dilated cardiomyopathy.

In patients with ischemic heart disease, an appropriate discharge of the ICD due to a recurrence of ventricular tachycardia or ventricular fibrillation occurs in a high proportion of patients (36%-57%) during a mean follow-up of 11-34 months [33-38]. This proportion is similar to that observed in patients with documented sustained ventricular tachyarrhythmias [36-38]. These findings suggest that electrophysiologic testing in undocumented syncope is effectively able to identify patients with potentially life-threatening ventricular tachyarrhythmias who need ICD implantation. It is noteworthy that the incidence of appropriate ICD interventions in patients with severe left ventricular dysfunction (EF ≤ 35%) is significantly higher than that in patients who are hemodynamically less compromised (EF > 35%): 82% vs 44% at 1 year [33]. This is in agreement with the results of two secondary analyses of the AVID and CIDS trials, which have demonstrated that the patients with ICD who benefit most from device implantation are those with a severely depressed left ventricular EF (≤ 35%) [39, 40]. Interestingly, patients with unexplained syncope and inducible sustained ventricular arrhythmias remain at high risk of dying, despite ICD implantation and the frequent appropriate delivery of ICD therapies [35]. The prognosis of these patients, as already found in studies performed in pre-ICD era, is significantly worse than that of noninducible patients [35] and similar to that of patients with documented ventricular tachyarrhythmias [37, 38], with 1-year and 2-year all-cause mortality rates of 33% and 55%, respectively [35].

Regarding idiopathic dilated cardiomyopathy, patients with unexplained syncope and negative electrophysiologic study have, according to Knight et al., the same incidence of appropriate ICD discharges (50% vs 42%) and overall mortality (28% vs 32%) than a matched group of patients with a cardiac arrest due to ventricular tachyarrhythmia [18]. This confirms that programmed ventricular stimulation has a low predictive value in patients with nonischemic cardiomyopathy and suggests that in these patients risk stratification based on clinical evaluation is superior to that based on the results of an electrophysiologic study. Implantation of ICD in these patients is associated with a high incidence of appropriate shocks (40%) and with a reduction of sudden death and overall mortality when compared to conventional therapy: 15% vs 33% at 2 years [41].

The value of ICD therapy in other clinical settings is less clear, but on the basis of indirect evidence it is likely that device implantation is useful in selected categories of patients with unexplained syncope and inducible ventricular arrhythmias, such as patients with hypertrophic cardiomyopathy, arrhythmogenic right ventricular cardiomyopathy, and Brugada syndrome.

Conclusions

Electrophysiologic study with programmed electrical stimulation is a valid diagnostic test in patients with ischemic heart disease and syncope of undetermined nature. Its utility is more questionable in patients with idiopathic dilated cardiomyopathy and other clinical conditions. The implantation of an ICD is certainly effective in inducible patients with ischemic cardiomyopathy. The device also seems to be useful in patients with idiopathic dilated cardiomyopathy regardless of the outcome of programmed ventricular stimulation. The role of ICD in other clinical situations needs to be clarified by future prospective studies.

References

1. Raviele A, Di Pede F, Piccolo E (1985) Protocollo di studio elettrofarmacologico seriato per la scelta della terapia antiaritmica cronica più efficace nei pazienti con tachicardie ventricolari sostenute e ricorrenti e nei sopravvissuti ad un arresto cardiaco secondario a tachiaritmie ventricolari. G Ital Cardiol 15/I:354-357
2. Bigger JT, Reiffel JA, Livelli FD, Wang PJ (1986) Sensitivity, specificity, and reproducibility of programmed ventricular stimulation. Circulation 73[Suppl II]:73-78
3. Morady F, Di Carlo L, Winston S et al (1984) A prospective comparison of triple extrastimuli and left ventricular stimulation in studies of ventricular tachycardia induction. Circulation 70:52-57
4. Brugada P, Green M, Abdollah H, Wellens HJJ (1984) Significance of ventricular arrhythmias initiated by programmed ventricular stimulation: the importance of the type of ventricular arrhythmia induced and the number of premature stimuli required. Circulation 69:87-92
5. Morady F, Shen E, Schwartz A et al (1983) Long-term follow-up of patients with recurrent unexplained syncope evaluated by electrophysiologic testing. J Am Coll Cardiol 2:1053-1059

6. Doherty JU, Pembrook-Rogers D, Grogane EW et al (1985) Electrophysiologic evaluation and follow-up characteristic of patients with recurrent unexplained syncope and presyncope. Am J Cardiol 55:703-708

7. Olshansky B, Mazuz M, Martins JB (1985) Significance of inducible tachycardia in patients with syncope of unknown origin: a long-term follow-up. J Am Coll Cardiol 5:216-223

8. Krol RB, Morady F, Flaker GC et al (1987) Electrophysiologic testing in patients with unexplained syncope: clinical and noninvasive predictors of outcome. J Am Coll Cardiol 10:358-363

9. Bass EB, Elson JJ, Fogoros RN et al (1988) Long-term prognosis of patients undergoing electrophysiologic studies for syncope of unknown origin. Am J Cardiol 62:1186-1191

10. Haïssaguerre M, Commenges D, Mathio JL et al (1989) Electrophysiologic study of syncope. Prediction of results. Presse Med 18:212-214

11. Linzer M, Prystowsky EN, Divine GW et al (1991) Predicting the outcomes of electrophysiologic studies of patients with unexplained syncope: preliminary validation of a derived model. J Gen Intern Med 6:113-120

12. Bachinsky WB, Linzer M, Weld L, Estes NAM III (1992) Usefulness of clinical characteristics in predicting the outcome of electrophysiologic studies in unexplained syncope. Am J Cardiol 69:1044-1049

13. Winters SL, Stewart D, Gomes JA (1987) Signal averaging at the surface QRS complex predicts inducibility of ventricular tachycardia in patients with syncope of unknown origin: a prospective study. J Am Coll Cardiol 10:775-781

14. Link MS, Kim KMS, Homoud MK et al (1999) Long-term outcome of patients with syncope associated with coronary artery disease and a nondiagnostic electrophysiologic evaluation. Am J Cardiol 83:1334-1337

15. Raviele A (1991) Aritmie ventricolari nella cardiomiopatia dilatativa. Significato clinico-prognostico e ruolo della stimolazione elettrica programmata. G Ital Cardiol 21:87-93

16. Middlekauff HR, Stevenson WG, Stevenson LW, Saxon LA (1993) Syncope in advanced heart failure: high risk of sudden death regardless of origin of syncope. J Am Coll Cardiol 21:100-116

17. Grimm W, Hoffmann J, Menz V et al (1998) Programmed ventricular stimulation for arrhythmia risk prediction in patients with idiopathic dilated cardiomyopathy and no sustained ventricular tachycardia. J Am Coll Cardiol 32:739-745

18. Knight BP, Goyal R, Pelosi F et al (1999) Outcome of patients with nonischemic dilated cardiomyopathy and unexplained syncope treated with an implantable defibrillator. J Am Coll Cardiol 33:1964-1970

19. Kuck KH (1997) Arrhythmias in hypertrophic cardiomyopathy. Pacing Clin Electrophysiol 20:2706-2713

20. Zhu DWX, Sun H, Hill R, Roberts R (1998) The value of electrophysiology study and prophylactic implantation of cardioverter defibrillator in patients with hypertrophic cardiomyopathy. Pacing Clin Electrophysiol 21:299-302

21. Fananapazir L, Epstein SE (1991) Value of electrophysiologic studies in hypertrophic cardiomyopathy treated with amiodarone. Am J Cardiol 67:175-182

22. Primo J, Geelen P, Brugada J et al (1998) Hypertrophic cardiomyopathy: role of the implantable cardioverter-defibrillator. J Am Coll Cardiol 31:1081-1085

23. Martinez-Rubio A, Schwammenthal Y, Schwammenthal E et al (1997) Patients with valvular heart disease presenting with sustained ventricular tachyarrhythmias or syncope. Circulation 96:500-508

24. Morady F, Shen E, Bhandari A et al (1984) Programmed ventricular stimulation in mitral valve prolapse: analysis of 36 patients. Am J Cardiol 53:135-138

25. Morady F, Higgins J, Peters RW et al (1984) Electrophysiologic testing in bundle branch block and unexplained syncope. Am J Cardiol 54:587-591
26. Englund A, Bergfeldt L, Rehnqvist N et al (1995) Diagnostic value of programmed ventricular stimulation in patients with bifascicular block: a prospective study of patients with and without syncope. J Am Coll Cardiol 26:1508-1515
27. Corrado D, Basso C, Thiene G (2000) Arrhythmogenic right ventricular cardiomyopathy: diagnosis, prognosis and treatment. Heart 83:588-595
28. Bhandari AK, Shapiro WA, Morady F et al (1985) Electrophysiologic testing in patients with the long QT syndrome. Circulation 71:63-71
29. Brugada J, Brugada R, Brugada P (1998) Right bundle-branch block and ST-segment elevation in leads V1 through V3. Circulation 97:457-460
30. Priori SG, Napolitano C, Gasparini M et al (2000) Clinical and genetic heterogeneity of right bundle branch block and ST-segment elevation syndrome. Circulation 102:2509-2515
31. Gulamhusein S, Naccarelli GV, Ko PT et al (1982) Value and limitations of clinical electrophysiologic study in assessment of patients with unexplained syncope. Am J Med 73:700-705
32. Silka MJ, Kron J, Cutler JE, McAnulty JH (1990) Analysis of programmed stimulation methods in the evaluation of ventricular arrhythmias in patients 20 years old and younger. Am J Cardiol 66:826-830
33. Militianu A, Salacata A, Seibert K et al (1997) Implantable cardioverter defibrillator utilization among device recipients presenting exclusively with syncope or near-syncope. J Cardiovasc Electrophysiol 8:1087-1097
34. Link MS, Costeas XF, Griffith JL et al (1997) High incidence of appropriate implantable cardioverter-defibrillator therapy in patients with syncope of unknown etiology and inducible ventricular arrhythmias. J Am Coll Cardiol 29:370-375
35. Mittal S, Iwai S, Stein KM et al (1999) Long-term outcome of patients with unexplained syncope treated with an electrophysiologic-guided approach in the implantable cardioverter-defibrillator era. J Am Coll Cardiol 34:1082-1089
36. Andrews NP, Fogel RI, Pelargonio G et al (1999) Implantable defibrillator event rates in patients with unexplained syncope and inducible sustained ventricular tachyarrhythmias. J Am Coll Cardiol 34:2023-2030
37. Pires LA, May LM, Ravi S et al (2000) Comparison of event rates and survival in patients with unexplained syncope without documented ventricular tachyarrhythmias versus patients with documented sustained ventricular tachyarrhythmias both treated with implantable cardioverter-defibrillators. Am J Cardiol 85:725-728
38. Menon V, Steinberg JS, Akiyama T et al (2000) Implantable cardioverter defibrillator discharge rates in patients with unexplained syncope, structural heart disease, and inducible ventricular tachycardia at electrophysiologic study. Clin Cardiol 23:195-200
39. Domanski MJ, Saksena S, Epstein AE et al (1999) Relative effectiveness of the implantable cardioverter-defibrillator and antiarrhythmic drugs in patients with varying degrees of left ventricular dysfunction who have survived malignant ventricular arrhythmias. J Am Coll Cardiol 34:1090-1095
40. Sheldon R, Connolly S, Krahn A et al (2000) Identification of patients most likely to benefit from implantable cardioverter-defibrillator therapy. Circulation 101:1660-1664
41. Fonarow GC, Feliciano Z, Boyle NG et al (2000) Improved survival in patients with nonischemic advanced heart failure and syncope treated with an implantable cardioverter-defibrillator. Am J Cardiol 85:981-985

Syncope and ICD: What Are the Implications and Recommendations for Driving?

A. JAUSSI, M. FROMER AND L. KAPPENBERGER

Introduction

Driving a motor car has become an essential part of modern life in all developed countries. People who live in remote areas, especially in rural communities, rely upon their vehicles for getting to work, as well as for many other daily activities, such as shopping and going to cultural and social events. Regardless the reason for it, being deprived of the right to drive may therefore represent a serious restriction of lifestyle, is always a major narcissistic wound and may impair social integration.

Obtaining (and keeping) a driving licence depends, in brief, on technical competence and medical fitness. Although there is a rather great variety, virtually all countries have some regulations, which in all cases seek to strike a balance between the liberty of the individual and the interests of the society, i.e., the threat that individual might pose to others as a potential cause of road accident. Road accidents are the commonest cause of death in young people and represent a substantial cause of morbidity and mortality throughout the individual's whole life, as well as a financial burden for society.

Medical condition is recognized as a rather rare causal factor in road accidents injuring other road users [1, 2], most accidents being due to multiple factors and especially to human error. Sudden incapacity at the wheel imputable to cardiovascular conditions accounts for a minority of accidents; it is clearly a less frequent medical cause than alcohol and fatigue. The epidemiological data are still scarce; European data suggest that 1.5%-3.4% of fatal accidents can be attributed to acute fatal cardiac conditions [3], a minority of them seeming to be directly arrhythmia-related.

The risk of harm to other road users posed by a driver with heart disease has been calculated by the Canadian Cardiovascular Society Consensus Conference [4] as a function of the time spent at the wheel (or distance driven), the type of vehicle used, the yearly risk of sudden cardiac death or sudden incapacity, and the probability that such an event will result in a fatal or injury-producing acci-

Division of Cardiology, CHUV-PMU, Lausanne, Switzerland

dent. A per annum risk of 1% of driver's cardiac death for commercial trucks is usually considered acceptable by society (the so-called 1%- rule). According to this calculated risk of harm to other road users, the acceptable risk of sudden death or sudden incapacity for a private driver with known heart disease equivalent to the 1% risk of a truck driver can easily be calculated.

Regulation and recommendations

Initiated mainly by the UK, regulations of medical aspects of driver licensing and re-licensing have been formulated and published since the early 1990s. At the European level, the Council Directive 1991/439/EEC sets out the basis of a common licensing practice. Regarding medical and especially cardiovascular fitness, it is stipulated that: "a licence should not be issued to anyone suffering any disease capable of exposing an applicant ... to a sudden failure of the cardiovascular system, such that there is a sudden impairment of the cerebral functions which constitutes a danger to road safety". For Group I drivers, i.e., private car drivers, the main obstacles are serious arrhythmias and angina during rest or emotion. For Group II drivers, professional drivers, the statement is more vague, stipulating that: "the competent medical authority shall give due consideration to the additional risk". Most European countries have now adopted these directives.

Contrary to other countries, Switzerland assigns the task of certifying medical aptitude to car driving to any practising physician who is asked to judge first licensing as well as re-licensing, for instance after an accident following (or due to) a syncope. Publishing recommendations and directives therefore has wide implications in terms of medical education as well as potential legal consequences.

The policy of notifying events to the licensing authority, especially cardiovascular disease and neurological disorders and specific treatments such as implantable cardioverter defibrillators, varies from country to country. The directives are strict in some countries such as the UK, while in Switzerland the system is particularly liberal, where physicians are allowed but not obliged to inform the authorities about medically unfit patients, especially if these patients are not willing to give up their licence themselves. Nevertheless, at least in theory, the physician could be sued for having omitted to inform the authorities [5] – a fact not yet encountered in Switzerland in cardiovascular situations but well known in other domains, such as Alzheimer's disease or alcoholism.

Current Situation

Licensing and re-licensing of cardiovascular patients are regulated by the ESC Task Force Report, *Driving and Heart Disease*, published in 1998 [6]. This report also incorporated the policy on ICD patients set up in the ESC Working Group Report, *Recommendations for Driving of Patients with Implantable Cardioverter Defibrillators*, published in 1997 [7]. Fundamentally, these recommendations seek to be in favour of those patients who might be able to drive in spite of their disease; in other words, their aim is to enable patients to stay at the wheel who otherwise might have been banned from driving by medically insufficiently informed authorities. Furthermore, the authors of the current recommendations recognize that medical guidance cannot totally prevent cardiovascular collapse as a cause of a road traffic accident.

While the regulation of management of patients with ischaemic heart disease seems to be quite easily applicable in daily practice, the scientific and technical evolution in the domains of syncope and ICD appears to call for continuous adaptation of the directives.

Currently, in the UK the guidelines are enforced. Elsewhere, the advising policy seems to be very heterogeneous throughout Europe [8, 9] and the USA [10].

Syncope

A patient having suffered from syncope, a sudden incapacity with loss of consciousness and spontaneous recovery, can resume private driving (Group 1) as soon as the cause is identified and symptoms are controlled [6]. For professionals (Group 2), a specialised evaluation is required including a neurological review if appropriate. Re-licensing may be permitted 3 months after "satisfactory results" of in-depth testing by provocation testing and investigation for arrhythmia [6].

Syncope due to arrhythmias implies generally malignant ventricular arrhythmias occurring on the grounds of other cardiac disease, but apparently benign arrhythmias, for example supraventricular tachycardia, may also sometimes cause incapacity in drivers, the best predictor of syncope in this case being a history of previous syncope.

"Trivial" vasovagal syncope is easy to recognize and does not constitute a real problem, given the fact that loss of consciousness is not abrupt. Thus, the appropriately informed patient does not present a hazard at the wheel. In contrast, neurally mediated syncope in older patients may well cause sudden loss of consciousness. Although there is agreement concerning the poor predictive value of even extensive investigation, provocative testing is usually needed after unexplained syncope [11]. The ESC Task Force recommends relying on clinical judgement by an experienced specialist. Re-examination of the guidelines in this area is currently being considered.

In Swiss practice, syncope at the wheel is a compulsory reason for the police to take away the victim's driving licence on the spot. Therefore, virtually all drivers who have experienced syncope at the wheel come to a medical investigation, as they do in many parts of the USA [5].

Implantable Cardioverter Defibrillators

Group I drivers are allowed to resume driving within 6 months of implantation of an ICD if no arrhythmia and no disabling symptoms at the time of ICD discharge have occurred. For patients benefiting from a prophylactic ICD implantation, no restrictions are imposed. For Group 2 an ICD is a permanently disqualifying reason [6].

These ESC Task Force recommendations are in keeping with the detailed recommendations of the ESC working group on cardiac pacing and arrhythmias published one year earlier [7]:

Class I patients, those treated with prophylactic ICD, have no restrictions. Class IIA patients are low-risk patients without recurrence of ventricular tachyarrhythmias who are subjected to a 6 month driving ban after ICD implantation. Class IIB patients are intermediate-risk patients with recurrence of haemodynamically well-tolerated ventricular tachyarrhythmias. They are subjected to an extended driving ban after ICD implantation until confirmation of the absence of disabling symptoms at the time of ICD therapy. Class III patients, suffering from total and generally permanent restriction, are high-risk patients with recurrence of unstable ventricular tachyarrhythmias and all commercial drivers (since it is unlikely that a commercial driver treated with an ICD has an annual risk of incapacity of 1% or less).

These recommendations, published 3 and 4 years ago, respectively, take into account the fact that patients treated with an ICD for major ventricular tachyarrhythmias have an ongoing risk of sudden incapacity that might cause harm to others while driving a car. Typically, those patients suffer from severe heart disease with often a poor ventricular function. Furthermore, there was initially serious concern about induction of involuntary movement, potential incapacity by device discharge and suboptimal device reliability.

Actually, it has been shown that involuntary movement is rare and that device reliability is good [11]. Patients with ICDs have approximately a 50% chance of a discharge in the first year, and approximately 15%-20% of patients will become syncopal. The initial 6 months are the period of highest risk for appropriate as well as inappropriate shock therapy [7]. Kou et al. [13] found that 15% of their patients who received shock therapy from their ICD had syncope. They did not find reliable predictors of syncope in these patients. At the time of publication of the cited recommendations [7], the available data did not convincingly demonstrate that patients who will suffer from syncope could be identified prospectively by any clinical parameter. More recently, Baensch et al. [14] were able to identify risk predictors of future syncope in their retrospective study of 421 patients. Amongst these patients, 54% had recurrent malignant ventricular arrhythmias and 62 patients (14.7%) had syncope. A low left ventricular ejection fraction (< 40%), induction of fast ventricular tachycardia (VT) with a cycle length of < 300 ms during programmed ventricular stimulation and chronic atrial fibrillation were indeed associated with an increased risk of syncope. Once patients had a VT recurrence, syncope during the first VT and a high VT rate were the strongest predictors of future syncope. Using the above-mentioned Canadian formula [4], they calculated that all patients with ICDs would cause 2.3 accidents per 100 000 patients in the first year, 1.2 in the second and 0.9 in the third. For professionals, these figures would be 50 accidents in the first year, 25 in the second and 20 in the third; 100 000 patients with none of the three mentioned risk factors would cause 0.9 accidents in the first and second years (professionals, 20) and less than 0.2 accidents in the third year (professionals, 5). In the first year, patients with low ejection fraction would cause three accidents (professionals, 65); patients with chronic atrial fibrillation, 3.7 (professionals, 65); and patients with inducible fast VT, 3.3 (professionals, 70). After the first syncope, 7.5 accidents should be expected in the first year (professionals, 160). Thus, the evaluation of ICD patients with syncope could be refined using these recent criteria, the cut-off, i.e., the "acceptable risk", being obviously an issue for the society. These figures bring the authors of this careful study to the following conclusions: if only one extra accident per 100 000 patient-years is acceptable, commercial driving could not be allowed at all. For private driving, patients with chronic atrial fibrillation should be advised never to drive again, patients with a low ejection fraction and inducible fast VTs should not drive for 1 year. After the first VT, patients should not drive for 2 years and after syncope for 1 year!

Current Advising Policy

In the UK the guidelines are enforced. In virtually all other countries throughout the world the advising policy and patients' compliance with the advices are very heterogeneous, at least it was so before the publication of the above-mentioned recommendations in 1997 and 1998. There has been no study published in this particular field since then. A European survey in 1996 [8, 9], reflecting about 10% of worldwide implanted ICDs at that time, showed that 77% of cardiologists advised their patients to cease driving after ICD implantation, nearly half of cardiologists (41%) gave advice only "sometimes". The recommended ban ranged from 3 months to "permanent". The criteria mainly applied were syncope, VT and ventricular fibrillation. Only 38% of the responding cardiologists knew their national law concerning arrhythmias and temporary loss of physical control or loss of consciousness; 13% of the cardiologists did not even know if any driving laws existed in their own country! Despite medical advice, the majority of patients resumed driving within a few months of ICD implantation. An American study published 4 years earlier [10] yielded similar results.

Evolving Policy?

The rapidly growing number of patients with implanted ICDs due to expanded therapeutic and prophylactic indications based on new scientific evidence [15-18], as well as impressive technical progress, will increase the importance of patient counselling and medical advice for ICD patients. A similar situation is encountered in syncope patients without ICDs, since clinical investigation has improved considerably.

Therefore, an adaptation of the published guidelines could well be useful, even if the basic elements, such as infrequency of events (road accidents due to syncope with or without ICD) and difficulty of prediction, remain. Special attention should be paid to patients with prophylactic ICDs and to those with ICDs implanted mainly for their antitachycardia function. Indeed, in patients who needed exclusively this function of their device, the concern of disabling symptoms and incapacity induced by the discharge of the device is no longer realistic for all of them, since this kind of discharge is often, though not always, asymptomatic. Remember, however, that approximately 10% of antitachycardia pacing results in acceleration and shock delivery, which is always painful and exceptionally leads even to loss of consciousness [19, 20].

Patient counselling and compliance with the advice given have been neglected in the past. Furthermore, medical advice has generally been incomplete and very heterogeneous throughout Europe and the USA. If the tremendous demand from patients is considered – questions about driving are in fact the most frequent concern of patients in the field of quality of life [21] – better coordination and better teaching of the physicians involved are mandatory.

Conclusions

Even if syncope and incapacitating events at the wheel causing road accidents are rare, the management of syncope and ICD patients with respect to driving a car remains difficult. Clear and uniform guidelines as well as optimal patient information and advice are essential.

Updating of the official ESC Working Group recommendations would be useful (every 5-10 years?), even if the current recommendations offer a helpful support in most cases. Nationally, some adaptations are of course possible without new European guidelines. For instance, due to the European experience described above, the required arrhythmia-free interval has already been reduced from 12 to 6 months in the UK.

Restrictions should probably be reduced on an individual basis for patients who need virtually only the antitachycardia part of their ICD. In these cases, advice similar to prophylactic use could seem reasonable.

Investigation of syncope of ICD patients should be extended and advice should take into account the importance of the now better-known risk factors, such as low ejection fraction, inducible fast VTs, previous syncope and chronic atrial fibrillation [14].

Last but not least, in order to improve medical advice given by the physicians involved – a still growing number – intensified teaching is essential. Indeed, one of the probably neglected issues is the legal obligation (at least in some countries, such as Germany) in these particular patients to note the advice given in the patient's record and/or in the report going to the general physician in charge. Every physician dealing with this issue should be clearly aware of the local laws regulating the certifying driver licence ability and the notifying policy of patients whose ability to drive safely is impaired. Welly- and uniformly-informed and closely followed-up patients presumably comply better with the medical advice given and are definitely much more confident!

References

1. Taylor J (1995) In: Medical aspects of fitness to drive. Medical Commission on Accident Prevention, London
2. Shephard RJ (1987) The cardiac patient and driving: the Ontario experience. In: Conference on cardiac disorders and commercial drivers. US Department of Transportation, Federal Highway Administration, Bethesda, MD, pp 85-94
3. Halinen MO, Jaussi A (1994) Fatal road accidents caused by sudden death of the driver in Finland and Vaud, Switzerland. Eur Heart J 15:888-894
4. Consensus Conference, Canadian Cardiovascular Society (1992) Assessment of the cardiac patients for fitness to drive. Can J Cardiol 8:406-411
5. Zucker MJ, Bloch JG (1998) Syncope and the law. In: Grubb BP, Ohlshansky B (eds) Syncope: mechanisms and management. Futura, Armonk, NY, pp 387-401
6. Petch MC (1998) Driving and heart disease. Eur Heart J 19:1165-1177
7. Jung W, Anderson M, Camm AJ et al (1997) Recommendations for driving of patients with implantable cardioverter defibrillators. Eur Heart J 18:1210-1219
8. Jung W, Grätz S, Wolpert Ch, et al (1996) Driving behaviour in implantable cardioverter-defibrillator recipients: a European survey. Pacing Clin Electrophysiol 19:605(abstr)
9. Lüderitz B, Jung W (1996) Driving restrictions after cardioverter/defibrillator implantation. In: Oto A (ed) Practice and progress in cardiac pacing and electrophysiology. Kluwer Academic, Dordrecht, pp 373-381
10. Di Carlo LA, Winston SA, Honoway S, Reed P (1992) Driving restrictions advised by midwestern cardiologists implanting cardioverter defibrillators: present practices, criteria utilized, and compatibility with existing state laws. Pacing Clin Electrophysiol 15:1131-1136
11. Epstein AE, Miles WM, Berdott DIG et al (1996) Personal and public safety issues related to arrhythmias that may affect consciousness: implications for regulation and physician recommendations. Circulation 94:1147-1166
12. Curtis AB, Conti JB, Tucker KJ et al (1995) Motor vehicle accidents in patients with an implantable cardioverter defibrillator. J Am Coll Cardiol 26:180-184
13. Kou WH, Calkins H, Lewis RR et al (1991) Incidence of loss of consciousness during automatic implantable cardioverter defibrillator shocks. Ann Intern Med 115:942-945

14. Bänsch D, Brunn J, Castrucci M et al (1998) Syncope in patients with an implantable cardioverter-defibrillator: incidence, prediction and implications for driving restrictions. J Am Coll Cardiol 31:608-615
15. Moss AJ, Hall WJ, Cannom DS et al (1996) Improved survival with an implanted defibrillator in patients with coronary disease at high risk for ventricular arrhythmia. N Engl J Med 335:1933-1940
16. AVID Investigators (1997) A comparison of antiarrhythmic drug therapy with implantable defibrillators in patients resuscitated from near-fatal ventricular arrhythmias: the antiarrhythmics versus implantable defibrillators (AVID) investigators. N Engl J Med 337:1576-1583
17. Buxton AE, Lee KL, Fisher JD et al (1999) A randomized study of the prevention of sudden death in patients with coronary artery disease: multicenter unsustained tachycardia trial investigators. N Engl J Med 341:1882-1890
18. Delacretaz E, Schlaepfer J, Metzger J et al (2000) Evidence rather than costs must guide use of the implantable cardioverter defibrillator. Am J Cardiol 86[Suppl]:52K-57K
19. Fromer M, Brachmann J, Block M et al (1992) Efficacy of automatic multiple device therapy for ventricular tachyarrythmia as delivered by a new implantable pacing cardioverter-defibrillator. Results of a European multicenter study incorporating 102 implants. Circulation 86:363-374
20. Fromer M, Schlaepfer J, Fischer A, Kappenberger L (1991) Experience with a new implantable pacer-, cardioverter-, defibrillator for the therapy of recurrent sustained ventricular tachyarythmies: a step forward toward a universal tachyarrythmia control device. Pacing Clin Electrophysiol 14:1288-1298
21. Sears SF, Todaro JF, Urizar G et al (2000) Assessing the psychosocial impact of the ICD: a national survey of implantable cardioverter defibrillator health care providers. Pacing Clin Electrophysiol 23:939-945

Therapy of Vasovagal Syncope: Is There a Role for Drugs Today?

R. SUTTON

Introduction

Treatment of vasovagal syncope usually demands no more than explanation and reassurance. However, if symptoms are frequent, severe and distressing and have not responded to the initial conservative measures, the physician's thoughts naturally turn to drugs.

The mechanism of vasovagal syncope is not fully understood, but it is known to be complex and involve many aspects of the neuroendocrine cardiovascular control system. Thus, it is possible to conceive that the application of a drug may have a favourable effect on one aspect and that this same drug could have an unfavourable effect on another aspect of the control system. This may explain why there is a myriad of anecdotal reports of drugs in the literature. Anecdotal reports of drug treatment are, of course, seldom unfavourable to the drug. This probability, when combined with the intermittent and cluster pattern behaviour of vasovagal syncope, offers a more complete explanation of lack of drug effects. Today, we live in an era of evidence-based medicine, and the medical community has started to respond to the need for provision of evidence of drug efficacy in the treatment of vasovagal syncope. However, relatively few controlled drug trials have been completed.

Randomized Controlled Drug Trials

The most often prescribed pharmaceutical agent in the treatment of vasovagal syncope is probably one of the β-blocker family. More trials of β-blockers have been performed than of any other single agent.

Royal Brompton and Chelsea & Westminster Hospitals, London, UK

β–Blocker Trials (Table 1)

The rationale in the use of β-blockers is to antagonise the epinephrine release which occurs prior to syncopal collapse [1, 2] and which has been shown to be associated with sinus tachycardia [3]. Also, β–blockers, at least those which cross the blood-brain barrier, may have some central action in reducing the frequency or occurrence of vasovagal syncope.

The first trial reported was that of Fitzpatrick et al. in 1991 [4] using atenolol in a dose of 50 mg/day. This was a three-arm randomised placebo-controlled study of short duration (1.5 months). The other drugs were transdermal scopolamine and clonidine in doses usually selected for migraine therapy. The trial can be criticised for its small number of patients ($n = 13$) and the brevity of the follow-up. No drug was effective.

The second trial published was performed by Brignole's group in 1992 [5]. The drug was again atenolol 50 mg/day but the number of patients was larger ($n = 22$) and the follow-up much longer (10 months). The paper presented data on many other drugs used on smaller numbers of patients. The result showed no significant benefit for any drug including atenolol. The basis of selection of drug for patient was not completely clear in this study.

The third and fourth trials were reported in 1995. Mahanonda et al. [6] conducted a study of 42 patients, a commendably large number, but follow-up was short, 1 month, and the end-point in most was repeat tilt testing. The study showed a benefit for atenolol 50 mg/day, but the trial design is now thought to be inadequate because of the relatively low reproducibility of tilt testing – a feature noted in the VASIS pacemaker trial [7], where paced and unpaced patients had tilt positivity of just over 60% at 2 weeks regardless of therapy.

Scott et al. [8] reported an open-label trial in paediatric patients with a positive result for atenolol. The trial limitations were both its open-label design and that β-blockers may be more effective in young patients. This is because they more frequently show sinus tachycardia before collapse, which is often a steep rate fall to asystole [9].

Table 1. Results of controlled trials with β-blockers in vasovagal syncope

Trial	First author	Year published	Drug	Dose (mg/day)	No. of patients	Follow-up (month)	Benefit
1	Fitzpatrick	1991	Atenolol	50	13	1.5	NS
2	Brignole	1992	Atenolol	100	15	10	NS
3	Mahanonda	1995	Atenolol	50	42	1	Positive
4	Scott	1995	Atenolol	25-100	29	6	Positive
5	Madrid	2001	Atenolol	50	50	12	NS

NS, not significant

The most recent report by Madrid et al. [10] is of a randomised placebo-controlled trial of atenolol 50 mg/day, which shows no benefit in 50 patients with a 1-year follow-up.

In summary, only two trials of five show benefit from atenolol; other β-blockers have not formally been studied. Any future trial of β-blockers should be directed toward an agent which crosses the blood-brain barrier, and only patients who show sinus tachycardia before collapse should be included. Table 1 summarises the results. The Prevention of Syncope trial (POST) is nearing the end of its recruitment of patients. It compares metoprolol with placebo (R. Sheldon, personal communication).

Drugs Other than β-Blockers (Table 2)

As might be expected from the complexity of vasovagal syncope, many other drugs have been considered in order to intervene at different sites in the neuroendocrine arc. Randomised trials have been performed using anti-arrhythmics, α- and β-agonists, fludrocortisone, scopolamine, clonidine, ACE inhibitors, and selective serotonin reuptake inhibitors.

The trial reported by Morillo in assessment of disopyramide [11], an anti-arrhythmic with important vagolytic and negative inotropic effects, was well designed and showed no benefit acutely or chronically from this drug. The vagolytic activity of the drug was considered less important than the negative inotropic effect by the original proponents of its use [12]. This hinged upon the dominance of ventricular baroreceptors in triggering the reflex. Their role has since been questioned [13, 14]. Morillo's report has been followed by a noticeable reduction in the use of disopyramide in vasovagal syncope.

The previously mentioned studies of Fitzpatrick et al. [4] and Brignole et al. [5] included other drugs than β–blockers. Fitzpatrick et al. [4] used clonidine and scopolamine. Clonidine was selected for its central action rather than its α-blockade and was used in doses usually advised for treatment of migraine. Scopolamine was chosen for its vagolytic activity. Neither drug offered any benefit. Brignole et al. [5] used dihydroergotamine, domperidone, and cafedrine. The numbers of patients studied on each drug were small and none showed benefit. Scopolamine, selected for its vagolytic effect, has also been studied by Lee et al. [15], but no benefit was demonstrated. Scott et al. [8], also mentioned above, looked at fludrocortisone to expand plasma volume as well as atenolol in their patients and found some benefit. However, fludrocortisone might be predicted to have least benefit for patients in the paediatric age group, bearing in mind that their typical collapse patterns do not include much hypotension until bradycardia ensues. These authors did not examine this feature in detail. Two studies have been performed using etilefrine. This is a weak α- and β-agonist. It was developed in the middle of the twentieth century for treatment of hypotension and it is available over the counter in Germany. The first study by Moya et al. in 1995 [16] had a good trial design but the lack of benefit shown could have been due to the 30 mg/day dosage of the

Table 2. Results of controlled trials with drugs other than β-blockers in vasovagal syncope

Trial	First author	Year published	Drug	Dose	No. of patients	Follow-up (months)	Benefit
1	Fitzpatrick	1991	Clonidine	25-75 µg/d	13	1.5	NS
			Scopolamine	133 mg/d	13	1.5	NS
2	Brignole	1992	Dihydroergotamine	18 mg/d	4	10	NS
			Domperidone	60 mg/d	4	10	NS
			Cafedrine	400 mg/d	2	10	NS
3	Morillo	1993	Disopyramide	800 mg/d	21	29	NS
4	Scott	1995	Fludrocortisone	100-200 µg/d	29	6	Positive
5	Moya	1995	Etilefrine	30 mg/d	60	12	NS
6	Lee	1996	Scopolamine	500 mg/d	60	0.18	NS
7	Ward	1998	Midodrine	15 mg/d	16	2	Positive
8	Zeng	1998	Enalapril	10 mg/d	30	13.4	Positive
9	Natale	1999	Midodrine	15-45 mg/d	61	6	Positive
10	Di Girolamo	1999	Paroxetine	20 mg/d	68	25.4	Positive
11	Raviele	1999	Etilefrine	75 mg/d	126	12	NS

NS, not significant

drug. A second, larger study, the largest so far reported in the field, of 126 patients and using 75 mg/day, the usually recommended dose, also showed no benefit for etilefrine [17].

Midodrine, a more powerful α-agonist anticipated to maintain peripheral resistance when it is expected to fall, has been studied by two groups with favourable outcomes [18, 19]. Ward et al. [18] concentrated on vasodepression in older patients and Natale et al. [19] showed benefit in a wider age group. The ACE inhibitor, enalapril, has been used in one study with reported benefit [20]. The mechanism of action of this drug in the neuroendocrine arc is unclear. The authors suggest that ACE inhibitors may inhibit catecholamine production.

Finally, the selective serotonin reuptake inhibitor (SSRI) paroxetine received an encouraging report in the study of Di Girolamo et al. [21]. With these drugs there is a presumed central action which is favourable on input to the vasomotor centre. These are somewhat conflicting pieces of evidence (Table 2) for use of any one of a large variety of drugs, leaving the physician without a clear impression of how to treat the patient. In the consulting room the drug, if a drug is really required, will be chosen on individual grounds. An algorithm for prescription is given in Fig. 1.

Fig. 1. Algorithm for treatment of vasovagal syncope with drugs

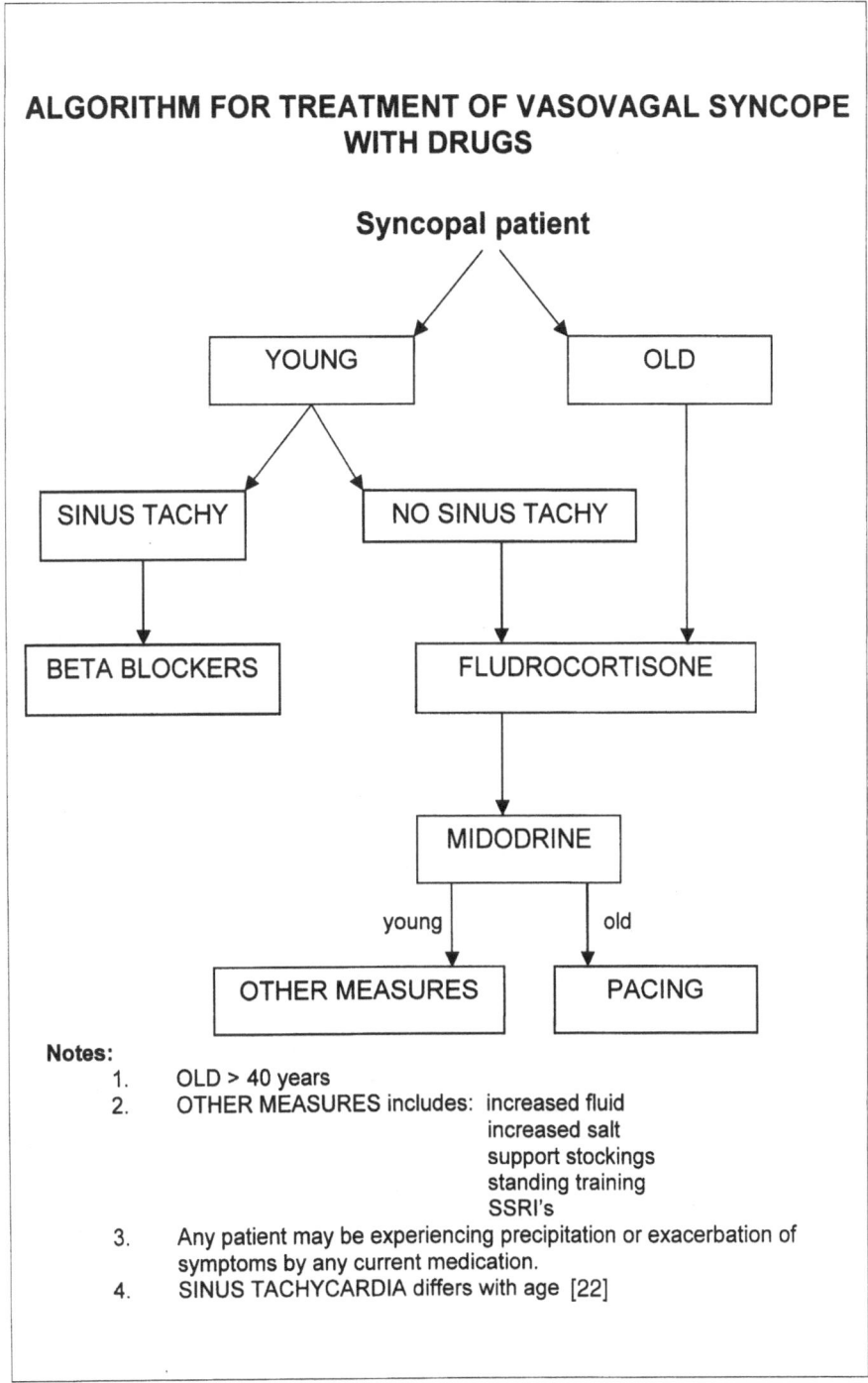

ALGORITHM FOR TREATMENT OF VASOVAGAL SYNCOPE
WITH DRUGS

Syncopal patient

YOUNG   OLD

SINUS TACHY   NO SINUS TACHY

BETA BLOCKERS   FLUDROCORTISONE

MIDODRINE

young   old

OTHER MEASURES   PACING

Notes:
1. OLD > 40 years
2. OTHER MEASURES includes: increased fluid
   increased salt
   support stockings
   standing training
   SSRI's
3. Any patient may be experiencing precipitation or exacerbation of symptoms by any current medication.
4. SINUS TACHYCARDIA differs with age [22]

The author uses β-blockers for patients who show some tachycardia on tilt testing before collapse. A recent study indicates what may be considered to be sinus tachycardia for a range of age groups [22]. If β-blockers are contraindicated on general grounds or there is an absence of tachycardia, fludrocortisone is chosen, and, if ineffective, is replaced by midodrine. In patients with very frequent attacks (e.g. > 1/month) or if a primary psychiatric disturbance is suspected, an SSRI is selected.

When drugs have clearly failed, the patient is over an arbitrary age limit of 40 years and some therapy is necessary, dual-chamber pacing with rate hysteresis is undertaken, for which there is some positive evidence [7, 23].

Role of Co-morbidity and Its Treatment

Patients with other cardiovascular conditions requiring treatment often present difficulties in management for the physician. These conditions are particularly hypertension and heart failure. Many of the the active drug treatments of vasovagal syncope involve raising the blood pressure, which is not compatible with control of hypertension. β-Blockade and, possibly, enalapril may offer a compromise in this situation. In patients with heart failure, drugs and diets which expand the plasma volume or raise the afterload cannot be prescribed. β-Blockers can often only be used in small doses. Reduction in diuretics may have to be undertaken.

End-Points of Trials

This subject has just been reviewed by Sheldon and Rose [24]. They point to four major outcome measures that can be used: quality of life, frequency of syncope, syncope-free actuarial survival, and intensity and frequency of presyncopal symptoms. They argue that time to first syncopal recurrence is the strongest end-point on the basis of their own work [25] and the basis of its ease of measurement together with its ability to retain patients in the trial. Trials involving syncopal frequency alone may lose many subjects from the study if they are expected to sustain many episodes. This has been the end-point used in the majority of trials. It should now be clear that, as a surrogate end-point, tilt-induced recurrence of syncope is unacceptable.

Conclusions

At this stage, the choice of drug and its effect cannot be determined from evidence-based medicine. The picture is unclear. It is hoped that future well-designed trials will bring the possibility of logical therapy rather than adopting the type of clinical algorithm shown in Fig. 1.

References

1. Sander-Jensen K, Secher NH, Astrup A et al (1986) Hypotension induced by passive head-up tilt: endocrine and circulatory mechanisms. Am J Physiol 251:R743-749
2. Fitzpatrick A, Williams T, Ahmed R et al (1992) Echocardiographic and endocrine changes during vasovagal syncope induced by prolonged head-up tilt. Eur J Card Pacing Electrophysiol 2:121-128
3. Klingenheben T, Kalusche D, Li Y-G et al (1996) Changes in plasma epinephrine concentration and in heart rate during head-up tilt testing in patients with neurocardiogenic syncope: correlation with successful therapy with β-receptor antagonist. J Cardiovasc Electrophysiol 7:802-808
2. Fitzpatrick AP, Ahmed R, Williams S, Sutton R (1991) A randomised trial of medical therapy in 'malignant vasovagal or neurally mediated bradycardia/hypotension syndrome'. Eur J Card Pacing Electrophysiol 1:99-102
5. Brignole M, Menozzi C, Gianfranchi L et al (1992) A controlled trial of acute and long-term medical therapy in tilt-induced neurally mediated syncope. Am J Cardiol 70:339-342
6. Mahanonda N, Bhuripanyo K, Kangkagate C et al (1995) Randomized double-blind, placebo-controlled trial of oral atenolol in patients with unexplained syncope and positive upright tilt table results. Am Heart J 130:1250-1253
7. Sutton R, Brignole M, Menozzi C et al (2000) Dual chamber pacing in the treatment of neurally mediated tilt-positive cardioinhibitory syncope. Pacemaker versus no therapy: a multicenter randomized study. Circulation 102:294-299
8. Scott W A, Giacomo P, Bromberg BI et al (1995) Randomized comparison of atenolol and fludrocortisone acetate in the treatment of pediatric neurally mediated syncope. Am J Cardiol 76:400-402
9. Kurbaan AS, Wijesekera N, Franzen A-C et al (2001) Age related differences in underlying pathophysiology of suspected vasovagal syncope. J Am Coll Cardiol 37:146A (abstr)
10. Madrid AH, Ortega J, Rebollo RG et al (2001) Lack of efficacy of atenolol for the prevention of neurally mediated syncope in a highly symptomatic population: a prospective double blind, randomised and placebo controlled study. J Am Coll Cardiol 37:554-559
11. Morillo C, Leitch J, Yee R, Klein GJ (1993) A placebo-controlled trial of intravenous and oral disopyramide for prevention of neurally mediated syncope induced by head-up tilt. J Am Coll Cardiol 22:1843-1848
12. Milstein S, Buetikofer J, Donnigan A et al (1990) Usefulness of disopyramide for prevention of upright tilt-induced hypotension-bradycardia. Am J Cardiol 65:1339-1344
13. Fitzpatrick A, Banner N, Cheng A et al (1993) Vasovagal reactions may occur after orthotopic heart transplantation. J Am Coll Cardiol 21:1132-1137
14. Dickinson CJ (1993) Fainting precipitated by collapse firing of venous baroreceptors. Lancet 342:970-972
15. Lee TM, Su SF, Chen MF et al (1996) Usefulness of transdermal scopolamine for vasovagal syncope. Am J Cardiol 78:480-482
16. Moya A, Permanyer-Miraldo G, Sagrista-Savleda J et al (1995) Limitations of head-up tilt test for evaluating the efficacy of therapeutic interventions in patients with vasovagal syncope: results of a controlled study of etilefrine versus placebo. J Am Coll Cardiol 25:65-69
17. Raviele A, Brignole M, Sutton R et al, for the Vasovagal Syncope International Study Investigators (1999) Effect of etilefrine in preventing syncopal recurrence in patients

with vasovagal syncope. A double-blind, randomised placebo-controlled trial. Circulation 99:1452-1457

18. Ward CR, Gray JC, Gilroy JJ, Kenny RA (1998) Midodrine: a role in the management of neurocardiogenic syncope. Heart 79:45-49

19. Natale A, Beheiry S, Tomassoni GF et al (1999) Randomized placebo control assessment of midodrine in the treatment of neurocardiogenic syncope. J Am Coll Cardiol 33:269A (abstr)

20. Zeng C, Zhu Z, Liu G et al (1998) Randomized, double-blind, placebo-controlled trial of oral enalapril in patients with neurally-mediated syncope. Am Heart J 136:852-858

21. Di Girolamo E, Di Forio C, Sabatini P et al (1999) Effects of paroxetine hydrochloride, a selective serotonin reuptake inhibitor, on refractory vasovagal syncope: a randomised, double-blind, placebo-controlled study. J Am Coll Cardiol 33:1227-1230

22. Petersen M, Williams TR, Gordon C et al (2000) The normal response to prolonged passive head-up tilt testing. Heart 84:509-514

23. Connolly SJ, Sheldon RS, Roberts RS, Gent M (1999) The North American Vasovagal Pacemaker Study. A randomised trial of permanent cardiac pacing for the prevention of vasovagal syncope. J Am Coll Cardiol 33:16-20

24. Sheldon R, Rose S (2001) Components of clinical trials for vasovagal syncope. Europace 3:233-240

25. Malik P, Koshman ML, Sheldon R, Malik P (1997) Timing of first syncope recurrence predicts syncope frequency following a positive tilt table test. J Am Coll Cardiol 29:1284-1289

Pacing for Vasovagal Syncope: Real Efficacy or Placebo Effect?

R.S. SHELDON

The American College of Cardiology/American Heart Association Task Force [1] and the British Pacing and Electrophysiology Group [2] recommend permanent pacing as treatment for neurally mediated syncope. What is the evidence that supports these recommendations? Unquestionably, fainting is a substantial problem for many of our patients and merits attempts at treatment. Although many believe that fainting is a transitory phase that passes, and that the severity of symptoms is minimal, this is far from the rule. Several studies reported that patients had medians of 5-15 syncopal spells, and had been fainting for of 2-10 years [3-9]. Many patients faint several times a year. Therefore vasovagal syncope can occur frequently, and it can be a problem that lasts many years. Not surprisingly, patients with frequent vasovagal syncope have a poor quality of life. Patients with recurrent syncope are impaired to a similar extent as those with severe rheumatoid arthritis or chronic low back pain, and as psychiatric inpatients [10]. The quality of life decreases as the frequency of syncopal spells increases [11]. Although some patients do respond to drug therapy, many do not, and for them treatment with a permanent pacemaker is often considered.

The Evidence for the Effectiveness of Pacing

Tilt testing commonly induces bradycardia around the time of syncope or presyncope. Prolonged passive tilt tests that are positive often induce heart rates well under 60 bpm. In contrast, positive tilt tests with isoproterenol usually have trough heart rates below 80 bpm. Most patients with positive tilt tests develop some degree of bradycardia at the time of presyncope or syncope, and pacing seems to be a plausible treatment. Indeed, temporary transvenous pacing is partially effective in reducing the proportion of patients who faint during tilt table

Cardiovascular Research Group, University of Calgary, Alberta, Canada

testing. The results of four reports taken together [12] showed that temporary dual chamber pacing prevented the development of syncope on tilt table testing in 24/41 subjects (57%), although most conscious subjects became lightheaded. These acute pacing studies suggested that permanent pacing might be helpful, but they were generally open-label, nonrandomized, sequential design studies.

Several groups reported studies of the usefulness of chronic pacing in the prevention of neurally mediated syncope. Petersen et al. [5] reported a pioneering study of dual chamber pacing in 37 syncope patients. The patients were moderately symptomatic, having had a median of 6 syncopal spells at a rate of about 2 spells per year, and had a positive tilt test with bradycardia. Of the 37 patients, 31 received pacemakers with rate hysteresis. Over a mean follow-up of 50 months, 62% of the patients remained free of syncope and 89% reported symptomatic improvement. The number of syncopal spells in the total population fell from an expected number of 136 to only 11. Several years later Benditt et al. [6] reported equally encouraging results in a study of 36 patients with predominantly vasovagal syncope. The patients were very symptomatic, with a median of 10 syncopal spells over about 24 months, or about 5 spells yearly. All patients received a novel pacemaker with rate drop responsiveness. This pacemaker can be programmed to sense small drops in heart rate and respond with temporary high rate pacing at rates of 100-120 bpm. They were followed for a mean of 6 months. During this time, syncope recurred in only 6 patients, compared to an expected rate of recurrences in about 30 patients. Therefore in this relatively short-term study, pacing may have benefited about 80% of patients. Finally, we studied 12 extremely symptomatic patients who had had a median syncope frequency of 3 spells/month [7]. All had had recurrent syncope after tilt testing and while on medical therapy. All received a pacemaker with a unique rate-smoothing feature that prevented abrupt drops in heart rate, but did not have a high rate response. Following implantation of the pacemaker, the actuarial syncope-free survival increased 20-fold, the syncope frequency dropped by 93%, and quality of life improved highly significantly. The patients had been selected on the basis of highly frequent syncope, and all had syncope early after tilt testing.

These were all sequential design studies, with no control for time-dependent effects. To address this concern two groups performed randomized clinical trials of pacing to prevent vasovagal syncope. The Vasovagal Pacemaker Study was a randomized clinical trial of permanent pacemaker in 54 patients with frequent vasovagal syncope [8]. All patients had fainted at least 6 times, and all had a positive tilt test with bradycardia. They had had a median of 14-35 syncopal spells before pacemaker insertion. Half received a dual chamber pacemaker with rate-drop responsiveness and half received conventional medical therapy. Of the 27 patients in each arm, 19 control patients fainted, and 6 paced patients fainted. There was a relative reduction in the risk of syncope of 85% in the paced patients ($p = 0.00002$). In contrast, pacing did not reduce the number of presyncopal spells.

The Vasovagal Syncope International Study investigators randomized 42 patients either to receive a dual chamber pacemaker with rate hysteresis or to continue with best noninvasive therapy [9]. The median number of historical syncopal spells was 6 and all patients had positive tilt tests with bradycardia. During a mean follow-up of 3.7 ± 2.2 years syncope occurred in 1/19 paced patients and 14/23 control patients ($p = 0.0006$).

Taken together, these observational and randomized open-label studies provide powerful evidence for the effectiveness of permanent pacemakers in the prevention of vasovagal syncope.

But do they?

Why the Benefit Might be Due to Placebo

The history of attempts to treat patients with implanted devices is replete with examples of initial promises of therapeutic success being dashed by subsequent well-controlled studies. For example, numerous small, open-label studies suggested that dual chamber pacing causes a marked improvement in the hemodynamics and functional status of patients with hypertrophic cardiomyopathy. Later randomized, controlled, blinded studies disappointingly revealed conflicting evidence of a much smaller effect size, and this therapy is no longer a prominent part of treatment for this disorder [13]. Similarly, much early open-label evidence suggested that atrially based pacing might prevent atrial fibrillation, but a tightly controlled, randomized, crossover clinical trial showed absolutely no benefit of conventional atrially based pacing in the prevention of atrial fibrillation [14, 15]. Finally, numerous large, open-label studies provided strong evidence for the ability of atrially based pacing to reduce stroke and death in patients with pacemakers. A large, randomized, blinded, controlled study showed that patients with atrially based pacemakers compared to those with single-lead ventricular pacemakers had no benefit with respect to death, stroke, quality of life, or exercise tolerance for several years after implantation [16]. From this experience we must draw the conclusion that great care should be taken in the assessment of open-label or nonrandomized pacemaker studies. The placebo effect can be substantial.

Although pacemakers may be helpful for patients with bradycardia at the time of syncope, there is relatively little direct evidence that this is common. Two studies attempted to determine whether there is sufficient symptomatic bradycardia during clinical syncope to make permanent pacing feasible. One Holter study of eight patients with very frequent vasovagal syncope detected no episodes of asystole or even marked bradycardia during syncope [17]. A complementary study assessed how often symptoms were associated with asystole. Pacemakers with sophisticated memories for bradycardic events were implanted in patients with frequent vasovagal syncope and documented asystole. Asystolic events a few seconds long were common, but only 0.7% of episodes 3-6 s long and 43% of episodes more than 6 s long resulted in presyncope or syncope [18]. Both studies were of highly selected patients and both were small. Long-lasting implantable digital loop recorders and pacemakers with large and patient-activated memories should provide a clearer estimate of the frequency and meaning of bradycardia and asystole in patients with vasovagal syncope. Other than anecdotal reports, there is surprisingly little evidence for symptomatic profound bradycardia in patients with very frequent vasovagal syncope.

Reasons Why Patients Might Improve After Intervention

There are several reasons why pacemaker therapy may seem favorable initially, but not be proven to be so with carefully controlled studies. The placebo effect is well known, but it is not the only cause. Patients receiving expensive or invasive therapy may be more inclined to report a benefit from it, possibly because they are loath to admit the possibility that such a therapy could be ineffective [19]. Finally, many patients with vasovagal syncope appear to improve spontaneously after tilt testing [3, 4]. This effect may be as much as 90%. The mechanism is unknown, but may include regression to the mean, the counseling received at the time of the clinic visit, and the sporadic nature of the timing of presentations of vasovagal syncope. This is a large effect, and about the same magnitude as the beneficial effect of pacing in sequential design trials.

Evidence for a Placebo Effect in Paced Patients

Ironically, the very success of all pacemaker studies in vasovagal syncope is an argument that some of the beneficial effect of pacing might be placebo. Given the difficulty in documenting profound bradycardia as a frequent cause of vasovagal syncope, many suspect that vasodepressor reactions may be a major cause. If so, then pacemakers with only conventional bradycardia support should not be very effective, and sophisticated presyncope detection algorithms might be more successful. The pacemakers that have been assessed most widely sense drops in heart rate as the sensed events. The three therapeutic options available now include rate smoothing, rate hysteresis, and rate drop sensing. All three options have been assessed clinically. Rate hysteresis was used by Petersen et al. and the VASIS investigators [5, 9]; rate-drop responsiveness by Benditt et al. and by the VPS I investigators [6, 8]; and rate smoothing was used in the third sequential design study [7]. All three modes gave roughly comparable results, with an approximate 80%-90% reduction of syncope in all the study populations. These are quite different approaches: rate smoothing simply prevents abrupt rate drops but does not provide a relative tachycardia; rate hysteresis is not activated until the rate drops below 45 bpm; and rate drop intervention affords a relative sinus tachycardia triggered by a small drop in heart rate. Interestingly, the three programming modes–rate hysteresis, rate-drop responsiveness, and rate smoothing–appeared to be comparably effective. This suggests that either a simple, transient, profound bradycardia causes much of vasovagal syncope, or that pacemakers have a beneficial effect on vasovagal syncope other than or as well as pacing.

Evidence for Mode-Specific Effects

Clearly these concerns can only be addressed with randomized, placebo-controlled clinical trials. Although these are under way, they are not yet completed. However, two small studies have included randomized comparisons between two or more pacing modes. If they showed a difference, it would suggest that something specific about the pacemaker programming is important, and therefore that not all of the beneficial effect is due to a placebo effect.

In a pivotal study McLeod et al. [20] reported the relative merits of single chamber ventricular pacing and dual chamber pacing in the prevention of vasovagal syncope in 12 highly symptomatic children with a median age of 2.9 years who had frequent syncope associated with asystolic pauses longer than 4 s. This was a three-way, double-blind, randomized crossover study in which the pacemakers were programmed to no pacing, ventricular pacing with rate hysteresis, or dual chamber pacing with rate-drop responsiveness. Each treatment exposure lasted 4 months. Both pacing modes were equivalent and more effective than no pacing in preventing syncope. However, dual chamber pacing was superior to ventricular pacing in preventing presyncope. This small study is critically important, since it directly and successfully addresses the role of pacing over and above any possible placebo effect.

Ammirati et al. performed a small, randomized clinical trial comparing rate hysteresis and rate-drop responsiveness [21]. Twenty patients with moderately frequent syncope received a pacemaker with either rate hysteresis or rate-drop responsiveness. Three patients with rate hysteresis fainted while no patients with rate-drop responsiveness fainted. Though small, this study suggests that rate-drop responsiveness is superior to rate hysteresis in preventing syncope, and therefore that not all of the pacemaker effect is due to placebo.

Vasovagal Syncope Pacemaker Study II

The second Vasovagal Pacemaker Study (VPS II) is a multinational randomized clinical trial that is assessing whether dual chamber pacing with rate-drop sensing is superior to placebo, and whether it is also superior to dual chamber pacing at an escape rate of 45 bpm. It is funded by the Canadian Institutes of Health Research and Medtronic. Patients are eligible if they have had six or more syncopal spells and have a positive tilt table test. Bradycardia need not be induced during the test. All patients receive a dual chamber pacemaker with rate-drop responsiveness, and half are double-blindly randomized to rate-drop sensing while the other half are randomized to a mode in which the pacemaker senses and records heart periods in a rolling loop recorder but does not pace. The primary outcome is the first syncope recurrence. Following the first phase (which lasts 6 months) they may enter the randomized crossover second phase in which they are randomized to pacing with or without rate-drop sensing. A total of 100 patients are being enrolled over 3 years at sites in Canada, the United States, and Columbia. Enrollment will be completed in September 2001, and the prespecified 6 months of follow-up completed in March 2002. When finished, the first phase of the study will demonstrate the magnitude of the pacemaker effect that is not attributable to placebo.

References

1. Derives LS, Fisch C, Griffin JC et al (1991) Guidelines for implantation of cardiac pacemakers and antiarrhythmia devices. A report of the American College of Cardiology/American Heart Association Task Force on Assessment of Diagnostic and Therapeutic Procedures (Committee on Pacemaker Implantation). J Am Coll Cardiol 18:1-13
2. Clarke M, Sutton R, Ward D et al (1991) Recommendations for pacemaker prescriptions for symptomatic bradycardia. British Pacing and Electrophysiology Group Working Party Report. Br Heart J 66:185-191
3. Sheldon R, Rose S, Flanagan P et al (1996) Risk factors for syncope recurrence after a positive tilt table test in patients with syncope. Circulation 93:973-981.
4. Natale A, Geiger MJ, Maglio C et al (1996) Recurrence of neurocardiogenic syncope without pharmacologic interventions. Am J Cardiol 77:1001-1003
5. Petersen MEV, Chamberlain-Webber R, Fitzpatrick AP et al (1994) Permanent pacing for cardioinhibitory malignant vasovagal syndrome. Br Heart J 71:274-281
6. Benditt DG, Sutton R, Gammage M and the Rate-drop Response Investigators (1997) Clinical experience with Thera DR rate drop response pacing algorithm in carotid sinus syndrome and vasovagal syncope. Pacing Clin Electrophysiol 20:832-839
7. Sheldon RS, Koshman ML, Wilson W et al (1997) Effect of dual-chamber pacing with automatic rate-drop sensing on recurrent neurally mediated syncope. Am J Cardiol 81:158-162
8. Connolly SJ, Sheldon RS, Roberts RS, Gent M (1999) The North American Vasovagal Pacemaker Study. A randomized trial of permanent cardiac for the prevention of vasovagal syncope. J Am Coll Cardiol 33:16-20
9. Sutton R, Brignole M, Menozzi C et al (2000) Dual chamber pacing in the treatment of neurally mediated tilt-positive cardioinhibitory syncope. Pacemaker versus no therapy: a multicentre randomized study. Circulation 102:294-299
10. Linzer M, Pontinen M, Gold DT et al (1991) Impairment of physical and psychosocial function in recurrent syncope. J Clin Epidemiol 44:1037-1043
11. Rose MS, Koshman ML, Spreng S, Sheldon RS (2000) The relationship between health related quality of life and frequency of spells in patients with syncope. J Clin Epidemiol 53:1209-1216
12. Sheldon RS (2000) Pacing to prevent vasovagal syncope. Cardiol Clin 18: 81-93
13. Sorijja P, Elliot PM, McKenna WJ (2000) Pacing in hypertrophic cardiomyopathy. Cardiol Clin 18:67-79
14. Gillis AM, Wyse DG, Connolly SJ et al (1999) Atrial pacing periablation for prevention of paroxysmal atrial fibrillation. Circulation 99:2553-2558
15. Gillis AM, Connolly SJ, Lacombe P et al (2000) Randomized crossover comparison of DDDR versus VDD pacing after atrioventricular junction for prevention of atrial fibrillation (PA^3) study investigators. Circulation 102:736-741
16. Connolly SJ, Kerr CR, Gent M et al (2000) Effects of physiologic pacing versus ven-

tricular pacing on the risk of stroke and death due to cardiovascular causes. Canadian Trial of Physiologic Pacing Investigators. N Engl J Med 342:1385-1391

17. Garred J, Wilson W, Koshman ML et al (1998) Heart periods during clinical syncope: Holter analysis of patients with neurally mediated syncope. Pacing Clin Electrophysiol 21:793

18. Menozzi C, Brignole M, Lolli G et al (1993) Follow-up of asystolic episodes in patients with cardioinhibitory, neurally mediated syncope and VVI pacemaker. Am J Cardiol 72:1152-1155

19. Redelmeier DA, Tu JV, Schull MJ et al (2001) Problems for clinical judgement: 2. Obtaining a reliable past medical history. Can Med Assoc J 164:809-813

20. McLeod KA, Wilson N, Hewitt J et al (1999) Cardiac pacing for severe childhood neurally mediated syncope with reflex anoxic seizures. Heart 82:721-725

21. Ammirati F, Colivicchi F, Toscano S et al (1998) DDI pacing with rate drop response function versus DDI with rate hysteresis pacing for cardioinhibitory vasovagal syncope. Pacing Clin Electrophysiol 21:2178-2181

Prevention of Vasovagal Syncope by Pacing: How to Select Patients and Which Pacing Mode to Choose

M. Brignole

Introduction

Despite the fact that vasovagal syncope is probably the most frequent of all causes of fainting, treatment strategies are as yet still based on an incomplete understanding of the pathophysiology of the faint. On the other hand, given the frequency with which the vasovagal syncope occurs, there is a wealth of clinical experience on which to draw. In the vast majority of cases, patients who seek medical advice after having experienced a vasovagal faint principally require reassurance and education regarding the nature of the condition. This assumption is derived from the knowledge of the benign nature of the disorder In particular, on the basis of a review of their medical history, patients should be informed of the likelihood of syncope recurrence. Initial advice should also include a review of typical premonitory symptoms, which may permit many individuals to recognize an impending episode and thereby avert a frank faint. Additional common sense measures such as avoidance of volume depletion and prolonged exposure to upright posture and/or hot, confining environments should also be discussed. In regard to these latter treatment concepts, formal randomized studies are not available, but physiological evidence and clinical experience are sufficient warrant.

Pacing in Vasovagal Syncope: it Works but Is it Worth It?

The results of the Vasovagal Syncope International Study (VASIS) [1] suggest that, when asystole is part of the mechanism of the vasovagal response, pacing is likely to be effective, and that this good result could be predicted by a cardioinhibitory response to tilt testing. Nevertheless, in the untreated group, no

Department of Cardiology and Arrhythmologic Center, Ospedali Riuniti, Lavagna, Italy patients had syncope-related injuries during the follow-up and the total burden of syncope was lower than expected, with a syncope recurrence rate of 0.44 per year during a follow-up period of more than 3 years (Table 1). Since this rate was lower than that observed in the 2 years before enrollment, there was obviously a spontaneous decrease of syncopal episodes even in the absence of any active or placebo treatment. This had been already observed in previous studies evaluating the outcome of patients after diagnostic tilt testing [2-4]. The reason for this is unclear. It might be that the simple fact that a patient was evaluated and diagnosed has a therapeutic effect, probably because the patient learns to recognize the onset of syncopal symptoms and to avoid loss of consciousness. Another explanation might be that syncopal episodes occur in clusters, with the maximum number of episodes at the time of evaluation [4]. At all events, the low recurrence rate and the low risk of related injury we observed suggest that the use of pacemaker therapy should be restricted to those patients who have frequent relapses after diagnostic evaluation or are at risk of associated injuries.

In the European Society of Cardiology guidelines on the management of syncope, [5], cardiac pacing is a class II indication in the case of patients with cardioinhibitory vasovagal syncope with a frequency of more than 5 attacks per year or severe physical injury or accident and age above 40 years.

Table 1. The main results of the VASIS study according to the "on treatment" analysis [1]

Outcome event	Pacemaker arm	No pacemaker arm	p value
Number in analysis	22	20	
Syncopal recurrence	1 (5%)	14 (70%)	0.0001
Total number of syncopes	2	24	
Mean no. per patient		1.7 ± 0.9	
Median time to first recurrence, months (interquartile range)	15	5 (2-20)	
Follow-up, years	77.8	54.7	
Rate per year	0.03	0.44	

The Role of Head-Up Tilt Test in Treatment Selection for Vasovagal Syncope

Pacemaker therapy was more effective in the VASIS [1] than in the North American trial [6]. There are some important differences between the two studies. Firstly, two different tilt protocols – long passive phase plus eventual trinitrin challenge versus isoproterenol challenge – were used. Secondly, in the VASIS study all the patients had had a severe cardioinhibitory response of type

2A or 2B during tilt testing, and 86% of these had a very long ventricular pause at the time of induced syncope (mean asystole 13.9 ± 10.2 s). The magnitude of the cardioinhibitory reflex can hardly be evaluated with the isoproterenol challenge, and, indeed, in the North American trial cardioinhibitory response was broadly defined as a relative bradycardia of less than 60-80 bpm. This suggests that pacing is likely to be effective when asystole is part of the mechanism of the vasovagal response, and that the better results of the VASIS trial could be predicted by a cardioinhibitory response to tilt testing. In this respect the study validates the usefulness of the passive-trinitrin protocol of tilt testing and of the VASIS classification. In 1992, Sutton et al. [7], using the details of hemodynamic responses to tilt testing, proposed the VASIS classification of the positive responses, which has been recently modified [8]. This classification is shown in Table 2.

Finally, in the VASIS trial a conventional DDI pacemaker programmed for prevention of extreme bradycardia and asystole was used, whereas in the other study a specifically designed device with a rate response feature and a higher pacing rate (100 bpm) was implanted. Given the good results of the VASIS trial, when asystole is the likely cause of syncope, a conventional dual-chamber pacemaker seems to be very effective, and special features may not add significant benefit. This is in contrast with some other preliminary data from an ongoing study of comparison between DDI pacing with hysteresis and rate-drop response function, which showed superiority of the latter mode of pacing [9]. The study population of that study, 20 patients with cardioinhibitory responses during two head-up tilt tests, was randomized to receive either DDI pacing with rate hysteresis (8 patients) or DDD pacing with a rate-drop response function (11 patients). During follow-up no patients with a DDD pacemaker with rate-drop response function had syncope, while 3 of 8 patients with a DDI pacemaker with rate hysteresis experienced recurrence of syncope ($p < 0.05$).

Table 2. The new VASIS classifications of positive responses to tilt testing [9]

Type 1: Mixed. Heart rate falls at the time of syncope but the ventricular rate does not fall to less than 40 bpm or falls to less than 40 bpm for less than 10 s with or without asystole of less than 3 s. Blood pressure falls before the heart rate falls.

Type 2A: Cardioinhibition without asystole. Heart rate falls to a ventricular rate less than 40 bpm for more than 10 s but asystole of more than 3 s does not occur. Blood pressure falls before the heart rate falls.

Type 2B: Cardioinhibition with asystole. Asystole occurs for more than 3 s. Blood pressure fall coincides with or occurs before the heart rate fall.

Type 3: Vasodepressor. Heart rate does not fall more than 10% from its peak at the time of syncope.

Exception 1: Chronotropic incompetence. No heart rate rise during the tilt testing (i.e., less than 10% from the pre-tilt rate).

Exception 2: Excessive heart rate rise. An excessive heart rate rise both at the onset of upright position and throughout its duration before syncope (i.e., greater than 130 bpm).

In order to investigate this hypothesis in more depth, the results of the published articles on pacing treatment of tilt-induced vasovagal syncope have been reviewed and pooled together in Tables 3. The data have been subdivided in two groups: the top part shows the results of 60 patients who had a dominant asystolic response during the index tilt testing, while the lower part gives the results of the 107 patients who had a nonasystolic response. After pacemaker treatment, the patients of the asystolic group showed a significantly lower syncope recurrence rate than those of the nonasystolic group (8% vs 30%; $p = 0.0007$).

These results suggest that pacing therapy is effective in patients with vasovagal syncope and asystolic response during the index tilt testing. The usefulness of pacing therapy in the patients with nonasystolic response is more controversial. Many cardiologists probably do not accept such a high risk of failure of therapy for their patients and wish to perform further tests in order to increased the likelihood of success. In this context, an implantable loop recorder seems a useful means to substantiate the diagnosis of dominant cardioinhibitory vasovagal syncope.

Table 3. Pooled data of articles concerning pacemaker therapy in patients with vasovagal syncope according to the results of tilt test

	No. of patients	Asystole > 3s (% of patient)	Tilt protocol [months]	Follow-up [recurrence]	Syncope [n	%]
Asystolic tilt						
- Brignole et al. [10]	6	70	Passive-- trinitrin	22	0	0
- Shah et al. [11]	12	100	Passive-- isoproterenol	19	1	8
- Ammirati et al [1]	20	VASIS 2B	Passive-- trinitrin	18	3	15
- Sutton et al. VASIS [1]	22	86	Passive trinitrin	44	1	5
Total	60				5	8
Non-asystolic tilt						
- Petersen et al. [12]	37	30	Passive	50	14	38
- Benditt et al. [13]	31	n.d.	n.d.	7	6	19
- Sheldom et al. [14]	12	0	ISO	12	6	50
- Connolly et al. VPS [6]	27	0	ISO	0-15	6	22
Total	107				32	30

Role of the Implantable Loop Recorder in "Isolated" Syncope and Tilt-Positive Syncope

Although the asystolic response during tilt testing seems to predict that spontaneous attacks are likely to be asystolic also (as demonstrated indirectly by the effectiveness of pacing), we do not know whether the other types of response induced during tilt testing – vasodepressor, mixed, and cardioinhibitory without asystole – correlate with the spontaneous vasovagal attacks. Knowing the exact mechanism of the spontaneous attack is of course of great practical importance in choosing the best treatment.

The International Study on Syncope of Uncertain Etiology (ISSUE) is an ongoing prospective study which aims to analyze the diagnostic yield of the implantable loop recorder in specific subgroups of patients with syncope of uncertain etiology; the groups were predefined and the patients assigned to their groups at the time of enrollment [15]. Overall, more than 200 patients have been enrolled and are being followed up. To date, we have results on the subgroup of patients with isolated syncope, i.e., no heart disease and complete negative work-up including tilt testing, and on the subgroup of patients with a positive response to tilt testing and no heart disease. The main findings are the following:

1. In both groups, about two-thirds of patients had no recurrence of syncope during follow-up; of those who had recurrences, none suffered trauma or consequences caused by syncope. The low recurrence rate and the low risk of related injury observed in the "real world" suggest that treatment, in particular pacemaker therapy, could be restricted only to those patients who have relapses after diagnostic evaluation or are at very high risk of injury.
2. Among the patients with isolated syncope who had syncopal recurrences, three-quarters had progressive sinus bradycardia most often followed by

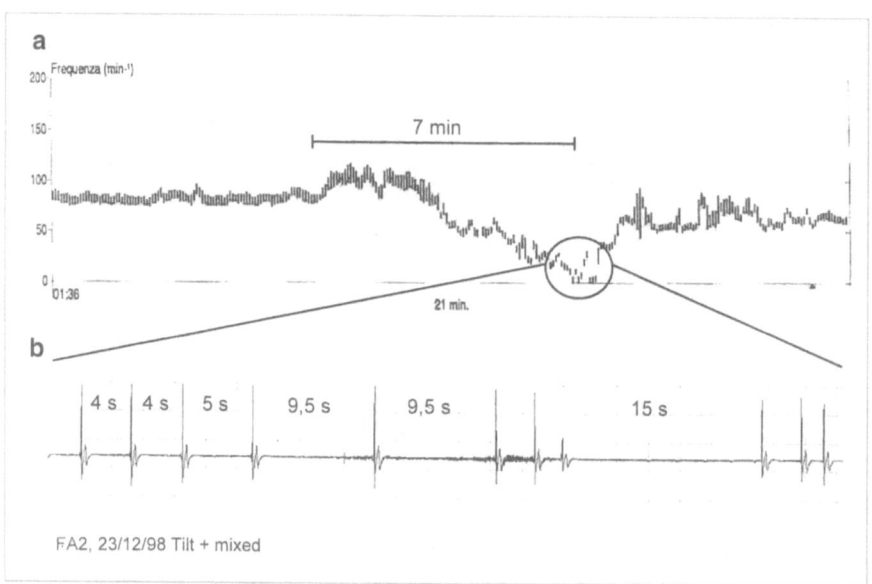

Fig. 1. Tilt-positive patient. During the test the patient had had a mixed response. **a** Heart rate trend during 21 min loop recording. Initially, the heart rate is stable at approximately 80 bpm; at the beginning of the episode the heart rate increases to 120 bpm, then progressively decreases to a very low rate. **b** The expanded electrocardiogram at the time of syncope shows prolonged multiple pauses due to sinus arrest

asystole, or progressive tachycardia followed by progressive bradycardia and most often asystole (with or without concomitant blocked P waves). These findings strongly suggest that the likely etiology of syncope is neurally mediated and the most frequent mechanism is a dominant cardioinhibitory reflex with prolonged asystolic pauses.

3. In the tilt-positive patients, the results were very similar to those in the isolated syncope group, suggesting that the two groups have similar etiologies of syncope (Fig. 1). Furthermore, in this group, an asystolic syncope was also recorded when the type of response to tilt testing was vasodepressor or mixed. Thus, it seems that spontaneous syncope is much more frequently asystolic than one would expect on the basis of the results of tilt testing, which cannot be used to predict the type of response of spontaneous attacks. This explains why pacemaker therapy is more efficacious in preventing syncopal recurrences than expected [1].

In both groups, apart from the pattern described above, a normal sinus rhythm was frequently recorded at the time of syncope. Though not diagnostic, this finding allows us definitely to exclude an arrhythmia as the cause of syncope.

Conclusions

The benign course of the disorder suggests that the use of pacemaker therapy should be restricted only to those very few patients who have frequent relapses after diagnostic evaluation or are at high risk of associated injuries.

An asystolic response during diagnostic tilt testing seems to be able to predict a high success rate of pacemaker therapy in reducing syncopal recurrences.

When the response to diagnostic tilt testing is not asystolic, the effectiveness of pacemaker therapy is lower. In these cases, the indication for pacing probably needs to be confirmed by further investigations. An implanted loop recorder is a very promising tool for discovering the exact mechanism of the spontaneous syncope and thus guiding the pacemaker implantation.

Dual-chamber pacing is the mode of pacing of which most experience exists. In the absence of large comparison data between modes of dual-chamber pacing, no one algorithm has been definitely proven to be superior to another. Asystolic syncope seems to be the major predictor of pacing effectiveness, rather than pacing modality.

References

1. Sutton R, Brignole M, Menozzi C et al (2000) Dual-chamber pacing is efficacious in treatment of neurally-mediated tilt-positive cardioinhibitory syncope. Pacemaker versus no therapy: a multicentre randomized study. Circulation 102:294-299

2. Brignole M, Menozzi C, Gianfranchi L et al (1992) A controlled trial of acute and long-term medical therapy in tilt-induced neurally mediated syncope. Am J Cardiol 70:339-342
3. Sheldon R, Rose S, Flanagan P et al (1996) Risk factors for syncope recurrence after a positive tilt-table test in patients with syncope. Circulation 93:973-981
4. Natale A, Geiger MJ, Maglio C et al (1995) Recurrence of neurocardiogenic syncope without pharmacologic interventions. Am J Cardiol 77:1001-1003
5. Brignole M, Alboni P, Benditt D et al (2001) Task Force on Syncope, European Society of Cardiology: guidelines on management (diagnosis and treatment) of syncope. Eur Heart J (in press)
6. Connolly SJ, Sheldon R, Roberts RS, Gent M (1999) Vasovagal pacemaker study investigators. Cardiac pacing for the prevention of vasovagal syncope. J Am Coll Cardiol 33:16-20
7. Sutton R, Petersen M, Brignole M et al (1992) Proposed classification for tilt induced vasovagal syncope. Eur J Cardiac Pacing Electrophysiol 3:180-183
8. Brignole M, Menozzi C, Del Rosso A et al (2000) New classification of haemodynamics of vasovagal syncope: beyond the VASIS classification. Analysis of the pre-syncopal phase of the tilt test without and with nitroglycerin challenge. Europace 2:66-76
9. Ammirati F, Colivicchi F, Toscano S et al (1998) DDD pacing with rate drop response function versus DDI with rate hysteresis pacing for cardioinhibitory vasovagal syncope. Pacing Clin Electrophysiol 21:2178-2181
10. Brignole M, Menozzi C (1997) Methods other than tilt testing for diagnosing neurocardiogenic (neurally mediated) syncope. Pacind Clin Electrophysiol 20:795-780
11. Shah CD, Thakur R, Xie B, Patrak P (1999) Dual chamber pacing for neurally mediated syncope with a prominent cardioinhibitory component. Pacing Clin Electrophysiol 22:999-1003
12. Petersen MEV, Chamberlain-Webber R, Fizpatrick AP et al (1994) Permanent pacing for cardio-inhibitory malignant vasovagal syndrome. Br Heart J 71:274-281
13. Benditt D, Sutton R, Gammage M et al (1997) Clinical experience with Thera DR rate-drop response pacing algorithm in carotid sinus syndrome and vasovagal syncope. Pacing Clin Electrophysiol 20 (part II):832-839
14. Sheldon R, Koshman ML, Wilson W et al (1998) Effect of dual-chamber pacing with automatic rate-drop sensing on recurrent neurally-mediated syncope. Am J Cardiol 81:158-162
15. Moya A, Brignole M, Menozzi C et al (2001) The mechanism of syncope in patients with isolated syncope and in patients with tilt-positive syncope. Circulation (in press)

CARDIAC RESYNCHRONIZATION THERAPY: WHEN, HOW AND WHY

How Many Patients Really Need Ventricular Resynchronization Therapy?

A. Boccanelli and G. Cacciatore

It has been estimated that heart failure affects 4.6 million patients in the United States and 22.5 million patients all over the world, and an equal number of patients have asymptomatic left ventricular dysfunction with a high risk of developing heart failure [1]. This condition is the primary discharge diagnosis from hospitals in Western countries. Prognosis is poor, with annual mortality ranging from approximately 10% in NYHA class I-II to 25% in NYHA class III-IV. Heart failure is a condition that principally affects the elderly, and with the progressive ageing of the population it is likely that the prevalence of heart failure will continue to increase during the coming years in both developed and developing countries.

Heart failure is currently viewed as a progressive disorder triggered by an index event that causes loss of myocytes or reduces the ability of myocardium to contract adequately [2]. In most cases, the patient will initially remain asymptomatic for a period of years. After the cardiac injury has occurred, many compensatory mechanisms are activated to sustain left ventricular function: the sympathetic nervous system, the renin-angiotensin-aldosterone system, natriuretic peptides, prostaglandins, and nitric oxide. However, sooner or later patients become symptomatic, with a resultant increase in morbidity and mortality. Because of the toxic effects exerted by these active molecules on the heart and circulation, progression of heart failure is independent of the hemodynamic status of the patient. It has been widely shown that interventions aimed solely at the correction of low cardiac output offer symptomatic benefit, but do not slow the progression of heart failure nor reduce mortality [3, 4]. By contrast, treatment with drugs capable of antagonizing the effects of neuroendocrine activation, such as angiotensin-converting enzyme inhibitors, β-blockers, and antialdosterone agents, has induced significant reductions of morbidity and mortality among heart failure patients [5-7]. However, the available data suggest that pharmacological therapy does not alter the incidence of cardiac events associated with heart failure, but merely postpones them. Nonpharmacological therapies such as implantable devices and cardiac transplantation are considered only in the most advanced stages of heart failure and are of limited availability.

U.O.D. Cardiologia, Azienda Ospedaliera San Giovanni-Addolorata, Rome, Italy

On these grounds a conceptually new and promising therapeutic strategy has been proposed: resynchronization therapy by means of biventricular pacing, aimed at bringing about more effective mechanical performance of the heart through better ventricular synergy [8]. This could be the first treatment for heart failure to act exclusively on the heart. Theoretically it has some advantages and disadvantages: the changeability over time of some variables such as the atrioventricular interval, the certainty of compliance, the measurability of the direct effects of the therapy in individual patients and their variations over time. The main disadvantages are the invasiveness of the procedure, its risk and cost, as well as the necessity of systematic follow-up over time. The rationale of this therapy resides in the detrimental effects on mechanical efficiency of left ventricular contraction in the presence of left ventricular conduction delay, the prevalence of which is high (30%-50%) in patients with heart failure [9]. Recent data have shown that patients with chronic heart failure and conduction defects have a higher risk of cardiovascular events and a poor prognosis [10]. A variety of studies have supported the concept that electrical stimulation of the left ventricle or both the left and right ventricles in combination may reduce the degree of dyssynchrony of left and right ventricular contraction in patients with disordered intraventricular conduction [11]. Short-term studies have shown that atrio-biventricular pacing improves hemodynamics by reducing dyssynchrony, improving symptoms, exercise tolerance, and functional class [12, 13].The main characteristics of the populations enrolled in the non-randomized observational studies performed so far are similar: high functional class (NYHA III–IV), prolonged QRS (> 120 ms), dilated left ventricle with ejection fraction below 35%, clinical stability, and the absence of a standard indication for cardiac pacing. The importance of baseline QRS duration in particular is underlined by Auricchio et al. who showed that the majority of acute responders had a QRS complex greater than 150 ms, while in patients with a QRS duration of 120-150 ms left ventricular function did not improve with pacing averaged over all sampled atrioventricular delays [14]. The role of QRS shortening after pacing as a predictor of improvement is not yet clear. Kass et al. did indeed report that mechanical improvement with pacing was not associated with QRS narrowing [12]. However, the same authors found a positive linear relationship between the baseline QRS duration during intrinsic conduction and the percentage of increase in left ventricular dP/dt during biventricular or left ventricular VDD pacing compared with baseline or no pacing [12]. This supports the notion that the more dyssynchronous the heart at baseline, the more likely it is that pacing will acutely benefit function. A potential explanation of this discrepancy is that acute studies may not reflect long-term responses. In the reported series patients are usually in NYHA class III, with relative stability of symptoms and optimal pharmacological therapy including ACE-inhibitors, digitalis, diuretics, and in some cases β-blockers, and have sinus rhythm. The observations of Leclercq et al. suggest that the extremely high mortality rate of patients in NYHA class IV is unlikely to be significantly improved by ventricular resynchronization therapy [15]. In this study the 12-month mortality rate for NYHA class IV patients was 55% – strikingly similar to that of the placebo arm of the CONSENSUS study for patients receiving vasodilators at the time of randomization [15]. Because patients with advanced heart failure are at high risk of sudden cardiac death, it is possible that biventricular pacing would offer the greatest survival benefit when combined with antitachycardia therapy via an implantable cardioverter-defibrillator. Indeed, randomized trials are underway that aim to determine the independent effects of biventricular pacing combined with the features of an implantable cardioverter-defibrillator. Overall the results so far are promising: left ventricular function appears to be improved and the end-diastolic diameter reduced. Physical performance, measured by peak VO_2 during a maximal symptom-limited exercise test or with a submaximal exercise test such as the 6-min walking test, is consistently improved. Quality of life, measured by the Minnesota Living with Heart Failure questionnaire, also improves.

None of these results, however, demonstrates the efficacy of ventricular stimulation as a therapy for heart failure. How many patients may benefit from resynchronization therapy? If we limit our consideration to the currently accepted indications, as described above, it is likely that in Europe, in a population of 6,500,000 heart failure patients, about 30% (1,950,000) have left bundle branch block. About 30% of these patients are in NYHA class III and might benefit from biventricular pacing. How many of these 650,000 patients are in sinus rhythm? How many patients have really drug-refractory heart failure? The promising results reported above have prompted a rapid rise in the number of implants worldwide, outside any study protocol, together with proposals to extend the indications to patients with less severe degrees of heart failure, or to patients with severe heart failure regardless of QRS morphology and duration, and to patients with atrial fibrillation.

Some randomized trials of biventricular stimulation in heart failure with surrogate end-points have been completed (PATH-CHF, MUSTIC, MIRACLE) or are drawing to an end (VIGOR, VENTAK-CHF, Contak-CD, PACMAN), and their results seem encouraging. We believe that trials with hard end-points (mortality and morbidity) that have been started in the last few months (COMPANION, CARE-HF) will be able to define more precisely the characteristics of heart failure patients who will benefit from biventricular pacing. It will then be possible to answer the question of how many patients may benefit from resynchronization therapy.

References

1. Braunwald E, Bristow MR (2000) Congestive heart failure: fifty years of progress. Circulation 102:IV-14-IV-23
2. Mann DL (1999) Mechanisms and models in heart failure. A combinatorial approach. Circulation 100:999-1008
3. Packer M, Carver JR, Rodeheffer RJ et al (1991) Effect of oral milrinone on mortality in severe chronic heart failure. N Engl J Med 325:1468-1475

4. Massie BM (1998) 15 years of heart-failure trials: what have we learned? Lancet. 352[Suppl]:29-33
5. The SOLVD Investigators (1991) Effect of enalapril on survival in patients with reduced left ventricular ejection fraction and congestive heart failure. N Engl J Med 325:293-302
6. Packer M, Bristow MR, Cohn JN et al (1996) The effect of carvedilol on morbidity and mortality in patients with chronic heart failure. N Engl J Med 334:1350-1355
7. Pitt B, Zannad F, Remme WJ et al (1999) The effect of spironolactone on morbidity and mortality in patients with severe heart failure. N Engl J Med 341:709-717
8. Blanc JJ, Etienne Y, Gilard M et al (1997) Evaluation of different ventricular pacing sites in patients with severe heart failure: results of an acute hemodynamic study. Circulation 96:3273–3277
9. Zaidi M, Robert A, Fesler R et al (1997) Dispersion of ventricular repolarization in dilated cardiomyopathy. Eur Heart J 18:1129-1134
10. Shamin W, Francis DP, Yousufuddin M et al (1999) Intraventricular conduction delay: a prognostic marker in chronic heart failure. Int J Cardiol 70:171-178
11. Cazeau S, Ritter P, Lazarus A et al (1996) Multisite pacing for end-stage heart failure: early experience. Pacing Clin Electrophysiol 19:1748–1757
12. Kass DA, Chen C-H, Curry C et al (1999) Improved left ventricular mechanics from acute VDD pacing in patients with dilated cardiomyopathy and ventricular conduction delay. Circulation 99:1567–1573
13. Alonso C, Leclercq C, Victor C et al (1999) Electrocardiographic predictive factors of long-term clinical improvement with multisite biventricular pacing in advanced heart failure. Am J Cardiol 84:1417-1421
14. Auricchio A, Klein H, Spinelli J (1999) Pacing for heart failure: selection of patients, techniques and benefits. Eur J Heart Failure 1:275-279
15. Leclercq C, Cazeau S, Ritter P et al (2000) A pilot experience with permanent biventricular pacing to treat advanced heart failure. Am Heart J 140:862-870

What Are the Clinical Benefits of Biventricular Pacing in Heart Failure Patients?

S. Garrigue, S. Reuter, P. Bordachar, M. Hocini, P. Jaïs, M. Haïssaguerre
and J. Clémenty

Introduction

The conventional DDD mode of pacing, using the right ventricular (RV) apex as the usual site of depolarization, results in retrograde activation of the left ventricle (LV). This opposite electrical sequence produces deleterious hemodynamic effects as well as the left bundle branch block regularly associated with dilated cardiomyopathy [1]. Optimization of the atrioventricular delay (AVD) provides a better LV filling pattern but does not always compensate RV pacing consequences [2]. Biventricular (BV) pacing was therefore developed to prevent interventricular dyssynchrony and, potentially, intraventricular dyssynchrony. BV pacing was initially demonstrated to provide acute hemodynamic improvement in patients with severe congestive heart failure (CHF) with prolonged QRS duration [3-5]. With BV pacing, the first clinical studies revealed an acute diminution of the capillary wedge pressure associated with an improvement in the cardiac index, suggesting regression of heart failure symptoms. However, potential clinical benefits were only confirmed at a mid-term follow-up.

Does Biventricular Pacing Provide Durable Clinical Improvement in Heart Failure Patients ?

In 1996, Cazeau et al. reported a substantial clinical improvement from class IV to class II of the New York Heart Association (NYHA) classification in four patients after a 6-month period of chronic BV pacing [4]. In 1998, Leclercq et al. presented mid-term results (15.4 ± 10.2 months) of a multicenter study and demonstrated a functional improvement in NYHA class (2.37 vs 3.7; $p < 0.01$) [6]. With regard to the treadmill test, duration and exercise capacity were significantly better, associated with a maximal VO_2 improvement. The InSync study (68 patients) also reported a significant improvement in NYHA function-

Hôpital Cardiologique du Haut-Lévêque, University of Bordeaux, France

al class associated with higher performances during the 6-min walking test [7]. The MUSTIC study (MUltisite StimulaTion In Cardiomyopathies) [8], the first randomized single-blinded multicenter study with crossover, was performed to assess the clinical efficacy and safety of BV pacing in 67 patients with severe heart failure and sinus rhythm and QRS greater than 150 ms. The Minnesota score (quality of life questionnaire) decreased by 32%, and the mean 6-min walking distance increased by 23% associated with a significantly higher peak VO_2. At the same time, the number of hospitalizations related to heart failure was reduced by two-thirds. Recently, two long-term studies of the clinical benefits of BV pacing have confirmed data reported by the MUSTIC protocol [9, 10].

Our clinical experience [11] is based on a population of 102 patients (mean age 65 ± 9.9 years, 19% females) with severe CHF and a low left ventricular ejection fraction (LVEF; 23.6 ± 7.8%). Sixty-two patients (60%) were in NYHA class III, 32 (30%) were in class IV, and 8 (10%) in class II despite maximal medical treatment including diuretics and angiotensin-converting enzyme (ACE) inhibitors. All patients presented with prolonged QRS duration (183 ± 37 ms). Thirty-two patients (31%) were in chronic atrial fibrillation. The LV was paced via the coronary sinus with specifically designed endovenous pacing leads in 89 patients (87.2%). The lead was placed in the anterobasal region of the LV in 8.8% of the patients, in a posterolateral tributary vein in 4.9%, and in an antero-lateral tributary vein in 73.5%. In 13 patients (12.8%), the LV lead was actively affixed to the endocardial surface of the LV via a transseptal procedure because of inability to cannulate the coronary sinus and/or one of its venous tributaries [12]. Patients with chronic atrial fibrillation systematically underwent a His bundle ablation. Clinical, echocardiographic, and hemodynamic data were collected before and immediately after implantation of a definitive BV pacing device, and then every 3 months afterwards. NYHA functional class, VO_2, and drug regimens were also recorded.

Over a 12-month period of BV pacing, we observed a significant reduction of the proportion of patients in NYHA class IV compared to before implantation (30% vs 7%; $p < 0.001$), and the same was true for class III (60% vs 14%; $p = 0.01$). In 36 patients (35%), dosages of diuretics could be reduced in association with initiation of β-blockers, which could not be done before implantation due to low blood pressure. QRS duration significantly decreased from 184 ± 38 to 170 ± 28 ms ($p < 0.01$) at 3 months' follow-up, and 168 ± 25 ms ($p < 0.01$) at 12 months' follow-up (Fig. 1). Simultaneously, performance at the maximal treadmill test was significantly higher at 8 months and 12 months after implantation than it was before (71 ± 26 W before vs 88 ± 29 W at 8 months and 83 ± 28 W at 12 months; $p = 0.003$) with no change in terms of maximum VO_2 (respectively 16 ± 4 vs 16 ± 5 vs 14 ± 5 ml/kg min; n.s.). The radionuclide LVEF remained unchanged from baseline to 8 months and was slightly higher at 12 months of BV pacing (respectively 23 ± 7% vs 26 ± 11% vs 26 ± 10%). In contrast, the aortic velocity-time integer increased from 13.9 ± 4.9 cm at baseline to 15 ± 4.2 cm at 3 months after implantation ($p = 0.024$) and to 17 ± 6.1 cm at 8 months ($p < 0.01$) (Fig. 2). At 1 year follow-up, 11 patients had died: 4 in the subgroup of improved patients from ventricular tachycardia and 7 (2 from ven-

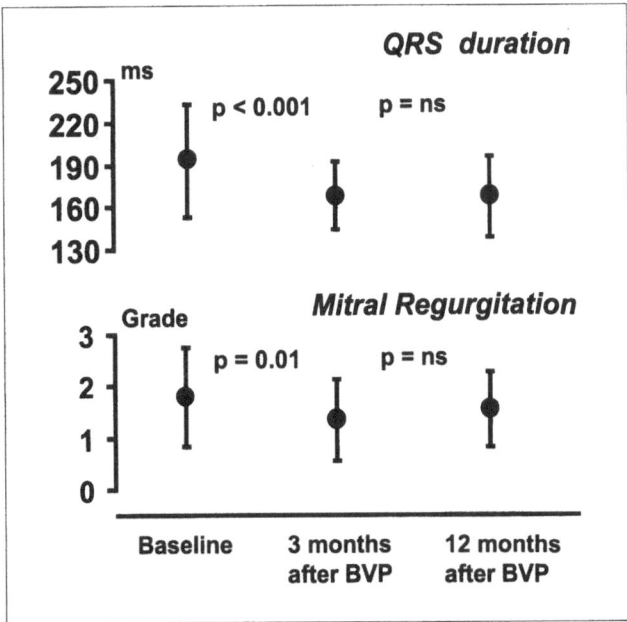

Fig. 1. Evolution of QRS duration and mitral regurgitation during 12 months of BV pacing (BVP)

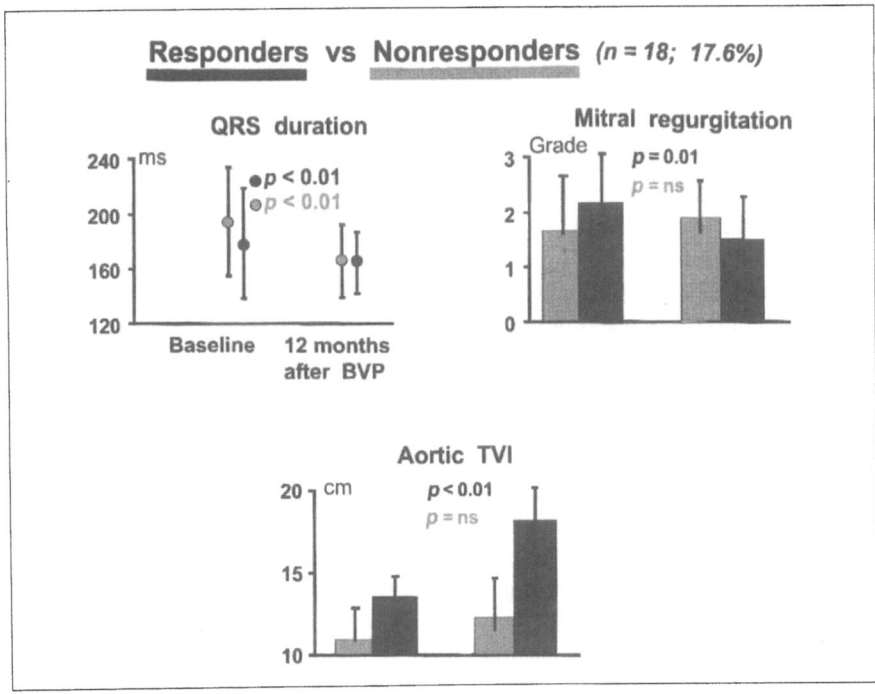

Fig. 2. QRS duration, mitral regurgitation, and aortic velocity-time integer in responders and nonresponders

tricular tachycardia) in the nonimproved patient subgroup. While 8% of patients showed no clinical improvement after 1 month of BV pacing, this percentage increased to 17% after 12 months of follow-up ($p = 0.02$). An intermediate multivariate statistical analysis showed that at 8 months the absence of regression of mitral regurgitation ($p = 0.01$) and the presence of ischemic disease ($p = 0.025$) were independent risk factors for failure of BV pacing.

What Are the Potential Mechanisms Involved in Clinical Improvement with BV Pacing?

The capacity of conventional dual-chamber cardiac pacing for optimization of the AV timing promoted pacing therapy as a promising treatment for drug-refractory heart failure patients in the early 1990s [13]. It is true that optimization of AVD, reduction of atrial arrhythmias by atrial overdrive, and heart rate modulation during exercise, allowing more sustained medical treatment, are beneficial effects of dual-chamber pacing to improve heart failure. However, atrial-synchronized RV pacing induces a reversal of the electrical and mechanical activation sequence from the apex to the base of the heart [1], even though it has been demonstrated that some CHF patients with complete left bundle branch block could be clinically improved with RV pacing [14]. The latter is consistent with the first studies showing clinical benefits of short AVD with DDD pacing in such patients [13, 15]. However, the effect was limited and was not reported in numerous other studies [2, 16, 17].

Our experience reveals a sustained therapeutic effect of multisite ventricular pacing but with discrepancies between clinical improvement and BV pacing-induced hemodynamic changes throughout follow-up. We did not find any correlation between the QRS duration and clinical improvement. At 8 months of follow-up, of nine patients with a BV pacing-induced increase in QRS duration, only two were not clinically improved. These data are consistent with short-term studies showing that LV pacing provides a significant hemodynamic improvement despite prolonging the QRS duration compared with spontaneous rhythm [18, 19]. Therefore, changes in QRS duration are not the only predictor of BV pacing efficacy: the electromechanical RV-LV resynchronization may not be always apparent on the surface electrocardiogram.

In our study, improved patients, irrespective of their QRS width after BV pacing, had a significant decrease of the mitral regurgitation (see Fig. 2). The fact that LV end-diastolic diameters remained unchanged before and 8 months after BV pacing (71 ± 8 vs 73 ± 10 mm) suggests that mitral regurgitation regression might result from a more homogeneous LV wall activation, especially around the mitral annulus. Doppler tissue imaging (DTI) echocardiography clearly demonstrates that BV pacing results in significantly more homogeneous LV regional electromechanical delays and visualizes the potential mechanisms of BV pacing on clinical improvement [20].

The multivariate analysis suggests that patients with ischemic cardiomyopathy are less likely to benefit from BV pacing. Indeed, the regional ischemia around the mitral annulus might be an obstacle for pacing-induced LV wall resynchronization and regression of mitral regurgitation. Although we did not find any significant increase in LVEF, our data suggest that mitral regurgitation regression results in an increase in the aortic velocity time integer and consequently, an increase in cardiac output.

Conclusions

Mid- and long-term improvement of NYHA functional class, quality of life score, and exercise capacity support the use of BV pacing as a primary treatment for patients with severe heart failure and wide QRS despite maximal medical treatment. However, our preliminary results showed discrepancies between clinical benefits and BV pacing-induced hemodynamic changes. No significant LVEF increase was observed in our population although more than 75% of the patients reported being clinically improved, irrespective of the paced QRS duration.

The final goal of BV pacing might be to restore more homogeneous LV regional electromechanical delays, which cannot always be seen on the surface ECG. The presence of an ischemic area might counteract this process and could explain the nonnegligible proportion of nonresponders. In this case, the location of the LV pacing lead is determinative and needs to be more deeply investigated.

References

1. Rosenquist M, Isaaz K, Botvinik et al (1991) Hemodynamic importance of activation sequence compared to atrioventricualr synchrony in left ventricular function. Am J Cardiol 67:148-156
2. Nishimura RA, Hayes DL, Holmes DR, Tajik AJ (1995) Mechanism of hemodynamic improvement by dual-chamber pacing for severe left ventricular dysfunction: an acute Doppler and catheterisation hemodynamic study. J Am Coll Cardiol 25:281-288
3. Foster AH, Gold MR, McLaughlin JS (1995) Hemodynamic effects of atrio-biventricular pacing in humans. Ann Thorac Surg 59:294-300
4. Cazeau S, Ritter P, Lazarus A et al (1996) Multisite pacing for end-stage heart failure: early experience. Pacing Clin Electrophysiol 19:1748-1757
5. Leclercq C, Cazeau S, Le Breton H et al (1998) Acute hemodynamic effects of biventricular DDD pacing in patients with end-stage heart failure. J Am Coll Cardiol 32:1825-1831
6. Leclercq C, Cazeau S, Victor F et al (1998) Long-term results of permanent biventricular pacing in patients with refractory heart failure. Eur Heart J 19:573 (abstr)

7. Gras D, Mabo P, Tanr T et al (1998) Multisite pacing as a supplemental treatment of congestive heart failure: preliminary results of the Medtronic Inc InSync study. Pacing Clin Electrophysiol 21:2249-2255

8. Cazeau S, Leclercq C, Lavergne T et al (2001) Effects of multisite biventricular pacing in patients with heart failure and intraventricular conduction delay. N Engl J Med 344:873-880

9. Alonso C, Leclercq C, Victor F et al (1999) Electrocardiographic predictive factors of long-term clinical improvement with multisite biventricular pacing in advanced heart failure. Am J Cardiol 84:1417-1421

10. Leclercq C, Victor F, Alonso C et al (2000) Comparative effects of permanent biventricular pacing for refractory heart failure in patients with stable sinus rhythm or chronic atrial fibrillation. Am J Cardiol 85:1154-1156

11. Reuter S, Garrigue S, Bordachar P et al (2000) Intermediate-term results of biventricular pacing in heart failure: correlation between clinical and hemodynamic data. Pacing Clin Electrophysiol 23:1713-1717

12. Jais P, Takahashi A, Garrigue S et al (2000) Mid-term follow up of endocardial biventricular pacing. Pacing Clin Electrophysiol 23:1744-1747

13. Hochleitner M, Hortnagl H, Fridich L et al (1990) Usefulness of physiologic dual-chamber pacing in drug-resistant idiopathic dilated cardiomyopathy. Am J Cardiol 66:198-202

14. Garrigue S, Barold SS, Valli N et al (1999) Effect of right ventricular pacing in patients with complete left bundle branch block. Am J Cardiol 83:600-604

15. Brecker S, Xiao H, Sparrow J, Gibson G (1992) Effects of dual-chamber pacing with short atrioventricular delay in dilated cardiomyopathy. Lancet 340:1308-1312

16. Linde C, Gadler F, Edner M et al (1995) Results of atrioventricular synchronous pacing with optimized delay in patients with severe congestive heart failure. Am J Cardiol 75:919-923

17. Gold MR, Feliciano Z, Gottlieb SS et al (1995) Dual-chamber pacing with a short atrioventricular delay in congestive heart failure: a randomised study. J Am Coll Cardiol 26:967-973

18. Blanc JJ, Etienne Y, Gilard M et al (1997) Evaluation of different ventricular pacing sites in patients with severe heart failure: results of an acute hemodynamic study. Circulation 96:3273-3277

19. Kass DA, Chen CH, Curry C et al (1999) Improved left ventricular mechanics from acute VDD pacing in patients with dilated cardiomyopathy and ventricular conduction delay. Circulation 99:1567-1573

20. Garrigue S, Lafitte S, Hocini M et al (2000) Mechanisms of left ventricular wall resynchronisation during multisite ventricular pacing: direct effects on the variations of the regional electromechanical delays and wall motion velocities. Pacing Clin Electrophysiol 23:682

Neurohormonal and Anatomical Remodeling After Ventricular Resynchronization Therapy: Does It Really Happen?

J.P. Boehmer, J.C. Luck, D.L. Wolbrette and G.V. Naccarelli

Chronic heart failure is a global public health problem. The incidence of heart failure is very high among developed nations and contributes significantly to the cost of medical care. It is a very common cause of hospitalization for elderly patients [1]. In addition to the morbidity associated with heart failure, it remains very lethal. Despite advances in the medical therapy of heart failure, the projected 5-year mortality remains greater than 50% at 5 years [2]. Accordingly, new treatments are needed.

Recently, attention has been drawn to the potential of cardiac resynchronization therapy (CRT) to improve the symptoms and functional capacity of patients with heart failure. CRT is the use of ventricular pacing at either specific sites or multiple sites to improve contractile performance in patients with intraventricular conduction delays and discoordinated ventricular contraction. CRT has been studied in selected patients and produced improvement in acute hemodynamics, exercise capacity, symptoms, quality of life, and left ventricular size and function [3-5]. However, long-term effects of CRT are not yet known.

Activation of the Sympathetic Nervous System in Heart Failure

One of the hallmarks of heart failure is an increase in sympathetic nervous system activity. Originally believed to simply be a compensatory mechanism in heart failure, the increase in sympathetic nervous system activity is now believed to play a pathologic role in the progression of heart failure. Activation of the sympathetic nervous system perpetuates a continuing cycle of adverse hemodynamic and metabolic events that lead to worsening heart failure. After a myocardial injury occurs, there is a drop in cardiac output. This decrease in cardiac output leads to activation of a number of compensatory mechanisms including the sympathetic nervous system. Activation of the sympathetic nervous system is known to have a myriad of effects that could be detrimental to

Division of Cardiology, Penn State College of Medicine, The Milton S. Hershey Medical Center, Hershey, Pennsylvania, USA

the heart failure patient. These include decreased coronary blood flow, increased automaticity, progressive cardiac remodelling with maladaptive hypertrophy, cytokine activation, activation of the renin-angiotensin-aldosterone system, decreased myocardial reserve and, with chronic stimulation, decreased contractility. The degree of sympathetic nervous system activation is proportional to the severity of heart failure. As further evidence of this relationship, serum norepinephrine levels are associated with prognosis in heart failure patients [6].

CRT and the Sympathetic Nervous System in Heart Failure

Because of the known mechanisms by which the sympathetic nervous system may lead to progressive heart failure, new treatments are evaluated to determine whether they may reduce sympathetic nervous system activity. There are several ways to evaluate the activation of the sympathetic nervous system. The most direct method is to measure sympathetic nervous system activity by means of muscle sympathetic nerve activity (MSNA). This technique involves the use of microneurography to isolated sympathetic traffic to muscle, typically using the peroneal nerve. We have evaluated the acute effects of CRT on MSNA. Figure 1 presents the effects of CRT on MSNA in two patients with advanced heart failure. The patients were evaluated over a series of heart rates, and in each instance MSNA was lower with CRT than without CRT. In a larger series a statistically significant difference was found between no CRT and CRT via either left ventricular pacing or biventricular pacing [7].

The most common method used to assess sympathetic nervous system activity is measurement of serum norepinephrine. Although limited by issues of reuptake, spillover, and the influence of methods of obtaining and handling specimens, serum norepinephrine measurement have been proven to correlate well with prognosis in heart failure patients [8]. Serum norepinephrine was measured in a series of patients participating in the VIGOR CHF study [9]. This study involved the use of a CRT device implanted using an epicardial left ventricular lead via a small lateral thorocotomy [10]. The study was designed for the patients to serve as their own control, although there was a blinded, controlled 6-week period where patients were programmed either to no ventricular pacing (ODO mode) or to CRT (VDD mode). Prospectively, a significant decrease in norepinephrine was defined as a decrease of 40% in serum norepinephrine concentration. The proportion of patients experiencing this decrease progressively grew over the 18 weeks of study (Fig. 2). The mean decrease in norepinephrine was both statistically significant and clinically impressive at 283 pg/ml. However, long-term parallel group data are needed to confirm these findings.

A third method of assessing sympathetic nervous system activity is by the heart rate variability. Although this method does not give a direct assessment of sympathetic nervous system activity, higher heart rate variability is believed to be associated with a favorable balance between sympathetic and parasympa-

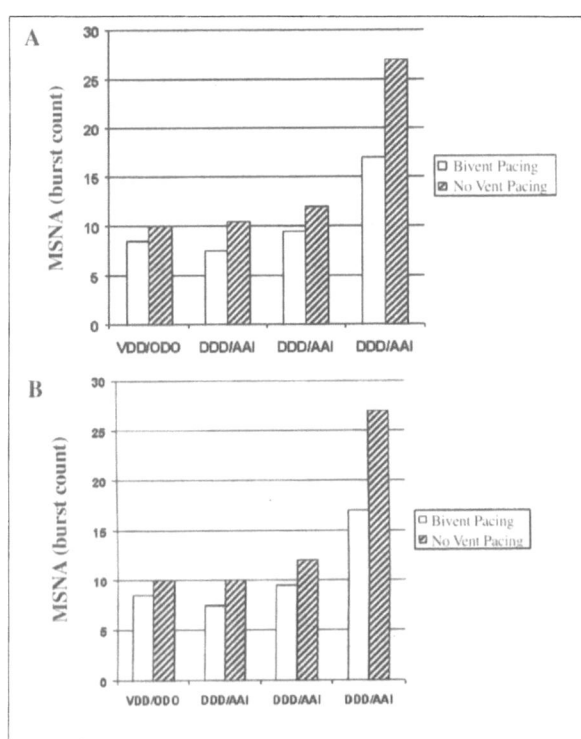

Fig. 1A,B. Muscle sympathetic nerve activity (MSNA) in two patients (**A, B**) at various heart rates in each. Both patients had chronic heart failure with severe left ventricular systolic dysfunction and a left bundle branch block. The *open bars* represent time of biventricular pacing (CRT) and the *hatched bars* times when there is no ventricular pacing. In each instance, the MSNA is lower with CRT than with intrinsic conduction

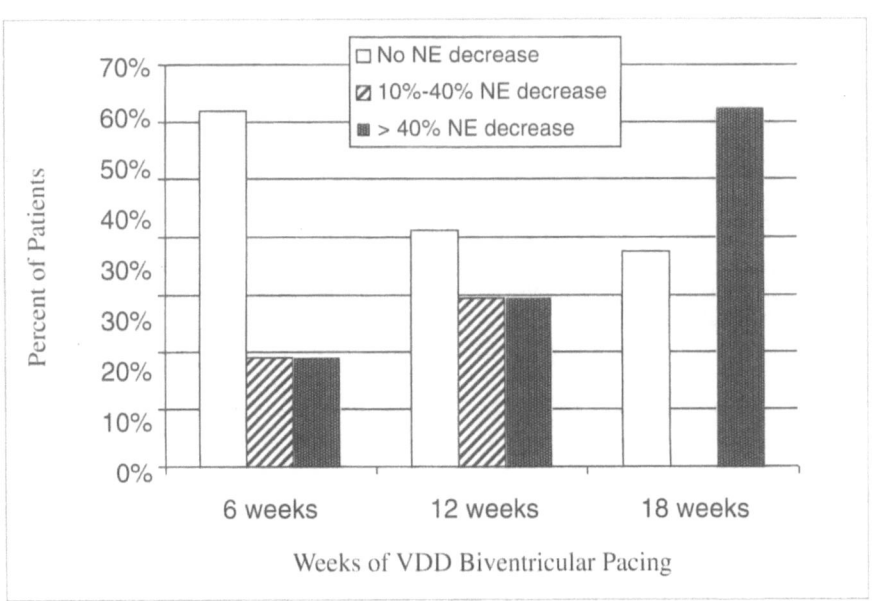

Fig. 2. Percentages of patients who had either no decrease in serum norepinephrine (*open bars*), a 10%-40% decrease in serum norepinephrine (*hatched bars*) or a > 40% decrease in serum norepinephrine (*shaded bars*). After 18 weeks of CRT, the majority of the patients had a > 40% decrease in serum norepinephrine

thetic nervous system activity. This technique was used in the European PATH-CHF study. In this study, patients received a biventricular pacemaker and were programmed to a CRT mode for 4 weeks, then no pacing for 4 weeks followed by another 4 weeks of CRT [3]. In this study heart rate variability increased with pacing therapy and returned towards baseline with the no pacing period [11] (Fig. 3). This is consistent with other findings suggesting a beneficial effect of CRT on sympathetic nervous system activity.

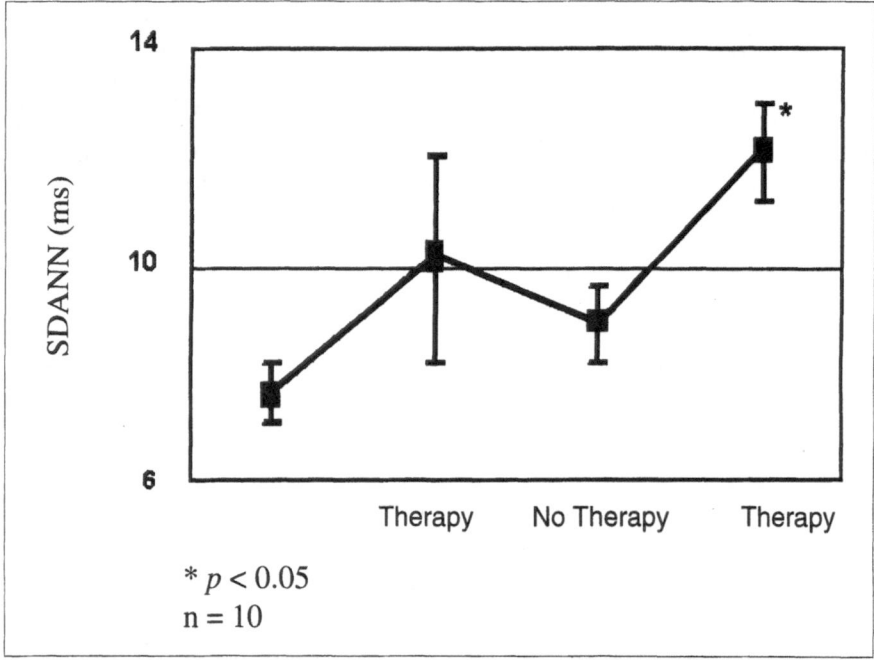

Fig. 3. Heart rate variability in ten patients from the PATH-CHF study of CRT. The time points are at baseline prior to CRT, after 4 weeks of CRT, after an additional 4 weeks of no CRT, and, finally, after 4 more weeks of CRT. CRT resulted in a significant increase in heart rate variability, suggesting an improvement in the balance of sympathetic to parasympathetic nerve activity

Structural Remodeling

Heart failure is also characterized by progressive left ventricular dilation and a decrease in ejection fraction. Intraventricular conduction defects can cause abnormal wall stress in unusual patterns. These abnormal wall stresses may contribute to abnormal left ventricular remodeling [12]. CRT has the potential to improve the distribution and wall stress and may, therefore, have a beneficial effect on left ventricular structure. Observational studies of this therapy have revealed an improvement in left ventricular ejection fraction [3, 13]. An uncontrolled observation in the VIGOR CHF and VENTAK trials revealed a decrease in left ventricular volumes. More recently, both the MIRACLE trial and CON-TAK CD trial have reported randomized, parallel group data that revealed clinically important reductions in left ventricular diastolic volumes [5, 14]. This reverse remodeling has only previously been seen with β-blockers and holds hope for beneficial long-term effects of this therapy.

References

1. American Heart Association (2000) 2001 Heart and stroke statistical update. American Heart Association, Dallas, TX
2. Levy D, Vasan RS, Benjamin EJ et al (2000) Temporal trends in heart failure risk factors from 1950-1998. American Heart Association Scientific Sessions, New Orleans, November 2000
3. Auricchio A, Stellbrink C, Block M et al (1999) Effect of pacing chamber and atrioventricular delay on acute systolic function of paced patients with congestive heart failure. Circulation 99:2993-3001
4. Cazeau S, Leclercq C, Lavergne T et al (2001) Effects of multisite biventricular pacing in patients with heart failure and intraventricular conduction delay. N Engl J Med 344:873-880
5. Abraham WT (2001) Multicenter InSync randomized clinical evaluation. Results of a randomized, double-blind, controlled trial to assess cardiac resynchronization therapy in heart failure patients. American College of Cardiology Scientific Sessions, Orlando, FL, March 2001
6. Thomas JA, Marks BH (1978) Plasma norepinephrine in congestive heart failure. Am J Cardiol 41:233-243
7. Hamdan MH, Zagrodzky JD, Joglar JA et al (2000) Biventricular pacing decresases sympathetic activity compared with right ventricular pacing in patients with depressed ejection fraction. Circulation 102:1027-1032
8. Francis G (1993) Plasma norepinephrine, plasma renin activity and congestive heart failure. Circulation 87[Suppl VI]:40-47
9. Saxon L, DeMarco T, Chatterjee K, Boehmer J (1998) The magnitude of sympathoneural activation in advanced heart failure is altered with chronic biventricular pacing. Pacing Clin Electrophysiol 21 (part II):914
10. Saxon LA, Boehmer JP, Hummel J et al (1999) Biventricular pacing in patients with congestive heart failure: two prospective randomized trials. The VIGOR CHF and VENTAK CHF Investigators. Am J Cardiol 83:120D-123D
11. Auricchio A (1999) Pacing therapy reduces heart rate and increases heart rate variability in CHF patients. J Card Failure 5[Suppl 1]:44
12. Curry CW, Nelson GS, Wyman BT et al (2000) Mechanical dyssynchrony in dilated cardiomyopathy with intraventricular conduction delay as depicted by 3D tagged magnetic resonance imaging. Circulation 101:e2
13. Nelson GS, Berger RD, Fetics BJ et al (2000) Left ventricular or biventricular pacing improves cardiac function at diminished energy cost in patients with dilated cardiomyopathy and left bundle-branch block. Circulation 102:3053-3059
14. The CONTAK CD Investigators (2001) The results of the CONTAK CD trials. North American Society of Pacing and Electrophysiology, Boston, May 2001

Is Echocardiography Useful for Selecting Patients with Heart Failure as Candidates for Ventricular Resynchronization Therapy?

B. De Piccoli, C. Zanella and P. Della Valentina

Introduction

In recent years cardiac resynchronization by biventricular pacing (Bi-Ve) has been proposed as an adjunctive therapy for patients with chronic heart failure and conduction delays [1, 2]. Clinical studies concluded that the new tool improves symptoms and exercise capacity. Furthermore, acute hemodynamic investigations [3, 4] demonstrated that it increases the cardiac index and lowers the wedge pressure, with an overall improvement of left ventricular function.

Many studies have utilized echocardiography for the management of patients assigned to Bi-Ve; the tool has proved to be effective for quantifying the desynchronization of ventricles [5] and the impairment of ventricular filling [6], as well as on selecting the optimal A-V delay of the stimulation [7,8]; furthermore, it demonstrated that Bi-Ve can reverse ventricular remodeling [9] and improve the synchronization of the electromechanical activity of the ventricles [10]. Thus, echocardiography constitutes an adequate method for evaluating patients candidated to biventricular stimulation and for recording changes of cardiac anatomical and functional parameters during follow-up of the treated patients.

We have utilized echo-Doppler for the management of patients affected by heart failure refractory to optimal pharmacological therapy, and we have considered the echo-Doppler parameters of cardiac morphology and function before implantation of the biventricular stimulator and at two follow-up steps.

Study Population

Twenty patients, 14 males, and 6 females, mean age 70.10 ± 5.38 years (range 59-78), with left branch block on ECG and with NYHA Class III and IV heart failure refractory to optimal tritration of digoxin, diuretics, carvedilol and angiotensin-converting enzyme inhibitors, who received a biventricular pace-

Cardiovascular Department, Division of Cardiology, Umberto I Hospital, Mestre-Venice, Italy

maker (Contak system by Guidant Corporation, 12 patients; Insync system, by Medtronic Corporation, eight patients).

The underlying heart disease was: ischemic cardiomyopathy in 13 patients; idiopathic dilated cardiomyopathy in five patients; hypertensive cardiomiopathy in two patients. All patients exhibited a dilated left ventricle (LV) with an ejection fraction (EF) < 35%.

Method

In each subject, an atriosynchronized Bi-Ve was implanted; the left ventricular pacing lead was transvenously inserted through the coronary sinus and was advanced into the lateral or posterolateral cardiac vein. The atrioventricular interval was optimized for maximal diastolic filling and/or maximal aortic flow calculated by Doppler: it was settled in 105.33 ± 10.85 ms. A clinical and echo-Doppler evaluation was performed in each patient before pacemaker implantation and after 1 and 3 months.

The morphological indices were evaluated by the calculation of LV internal dimensions and volumes and by the calculation of the anteroposterior dimension of the left atrium (LA). The indices of the systolic function of LV were evaluated by the calculation of its ejection fraction (EF) and of the velocity-time integral of the Doppler aortic flow (VTI-A0). For the evaluation of the diastolic function of LV, we calculated the overall diastolic mitral flow (VTI-Global), the ratio of the early and late diastolic mitral flow (VTI-E/VTI-A), the deceleration time of the E wave (DT-E) and the ratio of the durations of mitral A wave and of the reverse flow of the pulmonary venous flow (dur. A_M / dur. RF).

The mitral regurgitation area, the systolic pulmonary artery pressure (SPAP), the difference between the electromechanical intervals of aortic and pulmonary output ($qA_2 - qP_2$) and the electromechanical interval of the LV lateral wall (q-LW), which is settled near the site of stimulation of the left lead of Bi-Ve, were also calculated.

Statistical Analysis

The parametric variables calculated at the three different time points were compared to each other using a paired sample *t*-test with Bonferroni correction. All data were expressed as mean ± standard deviation (SD); a *p* value < 0.05 was considered as statistically significant.

Results

Table 1 outlines the basal morphological echocardiographic parameters, as well as their trend during the 3 month follow-up. The internal diastolic dimensions of the LV slightly decreased; the difference among the three steps did not produce significant results, considering the overall study population, but if we took into account only patients with an end-diastolic LV diameter (EDLVD) ≤ 70 mm, we could then demonstrate a significant reduction of the internal dimensions of the LV at the 3 months control. On the other hand, patients with an EDLVD > 70 mm did not exhibit a significant change during follow-up.

The change of LV volumes paralleled the trend of LV dimensions; in fact only volumes ≤ 200 ml exhibited a significant reduction after 3 months.

Table 2, which summarizes the changes of echo-Doppler functional parameters of the LV during follow-up, shows a significant increase of the following indices: EF; mitral forward flow (VTI-Global); aortic flow (VTI-A$_0$); the deceleration time of the E wave of mitral flow; and finally, the ratio of the durations of mitral A wave and reverse flow (RF) of the venous pulmonary flow, which is correlated with the end-diastolic LV pressure [11]. On the other hand, the MR area, ratio VTI-E/VTI-A of the mitral flow, the systolic pul-

Table 1. Trend of the morphological parameters during follow-up

Morphological Parameters	Basal	1 Month	3 Months	p
EDLVD (mm)	67.50 ± 7.5	65.30 ± 8.11	61.58 ± 9.3	1→ 2: NS 1→ 3: NS 2→ 3: NS
EDLVD>70 mm	75.25 ± 4.11	74.00 ± 2.71	71.50 ± 7.68	1→ 2: NS 1→ 3: NS 2→ 3: NS
EDLVD ≤ 70 mm	65.44 ± 4.28	62.67 ± 5.85	57.22 ± 4.94	1→ 2: NS 1→ 3: 0.002 2→ 3: 0.049
EDLVV (ml)	202.75 ± 55.95	199.58 ± 63.12	170 ± 58.66	1→ 2: NS 1→ 3: NS 2→ 3: NS
EDLVV>200 ml	253.50 ± 35.40	248.33 ± 38.82	224.17 ± 34.70	1→ 2: NS 1→ 3: NS 2→ 3: NS
EDLVV ≤ 200 ml	152.00 ± 37.06	142.50 ± 31.26	108.33 ± 25.63	1→ 2: NS 1→ 3: 0.039 2→ 3: 0.06
LA (mm)	48.82 ± 4.79	46.33 ± 4.25	45.42 ± 2.82	1→ 2: NS 1→ 3: NS 2→ 3: NS

EDLVD, end diastolic left ventricle dimension; *EDLVV*, end diastolic left ventricle volume; *LA*, left atrium

Table 2. Trend of the functional parameters during follow-up

Functional Parameters	Basal	1 Month	3 Months	p
EF (%)	28.00 ± 3.74	34.08 ± 5.92	38.83 ± 5.20	1→2: 0.006 2→3: 0.048
MR area (cm^2)	6.36 ± 3.99	3.71 ± 1.72	2.40 ± 1.19	1→2: 0.036 2→3: 0.048
VTI-E/VTI-A	2.62 ± 0.97	1.37 ± 0.69	1.15 ± 0.52	1→2: 0.0001 2→3: NS
VTI-Global (cm)	11.45 ± 1.12	14.9 ± 1.22	16.10 ± 1.16	1→2: 0.0001 2→3: NS
DT-E (ms)	138.64 ± 18.85	190.91 ± 47.11	233 ± 34.97	1→2: 0.003 2→3: 0.042
SPAP (mmHg)	51.08 ± 13.32	40.92 ± 8.77	34.25 ± 3.22	1→2: 0.044 2→3: 0.049
VTI-A$_0$ (cm)	14 ± 3.39	18.49 ± 4.77	19.94 ± 5.74	1→2: 0.019 2→3: NS
dur.A$_M$ / dur.RF	0.82 ± 0.19	1.08 ± 0.13	1.22 ± 0.09	1→2: 0.0001 2→3: 0.046
qA$_2$ – qP$_2$ (ms)	54.33 ± 13.38	19.58 ± 14.37	14.55 ± 13.50	1→2: 0.0001 2→3: NS
q-LW (ms)	153.00 ± 50.18	112.50 ± 21.89	104.00 ± 16.96	1→2: 0.031 2→3: NS

EF, ejection fraction of left ventricle; *MR*, mitral regurgitation; *VTI-E/VTI-A*, ratio of the time integrals of E and A waves of the mitral flow; *VTI-Global*, velocity-time integral of the global mitral flow; *DT-E*, deceleration time of E wave of the mitral flow; *SPAP*, systolic pulmonary artery pressure; *VTI-A$_o$*, velocity-time integral of the aortic flow; *dur.A$_M$/dur. RF*, ratio of the durations of A wave of the mitral flow (A$_M$) and the reverse flow (RF) of the venous pulmonary flow; *qA$_2$ - qP$_2$*, difference of the time intervals between q wave of ECG and aortic (A$_2$) and pulmonary (P$_2$) valve opening; *q-LW*, time interval between q wave of ECG and the start of the lateral wall motion of left ventricle

monary artery pressure, and the time intervals qA$_2$ - qP$_2$ and q-LW, exhibit a significant decrease.

Thus, we can realise that there was a definite improvement of the functional echo-Doppler parameters of the patients considered; the most beneficial change took place during the first month of follow-up and was maintained or further improved during the following 2 months. Moreover, the symptoms of patients also improved and each subject shifted to at least one lower NYHA class.

Finally, Table 3 outlines that the rate of variation of EF parallels the rate of variation of mitral VTI-Global as well as of qA$_2$ - qP$_2$ and q-LW time intervals; the first parameter is related to the filling pattern of the LV, while the two latter

Table 3. Comparison between basal echo-Doppler parameters, or their change during the follow-up, and the increase of EF at 3 months evaluation

Basal $qA_2 - qP_2$ (ms)	62.00 ± 9.27	13.00 ± 3.46	3 Months Δ EF (%)
	43.33 ± 6.83	7.00 ± 3.41	
	$p = 0.003$	$p = 0.013$	
3 Months $\downarrow qA_2 - qP_2$ (ms)	48.33 ± 8.16	12.50 ± 4.14	3 Months Δ EF (%)
	31.83 ± 4.96	7.17 ± 3.19	
	$p = 0.002$	$p = 0.013$	
Basal VTI-Global (cm)	10.92 ± 0.78	12.33 ± 4.37	3 Months Δ EF (%)
	12.27 ± 0.54	7.17 ± 3.60	
	$p = 0.006$	$p = 0.049$	
3 Months $\uparrow$ VTI-Global (cm)	4.67 ± 0.37	13.05 ± 3.64	3 Months Δ EF (%)
	3.62 ± 0.44	6.67 ± 2.88	
	$p = 0.001$	$p = 0.007$	
Basal q-LW (ms)	198 ± 16.43	12.14 ± 3.89	3 Months Δ EF (%)
	137 ± 46.58	7.43 ± 4.2	
	$p = 0.025$	$p = 0.05$	
3 Months $\downarrow$ q-LW (ms)	67.00 ± 11.51	12.00 ± 4.10	3 Months Δ EF (%)
	35.00 ± 19.36	7.00 ± 3.41	
	$p = 0.013$	$p = 0.044$	

$qA_2 - qP_2$, difference of the time intervals between the q wave of ECG and aortic (A_2) and pulmonary (P_2) valve opening; $\downarrow$, decrease; *VTI-Global*, velocity-time integral of the global mitral flow. $\uparrow$, increase; *q-LW*, time interval between the q wave of ECG and the start of the lateral wall motion of the left ventricle

are related to ventricular desynchronization [8, 10]. Furthermore, the table shows that the worst basal values of those parameters are associated with the best increase of EF during the follow-up.

Discussion

In agreement with previous reports [8-10, 12] our study confirms that biventricular pacing in patients with advanced heart failure improves systolic function and filling of the LV; moreover, the pacing decreases mitral regurgitation and lowers arterial pulmonary pressure. These improvements are associated with a ventricular resynchronization, as documented by a shortening of the electromechanical delay of LV; in fact, after Bi-Ve we documented a reduction of the time interval from the pulmonary and aortic valve opening, as well as a reduction of the time from the q wave of ECG and the start of the contraction of the lateral wall of the LV. The increase of ventricular filling time was associated with such changes of the mitral flow as the prolongation of the deceleration time of the E wave and the relative enhancement of the velocity-time integral of the A wave, consistent with a lowering of the LV filling pressure [6]. Moreover, we documented a shortening of the duration of the pulmonary venous reverse flow and a consequent increase of the ratio A_M/RF, which further confirms the improvement of the diastolic function of LV [11].

Decreases of mitral regurgitation and ventricular filling pressure are probably the leading factors in reduction of the dimensions and volumes of the LV, although all echo-Doppler functional parameters exhibited a significant improvement at the first control after 1 month, while LV morphology changed significantly only after 3 months. Thus, in our study, as previously reported by Lau and Coll [9], we documented that the reversal of LV remodeling takes place later in comparison with the functional parameters. Heart size change is probably consequent to structural variations of myocardial fibers, therefore it is time-dependent; while such parameters as EF, LV filling time and pressure, as well as mitral regurgitation, can be improved more quickly by synchronous biventricular pacing.

In the present study we also documented that highly impaired LVs with internal end-diastolic dimensions > 70 mm or volumes > 200 ml have a low chance of improving by Bi-Ve, at least during a short follow-up of 3 months. This observation agrees with previous reports about patients treated by Bi-Ve [13] or medical therapy [14].

By contrast, poor functional parameters documented at the basal evaluation do not predict a poor outcome; in fact, patients with a reduced LV filling pattern, represented by a low VTI-Global, or patients with prolonged electro-mechanical time intervals, outlined by long qA_2 - qP_2 or q-LW intervals, exhibited the best variations of LV EF during follow-up. Thus, these indices of impaired LV function appear to be useful in selecting people who can benefit from biventricular stimulation.

Conclusions

From analysis of the data achieved in our study population, we can conclude that:
1. Echocardiography is an adequate tool for selecting patients assigned to resynchronization ventricular therapy and for evaluating them during follow-up.
2. Bi-Ve has a beneficial impact on the functional and anatomical parameters of the LV.
3. Functional indices exhibit a strong and rapid improvement, while the change of anatomical parameters is lower and later.
4. Poorer indices of LV filling pattern and LV desynchronization seem to predict a greater benefit by Bi-Ve.
5. Most enlarged LVs look to be less susceptible to future improvement of their remodeling by Bi-Ve.

References

1. Cazeau S, Ritter P, Bakdach S et al (1994) Four chamber pacing in dilated cardiomyopathy. Pacing Clin Electrophysiol 17:1974-1979
2. Leclercq C, Cazeau S, Ritter P et al (2000) A pilot experience with permanent biventricular pacing to treat advanced heart failure. Am Heart J 140:862-870
3. Blanc J-J, Etienne Y, Gilard M et al (1997) Evaluation of different ventricular pacing sites in patients with severe heart failure: results of an acute hemodynamic study. Circulation 96:3273-3277
4. Kass DA, Chen C-H, Curry C et al (1999) Improved left ventricular mechanics from acute VDD pacing in patients with dilated cardiomyopathy and ventricular conduction delay. Circulation 99:1567-1573
5. Bordachar P, Garrigue S, Reuter S et al (2000) Hemodynamic assessment of right, left, and biventricular pacing by peak endocardial acceleration and echocardiography in patients with end-stage heart failure. Pacing Clin Electrophysiol 23 (2):1726-1730
6. Nishimura RA, Hayes DL, Holmes DR, Tajik J (1995) Mechanism of hemodynamic improvement by dual-chamber pacing for severe left ventricular disfunction: an acute Doppler and catheterization hemodynamic study. J Am Coll Cardiol 25:281-288
7. Guardigli G, Ansani L, Percoco GF et al (1994) AV delay optimization and management of DDD paced patients with dilated cardiomyopathy. Pacing Clin Electrophysiol 17(2):1984-1988
8. Breithardt OA, Stellbrink C, Franke A et al (2000) Echocardiographic evidence of hemodynamic and clinical improvement in patients paced for heart failure. Am J Cardiol 86[Suppl]:133K-137K
9. Lau C-P, Yu C-M, Chau E et al (2000) Reversal of left ventricular remodeling by synchronous biventricular pacing in heart failure. Pacing Clin Electrophysiol 23(2):1722-1725
10. Verlato R, Turrini P, Baccillieri MS et al (2000) Biventricular pacing and atrioventricular junction ablation as treatment of low output syndrome due to refractory congestive heart failure and chronic atrial fibrillation. Ital Heart J 12:844-847
11. Appleton CP, Galloway JM, Gonzales MS et al (1993) Estimation of left ventricular filling pressures using two-dimensional and Doppler echocardiography in adult cardiac patients: additional value of analyzing left atrial size, left atrial ejection fraction and the difference in the duration of pulmonary venous and mitral flow velocity at atrial contraction. J Am Coll Cardiol 22:1972-1982
12. Alonso C, Leclercq C, Victor F et al (1999) Electrocardiographic predictive factors of long-term clinical improvement with multisite biventricular pacing in advanced heart failure. Am J Cardiol 84:1417-1421
13. Auricchio A, Stellbrink C, Sack S et al (1999) The pacing therapies for congestive heart failure (PATH-CHF) study: rationale, design, and endpoints of a prospective randomized multicenter study. Am J Cardiol 83[Suppl 5B]:130D-135D
14. Levine TB, Levine AB, Bolenbaugh J, Stomel RJ (1999) Impact of left ventricular size on pharmacological reverse remodeling in heart failure. Circulation 100:I-678 (abstr)

Is Acute Hemodynamic-Angiographic Evaluation Necessary Before Implantation of a Left Ventricular-Based Pacemaker?

J.J. Blanc, M. Gilard, Y. Etienne, K. Touiza, M. Fatemi and J. Mansourati

Left ventricular-based (LV) pacing is considered an effective adjunct to pharmacological treatment in patients with severe chronic heart failure (CHF) [1, 2]. However, many questions related to this new therapeutic option remain open. One of these is the utility of acute hemodynamic-angiographic evaluation prior to the permanent implantation. The aim of this review is to attempt to summarize our knowledge on this topic.

Hemodynamic Evaluation

There is no question but that acute hemodynamic evaluations were the precursors of permanent LV-based pacing [3-6]. In fact, these preliminary acute evaluations have demonstrated many major data which made it possible to take the next step to permanent pacing. The most important result was that among patients with severe CHF and left bundle branch block (LBBB), acute epicardial or endocardial pacing of the lateral part of the LV resulted in clear hemodynamic improvement in a majority. The most striking feature was that this improvement occurred on an "on-off" basis: as soon as LV-based pacing was initiated, a decrease in capillary wedge pressure (CWP) was observed, which immediately returned to its initial value when LV pacing was turned off (see Fig. 2 in [3]). Initially, it was shown that only CWP and V wave were improved [6], but subsequent series demonstrated that systolic blood pressure [3] and dP-dT [4] were also significantly increased by acute LV-based pacing. Of note all the series which have compared LV pacing alone and biventricular (BIV), pacing concluded either that these two pacing modalities achieved either similar improvements [3] or that LV pacing alone was even more effective than BIV pacing [4, 5].

Further analysis of the results of these acute hemodynamic evaluations concluded that sinus rhythm was not mandatory and that improvement was

Department of Cardiology, Brest University Hospital, Brest, France

also achieved in patients with atrial fibrillation (AF) [7]. The same observation was made when patients were divided into two groups according to their underlying heart disease: there was no difference between groups of patients with ischemic versus dilated cardiomyopathies [8]. These studies brought another finding concerning patient selection: those with the longest QRS duration were those with the most significant improvement, indicating that a wide LBBB was probably one of the conditions to fulfill prior to permanent pacing [4]. However, another important finding drawn from these studies was somewhat underestimated: that not all the patients during these acute evaluations were improved. Although the patient without improvement represent a minority, their percentage was estimated at around 30% in a trial by the present anthors. A subsequent study of permanent LV-based pacing also reported patients who did improve (they represented approximately 30% in the recently reported MIRACLE trial [2]). So besides its "historical" role to demonstrating that LV-based pacing effective, acute hemodynamic evaluation might play a role in identifying patients in whom long-term pacing will be ineffective. Unfortunately, we have very few data on this subject. The reasons for this are multiple and may be summarized as follows: (1) as we are unable to distinguish responders to non responders, all patients have to be implanted; (2) lack of improvement in some patients is due to an inappropriate pacing site; (3) acute hemodynamic testing is invasive, so other techniques such as echocardiography should be tested.

Finally, we know that all the patients who show improvement during acute hemodynamic studies are not necessarily improved during permanent pacing with the present technical procedures (personal observations). We tried to evaluate which parameters could be of value in identifying long-term responders and found that increase in systolic blood pressure during LV-based pacing was the most useful parameter [9], but this result was based on a limited number of patients and of course the criteria by which a patient was defined as a responder on nonresponder to long-term pacing could be debated. The only way to assess the ability of acute hemodynamic testing to distinguish long-term responders from nonresponders would be systematically to perform an acute hemodynamic evaluation, implant the patients regardless of the result and then follow them for several months. Such a study has not been performed and to our knowledge has not yet been designed.

Angiographic Evaluation

Although there are some alternatives, the transvenous route is the most generally used to pace the left ventricle epicardially. To achieve this, the coronary sinus (CS) has to be cannulated and the lead placed, generally through a long guiding sheath, in a tributary of the CS [10]. However, the anatomy of the tributaries of the CS varies greatly from one patient to another [11], and in some instances (around 7%) there is no tributary except the great and the mid cardiac veins, which are constant. Although no hard data exist, it seems that the optimum position for pacing the LV is in its posterolateral part. The presence of a lateral vein is therefore mandatory, and only angiography of the CS including its tributaries can give a precise idea of its anatomy.

There are two possibilities for obtaining the venogram: to perform coronary angiography and wait for the venous phase, or to inject dye retrogradely in a CS occluded for some seconds. The latter option yields more suitable images for the purpose. Whether direct CS angiography should be performed a few days or hours before the implantation of the permanent lead or in the same session remains a subject of debate. Table 1 summarizes the advantages of both techniques.

Table 1. Respective advantages of carrying out angiographic evaluation before or at the time of implantation of a permanent pacemaker lead

Before permanent pacing	At the time of permanent pacing
Allows acute hemodynamic evaluation of "different" pacing sites	Does not require two procedures, so saves time and money
Gives an idea of the difficulties to be encountered in cannulating the CS	
Gives an idea of the difficulties of placing the lead in a tributary of the CS	
Gives time to discuss the most appropriate lead for the patient	

Conclusions

There are no data on the basis of which to recommend systematically a hemo-dynamic-angiographic evaluation prior to implantation of a permanent LV-based pacing system, but there are at least some arguments that it may be useful at least in some cases. Investigations and further experience over the next few months and years will give a more precise estimate of its exact utility, if any.

References

1. Cazeau S, Leclercq C, Lavergne T et al (2001) Effects of multisite biventricular pacing in patients with heart failure and intraventricular conduction delay. N Engl J Med 344:873-880
2. Abraham W for the MIRACLE Study Group. ACC Meeting, March 2001
3. Blanc JJ, Etienne Y, Gilard M et al (1997) Evaluation of different ventricular pacing sites in patients with severe heart failure: results of an acute hemodynamic study.

Circulation 96:3273-3277

4. Kass DA, Chen CH, Curry C et al (1999) Improved left ventricular mechanics from VDD pacing in patients with dilated cardiomyopathy and ventricular conduction delay. Circulation 99:1567-1573

5. Auricchio A, Stellbrink C, Block M et al (1999) Effect of pacing chamber and atrio-ventricular delay on acute systolic function of paced patients with congestive heart failure. Circulation 99:2993-3001

6. Cazeau S, Ritter P, Lazarus A et al (1996) Multisite pacing for end-stage heart failure. Early experience. Pacing Clin Electrophysiol 19:1748-1757

7. Etienne Y, Mansourati J, Gilard M et al (1999) Evaluation of left ventricular-based pacing in patients with congestive heart failure and atrial fibrillation. Am J Cardiol 83:1138-1140

8. Mansourati J, Etienne Y, Gilard M et al (2000) Left ventricular-based pacing in patients with chronic heart failure: comparison of acute hemodynamic benefits according to underlying heart disease. Eur J Heart Failure 2:195-199

9. Touiza A, Etienne Y, Gilard M et al (2000) Does acute hemodynamic evaluation predict long-term benefit of left ventricular-based pacing in patients with severe heart failure? Circulation 102:II 693 (abstr)

10. Blanc JJ, Benditt DG, Gilard M et al (1998) A method for permanent transvenous left ventricular pacing. Pacing Clin Electrophysiol 21:2015

11. Gilard M, Mansourati J, Etienne Y et al (1998) Angiographic anatomy of the coronary sinus and its tributaries. Pacing Clin Electrophysiol 21:2280-2284

Cardiac Resynchronization Therapy: Is There Any Correlation Between Pacing Site and Hemodynamic Improvement?

C.M.C. van Campen and H.S. Vos

Introduction

With the start of the pacing era, the right ventricular apex was used as a pacing site due to the stable position and ease of implantation [1]. With the importance of hemodynamics in the 1980s AV sequential pacing was introduced [2]. With the introduction of active fixation leads, other stimulation sites, such as the right ventricular outflow tract, were studied for hemodynamic results because of the impaired hemodynamic function of stimulating the right ventricular apex [3-5].

After showing a hemodynamic improvement in end-stage dilated cardiomyopathy by AV sequential pacing, the era of pacing for heart failure was opened [6]. This way of treating heart failure patients is pursued because, despite recent developments in pharmacological intervention with ACE inhibitors, β-blockers and spironolactone in heart failure patients, overall prognosis nevertheless remains poor. The Framingham study showed a 5 year survival from the time of diagnosis of less than 40%. Several studies showed that in patients with a severe intraventricular conduction delay, mortality was even higher than in patients without [7-10]. Hochleitner [6, 11] suggested for the first time that electrical stimulation might improve cardiac function, as he showed a significant improvement in left ventricular ejection fraction and systolic blood pressure. He also showed in his group of end-stage dilated cardiomyopathy a decrease in left atrial size and in LV end-diastolic and end-systolic volumes by pacing. After the initial positive results of Bakker et al. [12] in the last 5-6 years, more studies on biventricular pacing are ongoing.

In this article we give a short review of a possible improvement in hemodynamics in pacing in general and of multisite pacing in heart failure with respect to hemodynamics.

Department of Cardiology, VU Medical Center, Amsterdam, The Netherlands

Right Ventricular Outflow Tract Pacing

Since the 1960s several studies have been carried out with right ventricular outflow tract pacing [13-28]. Despite multiple positive results with respect to
hemodynamics, this type of treatment still is not used regularly. De Cock et al.
showed a significant increase in cardiac index when pacing occurred from the
right ventricular outflow tract compared to the apex (see Table 1) [29]. An
increase in cardiac index of 20% was seen at 85 beats/min (bpm), 19% increase
at 100 bpm and 14% increase at 120 bpm. Giudici et al. showed a similar
increase in cardiac index in 89 patients (see Table 2) [17]. Table 3 summarizes
all prospective studies dealing with left ventricular function when studying
right ventricular outflow tract pacing compared to right ventricular apex pacing. When pooling the data from these studies, a modest but definite effect in
favor of right ventricular outflow tract pacing, as compared to apex pacing, is
demonstrated (95% CI, 0.13-0.49). The divergence in study results is probably at
least partly the result of differences in patient selection. Right ventricular out-

Table 1. Hemodynamic outcome when comparing right ventricular outflow tract pacing
and right ventricular apical pacing in a patient population with an indication for
pacing [29]

	RVOT	RVAP	p value
85 bpm			
MAP	97 ± 13	99 ± 12	< 0.002
CI	2.42 ± 1.2	2.04 ± 1.0	< 0.002
100 bpm			
MAP	102 ± 10	100 ± 11	< 0.01
CI	2.78 ± 1.4	2.35 ± 1.1	< 0.01
120 bpm			
MAP	99 ± 13	99 ± 12	< 0.01
CI	3.00 ± 1.5	2.61 ± 0.9	< 0.01

CI, cardiac index; *bpm*, beats/min; *MAP*, mean arterial pressure; *RVOT*, right ventricular outflow tract pacing; *RVAP*, right ventricular apex pacing

Table 2. Hemodynamic outcome in comparing outflow tract and apical pacing in a larger
group with the need for pacing therapy [17]

	RVOT	RVAP	p value
Cardiac output	7.8 ±2.9	6.6 ± 2.4	< 0.001
Cardiac index	4.1 ±1.5	3.5 ± 1.3	< 0.001

Delta cardiac index, 21%

Table 3. Summary of studies performed with outflow tract and apical pacing

Reference	Publication	No. patients	Parameter	Outcome
[13]	Circulation 1966	6	CO[T]	±
[14]	Am J Cardiol 1969	52	CO[T]	±
[15]	Circulation 1984	18	CO[T]	-
[16]	Pacing Clin Electrophysiol 1994	15	CO[T]	+
[17]	Am J Cardiol 1997	98	CO[T]	+
[18]	Am J Cardiol 1997	13	CO[T]	±
[19]	Pacing Clin Electrophysiol 1997	22	LVEDP	+
[20]	Circulation 1997	14	PCWP	±
[21]	Pacing Clin Electrophysiol 1997	11	CO[E]	±
[29]	Pacing Clin Electrophysiol 1998	17	CO[E]	+
[24]	J Cardiac Electr 1998	11	FAC[E]	+
[22]	Pacing Clin Electrophysiol 1998	14	CO[T]	±
[25]	Pacing Clin Electrophysiol 1999	12	EF[N]	+
[23]	Pacing Clin Electrophysiol 1999	37	CO[T]	±
[26]	J Am Coll Cardiol 1999	14	EF[N]	+
[27]	J Am Coll Cardiol 1999	16	CO[T]	±
[28]	Chest 2000	20	CO[E]	+
[41]	Progr Biomed Res 2001	19	CO[E]	+

CO, cardiac output; *T*, thermodilution; *PCWP*, pulmonary capillary wedge pressure; *E*, echo-Doppler study; *FAC*, fractional area change; *N*, nuclear study; *EF*, ejection fraction.
Outcome: +, positive effect; -, negative effect; ±, no effect for outflow tract pacing as compared with apex pacing

flow tract pacing showed a modest but significant improvement in hemodynamics and should therefore be considered as a valid alternative to apex pacing, especially in patients with an impaired left ventricular function, but maybe in all patients.

Biventricular Pacing

Heart failure is a remarkably common but complex syndrome and worldwide a large and growing population suffers from this disease. Prognosis is still poor, particularly in the presence of a wide QRS complex on the ECG [7-10]. With the progression of heart failure, QRS duration increases because of inter- and intraventricular conduction delays. This leads to ventricular dyssynchrony, leading to paradoxical septal wall motion, nonuniform wall stress, increase in mitral regurgitation and reduced diastolic filling times [30, 31]. These findings have huge hemodynamic consequences in the heart failure patient, but despite significant progress in pharmacological treatment in this patient group, little could be done to improve these abnormalities. In the early 1990s several studies were done in this patient population on conventional right-sided DDD pacing, with equivocal results (see Table 4) [6, 11, 32-35]. Bakker et al., in a pilot study, showed the possibility of improving this patient population with biventricular pacing [12]. In 12 patients with an ejection fraction of 15 ± 6 % and a QRS duration of 190 ± 20 ms, there was a significant improvement after 3 months follow-up in ejection fraction and peak oxygen consumption. Furthermore, there was a significant decrease in use of diuretics.

After this attempt, several registries and studies were performed which will be discussed below.

Table 4. Hemodynamic benefit of conventional AV sequential pacing in patients with heart failure

Reference	Publication/year	Acute/chronic	No. of patients	Outcome
[32]	Lancet 1992	Acute	12	+
[33]	Pacing Clin Electrophysiol 1994	Acute	12	-
[34]	J Am Coll Cardiol 1995	Acute	15	-
[6]	Am J Cardiol 1990	Chronic	16	+
[11]	Am J Cardiol 1992	Chronic	17	-
[35]	Pacing Clin Electrophysiol 1995	Chronic	10	-

French Feasibility Study by Daubert et al. [36]

This study describes the feasibility of epicardial pacing by the transvenous route with electrodes selectively inserted in the cardiac veins over the LV free wall in patients with NYHA (New York Heart Association) Class III or IV drug-refractory congestive heart failure. The LV ejection fraction had to be < 35% and the echocardiographic LVEDD > 60 mm, with a QRS duration of > 150 ms. Patients with atrial fibrillation were included. Included were 47 patients (42 male) with a mean age of 68 ± 9 years. Mean LVEF was 17 ± 4% and 41 patients were in NYHA Class IV. Twenty-five patients had an ischemic etiology. Mean QRS duration was 187 ± 27 ms. The implantation success rate was 75% (35/47) with failures due to no entrance in the coronary sinus, no entrance in the LV cardiac veins and unacceptable pacing thresholds. Of 35 successful implants, the lead was positioned in the anterior wall through the great cardiac vein in 8 patients, in the middle cardiac vein in 1 patient and in the lateral or posterolateral wall in 26 patients. As to pacing and sensing characteristics, no differences were seen between the different sites. About 6% early dislocation rate occurred. After a follow-up of about 10 months, 34/35 leads remained functional, with effective LV pacing. The transvenous approach is therefore feasible for pacing the left ventricle.

PATH-CHF Study [37, 38]

This study enrolled NYHA Class III or IV heart failure patients of any etiology, with optimal medical treatment, PR ≥ 150 ms, QRS ≥ 120 ms and without an indication for pacemaker implantation. In this study, 42 patients were included, with a mean age of 60 ± 7 years (50% male patients) with 71% having an idiopathic cardiomyopathy and 93% a left bundle branch block. The mean QRS duration was 175 ± 32 ms and the mean ejection fraction 23 ± 7. The study consisted of four phases: an evaluation phase before implant; an acute testing phase at the implantation procedure; a randomized crossover protocol with two different pacing modes (best chamber and biventricular) with a no pacing (washout) period in between; and a chronic pacing phase. Each patient was implanted with two Vigor pacemakers: one right-sided and the other one with a left ventricular epicardial lead. One pacemaker was in the DDD mode and the other in VVT mode [37]. Looking at the hemodynamics, pacing significantly increased LV + dP/dt, whereas biventricular and left ventricular pacing significantly increased aortic systolic pressure and pulse pressure [38]. In this study, patients with a broad QRS complex especially improved, whereas patients with a small QRS complex did not. In 27 patients chronic follow-up was present. A significant improvement was seen in peak oxygen consumption and 6 min walking test, with no improvement in the no-pacing period. There was also a significant decrease in hospitalizations for chronic heart failure after 1 year ($p < 0.001$). Biventricular pacing therefore shows a clinical improvement in heart failure patients.

INSYNC Multicenter Study [39]

This study enrolled Class III or IV heart failure patients of any etiology with optimal medical treatment, QRS duration > 150 ms, LV ejection fraction < 35% and LV end diastolic diameter > 60 mm. Of 81 patients, 68 were successfully implanted (84%; no catheterization of the coronary sinus [3], no introduction into a cardiac vein [5] or unacceptable high pacing threshold [3] or unstable lead position [2]). In 62% a lateral position was reached, in 32% the great cardiac vein and in 6% the middle cardiac vein. Patients were studied after 1, 3, 6 and 12 months. The mean age was 66 ± 10 years (52 male), 43 patients (63%) were in Class III and 28 (41%) had an ischemic etiology of heart failure. At baseline, LVEF was 21% ± 9%, mean QRS duration 177 ± 29 ms and mean distance of 6 min walk 177 ± 121 m. Eleven patients left the study during follow-up, of whom seven died (four suddenly and three because of progression in heart failure). Reintervention for the LV lead was needed in three patients. The LV ejection fraction showed a trend to improvement at 1 and 3 months. Six min walking distance improved significantly from 299 m to 360 m at 1 month and 418 m at 3 months ($p = 0.001$ and $p < 0.04$, respectively). NYHA Class decreased significantly from 3 to 2 during follow-up ($p < 0.001$). QRS duration decreased from 179 to 149 and 143 ms ($p < 0.001$). These improvements remained during the 6 and 12 month follow-up.

In conclusion, this study confirms the feasibility and reliability of biventricular pacing using a conventional venous access route to lead introduction.

MUSTIC Trial [40]

This study enrolled Class III or IV heart failure patients of any etiology with optimal medical treatment, an ejection fraction < 35%, LV end-diastolic diameter > 60 mm. All patients were in sinus rhythm with a QRS duration > 150 ms, without an indication for pacemaker implantation. The study design was a single-blind, randomized, controlled crossover study to assess the clinical efficacy and safety of atriobiventricular pacing. Sixty-seven patients (50 males) with a mean age of 63 ± 10 years were included. All were in Class III and 25 (37%) had heart failure due to ischemic heart disease. The mean LVEF was 23 ± 7%, mean LVEDD 73 ± 10 mm, mean QRS duration 176 ± 19 ms and mean 6 min walking distance 320 ± 97 m. In total, nine patients dropped out of the study for several reasons. The implantation success rate was 92% and a lateral position was reached in 80% of the patients with a mean threshold of 1.4 ± 1.1 V. Early dislodgement occurred in eight patients (12.5%). Ten patients did not complete the second crossover period (no consent, no LV pacing, worsening heart failure, death). After 3 months active or inactive pacing, the 6 min walking distance increased from 326 ± 134 m to 399 ± 100 m ($p < 0.001$) with pacing (increase of 23%), quality of life score decreased from 43 ± 23 to 30 ± 21 ($p < 0.001$) with pacing (decrease of 32%), and peak oxygen uptake increased from 15 ± 5 ml/kg/min to 116 ± 5 ml/kg/min ($p < 0.03$). In conclusion, therefore, ventricular resynchronization in this patient group significantly improved exercise tolerance and quality of life. Studies on long-term results and mortality still need to be performed.

Conclusions

As improvement in hemodynamics is getting more and more important in clinical management, not only in heart failure patients but also in conventional pacing, it may be that choosing the right ventricular outflow tract as a definite place for pacing might be the future for patients with a conventional need for pacing. With current developments, lead position is stable and the introduction and localization of the lead is easy. In heart failure patients, biventricular pacing can be of use. The problem still is that lead and generator technology is still in development and there is little knowledge about the long-term efficacy and clinical results or the effect on mortality. In addition there is a high proportion (about 15-20%) of non-responders to biventricular pacing. We have still to discover how to identify this group of patients and to resolve how to treat this subgroup.

References

1. Charles RG, Clarke LM, Drysdale M, Sequeira RF (1977) Endocardial pacing electrode design and rate of displacement. Br Heart J 39:515-516
2. Sutton R, Perrins J, Citron P (1980) Physiological cardiac pacing. Pacing Clin Electrophysiol 3:207-219
3. Heyndrickx GR, Vilaine JP, Knight DR, Vatner SF (1985) Effects of altered site of electrical activation on myocardial performance during inotropic stimulation. Circulation 71:1010-1016
4. Little WC, Reeves RC, Arciniegas J et al (1982) Mechanism of abnormal interventricular septal motion during delayed left ventricular activation. Circulation 65:1486-1491
5. Park RC, Little WC, O'Rourke RA (1985) Effect of alteration of left ventricular activation sequence on the left ventricular end-systolic pressure-volume relation in closed-chest dogs. Circ Res 57:706-717
6. Hochleitner M, Hortnagl H, Hortnagl H et al (1992) Long-term efficacy of physiologic dual-chamber pacing in the treatment of end-stage idiopathic dilated cardiomyopathy. Am J Cardiol 70:1320-1325
7. Schoeller R, Andresen D, Buttner P et al (1993) First- or second-degree atrioventricular block as a risk factor in idiopathic dilated cardiomyopathy. Am J Cardiol 71:720-726
8. Aaronson KD, Schwartz JS, Chen TM et al (1997) Development and prospective validation of a clinical index to predict survival in ambulatory patients referred for cardiac transplant evaluation. Circulation 95:2660-2667
9. Wilensky RL, Yudelman P, Cohen AI et al (1988) Serial electrocardiographic changes in idiopathic dilated cardiomyopathy confirmed at necropsy. Am J Cardiol 62:276-283
10. Xiao HB, Roy C, Fujimoto S, Gibson DG (1996) Natural history of abnormal conduction and its relation to prognosis in patients with dilated cardiomyopathy. Int J Cardiol 53:163-170
11. Hochleitner M, Hortnagl H, Ng CK et al (1990) Usefulness of physiologic dual-chamber pacing in drug-resistant idiopathic dilated cardiomyopathy. Am J Cardiol 66:198-202
12. Bakker P, Chin A, Sen K et al (1995) Biventricular pacing improves functional capacity in patients with end-stage congestive heart failure. Pacing Clin Electrophysiol 18(part II):825
13. Benchimol A, Liggett MS (1966) Cardiac hemodynamics during stimulation of the right atrium, right ventricle, and left ventricle in normal and abnormal hearts. Circulation 33:933-944
14. Barold SS, Linhart JW, Hildner FJ, Samet P (1969) Hemodynamic comparison of endocardial pacing of outflow and inflow tracts of the right ventricle. Am J Cardiol 23:697-701
15. Raichlen JS, Campbell FW, Edie RN et al (1984) The effect of the site of placement of temporary epicardial pacemakers on ventricular function in patients undergoing cardiac surgery. Circulation 70(3, part 2):I118-I123
16. Cowell R, Morris-Thurgood J, Ilsley C, Paul V (1994) Septal short atrioventricular delay pacing: additional hemodynamic improvements in heart failure. Pacing Clin Electrophysiol 17(part 2):1980-1983
17. Giudici MC, Thornburg GA, Buck DL et al (1997) Comparison of right ventricular outflow tract and apical lead permanent pacing on cardiac output. Am J Cardiol 79:209-212
18. Gold MR, Shorofsky SR, Metcalf MD et al (1997) The acute hemodynamic effects of right ventricular septal pacing in patients with congestive heart failure secondary to ischemic or idiopathic dilated cardiomyopathy. Am J Cardiol 79:679-681

19. Karpawich PP, Mital S (1997) Comparative left ventricular function following atrial, septal, and apical single chamber heart pacing in the young. Pacing Clin Electrophysiol 20(part 1):1983-1988
20. Blanc JJ, Etienne Y, Gilard M et al (1997) Evaluation of different ventricular pacing sites in patients with severe heart failure: results of an acute hemodynamic study. Circulation 96:3273-3277
21. Buckingham TA, Candinas R, Schlapfer J et al (1997) Acute hemodynamic effects of atrioventricular pacing at differing sites in the right ventricle individually and simultaneously. Pacing Clin Electrophysiol 20(part 1):909-915
22. Buckingham TA, Candinas R, Attenhofer C et al (1998) Systolic and diastolic function with alternate and combined site pacing in the right ventricle. Pacing Clin Electrophysiol 21:1077-1084
23. Buckingham TA, Candinas R, Duru F et al (1999) Acute hemodynamic effects of alternate and combined site pacing in patients after cardiac surgery. Pacing Clin Electrophysiol 22(part 1):887-893
24. Saxon LA, Kerwin WF, Cahalan MK et al (1998) Acute effects of intraoperative multi-site ventricular pacing on left ventricular function and activation/contraction sequence in patients with depressed ventricular function. J Cardiovasc Electrophysiol 9:13-21
25. Mera F, DeLurgio DB, Patterson RE et al (1999) A comparison of ventricular function during high right ventricular septal and apical pacing after his-bundle ablation for refractory atrial fibrillation. Pacing Clin Electrophysiol 22:1234-1239
26. Schwaab B, Frohlig G, Alexander C et al (1999) Influence of right ventricular stimulation site on left ventricular function in atrial synchronous ventricular pacing. J Am Coll Cardiol 33:317-323
27. Victor F, Leclercq C, Mabo P et al (1999) Optimal right ventricular pacing site in chronically implanted patients: a prospective randomized crossover comparison of apical and outflow tract pacing. J Am Coll Cardiol 33:311-316
28. Kolettis TM, Kyriakides ZS, Tsiapras D et al (2000) Improved left ventricular relaxation during short-term right ventricular outflow tract compared to apical pacing. Chest 117:60-64
29. de Cock CC, Meyer A, Kamp O, Visser CA (1998) Hemodynamic benefits of right ventricular outflow tract pacing: comparison with right ventricular apex pacing. Pacing Clin Electrophysiol 21:536-541
30. Grines CL, Bashore TM, Boudoulas H et al (1989) Functional abnormalities in isolated left bundle branch block. The effect of interventricular asynchrony. Circulation 79:845-853
31. Xiao HB, Brecker SJ, Gibson DG (1992) Effects of abnormal activation on the time course of the left ventricular pressure pulse in dilated cardiomyopathy. Br Heart J 68:403-407
32. Brecker SJ, Xiao HB, Sparrow J, Gibson DG (1992) Effects of dual-chamber pacing with short atrioventricular delay in dilated cardiomyopathy. Lancet 340:1308-1312
33. Innes D, Leitch JW, Fletcher PJ (1994) VDD pacing at short atrioventricular intervals does not improve cardiac output in patients with dilated heart failure. Pacing Clin Electrophysiol 17(part 1):959-965
34. Nishimura RA, Hayes DL, Holmes DR Jr, Tajik AJ (1995) Mechanism of hemodynamic improvement by dual-chamber pacing for severe left ventricular dysfunction: an acute Doppler and catheterization hemodynamic study. J Am Coll Cardiol 25:281-288
35. Linde C, Ryden L (1995) Pacing in dilated cardiomyopathy. Pacing Clin Electrophysiol 18:1341-1345

36. Daubert JC, Ritter P, Le Breton H et al (1998) Permanent left ventricular pacing with transvenous leads inserted into the coronary veins. Pacing Clin Electrophysiol 21(part 2):239-245

37. Auricchio A, Stellbrink C, Sack S et al (1999) The Pacing Therapies for Congestive Heart Failure (PATH-CHF) study: rationale, design, and endpoints of a prospective randomized multicenter study. Am J Cardiol 83:130D-135D

38. Auricchio A, Stellbrink C, Block M et al (1999) Effect of pacing chamber and atrio-ventricular delay on acute systolic function of paced patients with congestive heart failure. The Pacing Therapies for Congestive Heart Failure Study Group. The Guidant Congestive Heart Failure Research Group. Circulation 99:2993-3001

39. Gras D, Mabo P, Tang T et al (1998) Multisite pacing as a supplemental treatment of congestive heart failure: preliminary results of the Medtronic Inc InSync Study. Pacing Clin Electrophysiol 21(part 2):2249-2255

40. Cazeau S, Leclercq C, Lavergne T et al (2001) Effects of multisite biventricular pacing in patients with heart failure and intraventricular conduction delay. N Engl J Med 344:873-880

41. van Campen CMC, Vos DS, de Cock CC, Visser CA (2001) Mechanisms behind hemodynamic benefits of right ventricular outflow tract pacing compared to right ventricular apex pacing. Progr Biomed Res 6:137-141

Does Atrial Resynchronization Confer Further Benefit on Patients Undergoing Ventricular Resynchronization Therapy?

F. Di Pede, G. Gasparini, G. Zuin, A. Rossillo and A. Raviele

Congestive heart failure is considered to be one of the most important public health problems in cardiovascular medicine. In the United States, more than 3 million people are afflicted by the disease, with nearly 400 000 new cases diagnosed annually. Congestive heart failure is associated with increasing morbidity and high mortality and has overall 5-year survival rates of 25% and 38% for men and women respectively, with a median survival time of 1.7 years for men and 3.2 years for women. The therapeutic approach has evolved over the years as understanding of the disease and its associated compensatory mechanisms increased, and recently pacing therapy has been introduced into clinical practice. Patients with heart failure frequently have altered electrical activation which may lead to asynchronous contraction of the heart and to further impairment of their hemodynamic status. These data suggested the hypothesis that resynchronization of the electrical activity of the heart may improve the mechanics of the heart and, consequently, the performance of the whole cardiovascular system.

Ventricular Resynchronization Therapy

The first attempt to resynchronize the electrical activity of the heart was by shortening the atrioventricular interval during DDD pacing from the right ventricular apex to optimize left ventricular filling [1]. Since then, many authors have addressed this clinically relevant issue, with conflicting results [2, 3]. However a significant improvement was demonstrated with pacing at short atrioventricular delays in patients with wide QRS complexes and significant mitral regurgitation, and it was suggested that clinical improvement was due to a reduction in mitral and "presystolic" regurgitation and a concomitant increase in filling time [2]. Recently, ventricular resynchronization therapy performed with biventricular pacing has been recognized as one of the most promising techniques in the treatment of congestive heart failure patients [4-6]. Published papers demonstrate significant hemodynamic and clinical improve-

Cardiovascular Department, Division of Cardiology, Umberto I Hospital, Mestre-Venice, Italy

ment in dilated cardiomyopathy patients treated with VDD biventricular pacing and shortened atrioventricular delays [6]. It was hypothesized that biventricular pacing synchronizing contraction of the right and left ventricles may be a more effective pacing modality than right ventricular pacing alone, which may induce hemodynamically detrimental asynchrony between chambers. Permanent pacing of the left ventricle via the transvenous route is possible in most patients, with a success rate of over 80% when using electrodes specifically designed for pacing through the coronary sinus [7]. Some authors have emphasized the importance of optimization of the stimulation site during ventricular resynchronization therapy and concluded that a posterior/lateral/posterior-lateral left ventricle lead position in combination with a right ventricle apex lead position provided more consistent clinical improvements [8].

Optimization of Atrioventricular Delay

Nowadays the need for optimization of the atrioventricular delay used during ventricular resynchronization therapy on the basis of acute studies or echo measurements is widely recognized. Auricchio et al. [6] have clearly demonstrated that the greatest hemodynamic improvement occurs only within certain atrioventricular intervals. Ritter et al. [9] proposed a simple method based on Doppler echocardiography of transmitral flow to calculate the optimal atrioventricular delay in order to provide the longest left ventricular filling time. In clinical practice the optimal atrioventricular delay is determined on the basis of left ventricular performance; the optimization of right ventricular filling is not adequately addressed in the setting of ventricular resynchronization therapy. The importance of right ventricular function on exercise capacity and survival in heart failure patients arises from results of recently published studies. It is well known that right ventricular function depends on pulmonary artery pressure and, as a general rule, increased pulmonary artery pressure is coupled with reduced right ventricular systolic function and poor prognosis. Since pulmonary artery pressure depends on left ventricular function, right ventricular function seems mainly related to left ventricular function, which is a well known prognostic factor. However, Di Salvo et al. [10] observed that right ventricular ejection fraction predicts exercise capacity and is the only independent factor related to survival in a homogeneous population of advanced heart failure patients. De Groote et al. [11] expanded this observation to patients with moderate heart failure. This issue has been recently addressed by Ghio et al. [12], who demonstrated that, when pulmonary artery pressure is high at rest despite optimized medical therapy, the prognosis is strongly related to right ventricular function, while in patients with normal pulmonary artery pressure, right ventricular function does not add more information. These data emphasize the necessity of evaluating right heart hemodynamic variables to define the hemodynamic status of patients with heart failure and may be the background for studies aiming to improve right heart hemodynamics by optimizing right atrioventricular mechanical delay.

Interatrial Delay

Patients with congestive heart failure frequently have conduction delays at the atrial level in addition to the atrioventricular and intraventricular level. This may be the substrate for arrhythmias and may have hemodynamic consequences. Actually, in patients with prolonged interatrial and interventricular conduction time treated with DDD pacing, left and right atrioventricular mechanical delays may be substantially different, as shown by Porciani et al. [13]. In particular, in patients treated with biventricular stimulation, pacing at the right atrial appendage produced shorter left than right mechanical atrioventricular delay (left 142 ms, right 209 ms). Therefore, optimizing right mechanical atrioventricular delay may cause suboptimal left mechanical atrioventricular delay, and vice versa. Other authors [14] have observed that atrial pacing from conventional atrial sites may cause significant prolongation of the interatrial conduction time, potentially leading to further changes in left and right atrioventricular delays in comparison with the atrioventricular delays obtained during VDD pacing. Therefore, pacing at the right atrial appendage does not allow atrioventricular delay optimization of both the right and the left side of the heart in patients with spontaneous or induced interatrial conduction delay.

Atrial Septal Pacing

Multisite atrial pacing and septal atrial pacing have been performed in the attempt to synchronize atrial activation and contraction. Kindermann et al. [15] showed that single site right atrial septal pacing effectively shortens P wave duration. In unselected patients right atrial septal pacing reverses the physiological right-to-left atrial contraction sequence to a left-to-right sequence. Therefore, atrial septal pacing shortens the interatrial delay by anticipating left atrial activation, but does not synchronize right and left atrial contraction. On the basis of echo measurements, Porciani et al. [13] found that combined interatrial septum pacing and biventricular pacing produces similar left and right mechanical atrioventricular delays by reducing both interatrial and interventricular delays. In patients paced at the interatrial septum, left mechanical atrioventricular delay was 211 ms and right mechanical atrioventricular delay was 190 msec. The similarity of these atrioventricular delays was due to the greater delay in left mechanical atrioventricular delay in patients paced at the interatrial septum (211 ms) compared with that in patients paced at the right atrial appendage (142 ms). These data indicate that biventricular pacing with biatrial resynchronization can lead to similar right and left atrioventricular mechanical delays and probably makes feasible the optimization of atrioventricular delays on the right and left sides of the heart.

A further beneficial effect of atrial resynchronization can be expected from the prevention of recurrences of atrial fibrillation as suggested by recent papers

[16-18]. Permanent atrial pacing has been demonstrated to be effective in the prevention of atrial fibrillation or flutter in patients with vagal atrial fibrillation or flutter [19]. However, single site atrial pacing offers no clear benefit in the majority of atrial fibrillation patients. Recently, multisite atrial pacing or pacing at the interventricular septum has been proposed as an alternative therapy to prevent recurrences of atrial fibrillation. The rationale for this stimulation derives from the observation that intra-atrial and interatrial conduction disturbances are essential to the mechanisms that underlie atrial fibrillation, and therefore pacing techniques that reduce intra-atrial and interatrial conduction delays may be beneficial in this clinical setting. Pacing at the interatrial septum may have technical problems due to the limited operators experience. However Bens et al. [20] and Padeletti et al. [21], concluded that interatrial septum pacing is easy to perform, reliable, safe, and carried low costs. Long-term effectiveness and sensing and pacing thresholds are the same as for the other atrial sites. Thus, atrial resynchronization therapy seems to be advantageous in patients with interatrial conduction block from an electrophysiologic point of view, but its hemodynamic consequences have still to be elucidated. The translation of the electrophysiologic concept of atrial resynchronization to the hemodynamic needs some caution because of the nonphysiologic character of activation of atria by septal or multisite stimulation. In patients with sinus rhythm, impulses travel from the sinus node to the atrioventricular node, and consequently contraction follows a craniocaudal direction, while stimulation of another site of the atrium, such as the coronary sinus or low interatrial septum, may generate a different sequence of contraction leading to unpredictable hemodynamic effects. To date no study has investigated the hemodynamic effects of atrial resynchronization therapy on cardiac performance.

Future Perspectives

We have designed a study to investigate the acute hemodynamic effect on cardiac performance of atrial resynchronization therapy (performed by stimulation on the low interatrial septum) combined with biventricular stimulation in patients who need ventricular resynchronization therapy for congestive heart failure. The hypothesis underlying this study is that atrial stimulation at the interatrial septum provides a greater acute hemodynamic improvement than does pacing at the classical site (right atrial appendage), particularly in patients with interatrial conduction disturbances. The main objective of the study is to compare the acute effect on cardiac function of two different atrial pacing sites, right atrial appendage and low interatrial septum, during ventricular resynchronization therapy using DDD pacing. Therefore, the results of this study will answer the question whether atrial resynchronization may confer further acute hemodynamic benefits on patients undergoing ventricular resynchronization therapy. The results of this study, if positive, will form the background for long-term studies with clinical end-points, and will help to establish the requirements of optimal chronic DDD pacing in this patient population, especially those with sinus node dysfunction or drug-induced bradycardia who need chronic atrial pacing.

References

1.   Hochlertner M, Hortmagl H, Choi-keung NG et al (1999) Usefulness of physiologic dual-chamber pacing in drug-resistant idiopathic dilated cardiomyopathy. Am J Cardiol 66:198-202
2.   Brecker SJD, Xiao HB, Sparrow J, Gibson DG (1992) Effects of dual-chamber pacing with short atrioventricular delay in dilated cardiomyopathy. Lancet 340:1308
3.   Saxon LA, Stevenson WG, Middlekauff HR et al (1993) Increased risk of progressive hemodynamic deterioration in advanced heart failure patients requiring permanent pacemakers. Am Heart J 125:1306-1310
4.   Blanc JJ, Etienne Y, Gilard M et al (1997) Evaluation of different ventricular pacing sites in patients with severe heart failure. Circulation 93:3273-3277
5.   Leclercq C, Cazeau S, Le Breton H et al (1998) Acute hemodynamic effects of biventricular DDD pacing in patients with end stage heart failure. J Am Coll Cardiol 32:1825-1831
6.   Auricchio A, Stellbrink C, Block M et al (1999) Effect of pacing chamber and atrioventricular delay on acute systolic function of paced patients with congestive heart failure. Circulation 99:2993-3001
7.   Ritter PH, Gras D, Daubert C (2000) Implant success rate of the transvenous left ventricular lead in the MUSTIC trial. Pacing Clin Electrophysiol 23:580 (abstr)
8.   Auricchio A, Butter C, Stellbrink C et al (2000) Effect of left ventricular stimulation site on the systolic function of heart failure patients during ventricular resynchronization therapy. Pacing Clin Electrophysiol 23:589 (abstr)
9.   Ritter P, Dib JC, Lelievre T et al (1994) Quick determination of the optimal AV delay at rest in patients paced in DDD mode for complete AV block. European Journal Cardiac Pacing Electrophysiology 4:A163
10. Di Salvo TG, Mthier M, Semigran MJ, Dec GW (1995) Preserved right ventricular ejection fraction predicts exercise capacity and survival in advanced heart failure. J Am Coll Cardiol 25:1143-1153
11. De Groote P, Millaire A, Foucher-Hossein C et al (1998) Right ventricular ejection fraction is an indipendent predictor of survival in patients with moderate heart failure. J Am Coll Cardiol 32:948-954
12. Ghio S, Gavazzi A, Campana C et al (2001) Independent and additive prognostic value of right ventricular systolic function and pulmonary artery pressure in patients with chronic heart failure. J Am Coll Cardiol 37:183-188
13. Porciani MC, Colella A, Costoli A et al (2000) Left and right atrio-ventricular interval synchronization: a rising problem in new pacing techniques. Pacing Clin Electrophysiol 23:610
14. Parravicini U, Mezzani A, Bielli M (2000) DDD pacing and interatrial conduction block: importance of optimal AV interval setting. Pacing Clin Electrophysiol 23:1448-1450
15. Kindermann M, Schwaab B, Berg M, Fröhling G (2000) The influence of right atrial septal pacing on the interatrial contraction sequence. Pacing Clin Electrophysiol 23:1752-1753

16. Misier AR, Beukema WP, Luttikuis HAO, Willems R (2000) Multisite atrial pacing: an option for atrial fibrillation prevention? Preliminary results of the Dutch dual-site right atrial pacing for prevention of atrial fibrillation study. Am J Cardiol 86[Suppl]:20K-24K

17. D'Allones GR, Pavin D, Leclerque C et at (2000) Long-term effects of biatrial synchronous pacing to prevent drug-refractory atrial tachyarrhythmia: a nine-year experience. J Cardiovasc Electrophysiol 11:1081-1091

18. Prakash A, Saksena S, Hill M et al (1997) Acute effects of dual-site right atrial pacing in patients with spontaneous and inducible atrial flutter and fibrillation. J Am Coll Cardiol 29:1007-1014

19. Coumel PH, Attuel P, Leclerq JF, Friocourt P (1982) Arhytmie auricolaire d'origine vagale ou catécholagique: effets comparés du traitement béta-bloquant et phénomène d'échappement. Arch Mal Coeur 75:373-388

20. Bens JL, Pladys A, Gras E (2000) Interatrial septum stimulation and paroxysmal fibrillation prevention. Europace 1[Suppl D]:D127

21. Padeletti L, Porciani C, Colella A et al (2000) Comparison of interatrial septum pacing with right atrial appendage pacing for prevention on paroxysmal atrial fibrillation. Europace 1[Suppl D]:D14

Ventricular Resynchronization Therapy in Heart Failure Patients with Chronic Atrial Fibrillation: Is It Worthwhile ?

J. C. DAUBERT, C. LECLERCQ, C. ALONSO AND P. MABO

Ventricular resynchronization therapy (VRT) through biventricular pacing has recently been validated as a new treatment [1] for refractory heart failure in patients with chronic left ventricular systolic dysfunction and signs of discoordinated ventricular activation and contraction. Following positive results from several acute haemodynamic studies with temporary pacing [2-8] and those of two pilot studies with permanent pacing [10-12], controlled studies [1, 13] showed that atriobiventricular pacing with individually optimized AV synchrony significantly improved symptoms, exercise tolerance and quality of life in patients with severe heart failure (NYHA Classes III-IV) and stable sinus rhythm, without classical indication for permanent cardiac pacing. In addition, the number of hospitalizations for decompensated heart failure decreased significantly.

In patients in sinus rhythm, atriobiventricular pacing corrects atrioventricular asynchrony of the left heart - a very frequent occurrence, even if there is no PR interval prolongation on surface ECG [14] - as well as interventricular and left intraventricular dyssynchrony. The respective contribution of each of those various mechanisms of action probably varies from one patient to another, but many clinical and experimental facts [7-9] are consistent with the prevalence of ventricular resynchronization.

Is it realistic, therefore, to expect significant clinical benefit from biventricular pacing in patients with chronic atrial fibrillation (AF) who, by definition, have lost all atrial contribution to ventricular filling. The answer to that question is of utmost interest, both clinically and conceptually, because that experimental model is the only one that objectively assesses the effects of ventricular resynchronization *per se*. This paper sets out to synthesize current knowledge in that specific indication.

Département de Cardiologie et Maladies Vasculaires, Centre Cardio-Pneumologique, Hôpital Pontchaillou, Rennes, France

Atrial Fibrillation and Chronic Heart Failure

In all heart failure patients, the prevalence of permanent AF is relatively high at approximately 20% [15, 16], but may even reach 40% of patients with advanced heart failure [17, 18]. On the other hand, recent data from the Framingham study have suggested that chronic heart failure was associated with a 4.5-5.9-fold higher incidence of AF in women and men, respectively [19].

The prognostic value of AF in chronic heart failure patients remains controversial. In their first report [18] Middlekauf et al. reported higher mortality in heart failure patients with AF than in patients with stable sinus rhythm, although it was not confirmed in a recent study [20]. In contrast, Crijns et al. [21] report that AF, either present at heart failure diagnosis or occurring later in the course of illness is not associated with an adverse outcome during long-term follow-up *per se*. Likewise, Mahoney et al. [22] did not find any significant difference in event occurrence during survival between AF and non-AF heart failure patients.

None of those studies mentioned the existence or absence of intraventricular conduction delay associated with AF. The prognosis is probably very bleak in that subpopulation, as suggested by the data from the Italian Network on Heart Failure (Baldasseroni L, Maggioni A, et al., unpublished data, 2000), who found that chronic AF was associated with a significantly higher 1 year mortality rate in heart failure patients with intraventricular conduction delay than in those in sinus rhythm (26.5% vs 14.5%; $p < 0.001$). That can be related to Farwell et al.'s [23] recent findings that 40% of potential candidates for biventricular pacing were in chronic AF.

The interrelations that exist between AF and heart failure are complex. There are three main contributing factors: (1) the loss of atrial contribution to ventricular filling reduces the cardiac output in direct proportion to the level of left ventricular systolic dysfunction; (2) heart rate irregularity may also contribute to impaired cardiac function; and (3) frequent fast ventricular rate [24] may induce or enhance left ventricular systolic dysfunction in the context of tachycardia-induced cardiomyopathy [24-26]. It has now been accepted that rate control by AV node ablation and permanent VVIR pacing may improve, albeit partially, left ventricular systolic dysfunction and its clinical consequences in heart failure patients with persistent AF and fast ventricular rate [25-27]. Improvement usually takes less than 3 months [25].

Permanent and Full Ventricular Capture: a Prerequisite to the Objective Assessment of the Clinical Impact of Pacing in AF Patients

Because of heart rate irregularity and a usually fast ventricular rate, especially during exercise [15], the haemodynamic consequences of ventricular pacing, regardless of the pacing mode, can only be assessed in AF patients if heart rate is perfectly controlled, ensuring permanent pacing with full ventricular capture. Except for pre-existing or drug-induced atrioventricular block, that can only be achieved through total interruption of conduction by radiofrequency AV junction ablation. As previously mentioned, rate control alone can improve cardiac performance independently of the mode of ventricular pacing chosen. A lag phase of at least 3 months following ablation [25] is thus necessary to rule out possible tachycardia-induced tachycardiomyopathy and to allow for objective assessment of the benefits directly linked to the ventricular pacing mode being tested.

Non-controlled Studies on Permanent Biventricular Pacing in Heart Failure Patients with Chronic AF

The effects of biventricular or LV pacing in heart failure patients with AF have so far been little studied. In an acute haemodynamic study, Etienne et al. [28] compared the effects of left or biventricular pacing in 11 patients with AF and 17 with sinus rhythm, all with LVEF < 35% and left bundle branch block. An equal degree of improvement in pulmonary capillary wedge pressure and systolic arterial pressure was observed in both groups. In a noncontrolled pilot study, a French group [29] assessed the long-term clinical effects of permanent biventricular pacing in 22 patients with sinus rhythm (SR) and 15 with persistent AF. After a mean follow-up of 16 months, biventricular pacing was associated with a more pronounced improvement in AF patients. NYHA classification significantly improved in this subgroup of patients, decreasing from 3.3 ± 0.5 (mean ± SD) at baseline to 2.2 ± 0.7 at the end of follow-up ($p < 0.01$). Mean peak V_{O2} significantly increased from 11.2 ± 3.2 ml/min/kg at baseline to 16 ± 4.5 ml/min/kg (+34%; $p < 0.01$). Such an improvement can be explained by the fact that, in that pilot study, comparisons were made between baseline intrinsic rhythm with naturally fast ventricular rate, and the end of follow-up, after several months of VVIR pacing, with full and permanent biventricular capture resulting from the rate control imposed by AV node ablation. The results reflected the combined effects of rate control and biventricular pacing.

The MUSTIC-AF Trial

In contrast to these noncontrolled studies, the MUSTIC trial made crossover comparisons between two active pacing modes whose only differences were the ventricular pacing sites. Rate control was a prerequisite, to be effective 12 weeks before the beginning of crossover in patients who had been subject to AV-node ablation.

This single-blind, randomized, controlled, crossover study compared the patients' parameters, as monitored during two 3 month-treatment periods of conventional right univentricular vs biventricular pacing. The primary end-point was the 6 min walked distance, secondary end-points were peak oxygen uptake, quality of life, CHF-related hospitalizations, patients' preferred study period and mortality.

Sixty-four patients with severe heart failure (stabilized in NYHA Class III for at least 1 month under optimized drug treatment) due to left ventricular systolic dysfunction, with chronic AF, slow ventricular rate, either spontaneous or after AV junction ablation (64%) necessitating permanent ventricular pacing, and wide QRS complex (paced QRS duration $\geq$ 200 ms), were implanted with transvenous biventricular-VVIR pacemakers.

The results from this study are to be interpreted in consideration of the methodological limitations imposed by the investigational plan. The higher-than-expected dropout rate [27 patients or 42% withdrew before completing the 6 month crossover phase] and patient heterogeneity at baseline greatly limited the statistical power of the trial. That heterogeneity was reflected particularly by differences in the numbers of patients and in quality of life mean scores between the two treatment arms of the study. The fact that randomization order was determined at inclusion rather than at baseline probably explains these differences.

Seven of the study withdrawals were linked to technical difficulties with left ventricular pacing, including five LV lead implantation failures and two subsequent LV capture losses. Those might be interpreted as a relative failure of the transvenous route for LV permanent pacing. In fact, the 93% implantation success rate and 86% long-term effectiveness of this recently introduced technique [30] is very encouraging. Furthermore, the success rate may be further improved by the advances in implantation technique and device technology [31].

In addition, final core analysis identified two nonablated patients in whom > 50% intrinsic conduction occurred, regardless of programming mode. These two patients were therefore defined as not treated. Those observations illustrate the necessity, except in rare cases of chronic and perfectly stable AV block, for systematic AV node ablation in this type of heart failure patient with AF, so as to ensure permanent and full biventricular capture. Because of the high dropout rate, only 37 patients completed the two crossover phases. Despite these methodological limitations, the mean walked distance increased by 9.3% with biventricular pacing (374 $\pm$ 108 vs 342 $\pm$ 103 m in univentricular; $p = 0.05$). Peak oxygen uptake increased by 13% ($p = 0.04$). Hospitalizations decreased by 70% and 89% of the patients preferred the biventricular pacing period ($p < 0.001$). The overall mortality rate was 10.9%.

To summarize, those results were in favour of biventricular pacing. Their magnitude, however, was much less than that observed in patients in sinus rhythm who were treated by atriobiventricular pacing [1]. This was probably due to the fact that the concepts assessed by the two groups in the MUSTIC study were very different. In patients in sinus rhythm, full electrical resynchronization, atrioventricular and ventricular, was compared with no pacing at all. In patients with chronic atrial fibrillation, only the pacing sites differed, i.e.

right univentricular during one period and biventricular during the other. Otherwise, heart rate was identically controlled by active pacing in VVIR mode, with the same baseline and maximal sensor-driven pacing rates.

Further Orientations and Conclusions

The results reported leave hope for significant clinical effectiveness of biventricular pacing to treat refractory heart failure in patients with chronic AF, left ventricular systolic dysfunction and signs of ventricular discoordination.

Before recommending wider use of this novel treatment, large-scale controlled trials are still needed to assess the overall clinical impact of this technique (mortality, major morbidity, cost-effectiveness, etc.). Optimally, these studies should involve heart failure patients without any classical indication for permanent cardiac pacing, i.e. patients with chronic AF and fast ventricular rate, and compare between two or three treatment strategies: optimized medical treatment of both heart failure and ventricular rate control; standard right univentricular VVIR pacing following AV junction ablation in patients whose heart failure treatment has been optimized; and lastly, the same treatment protocol but under biventricular VVIR pacing.

References

1. Cazeau S, Leclercq C, Lavergne T et al (2001) Effects of multisite biventricular pacing in patients with heart failure and intraventricular conduction delay. N Engl J Med 344:873-880
2. Foster AH, Gold MR, McLaughlin JS (1995) Acute hemodynamic effects of atriobiventricular pacing in humans. Ann Thorac Surg 59:294-300
3. Cazeau S, Ritter P, Lazarus A et al (1996) Multisite pacing for end-stage heart failure. Pacing Clin Electrophysiol 19:1748-1757
4. Blanc JJ, Etienne Y, Gilard M et al (1997) Evaluation of different ventricular pacing sites in patients with severe heart failure. Circulation 96:3273-3277
5. Leclercq C, Cazeau S, Le Breton H et al (1998) Acute hemodynamic effects of biventricular DDD pacing in patients with end-stage heart failure. J Am Coll Cardiol 32:1825-1831
6. Kass D, Chen C, Curry C et al (1999) Improved left ventricular mechanics from acute VDD pacing in patients with dilated cardiomyopathy and ventricular conduction delay. Circulation 99:1567-1573
7. Auricchio A, Stellbrink C. Block M et al. for the Pacing Therapies for Congestive Heart Failure Study Group (1999) Effect of pacing chamber and atrioventricular delay on acute systolic function of paced patients with congestive heart failure. Circulation 99:2993-3001
8. Nelson GS, Curry CW, Wylan BT et al (2000) Predictors of systolic augmentation from left-ventricular pre-excitation in patients with dilated cardiomyopathy and intraventricular conduction delay. Circulation 101:2703-2709

9. Nelson GS, Berger RD, Fetics BJ et al (2000) Left ventricular or biventricular pacing improves cardiac function at diminished energy cost in patients with dilated cardiomyopathy and left bundle-branch block. Circulation 102:3053-3059

10. Gras D, Mabo P, Tang T et al (1998) Multisite pacing as a supplemental treatment of congestive heart failure: preliminary results of the Medtronic Inc. InSync study. Pacing Clin Electrophysiol 21:2249-2255

11. Leclercq C, Cazeau S, Ritter P et al (2000) A pilot experience with permanent biventricular pacing to treat advanced heart failure. Am Heart J 140:862-870

12. Alonso C, Leclercq C, Victor F et al (1999) Electrocardiographic predictive factors of long-term clinical improvement with multisite biventricular pacing in heart failure. Am J Cardiol 84:1417-1421

13. Auricchio A, Stellbrink C, Sack S et al (2000) Long-term benefit as a result of pacing resynchronization in congestive heart failure: results of the Path-CHF trial. Circulation 102: II-693 (abstr)

14. Daubert JC, Leclercq C, Pavin D, Mabo P (1998) Pacing therapy for congestive heart failure: present status and new perspectives. In: Barold SS, Mugica J (eds) Recent advances in cardiac pacing. Futura, Armonk, NY, pp. 51-88

15. CIBIS II Investigators and Committees (1999) The Cardiac Insufficiency Bisoprolol Study II (CIBIS II): a randomized trial. Lancet 353:9-13

16. MERIT-MF Study Group (1999) Effect of Metoprolol CR/XL in chronic heart failure: Metropolol CR/XL Randomized Intervention in Congestive Heart Failure (MERIT-HF). Lancet 353:2001-2007

17. The CONSENSUS Trial Study Group (1987) Effects of enalapril on mortality in severe congestive heart failure: results of the Cooperative North Scandinavian Enalapril Survival Study (CONSENSUS). N Engl J Med 316:1429-1435

18. Middelkauf HR, Stevenson WG, Stevenson LW (1991) Prognostic significance of atrial fibrillation in advanced heart failure. A study of 390 patients. Circulation 84:40-48

19. Kannel WB, Wolk PA, Benjamin EJ et al (1998) Prevalence, incidence, prognosis and predisposing conditions for atrial fibrillation: population-based estimates. Am J Cardiol 82:2N-9N

20. Stevenson WG, Stevenson LW, Middelkauf HR et al (1996) Improving survival for patients with atrial fibrillation and advanced heart failure. J Am Coll Cardiol 28:1458-1463

21. Crijns HJ, Tjeerdsma G, De Kam PJ et al (2000) Prognostic value of the presence and development of atrial fibrillation in patients with advanced heart failure. Eur Heart J 28:1238-1245

22. Mahoney P, Kimmel S, De Nofrio et al (1999) Prognostic significance of atrial fibrillation in patients at a tertiary medical center referred for heart transplantation because of severe heart failure. Am J Cardiol 83:1544-1547

23. Farwell D, Patel NR, Hall A et al (2000) How many people with heart failure are appropriate for biventricular resynchronization? Eur Heart J 21:1246-1250

24. Corbelli R, Masterson M, Maloney J et al (1988) Chronotropic response to exercise in patients with atrial fibrillation. Pacing Clin Electrophysiol 11:1823-1828

25. Edner M, Caidahl K, Bergfelt L et al (1995) Prospective study of left ventricular function after radiofrequency ablation of atrioventricular junction in patients with atrial fibrillation. Br Heart J 74:261-267

26. Rodriguez LM, Smeets RM, Baiyan X et al (1993) Improvement in left ventricular function by ablation of atrioventricular nodal conduction in selected patients with lone atrial fibrillation. Am J Cardiol 72:1137-1141

27. Brignole M, Menozzi C, Gianfranchi L et al (1998) Assessment of atrioventricular

junction ablation and VVIR pacemaker versus pharmacological treatment in patients with heart failure and chronic atrial fibrillation. Circulation 98:953-960

28. Etienne Y, Mansourati J, Gilard M et al (1999) Evaluation of left ventricular based pacing in patients with congestive heart failure and atrial fibrillation. Am J Cardiol 83:1138-1140

29. Leclercq C, Victor F, Pavin D et al (2000) Comparative effects of permanent biventricular pacing for refractory heart failure in patients with stable sinus rhythm or chronic atrial fibrillation. Am J Cardiol 85:1154-1156

30. Daubert C, Ritter P, Le Breton H et al (1998) Permanent left ventricular pacing with transvenous leads inserted into the coronary veins. Pacing Clin Electrophysiol 21:239-245

31. Alonso C, Leclercq C, Pavin D et al (2001) Six-year experience of transvenous left ventricular lead implantation for permanent biventricular pacing in patients with advanced heart failure. Heart (in press)

Ventricular Resynchronization Therapy: How to Follow Implanted Patients

E. Gronda, M. Mangiavacchi, B. Andreuzzi and A. Municinò

Resynchronization therapy is rapidly becoming widely used for treatment of heart failure in patients with intraventricular conduction delay, refractory to adequate medical therapy. In addition it is currently used to treat patients with an indication for pacemaker implantation in the presence of even moderate heart failure. Among the still-to-be-validated indications to resynchronization therapy may be the inability to adequately uptitrate "neurohormonal" drugs in severe heart failure patients: β-blockers (due to excessive bradycardia) or ACE inhibitors (due to hypotension).

A large number of patients may therefore be candidates for resynchronization therapy [1, 2]. New issues are related to the best way to follow up these patients to both evaluate the benefit (for investigational or prognostic purposes) and to decide how to implement other treatments with this innovative therapy.

"Historically", since the first appearance of this technique 7 years ago [3], both invasive and noninvasive methods have been used for evaluating the clinical usefulness of this pacing modality.

In patients responders to resynchronization therapy haemodynamic studies have demonstrated a rise in systemic arterial pressure, dP/dt, cardiac output and a decrease in pulmonary wedge pressure [4-6]. A decrease in myocardial oxygen consumption has been observed [7], as well as a decrease of neurohormonal activation [8]. A 6 min walking distance rise [9], as well as an improvement of the performance during a cardiopulmonary stress test, have been also demonstrated [10]. Reduction of cardiac volumes, sometimes of the degree of mitral regurgitation, and a rise in the left ventricular ejection fraction have been evaluated with echocardiography [11, 12]. Quality of life has been shown to improve as well as the NYHA class [9]. A reduction in the need for hospital re-admissions has been observed [13]. A shortening of the QRS duration is "the rule", and is usually considered to be a good index of a successful implantation, even if it may not strictly correlate with an improvement in interventricular myocardial delay [12].

Unità Operativa di Cardiologia Clinica ed Insufficienza Cardiaca, Dipartimento Cardiologico, Istituto Clinico Humanitas, Rozzano, Milan, Italy

To date, no data are available on the prognostic relevance of symptomatic or cardiac performance improvement, after biventricular pacing. Several ongoing trials are using some of these methods to further investigate the technique.

In the COMPANION trial, the performance on cardiopulmonary stress test is being investigated (this trial may prove to be of paramount importance, since its primary end-points are a combined death-rehospitalization and morbidity) [14].

In the MIRACLE study, a thorough noninvasive assessment has been planned: echocardiography, 6 minute walking test and cardiopulmonary stress test, in addition to clinical evaluation (NYHA class, quality of life assessment, plasma neuro-hormones levels), a cost-effectiveness evaluation (device cost plus other resources utilization: i.e. clinical procedures, office and emergency department visits, hospital re-admissions) [15]. Goals have been achieved in the published data.

In the VIGOR-CHF trial, echocardiography and cardiopulmonary performance assessment is planned, with evaluation of norepinephrine plasma levels [16].

However, the important task is to define how patients implanted should be followed up in order to: (1) monitor the device function; (2) be able to gain the most out of this new modality of treatment, or, to put this in the correct perspective, to integrate resynchronization therapy with all the other already well-established therapies.

We believe that no complicated approach should be used: invasive routine follow-up does not seem to be acceptable any longer (for both ethical-economical reasons and the fact that, during invasive assessment, displacement of the left ventricular stimulating catheter may occur).

First thing to be obtained is a 12 lead ECG to confirm a "biventricular pacemaker" pattern (i.e. the absence of the typical left bundle block pattern), possibly with a shortening of the QRS duration. This must be confirmed by electronic interrogation of the device. An echocardiogram should then be performed for both optimization of the AV delay and confirmation of the inter- and intra-ventricular dyssynchronization reduction.

At this point an uptitration of the medications can be started, which in turn may confirm the benefit obtained from the device: if improvement of the patient's condition allows us to lower the dose of loop diuretics, initiate or up titrate β-blockers and ACE inhibitors, this means that the biventricular pacer is working properly.

To substantiate clinical improvement, it is worthwhile to perform a functional test: a simpler 6 min walking test or a cardiopulmonary stress test. An echocardiogram should also be obtained on a regular basis. We usually perform these tests every 3 months.

Clinical follow-up timing is planned, taking into account the patient's condition and treatment regimen (e.g. NYHA Class IV patients, those started on a β-blocker post implant or those with a great reduction in the dose of diuretics, will be seen weekly in our outpatient clinic. In some low-output state patients, the immediate benefit of the implant may not be sufficient to wean them completely from inotropes, although it may allow discharging them on a program of outpatient inotropic infusion: these patients may even need to be seen twice a week at the beginning and then as frequently as necessary; in our experience this has happened in a minority of patients, 4 out of 92).

If clinical improvement after the implant does not reach the expected levels, in spite of optimization of the drug regimen, an electronic control of the device is mandatory (usually echo-assisted) to make sure that the pacemaker is working properly and there is no lead displacement (confirmed by a chest X-ray). If this is not the case, further therapeutic options have to be evaluated (e.g. mitral valve repair, ventricular assist device implantation, cardiac transplantation).

For the time being (awaiting data from ongoing trials, addressing also the prognostic relevance of symptomatic and cardiac performance improvement [14-16]) we believe the most relevant points are: (1) functional class improvement, confirmed by an increase in 6 min walking test distance; (2) improvement in echocardiographic parameters, e.g. left ventricular dimensions, ejection fraction, mitral regurgitation (more subtle parameters, such as right and left ventricular myocardial performance index, interventricular delay, right and left ventricular electromechanical delay, may be useful for investigational purposes but may not prove to add much to the more usual parameters for routine follow-up); (3) ability to modify the drug regimen; (4) opportunity to implement further therapeutic options in case clinical improvement after the implant is not as expected.

References

1. American Heart Association (1998) Heart and stroke statistical update. American Heart Association, Dallas, TX
2. Lamp B, Hammel D, Kerber S et al (1998) How many patients are eligible for multisite pacing in severe heart failure? Eur Heart J 19:572 (abstr)
3. Cazeau S, Ritter P, Bakdach S et al (1994) Four chamber pacing in dilated cardiomyopathy. Pacing Clin Electrophysiol 17:1974-1979
4. Blanc JJ, Etienne Y, Gilard M et al (1997) Evaluation of different pacing sites in patients with severe heart failure. Results of an acute hemodynamic study. Circulation 96:3273-3277
5. Kass DA, Chen CH, Curry C et al (1999) Improved left ventricular mechanics from acute VDD pacing in patients with dilated cardiomyopathy and ventricular conduction delay. Circulation 99:1567-1573
6. Auricchio A, Stellbrink C, Block M et al (1999) Effect of pacing chamber and atrioventricular delay on acute systolic function of paced patients with congestive heart failure. Circulation 99:2993-3001
7. Nelson GS, Berger RD, Fetics BJ et al (2000) Left ventricular or biventricular pacing improves cardiac function at diminished energy cost in patients with dilated cardiomyopathy and left bundle-branch block. Circulation 102:3053-3059
8. Saxon LA, DeMarco T, Chattergee K et al (1999) Chronic biventricular pacing decreases serum norepinephrine in dilated heart failure patients with the greatest sympathetic activation at baseline. Pacing Clin Electrophysiol 22:830 (abstr)
9. Gras D, Cazeau S, Mabo P et al (2000) Long-term benefit of cardiac resynchronization in heart failure patients: the 12 month results of the InSync Trial. J Am Coll Cardiol 359:230A (abstr)

10. Cazeau S, Leclercq C, Lavergne T et al (2001) Effect of multisite biventricular pacing in patients with heart failure and intraventricular conduction delay. N Engl J Med 344:873-880

11. Breithardt OA, Stellbrink C, Franke A et al (2000) Echocardiographic evidence of hemodynamic and clinical improvement in patients paced for heart failure. Am J Cardiol 86:K133-K137

12. Porciani MC, Puglisi A, Colella A et al (2000) Echocardiographic evaluation of the effect of biventricular pacing: the InSync Italian Registry. Eur Heart J Suppl 2[Suppl J]:J23-J30

13. Daubert JC, Linde C, Cazeau S et al (2000) Clinical effects of biventricular pacing in patients with severe heart failure and normal sinus rhythm: results from the Multisite Stimulation in Cardiomyopathy-MUSTIC-Group I. Circulation 102:694 (abstr)

14. Bristow MR, Feldman AM, Saxon LA et al (2000) Heart failure management using implantable devices for ventricular resyncronization: comparison of medical therapy, pacing, and defibrillation in chronic heart failure (COMPANION) trial. J Card Fail 6:276-285

15. Abraham WT (2000) Rationale and design of a randomized clinical trial to assess the safety and efficacy of cardiac resyncronization therapy in patients with advanced heart failure: the Multicentric InSync Randomized Clinical Evaluation. J Card Fail 6:369-380

16. Saxon LA, Boehmer JP, Hummel J et al (1999) Biventricular pacing in patients with congestive heart failure prospective randomized trials. The VIGOR CHF and VEN-TAK CHF investigators. Am J Cardiol 83:120D-123D

How Great Is the Arrhythmic Risk for Heart Failure Patients and Does Resynchronization Therapy Modify It?

M.R. GOLD AND R.W. PETERS

As our population progressively ages, congestive heart failure is emerging as a major public health problem [1]. There are currently almost 3 million people with congestive heart failure (CHF) in the United States and the number is rapidly increasing, with 400 000 new cases each year. Despite important advances in medical therapy, CHF is associated with a poor quality of life and carries an extremely high mortality [2-4]. Many of the deaths are sudden and presumed to be due to an arrhythmia. With recent developments in permanent pacing techniques and implantable cardioverter defibrillators (ICDs), there is growing interest in the use of these devices as a means of reducing the incidence of sudden cardiac death in the heart failure population.

Cardiac resynchronization (CRT), achieved with biventricular pacing, is emerging as an important nonpharmacologic adjunctive therapy in patients with advanced CHF, particularly those with marked intraventricular conduction delay. Most clinical studies have evaluated primarily subjects with NYHA class III or IV CHF symptoms and left bundle branch block. Acute studies have demonstrated improved hemodynamic function with either left ventricular or biventricular pacing in this cohort [5-7]. Increases in contractility (dP/dt) and cardiac output have been reported, as well as decreased filling pressures and reduction in the severity of mitral regurgitation. Chronic studies have shown improvements in functional status, exercise capacity, quality of life, and left ventricular ejection fraction, with a reduction of hospitalizations [8-10], but the impact upon mortality is less clear.

It is believed that about half of the mortality in the population with advanced CHF is due to arrhythmia [3, 4, 11, 12] causing sudden cardiac death. Most incidents of sudden cardiac death are due to ventricular tachyarrhythmias, although there may be an important component of bradyarrhythmic death in individuals with advanced heart failure [13]. Antiarrhythmic drugs, including amiodarone, have generally proved disappointing as a means of reducing mortality in the CHF population [14]. In contrast, the implantable

Division of Cardiology, Department of Medicine, University of Maryland School of Medicine and Department of Veterans Affairs Medical Center, Baltimore, Maryland, USA

defibrillator is emerging as primary therapy to prevent sudden death and to reduce total mortality in high-risk cohorts, particularly those with left ventricular dysfunction.

The emergence of CRT and ICDs represent two divergent applications of electrical therapy to treat patients with CHF. As expected, combined devices are now available that have both biventricular pacing and defibrillation capabilities. The impact of these therapies, either alone or combined, on the CHF population is the subject of the present review. Specifically, the role of ICDs will be summarized, as well as the possible impact of CRT on arrhythmic risk.

ICDs are now considered as initial therapy for the secondary prevention of sudden cardiac death. Specifically, in subjects who survived an episode of sustained ventricular tachycardia or aborted cardiac arrest, multiple prospective randomized trials have demonstrated improved survival with ICD therapy compared with antiarrhythmic drugs, primarily amiodarone [15-17]. A recent meta-analysis of these studies showed that the 28% reduction in total mortality is due almost entirely to a 50% reduction in arrhythmic death [18]. The authors also found that this benefit is most marked in the subgroup of patients with a reduced left ventricular ejection fraction ($\leq$ 35%). Unfortunately, the impact of CHF on the benefit of ICDs was not evaluated. However, on the average, about 46% of patients in these trials had clinical heart failure symptoms (Fig. 1). Assuming that about 30% of patients with CHF have QRS prolongation, then approximately 14% of patients with secondary prevention indications for ICDs would also be candidates for CRT and thus may benefit from combined devices.

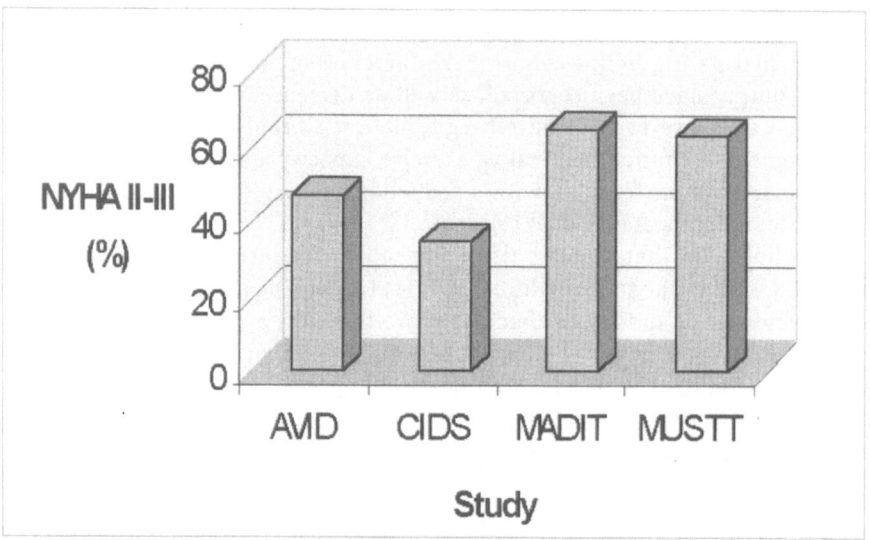

Fig. 1. Prevalence of CHF (NYHA class II or III) in primary and secondary trials of sudden death prevention. See text for further details

The potential role of CRT for patients with primary prevention indications for ICDs appears even greater. The incidence of CHF is greater in the MADIT and MUSTT cohorts than in the secondary prevention trials [19, 20]. Moreover, analysis of the MUSTT database showed that the presence of CHF is a strong predictor of the benefit of ICD therapy [21]. In fact, in patients with ischemic cardiomyopathy, nonsustained ventricular tachycardia (VT), CHF, and inducible sustained VT (using programmed stimulation), the mortality reduction with ICD implantation was 70% in this analysis, while no benefit was observed in those subjects without CHF.

Two large primary prevention studies, which are both close to completing enrollment, could have a large impact on the role of ICDs in the CHF population. The Sudden Cardiac Death Heart Failure Trial (SCDHeFT) study is evaluating patients with NYHA II or III CHF symptoms and left ventricular dysfunction (ejection fraction ≤ 35%). Patients are randomized to receive either ICD therapy, amiodarone, or placebo. The MADIT II trial is evaluating patients with ischemic heart disease and an ejection fraction of 30% or less. Although CHF symptoms are not required for entry, most patients with severe left ventricular dysfunction and coronary artery disease will have such symptoms. In this study, patients are randomized to receive ICD or medical therapy. If either or both of these studies show a mortality benefit for ICDs, then the requirement for combined ICD and CRT therapy would be expected to increase dramatically.

Despite the logical strategy of combining ICD and CRT therapy, it is not certain that such devices will completely replace ICDs or CRT pacemakers in the CHF population. At present, a vast majority of patients with CHF and left bundle branch block do not have an indication for ICD implantation. Moreover, the cost of ICDs may severely limit the dissemination of CRT therapy if only combined devices are available. Finally, the complexity of a combined device is likely to increase complication rates. The increased number and size of leads, the larger size of the device, and the prolongation of implantation times will probably result in more lead, pocket, and infectious complications. There is also a risk of inappropriate shocks resulting from sensing issues with two left ventricular leads and possible double counting of arrhythmias.

One of the more intriguing aspects of clinical trials of patients with CHF is the observation that treatment of heart failure may reduce the incidence of lethal ventricular arrhythmias [11, 22, 23]. Although the mechanisms remain to be fully elucidated, improvement in hemodynamics has been shown to reduce neurohormonal activation and decrease the circulating level of catecholamines (a known arrhythmogenic factor). It has also been suggested that wall motion abnormalities and ventricular dilatation may be involved in the genesis of arrhythmias and any improvement in ventricular function may have antiarrhythmic effects [24]. It is noteworthy that simply improving functional status may not reduce the risk of sudden cardiac death. In the MERIT study, which evaluated the effects of metoprolol in CHF, the proportion of sudden deaths increased as functional status improved [12].

Several of the factors which have been linked mechanistically with arrhythmias in CHF appear to improve with CRT. Preliminary studies of CRT demonstrated a reduction of serum catecholamines with chronic biventricular pacing

[25]. Moreover, the initial results from the MIRACLE trial indicated a decrease in left ventricular chamber size with CRT. CRT may also eliminate or decrease interventricular conduction delay, reducing the likelihood of reentry, and prevent pause-dependent ventricular tachyarrhythmias.

With this information in mind, the initial results of a study reported by Higgins and co-workers are of particular interest [26]. The authors analyzed data obtained from the datalogs of the ICDs of a subset of 32 patients from the Ventak-CHF trial. With patients serving as their own controls (using a randomized double-blind design), they found that CRT significantly reduced the incidence of antitachycardia therapy (shocks plus antitachycardia pacing) over a 3-month follow-up period. It is hoped that the completion of longer-term studies and larger numbers of subjects will confirm and extend these preliminary results. Of particular relevance is the COMPANION study, which is comparing CRT alone, CRT with ICDs (i.e., biventricular pacing defibrillators) and medical therapy in more than 2000 subjects with CHF and QRS prolongation. This study will provide the most comprehensive evaluation of the role of CRT and the need for defibrillation back-up for the prevention of sudden cardiac death.

In conclusion, CRT is a relatively new technique that has been demonstrated to improve hemodynamics, exercise capacity, and functional status in patients with CHF and marked intraventricular conduction delays. Preliminary data also suggest that it may decrease the incidence of serious ventricular arrhythmias. When combined with ICDs, CRT has the potential to significantly reduce the incidence of both tachy- and bradyarrhythmias. Ongoing studies will better define the role of CRT and the need for back-up defibrillation for the prevention of sudden cardiac death in the CHF population.

References

1. Steering Committee and Membership of the Advisory Council to Improve Outcomes Nationwide in Heart Failure (1999) Consensus recommendations for the management of chronic heart failure. Am J Cardiol 83:1A-38A
2. Zannad F, Briancon S, Juilliere Y et al (1999) Incidence, clinical and etiologic features, and outcomes of advanced chronic heart failure: the Epical Study. J Am Coll Cardiol 33:734-742
3. Garg RG, Yusuf S (1995) Overview of randomized trials of angiotensin-converting enzyme inhibitors on mortality and morbidity in patients with heart failure. J Am Med Assoc 273:1450-1456
4. The SOLVD Investigators (1991) Effect of enalapril on survival in patients with reduced left ventricular ejection fraction and congestive heart failure. N Engl J Med 325:293-302
5. Kass DA, Chen C-H, Curry C et al (1999) Improved left ventricular mechanics from acute VDD pacing in patients with dilated cardiomyopathy and ventricular conduction delay. Circulation 99:1567-1573
6. Blanc JJ, Etienne Y, Gilard M et al (1997) Evaluation of different pacing sites in patients with severe heart failure: results of an acute hemodynamic study. Circulation 96:3273-3277

7.   Auricchio A, Stellbrink C, Block M et al for the Pacing Therapies for Congestive Heart Failure Study Group (1999) The effect of pacing chamber and atrioventricular delay on acute systolic function of paced patients with congestive heart failure. Circulation 99:2993-3001

8.   Saxon LA, Boehmer JP, Hummel J et al (1999) Biventricular pacing in patients with congestive heart failure: two prospective randomized trials. The Vigor CHF and Ventak CHF investigators. Am J Cardiol 83:120D-123D

9.   Gras D, Mabo P, Bucknall C et al (2000) Responders and nonresponders to cardiac resynchronization therapy: results from the InSynch trial (abstract). J Am Coll Cardiol 35 (Suppl A) 230A

10. Cazeau S, Leclercq C, Laverne T et al for the Multisite Stimulation in Cardiomyopathy (MUSTIC) Investigators (2001) Effects of multisite biventricular pacing in patients with heart failure and intraventricular conduction delay. N Engl J Med 344:873-880

11. Pfeffer MA, Braunwald E, Moye LA et al (1992) Effect of captopril on mortality and morbidity in patients with left ventricular dysfunction after myocardial infarction: results of the survival and ventricular enlargement trial. N Engl J Med 327:669-677

12. MERIT-HF Study Group (1999) Effect of metoprolol CR/XL in chronic heart failure: metoprolol CR/XL randomized intervention trial in congestive heart failure (MERIT-HF). Lancet 353:2001-2007

13. Luu M, Stevenson WG, Stevenson LW et al (1989) Diverse mechanisms of unexpected cardiac death in advanced heart failure. Circulation 80:1675-1680

14. Singh SN, Fletcher RD, Fisher SG et al for the Survival Trial of Antiarrhythmic Therapy in Congestive Heart Failure (1995) Amiodarone in patients with congestive heart failure and ventricular arrhythmias. N Engl J Med 333:77-82

15. The Antiarrhythmics Versus Implantable Defibrillators (AVID) Investigators (1997) A comparison of antiarrhythmic drug therapy with implantable defibrillators in patients resuscitated from near-fatal ventricular arrhythmias. N Engl J Med 337:1576-1583

16. Connolly SJ, Gent M, Roberts RS et al (2000) Canadian implantable defibrillator study (CIDS): a randomized trial of the implantable cardioverter defibrillator against amiodarone. Circulation 101:1297-1302

17. Kuck KH, Cappato R, Siebels J, Ruppels R for the CASH Investigators (2000) Randomized comparison of antiarrhythmic drug therapy with implantable defibrillators in patients resuscitated from cardiac arrest. Circulation 102:748-754

18. Connolly SJ, Hallstrom AP, Cappato R et al for the AVID, CASH, and CIDS Investigators (2000) Meta-analysis of the implantable cardioverter defibrillator secondary prevention trials. Eur Heart J 21:2071-2078

19. Moss AJ, Hall WJ, Cannom DS et al for the Multicenter Automatic Defibrillator Implantation Trial Investigators (1996) Improved survival with an implanted defibrillator in patients with prior myocardial infarction, low ejection fraction and asymptomatic non-sustained ventricular tachycardia. N Engl J Med 335:1933-1940

20. Buxton A, Lee KL, Fisher JD et al for the MUSTT Investigators (1999) A randomized study of the prevention of sudden death in patients with coronary artery disease. N Engl J Med 341:1882-1890

21. Gold MR, O'Toole MF, Tang A et al (2000) The effect of ejection fraction and congestive heart failure on the benefit of implantable defibrillators in MUSTT. Pacing Clin Electrophysiol 23:559

22. McKenna W, Haywood G (1990) The role of ACE inhibitors in the treatment of arrhythmias. Clin Cardiol 13[6 Suppl 7]:49-52

23. Domanski MJ, Exner DV, Borkowf CB et al (1999) Effect of angiotensin converting enzyme inhibition on sudden cardiac death in patients following acute myocardial infarction. J Am Coll Cardiol 33:598-604

24. Stellbrink C, Auricchio A, Diem B et al (1999) Potential benefit of biventricular pacing in patients with congestive heart failure and ventricular tachyarrhythmia. Am J Cardiol 83:143D-150D

25. Saxon LA, DeMarco T, Chatterjee K, Boehmer J for the Vigor-CHF Investigators (1998) The magnitude of sympathoneural activation in advanced heart failure is altered with chronic biventricular pacing (abstract). Pacing Clin Electrophysiol 21:914

26. Higgins SL, Yong P, Scheck D et al for the Ventak CHF Investigators (2000) Biventricular pacing diminishes the need for implantable cardioverter defibrillator therapy. J Am Coll Cardiol 36:824-827

Does Cardiac Resynchronization Therapy Diminish the Need for Tachyarrhythmia Therapy?

S. Higgins, M. McDaniel, J. Putnam and R. Gillespie

Introduction

Heart failure, whether acute or chronic, is associated with an increased frequency of ventricular arrhythmias and, when these are present, implantable cardioverter-defibrillator (ICD) therapy [1-3]. With similar indications for an ICD, patients are more likely to receive an ICD shock if they have a lower ejection fraction or a higher New York Heart Association (NYHA) class [2, 3]. Cardiac resynchronization therapy (CRT) is a new and promising therapy for symptomatic improvement of heart failure in selected patients (e.g., low ejection fraction, intraventricular conduction delay). When first developed, this therapy required the insertion of left ventricular epicardial pacing leads via thoracotomy. In a previous study, we found that patients receiving CRT via thoracotomy had a significantly diminished incidence of ventricular arrhythmias and associated ICD therapy delivery [4].

Recent developments have resulted in the ability to provide left ventricular pacing and CRT via transvenous leads inserted through the coronary sinus [5]. Particularly since the mechanism for the purported antiarrhythmic benefit of CRT using epicardial leads is unknown, we elected to review the incidence of tachyarrhythmias in this newer population utilizing left ventricular pacing via coronary sinus leads. We compare these findings with the data from epicardial lead placement via thoracotomy.

Methods

Trial Design

Patients evaluated were all participants in the Contak CD trial enrolled at our one institution. The study is an as yet unpublished blinded, randomized comparison of biventricular pacing with "no" pacing (see protocol below) in candi-

Regional Cardiac Arrhythmia Center, Scripps Memorial Hospital, La Jolla, California, USA

dates for an ICD. Participants had to have symptomatic heart failure (NYHA class II or greater), an ejection fraction below 0.35, and a QRS width of 120 ms or greater. Although study patients had an intraventricular conduction delay, none was enrolled who had a requirement for a permanent pacemaker or had chronic atrial fibrillation.

Patient Characteristics

A total of 62 patients were evaluated, including 4 in whom an adequate left ventricular pacing site could not be achieved. Mean age was 67.2 ± 9.7 years; 84% were male. The mean QRS width of the enrollment electrocardiogram was 170.7 ± 30.9 ms, distributed as 38 (61%) left bundle branch block, 19 (31%) nonspecific intraventricular conduction delay, and 5 (8%) right bundle branch block. The mean left ventricular ejection fraction was 24.4 ± 6.0%. The etiology for the cardiomyopathies in 43 (69%) were ischemic and nonischemic (dilated) in 19 (31%).

After informed consent was obtained, all leads were placed transvenously via the left (preferably) or right subclavian vein. The left ventricular pacing leads were inserted via the coronary sinus with the aim of pacing the left ventricular posterolateral free wall (Fig. 1) [6]. The right atrial and right ventricu-

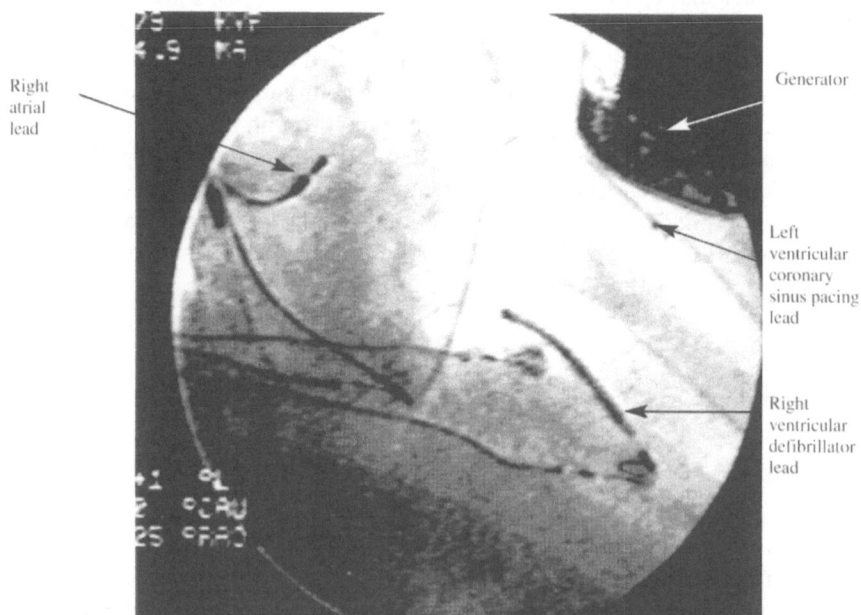

Fig. 1. Right anterior oblique fluoroscopic image of a cardiac resynchronization therapy system. The left ventricular lead is located in a lateral coronary sinus vein

lar pacing/ICD leads were inserted using standard insertion techniques and attached to a subpectoral ICD/CRT generator [7].

Protocol

After a 1-month postoperative recovery period, patients were randomized for 3- or 6-month periods to either atrial synchronous ventricular pacing (VDD) or "no pacing", which actually comprised biventricular pacing (VVI mode) at 40 pulses per minute (ppm), maintained for safety reasons. The patient was blinded to the pacing mode.

The trial required that the initial 24 patients, referred to as phase I, were enrolled in a randomized crossover trial with 3 months' exposure between biventricular VVI pacing at 40 bpm as a back-up and VDD mode pacing with the lower rate of 40 bpm. The time spent in VVI at 40 bpm is referred to as "no pacing" since it is likely that these patients had little to no exposure to biventricular pacing. The enrollment criteria excluded patients with a need for permanent pacing. Phase II consisted of the next 34 patients enrolled in a parallel design study with therapy randomized for 6 months to either of the two modes. Upon completion of the study-mandated 6-month observation, patients were randomized into a pacing mode left to the physicians' discretion. Exclusively, this included only VDD and DDDR pacing modes.

Upon completion of the 7-month trial phase, all patients were programmed with biventricular pacing activated. At 3-month intervals, patients underwent ICD interrogation including evaluation of episode frequency, antitachycardia pacing therapy history, shock therapy history, stored electrograms of therapy, histograms, percent paced, and other parameters.

Statistical Analysis

All tests were two-sided and p values below 0.05 were considered significant. Continuous paired variables were compared by means of a paired Student's t-test. Statistical tests were performed with Statview 5.0 for Windows (SAS Institute Inc., Cary, NC). Period effects, carryover effects, and other interactions between treatment and period were tested using the methodology described by Pocock [8]. Descriptive variables are reported as mean ± standard deviation.

Results

Of the 58 patients, 30 (52%) had therapy during the 18 months of enrollment and observation. The results are outlined in Table 1 and categorized by therapy delivery (antitachycardia pacing, shocks, and total therapy), programmed mode, and rhythm diagnosis determined by preshock electrogram review. As shown, a total of 65 episodes (9 VF, 56 VT) occurred while patients were programmed to no pacing compared to 14 (9 VF, 5 VT) in VDD mode (VF, $p = 0.54$, NS; VT, $p = 0.07$, NS).

To correct for the uneven months of exposure to activated biventricular pacing and no pacing, the total months of exposure for each of the three pacing modes are shown in Table 2. Again, there was no statistically significant difference between the episodes occurring in any of the three pacing modes.

Table 1. Antitachycardia episodes observed by pacing mode, with episodes divided into ventricular fibrillation (VF) and tachycardia (VT) as determined by electrogram review

	No Pacing	VDD	DDD(R)	Total
Shock therapy				
VF	9	9	11	
VT	8	4	20	
Total	17	13	31	61
Antitachycardia pacing				
VF	0	0	0	
VT	48	1	54	
Total	48	1	54	103
Combined antitachycardia therapy				
VF	9	9	11	
VT	56	5	74	
Total	65	14	85	164

Table 2. Antitachycardia episodes from Table 1, adjusted for days of exposure by pacing mode. See text for details

	No pacing	VDD	DDD(R)
Days of exposure by pacing mode			
	6724	3528	2638
Therapy adjusted for exposure			
VF	9	9	11
VT	56	5	74
Adjusted VF	0.001338	0.002551	0.00417
Adjusted VT	0.008328	0.001417	0.028052
Total	0.009667	0.003968	0.032221

Discussion

Previously, in a crossover study of epicardial CRT systems, we observed that ICD therapy was less common when biventricular pacing was active than when pacing was not active [4]. In the present study, such a difference was not observed. A trend to less tachycardia therapy was observed for antitachycardia pacing (ATP) therapy only, though this did not achieve statistical significance ($p = 0.07$).

Why was no difference observed? Several possible reasons are evident. The present study comprised a larger patient volume with a greater number of days of exposure (12 890 vs. 9720) than in the epicardial study. Thus, it appears that if there is significant difference underlying the trend toward less ATP when in biventricular pacing, the difference is small and would require a much larger study period to clarify. The research that resulted in the previous epicardial study achieving statistical significance ($p = 0.035$) was initiated by an anecdotal clinical observation [4]. This can lead to a type I statistical error when applied to a small study. For example, a total of 64 therapy episodes were observed in the previous study, but a single patient contributed 29 of these.

Could it be that epicardial left ventricular leads placed by thoracotomy provide an antiarrhythmic benefit not shared by transvenous left ventricular leads? While this is unexplored here, it is possible that the antiarrhythmic benefit observed with leads placed by thoracotomy is a result of the lead systems themselves. In an animal model, others have described prophylaxis of ventricular fibrillation with temporary epicardial electrodes [9]. However, other explanations exist.

Previously, we postulated that the beneficial effect of CRT on arrhythmia frequency could have been due to an improvement in ventricular hemodynamic performance. It is known that ICD therapy is less common when heart failure is clinically compensated [1-3]. Recent studies have shown that a posterior or lateral lead location of the left ventricular leads is associated with the greatest hemodynamic benefit [6]. This location is more likely to be achieved with the thoracotomy approach than the early transvenous experience.

Finally, it cannot be overlooked that there is a trend towards antiarrhythmic benefit of CRT in the present study. It is certainly possible that this benefit is too small to be determined by this study of a relatively small patient population (30 patients with therapy out of 58 studied). Interestingly, the Contak CD trial results have recently been reported but not yet published. In this presentation, 481 patients were reported to have received CRT with a 9% reduction in antitachycardia therapy noted when CRT was active - again, a non-statistically significant result. It is possible that a study of a far greater number of patients may be necessary before this small benefit is confirmed with statistical significance.

It is also possible, though admittedly unlikely, that the antiarrhythmic benefit of epicardial pacing demonstrated in the previous study is present only for a short period of time. Thus, the original epicardial study, which comprised 3-month follow-up intervals, produced significant results, while the present study, which included patients with up to 18 months of observation, did not.

From a clinical standpoint, these findings are of greater value than the statistical review may suggest. It is evident that CRT does *not* provide a strong antiarrhythmic benefit and thus demonstrates the continued need for ICD therapy. If it does provide any antiarrhythmic benefit, it cannot be disputed that life-threatening ventricular arrhythmias still occurred with frequency in the CRT treatment arm. Thus, it remains our recommendation that defibrillator therapy (ICD) be coupled to the CRT pacing system when patients are shown to be at risk of life-threatening arrhythmias.

Conclusions

The field of cardiac resynchronization therapy is evolving rapidly. Previously, we reported a possible antiarrhythmic benefit of CRT when applied via epicardial leads placed at thoracotomy. In the present study, that benefit was again noted only as a trend which did not achieve statistical significance. Possible explanations for these discrepant findings are offered. However, regardless of the explanation, it is clear that ICD back-up remains necessary in patients at risk of ventricular arrhythmias who are to receive a cardiac resynchronization system.

References

1.   Akhtar M, Jazayeri M, Sra J et al (1993) Implantable cardioverter defibrillator for prevention of sudden cardiac death in patients with ventricular tachycardia and ventricular fibrillation. Pacing Clin Electrophysiol 16:511-518
2.   Mehta D, Saksena S, Krol RB et al (1993) Device use patterns and clinical outcome of implantable cardioverter defibrillator patients with moderate and severe impairment of left ventricular function. Pacing Clin Electrophysiol 16:179-185
3.   Trappe HJ, Wenzlaff P, Pfitzner P, Fieguth HG (1997) Long term follow up of patients with implantable cardioverter-defibrillators and mild, moderate, or severe impairment of left ventricular function. Heart 78:243-249
4.   Higgins SL, Yong P, Scheck D et al for the Ventak CHF Investigators (2000) Biventricular pacing diminishes the need for ICD therapy. J Am Coll Cardiol 36:824-827
5.   Saxon LA, Kumar UN, De Marco T (2000) Heart failure and cardiac resynchronization therapies: U.S. experience in the year 2000. ANE 5:188-194
6.   Auricchio A, Klein H, Tockman B et al (1999) Transvenous biventricular pacing for heart failure: can the obstacles be overcome? Am J Cardiol 83:136D-142D
7.   Higgins SL (1997) The implantable cardioverter defibrillator. A videotape and manual. Futura, Armonk, NY
8.   Pocock SJ (1983) Clinical trials: a practical approach. Wiley, Chichester, pp 114-119
9.   Okishige K, Ohkubo T, Goseki Y et al (2000) Experimental study of the effects of multi-site sequential ventricular pacing on the prophylaxis of ventricular fibrillation. Jpn Heart J 4:193-204

Patients Undergoing ICD Implantation: How Many Need Biventricular Pacing?

G. Gasparini, F. Di Pede, A. Bonso, S. Themistoclakis, F. Giada, A. Corrado, A. Rossillo and A. Raviele

The goal of ICD therapy is to prevent premature sudden cardiac death (SCD) in patients who would otherwise have a long-term survival expectancy. The major challenge is to detect the greatest number of patients who might benefit from an ICD [1]. For instance, prevention of SCD in the general, unselected adult population requires an intervention in many individuals to prevent a few SCDs. On the other hand, to consider only very high-risk subgroups is much more efficient but the impact on the total number of SCDs is low. Heart failure patients and those with ventricular dysfunction and low left ventricular ejection fraction (LVEF) represent an intermediate but growing subgroup with an high incidence of SCD per year, in which a potentially effective intervention would be efficient; while the contribution of SCDs in congestive heart failure (CHF) patients to the total number of SCDs is high enough to predict a significant impact if an effective intervention could be applied. In this context, another important matter relating to CHF patients, in this era of implantable devices is the emerging data on the novel use of biventricular pacing to improve functional status and quality of life in such patients [2, 3].

The aim of this paper is to identify, on the basis of results from major trials, what kind of patient can benefit from an ICD either for secondary prevention (to prevent recurrence in patients with life-threatening arrhythmias) or for primary prevention (in patients without previous ventricular arrhythmias but at high risk of SCD); what kind of patient can benefit from biventricular pacing on the basis of recent data on this matter; and how many patients might benefit from a combined device able to pace both ventricles and to treat ventricular tachyarrhythmias.

ICD for Secondary Prevention

The natural history of patients who suffer from a cardiac arrest due to ventricular fibrillation (VF) or ventricular tachycardia (VT) not related to an acute

Cardiovascular Departement, Division of Cardiology, Umberto I Hospital, Mestre-Venice, Italy myocardial infarction or reversible causes is to be at high risk of recurrent SCD (30%-50% at 2 years follow-up) [4].

In the Antiarrhythmic Versus Implantable Defibrillators (AVID) trial, the first and largest randomized trial of ICDs for secondary prevention, 1016 patients with VF or symptomatic VT and LVEF ≤ 0.40 were randomized to receive ICD (transvenous in 93%) or antiarrhythmic drug treatment (empirical amiodarone in 96%) [5]. At 3 years' follow-up, mortality was reduced by 29% in ICD patients. It was interesting to note that in a post-hoc subgroup analysis the improved survival in the ICD group was limited to patients with LVEF ≤ 0.35 [6].

The Canadian Implantable Defibrillator Study (CIDS) compared secondary prevention by ICD with amiodarone in 659 patients with clinical characteristics similar to those in the AVID trial. In the ICD group there was a 20% decrease in all-cause mortality and a 33% decrease in arrhythmic mortality over 5 years, which was not significant ($p = 0.14$ and 0.09 respectively) [7]. However, again, a post-hoc subgroup analysis showed ICD benefit only in the older patients with LVEF ≤ 0.35 or in NYHA class III [8].

Finally, in the Cardiac Arrest Study Hamburg (CASH), 288 patients resuscitated from cardiac arrest were randomized to receive an ICD or amiodarone or metoprolol (or propafenone only at the beginning of the study). There was a 23% decrease in all-cause mortality with ICD during a 57-month follow-up ($p = 0.08$). It should be pointed out that the mean LVEF was higher than in previous reports (0.46), about 10% of the CASH patients had no structural heart disease, and over half the CASH patients received an epicardial lead system, resulting in higher perioperative mortality [9].

These studies confirm that ICD implantation is more effective than medical treatment in patients with life-threatening arrhythmias, but patients with a low ventricular function and more advanced heart failure derive the greatest benefit.

ICD for Primary Prevention

While in some specific cardiac diseases we know methods for assessing the risk of developing life-threatening arrhythmias, for many others we have little knowledge of predictors of arrhythmic events and appropriate therapy is still a matter of controversy. However, the underlying cardiac disease has an important role in prognosis, helping in the choice of better treatment. It is known that patients with a previous myocardial infarction, low LVEF (≤ 0.35), and nonsustained VT have an increased risk of life-threatening arrhythmias, with a 2-year mortality of about 30% [4].

In the Multicenter Automatic Defibrillator Implant Trial (MADIT) such patients underwent electrophysiological study for risk stratification. Patients in whom sustained ventricular arrhythmias were inducible but not suppressed by procainamide were randomly assigned to ICD or conventional treatment (amiodarone in 80%). At 2 years' follow-up the ICD group had a significant decrease

(54%) in risk of all-cause mortality [10]. A post-hoc analysis showed greatest benefit in the patients with lower ventricular function (LVEF < 0.26) [11].

In the Multicentre UnSustained Tachycardia Trial (MUSTT) there was a comparison of an electrophysiological study-guided approach with no specific treatment in symptom-free patients with a previous myocardial infarction, a LVEF ≤ 0.40, and nonsustained VT. In 2202 patients an electrophysiological study was performed: 65% of these patients were not inducible and were followed-up in a registry, while 765 patients (35%) with inducible sustained ventricular arrhythmias were randomized to either no antiarrhythmic treatment (353 patients) or electrophysiologically guided treatment (351 patients). This second group was further randomized to an effective antiarrhythmic drug or to ICD. Therefore, in the end, patients randomized to electrophysiologically guided treatment received either an ICD or an effective drug. At 5 years' follow-up, arrhythmia-related mortality was 32% in patients receiving no antiarrhythmic therapy and 25% in patients receiving electrophysiologically guided therapy (p = 0.04). However, 5-year mortality was 9% in inducible patients who received an ICD compared with 34% in inducible patients treated with drugs and 32% in those not treated with antiarrhythmic drugs ($p < 0.001$) [12].

The CABG-Patch trial randomized to receive ICD or no treatment 900 patients who were candidates for coronary bypass surgery with LVEF ≤ 0.35 and abnormal signal-averaged ECG. At 32 months' follow-up there was no difference in overall or cardiac mortality. It should be pointed out that this study enrolled patients who had no spontaneous or induced ventricular arrhythmias and who were undergoing revascularization [13].

The MADIT and MUSTT studies confirm that in patients with a previous myocardial infarction, low ventricular function, symptomless unsustained VT, and inducible sustained ventricular arrhythmias, ICD is better than medical treatment.

What comes out of all these studies, both for secondary and for primary prevention, is that the sickest patient fares better with treatment based on an implantable device than on pharmacological treatment.

The incidence of CHF is increasing due to the aging of the population and the improvement in survival after myocardial infarction. The contribution of SCD to overall deaths among CHF patients shows an inverse relation to functional class and total mortality. In NYHA class II patients, the annual mortality rate is 5%-15%, and 50%-80% of these deaths are estimated to be sudden. In NYHA class III patients the respective estimates for annual mortality and percentage of SCD are 20%-50% and 30%-50% while in NYHA class IV patients the estimated figures are 30%-70% and 5%-30% [14]. An interesting fact emerges from six different trials of amiodarone [15-20]: there is a relation between annual SCD rate and LVEF, with a higher incidence of SCD in patients with lower LVEF; but if we consider the contribution of SCD to overall mortality (percentage of all deaths that are sudden), this is *greater* in patients with *less* depressed left ventricular function. The implications of this are of great relevance to clinical practice. In fact, in patients with a mild degree of functional impairment or only mildly depressed ventricular function, the mortality rate expected within 1 year is relatively low, but a significant proportion of these deaths will be sudden. The detection of patients at higher risk of sudden death is important because by preventing sudden death we may be able to offer increased life expectancy to these patients who still enjoy a reasonable quality of life.

Until some years ago, prevention of SCD in NYHA class III-IV patients was considered to change the form of death without significantly increasing life expectancy. However, recent data [2, 3] suggest that biventricular pacing therapy may improve the functional status and quality of life in patients with advanced CHF. The rationale for this therapy is based on the high prevalence (30%-50%) [21, 22] of intraventricular conduction delay among patients with heart failure. The electromechanical consequences of this are prolongation of isovolumetric contraction time and relaxing time of the left ventricle, worsening of mitral regurgitation, and shortening of left ventricular filling time with reduction of pump function. Thus, in patients with a cardiomyopathy, LVEF $\leq$ 0.35, NYHA functional class $\geq$ II, and QRS duration $\geq$ 120 ms, it has been proposed that biventricular pacing would resynchronize ventricular contraction. Initial short-term studies have demonstrated acute hemodynamic improvements by reducing ventricular asynchrony [23-26]. Results from uncontrolled studies of permanent biventricular pacing have shown prolonged improvement in terms of symptoms, exercise tolerance, and well-being [27]. This is confirmed in single-blind, randomized, controlled crossover studies, as recently published [28, 29].

So, the availability of an ICD with biventricular pacing capability may also be an interesting therapy for patients with advanced CHF at risk for ventricular arrhythmias.

But, among patients undergoing ICD implantation, how many need biventricular pacing?

Stellbrink and coworkers [30] retrospectively analyzed the number of patients with an ICD indication who might be candidates for biventricular pacing as an adjunct therapy for CHF. They considered 384 consecutive patients who underwent ICD implantation. The incidence of symptomatic CHF (NYHA class $\geq$ II) was 82% (315 patients). The inclusion and some of the exclusion criteria of the PATH-CHF study were chosen [30] to identify candidates for biventricular pacing at the time of ICD implantation. There were 106 patients with NYHA class III disease or worse; of these, 56 had a QRS > 120 ms. Twenty-eight patients were excluded on the basis of a recent myocardial infarction (3 patients), planned surgical revascularization (5 patients), atrial fibrillation within the last 6 months (16 patients), and associated noncardiac reasons (4 patients). Thus, 28 patients (7.3%) were candidates for biventricular pacing. If patients with NYHA class II disease and a very low LVEF ($\leq$ 0.30) were included, the number increased to 48 patients (12.5%).

This study gives us an idea of the consistent percentage of the growing population of heart disease patients who would potentially be candidates for a combined device – ICD plus biventricular pacing – in order to reduce SCD and, perhaps, death due to progressive CHF. Moreover, it seems that better synchronized ventricles may diminish the need for appropriate ICD interventions, probably due to the improvement in left ventricular performance achieved with biventricular pacing [31]. However, we need more data from ongoing and planning trials to understand (1) whether the combined therapy with ICD and biventricular pacing really improves survival in addition to functional status and quality of life in CHF patients; (2) what kind of patient can most benefit from this therapy, and (3) how to identify beforehand patients who will respond to this treatment. Today, to have a safe and effective automatic implantable device for CHF patients with malignant arrhythmias means to have a powerful therapeutic tool, with 100% patient compliance.

References

1. Myerburg RJ, Kessler KM, Castellanos A (1992) Sudden cardiac death: structure, function and time-dependence of risk. Circulation 85[Suppl 1]: I2-I10
2. Bakker P, Meijburg H, de Jonge N et al (1994) Beneficial effects of biventricular pacing in congestive heart failure. Pacing Clin Electrophysiol 17:820
3. Cazeau S, Ritter P, Lazarus A (1996) Multisite pacing for end-stage heart failure: early experience. Pacing Clin Electrophysiol 19:1748-1757
4. Gregoratos G, Cheitlin MD, Conill A et al (1998) ACC/AHA guidelines for implantation of cardiac pacemakers and antiarrhythmia devices: executive summary – a report of the American College of Cardiology/American Heart Association Task Force on Practice Guidelines (Committee on Pacemaker Implantation). Circulation 97:1325-1335
5. The Antiarrhythmic Versus Implantable Defibrillator (AVID) Investigators (1997) A comparison of antiarrhythmic-drug therapy with implantable defibrillators in patients resuscitated from near-fatal ventricular arrhythmias. N Engl J Med 337:1576-1583
6. Domanski MJ, Sakseena S, Epstein AE et al (1999) Relative effectiveness of the implantable cardioverter-defibrillator and antiarrhythmic drugs in patients with varying degrees of left ventricular dysfunction who have survived malignant ventricular arrhythmias: AVID Investigators. J Am Coll Cardiol 34:1090-1095
7. Connolly SJ, Gent M, Roberts RS et al (2000) Canadian implantable defibrillator study (CIDS): a randomized trial of the implantable defibrillator against amiodarone. Circulation 101:1297-1302
8. Sheldon R, Connolly S, Krahn A et al (2000) Identification of patients most likely to benefit from implantable cardioverter-defibrillator therapy: the Canadian Implantable Defibrillator Study. Circulation 101:1660-1664
9. Kuck KH, Cappato R, Siebels J, Ruppel R (2000) Randomized comparison of antiarrhythmic drug therapy with implantable defibrillators in patients resuscited from cardiac arrest – The Cardiac Arrest Study Hamburg (CASH). Circulation 102:748-754
10. Moss AJ, Hall WJ, Cannom DS et al (1996) Improved survival with an implantable defibrillator in patients with coronary disease at high risk for ventricular arrhythmias: Multicenter Automatic Defibrillator Implantation Trial Investigators. N Engl J Med 335:1933-1940
11. Moss AJ (2000) Implantable cardioverter defibrillator therapy: the sickest patients benefit the most. Circulation 101:1638-1640
12. Buxton AE, Lee KL, Fisher JD et al (1999) A randomized study of the prevention of sudden death in patients with coronary artery disease: Multicenter Unsustained Tachycardia Trial Investigators. N Engl J Med 341:1882-1890
13. Bigger JT Jr (1997) Coronary Artery Bypass Graft (CABG) Patch Trial Investigators. Prophylactic use of implanted cardiac defibrillators in patients at high risk for ven-

tricular arrhythmias after coronary-artery bypass graft surgery. N Engl J Med 337:1569-1575

14. Uretsky BF, Sheahan RG (1997) Primary prevention of sudden cardiac death in heart failure: will the solution be shocking? J Am Coll Cardiol 30:1589-1597

15. Burkart F, Pfisterer M, Kiowski W et al (1990) Effect of antiarrhythmic therapy on mortality in survivors of myocardial infarction with asymptomatic complex ventricular arrhythmias: Basel Antiarrhythmic Study of Infarct Survival. J Am Coll Cardiol 6:1711-1718

16. Ceremuzynski L, Kleczar E, Krzeminska-Pakula M et al (1992) Effect of amiodarone on mortality after myocardial infarction: a double-blind, placebo controlled, pilot study. J Am Coll Cardiol 10:1056-1062

17. Navarro-Lopez F, Cosin J, Marrugat J et al (1993) Comparison of the effect of amiodarone versus metoprolol on the frequency of ventricular arrhythmias and on mortality after acute myocardial infarction. SSSD Investigators. Spanish Study on Sudden Death. Am J Cardiol 72:1243-1248

18. Julian DG, Camm AJ, Frangin G et al (1997) Randomized trial of effect of amiodarone on mortality in patients with left-ventricular dysfunction after recent myocardial infarction: EMIAT. European Myocardial Infarction Amiodarone Trial Investigators. Lancet 349:667-674

19. Doval HC, Nul DR, Grancelli HO et al (1994) Grupo de Estudio de la Sobrevida en la Insuficiencia Cardiaca en Argentina: randomised trial of low-dose amiodarone in severe congestive heart failure. Lancet 344:493-498

20. Singh SN, Fletcher RD, Fisher SG et al, and the CHF STAT Investigators (1993) Veterans Affairs congestive heart failure antiarrhythmic trial. Am J Cardiol 72:99F-102F

21. Aaronson KD, Schwartz JS, Chen TM et al (1997) Development and prospective validation of a clinical index to predict survival in ambulatory patients referred for cardiac transplant evaluation. Circulation 95:2660-2667

22. Shamim W, Francis DP, Yousufuddin M et al (1999) Intraventricular conduction delay: a prognostic marker in chronic heart failure. Int J Cardiol 70:171-178

23. Blanc JJ, Etienne Y, Gilard M et al (1997) Evaluation of different ventricular pacing sites in patients with severe heart failure. Circulation 96:3273-3277

24. Leclercq C, Cazeau S, Le Breton H et al (1998) Acute hemodynamic effects of biventricular DDD pacing in patients with end-stage heart failure. J Am Coll Cardiol 32:1825-1831

25. Kass DA, Chen CH, Curry C et al (1999) Improved left ventricular mechanics from acute VDD pacing in patients with dilated cardiomyopathy and ventricular conduction delay. Circulation 99:1567-1573

26. Auricchio A, Stellbrink C, Block M et al (1999) Effect of pacing chamber and atrioventricular delay on acute systolic function of paced patients with congestive heart failure. Circulation 99:2993-3001

27. Gras D, Mabo P, Tang T et al (1998) Multisite pacing as a supplemental treatment of congestive heart failure: preliminary results of the Medtronic Inc. InSync Study. Pacing Clin Electrophysiol 21:2249-2255

28. Auricchio A, Stellbrink C, Block M, Mortensen P, on behalf of the PATH-CHF Investigators (1998) Clinical and objective improvements in severe congestive heart failure patients using univentricular or biventricular pacing: preliminary results of a randomized prospective study. J Am Coll Cardiol 31[2 Suppl A]: 31A

29. Cazeau S, Leclercq C, Lavergne T et al, for the Multisite Stimulation in Cardiomyopathies (MUSTIC) Study Investigators (2001) Effects of multisite biventri-

cular pacing in patients with heart failure and intraventricular conduction delay. N Engl J Med 344:873-880

30. Stellbrink C, Auricchio A, Diem B et al (1999) Potential benefit of biventricular pacing in patients with congestive heart failure and ventricular tachyarrhythmias. Am J Cardiol 83:143D-150D

31. Higgins SL, Yong P, Scheck D et al (2000) Biventricular pacing diminishes the need for implantable cardioverter defibrillator therapy. J Am Coll Cardiol 36:824-827

Multisite Pacing in ICD Patients: Which Benefits?

B. Merkely and H. Vágó

A number of innovative multisite pacing modalities have recently been developed for the optimization of cardiac function [1-5]. These new techniques aim to decrease the degree of atrial and/or ventricular electromechanical asynchrony by modifying the pathways of depolarization provided by standard pacemakers [6]. Multisite pacing may become useful in a variety of conditions to achieve either hemodynamic or antiarrhythmic results. Pacing from both the right and left ventricles (or atria) is often called "biventricular" (or "biatrial") pacing [7]. While biatrial or biventricular pacing is proposed to be effective in the prevention of special arrhythmias, implantable cardioverter defibrillators (ICDs) are accepted in the therapy of a wide range of arrhythmias.

Management of Atrial Fibrillation: Prevention and Therapy

Up to 50% of patients treated with antiarrhythmic drugs for converting atrial fibrillation (AF) and maintaining sinus rhythm experienced recurrences during long-term treatment [8]. In addition, the proarrhythmic effects of these agents limited their widespread use, especially in patients with poor ventricular function [9, 10]. The limited efficacy and proarrhythmic risks of antiarrhythmic drug therapy has led to the exploration of nonpharmacologic therapeutic approaches [11].

The first implantable atrial cardioverter defibrillator consisted of a three-lead system with right atrial and distal coronary sinus shock coils and a ventricular lead to allow R-wave synchronization and post-shock ventricular pacing.

Right atrial pacing has been shown to reduce recurrences of atrial fibrillation when compared with ventricular demand pacing in observational and controlled clinical trials [12, 13]. More recently, multisite atrial pacing modes

Department of Cardiovascular Surgery, Semmelweis University, Budapest, Hungary have been reported to be effective in the prevention of AF, including biatrial pacing and dual-site right atrial (RA) pacing [14-17]. Saksena [14, 15] and Prakash [18] demonstrated that multiple-site atrial pacing showed a trend to be superior to single RA pacing in the prevention of recurrent AF. Biatrial pacing has been shown to be similarly effective in patients with AF and advanced interatrial block [2]. The mechanism of antiarrhythmic benefit of these modes of atrial pacing is not completely understood [18].

The use of several modalities of treatment in a single patient with atrial fibrillation may provide additional benefits beyond single therapy. The concept of hybrid therapy may take the form of varying combinations of ablation, pacing (including preventive and antitachycardia pacing), atrial defibrillators and drugs. Certain combinations may prove to be synergistic for specific types of AF [19].

Biatrial Pacing and ICD

The antiarrhythmic mechanisms of multisite atrial pacing are unknown but could be related to altered electrophysiologic parameters (atrial resynchronization) and improved hemodynamics as the left atrioventricular interval is decreased [20]. Interatrial conduction block with retrograde activation of the left atrium was reported to be associated with a high incidence of atrial tachyarrhythmias [21].

Biatrial pacing resynchronizes the electrical activity of the atria, expressed as normalization of P wave morphology and duration in contrast to single right atrial or coronary sinus pacing [5] (Fig. 1). Prakash et al. [18] observed that single-site pacing was associated with an increase in P wave duration as well as regional activation times, suggesting a true prolongation of global atrial activation. Dual-site right atrial and biatrial pacing resulted in its abbreviation, reflecting improved global conduction.

There is preliminary evidence that simultaneous right and left atrial pacing increases atrial refractoriness and decreases the intra-atrial conduction delay after a low right atrial ectopic beat [22]. Previous studies have demonstrated that dispersion of refractoriness and anisotropic conduction were two essential elements for sustaining atrial arrhythmia [23, 24]. Biatrial pacing might change the dispersion of refractoriness or anisotropic conduction; thus, it could prevent recurrence of atrial fibrillation. Wood et al. [25] showed that dispersion of atrial repolarization could be minimized by left atrial pacing only or by biatrial pacing in the isolated rabbit heart. By homogenizing atrial repolarization, dispersion of refractoriness will also be decreased.

For many patients, the natural history of paroxysmal AF is a process of degeneration to the chronic form of the disease [26]. Since "AF begets AF", recurrences of AF may lead to a pathologic process of electrical remodeling and/or structural changes, which is thought to promote the persistence of the arrhythmia and make maintenance of sinus rhythm more difficult [27, 28].

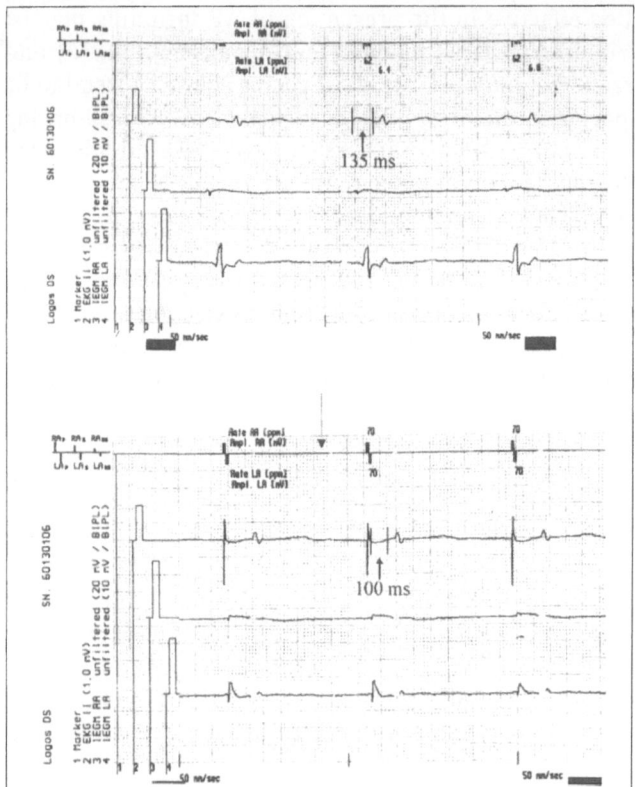

Fig. 1 a, b. Effect of biatrial pacing on P wave duration. Intracardiac electrograms: **a** spontaneous rhythm; **b** during biventricular pacing P wave duration is abbreviated

The possible role of inhibition of atrial remodeling in the antiarrhythmic mechanism could also be taken into account. By reducing the number of atrial premature beats, the trigger of AF will be eliminated (reentry and focal activity) and the progressive electrophysiological and/or structural atrial remodeling will be limited (Fig. 2). Premature beats may enhance the inhomogenity of atrial refractoriness. There is a complex situation in AF with multiple, ever-changing wavelets and a marked functional inhomogenity of the atrial tissue [29]. Regional control of atrial tissue by rapid pacing is feasible during AF, and through a multisite approach this pacing modality might lead to a situation where the remaining non-entrained atrial tissue is just no longer reaching the critical mass [29]. Interestingly, rapid pacing (with bursts) may be effective in the termination of AF or atrial flutter in some cases, not only in the right but also in the left atrium, depending on the origin of the tachyarrhythmia (Fig. 3).

Up to 30% of ICD patients have paroxysmal AF. Special multichamber cardioverter defibrillators give us the possibility for both synchronous dual-chamber and biatrial pacing and dual-chamber tachyarrhythmia detection and therapy. Thus, the duration and possibly also the number of AF episodes are reduced [30]. A high-frequency burst and a low-energy cardioversion using a coronary sinus shock coil can reduce the duration of AF. Shortening the attacks of AF may exert an antiarrhythmic effect by limiting electrical, anatomical and neurohumoral remodeling [31]. Serial increase in post-shock sinus rhythm duration has been seen in some patients treated with repeated endocardial defibrillation [32]. Therefore, sinus rhythm should be restored as rapidly as possible to avoid adverse electrophysiological remodeling.

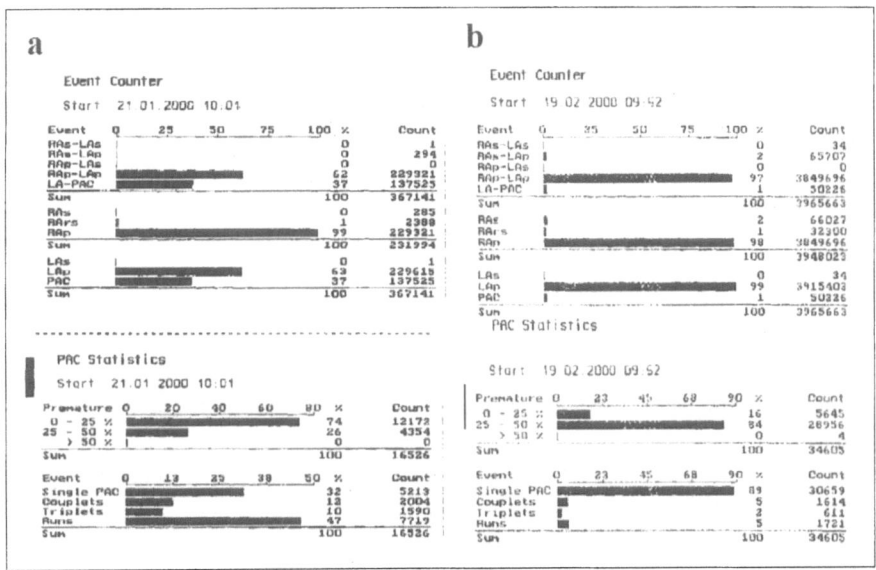

Fig. 2 a, b. Reduction of the number of atrial premature beats using biatrial stimulation. Event counter and premature atrial beat statistics, **a** 2 days after the implantation, **b** 1 month after the implantation

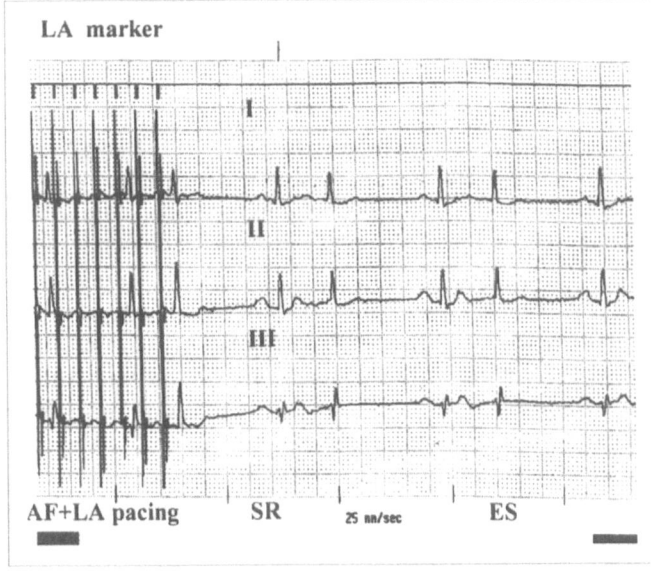

Fig. 3. Termination of atrial fibrillation using left atrial burst stimulation. *LA*, left atrial; *AF*, atrial fibrillation; *SR*, sinus rhythm; *ES*, extrasystole

Biventricular Pacing

Biventricular pacing has recently been proposed for treating patients with drug-refractory heart failure associated with severe left ventricular systolic dysfunction and intraventricular conduction delay [33]. The rationale of multisite biventricular pacing in advanced heart failure is based on the high incidence and gradual deterioration of conduction disorders, especially intraventricular conduction delay [34, 35]. These conduction disorders are responsible for major electromechanical abnormalities, which mainly affect left atrioventricular (AV) synchrony and the ventricular contraction/relaxation sequence [36].

The purpose of multisite, biventricular pacing is to restore ventricular relaxation and contraction sequences by simultaneously pacing both ventricles at specific sites [37].

The potential interest in biventricular pacing to treat refractory heart failure was first investigated in studies of acute hemodynamics using temporary leads. Some investigators were able to find significant improvement in hemodynamic parameters [increased cardiac output, lower pulmonary capillary wedge pressure (PCWP) and V wave] in patients with advanced heart failure and left ventricular systolic dysfunction under biventricular pacing, relative to intrinsic conduction or single-site DDD right ventricular pacing [4]. As Cazeau et al. demonstrated, this acute hemodynamic improvement was independent of AV delay optimization [33]. Biventricular pacing decreased mitral valve regurgitation, which was confirmed by scintigraphic and echo-Doppler examinations. Most of the patients examined showed an abnormal activation sequence during standard pacing, which was corrected by biventricular pacing. Therefore, biventricular pacing improved not only the electrical but also the mechanical activation sequence.

The MUSTIC study investigated the clinical efficacy and safety of transvenous atrio-biventricular pacing in patients with severe heart failure and major intraventricular conduction delay, but without standard indications for a pacemaker. This single-blind, randomized, controlled crossover study compared the responses of the patients during two periods: a 3 month period of active (atrio-biventricular) and inactive (ventricular inhibited pacing at a basic rate of 40 bpm) treatment. The results demonstrated that the mean distance walked in 6 min was greater with active pacing, the quality-of-life score improved, peak oxygen uptake increased, hospitalizations were decreased, and active pacing was preferred by 85% of the patients [38].

The results of one study demonstrated that the long-term benefits of biventricular pacing were correlated with the quality of ventricular resynchronization, as assessed from shorter QRS duration and the tendency for QRS axis normalization [37]. However, other experiences are conflicting. The results of one clinical study demonstrated [39] that the reduction of QRS duration did not predict the best hemodynamic results, which was also strongly supported by our experiences with biventricular pacing. Figure 4 shows an intracardiac electrogram with a QRS duration of 120 ms with biventricular pacing, which is profoundly shorter in comparison with the 180 ms QRS duration for a patient without pacing.

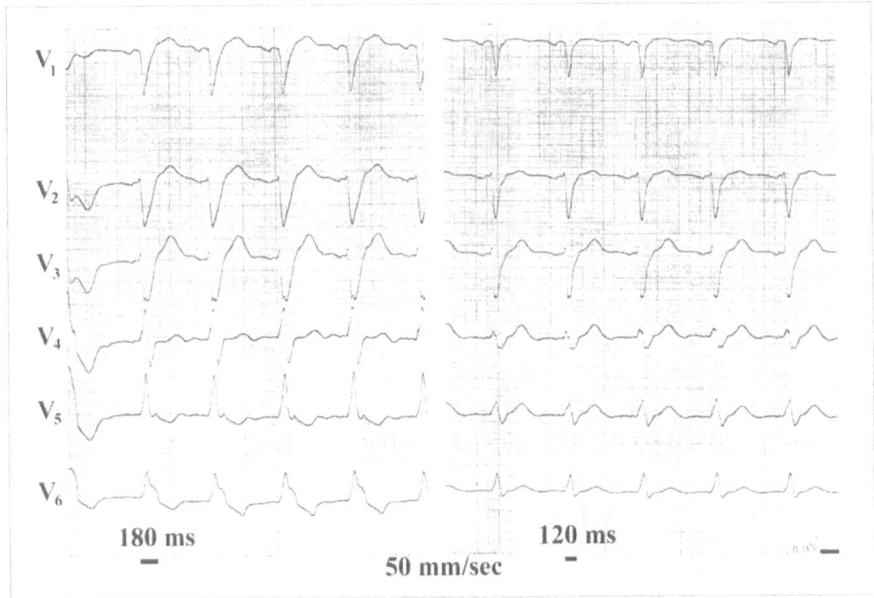

Fig. 4. Reduction of QRS duration by biventricular pacing

In patients with end-stage heart failure, multisite pacing may be associated with a rapid and sustained hemodynamic improvement. In this way arrhythmogenic factors may also be attenuated.

A randomized crossover study investigated the effects of biventricular pacing on ventricular arrhythmogenesis [40]. The investigators concluded that biventricular pacing significantly decreased the 24 h ventricular ectopic count and the ventricular salve count, as measured by Holter monitoring, without altering the mean daily heart rate, when compared to no pacing. Ventricular extrasystoles can trigger ventricular tachycardia based on different mechanisms. This has important indications concerning the potential safety and antiarrhythmic potential of this novel therapy.

Biventricular Pacing and ICD

A leading cause of death in patients suffering from severe heart failure is sudden death mediated by malignant ventricular arrhythmia [41]. Antiarrhythmic drug therapies have failed to influence this risk [42], whereas the ICD has been shown to be beneficial for the prevention of arrhythmic sudden death in certain patient groups [43]. Therefore, the use of ICDs is increasingly accepted as a standard therapy for patients with heart failure who are at high risk of sudden death [44]. In addition to their poor prognosis, heart failure patients also suffer from a poor quality of life [45]. ICD implantation does not alter this impaired quality of life, whereas biventricular pacing has been advocated for the symptomatic management of medically refractory New York Heart Association (NYHA) Class III-IV heart failure. There is no evidence that this pacing technique will affect the prognosis in this patient group. It is increasingly likely that heart failure patients with poor functional status at high risk of sudden death will be considered for both an ICD and a biventricular pacemaker [46]. Figure 5 shows a biventricular ICD with right atrial and ventricular leads, whereas the left ventricle is paced by a lead inserted in a coronary sinus tributary vein.

Walker et al. reported their preliminary experiences with the combined use of an ICD and a biventricular pacemaker in six patients with heart failure and a malignant ventricular arrhythmia [47]. Four patients underwent both ICD and biventricular pacemaker implantation and two patients underwent a single-device implantation. It was concluded that implantation of combined devices may be feasible with currently available pacing technology.

One study evaluated the number of ICD patients (n = 360) presenting a biventricular pacing indication [48]. These investigators predefined possible indications for biventricular pacing as follows: complete bundle branch block, left ventricular ejection fraction < 35% and NYHA Class > II. They concluded that about 10% of their ICD patients had an indication for biventricular pacing at the time of implantation. During the mean follow-up of 34 months, 16% of all

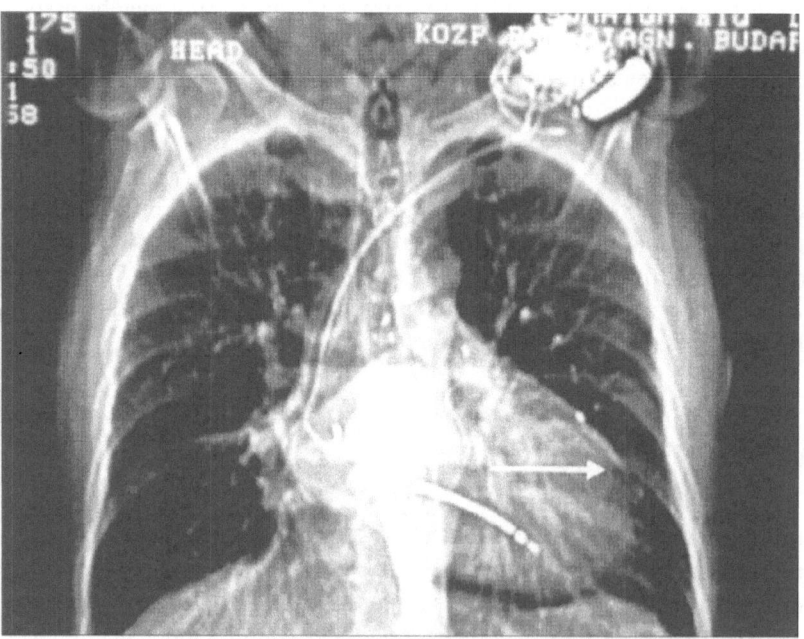

Fig. 5. Biventricular ICD with right atrial, right ventricular and coronary sinus electrodes. *Arrow* shows the distal end of coronary sinus electrode (computer tomography image)

patients presented an indication for biventricular pacing. Furthermore, patients with an indication for biventricular pacing had a higher mortality rate and more frequent atrial fibrillation than patients without [48].

In one study, cardioverter defibrillator systems were implanted with the option for transvenous bi- or univentricular stimulation in eight patients [49]. Four weeks after the onset of AV delay, optimized pacing heart failure symptoms and functional parameters improved markedly. It was concluded that electric resynchronization in ICD patients with advanced chronic heart failure and left bundle branch block leads to a striking improvement of symptoms and functional parameters shortly after implantation.

The results of one study demonstrated that, in patients with standard ICD indication who also have congestive heart failure, left ventricular dysfunction and an intraventricular conduction delay, ICD shocks are less common with biventricular pacing. Although biventricular pacing does not obviate the need for an ICD, it does diminish the need for appropriate tachyarrhythmia therapy in selected patients [50].

The potential antiarrhythmic effect of biventricular pacing may be associated with both improving hemodynamic status and direct electrophysiological effects. There are several potential mechanisms, a decrease in ventricular conduction delays with biventricular pacing, contributing to a decrease in macrore-entry, avoidance of pause-dependent tachyarrhythmias and a decrease in plasma catecholamine levels with biventricular pacing [50].

The future potential for the combination of these devices is of importance, as medically refractory heart failure is associated with a poor prognosis and an impaired quality of life, and there are no other therapies with widespread availability that address both of these problems. Patients who are suffering from severe drug refractory congestive heart failure, having a Class I or IIB indication for ICD, NYHA Class III or IV, low left ventricular ejection fraction (< 35%) and significant intraventricular conduction disturbance and typical dyssynchronization of left ventricular contraction due to left bundle branch block, could have most benefit from biventricular ICDs. Potential benefits include long-term left ventricular remodeling (secondary to biventricular pacing) with a consequent reduction in arrhythmogenesis, a further improvement in patients' quality of life, and a reduction in the long-term risk of mortality [51]. Among patients with congestive heart failure requiring ventricular resynchronization, it becomes more difficult to identify those without clear ICD indications who are at high risk of sudden arrhythmic death. Both noninvasive and invasive tests have many limits with regard to stratifying sudden death risk. Implanting ICDs combined with biventricular pacing has proved to be safe, without major complications [52]. The only objection to defibrillation backup is the higher cost of the device compared to the triple-chamber pacemaker. However, long-term randomized studies are needed to better identify the subgroup of patients that will most benefit from this kind of stimulation and to demonstrate whether the survival of these patients could really be prolonged [52].

References

1. Cazeau S, Ritter P, Bakdach S et al (1994) Four-chamber pacing in dilated cardiomyopathy. Pacing Clin Electrophysiol 17:1974-1979
2. Daubert C, Gras D, Berder V et al (1994) Permanent atrial resynchronization by synchronous biatrial pacing in the preventive treatment of atrial flutter associated with high degree interatrial block. Arch Mal Coeur Vaisseaux 87:1535-1546
3. Daubert C, Gras D, Ritter P et al (1995) Experience with a new coronary sinus lead specifically designed for left atrial pacing. Pacing Clin Electrophysiol 18:825
4. Daubert C, Pavin D, Baisset JM et al Pacing therapy in congestive heart failure: present status and new perspectives. In: Barold SS, Mugica J (eds) Recent advances in cardiac pacing. Goals for the 21st century. Futura, Armonk, NY, pp 51-81
5. Daubert JC, Leclerq C, Pavin D et al (1997) Biatrial synchronous pacing. A new approach to prevent arrhythmias in patients with atrial conduction block. In: Dauber JC, Prystowsky EN, Ripart A (eds) Prevention of tachyarrhythmias with cardiac pacing. Futura, Armonk, NY, pp 99-119
6. Barold SS, Cazeau S, Mugica J et al (1997) Permanent multisite cardiac pacing. Pacing Clin Electrophysiol 20:2725-2729
7. Bakker PF, Meijburg H, de Jonge N et al (1994) Beneficial effects of biventricular pacing in congestive heart failure. Pacing Clin Electrophysiol 17:820(abstr)
8. Fuchs T, Podrid PJ (1992) Pharmacologic therapy for revision of atrial fibrillation and maintenance of sinus rhythm. In: Falk RH, Podrid PJ (eds) Atrial fibrillation: mechanisms and management. Raven, New York, NY, pp 253-254
9. Coplen SE, Antman EM, Berlin JA et al (1990) Efficacy and safety of quinidine therapy for maintenance of sinus rhythm after cardioversion. A meta-analysis of randomized controlled trials. Circulation 82:1106-1116
10. Feld GK, Chen PS, Nicod P et al (1990) Possible atrial proarrhythmic effects of Class IC antiarrhythmic drugs. Am J Cardiol 66:378-383
11. Waldo AL, Prystowsky EN (1998) Drug treatment of atrial fibrillation in the managed care era. Am J Cardiol 81:23-29
12. Andersen HR, Nielsen JC, Thomsen PE et al (1997) Long-term follow-up of patients from a randomised trial of atrial versus ventricular pacing for sick-sinus syndrome. Lancet 350:1210-1216
13. Andersen HR, Thuesen L, Bagger JP et al (1994) Prospective randomized trial of atrial versus ventricular pacing in sick-sinus syndrome. Lancet 344:1523-1528
14. Saksena S, Delfaut P, Prakash A et al (1998) Multisite electrode pacing for prevention of atrial fibrillation. J Cardiovasc Electrophysiol 9:155-162
15. Saksena S, Prakash A, Hill M et al (1996) Prevention of recurrent atrial fibrillation with chronic dual-site right atrial pacing. J Am Coll Cardiol 28:687-694
16. Ramdat Misier AR, Beukema WP, Oude Luttikhuis HA (1999) Multisite or alternate site pacing for the prevention of atrial fibrillation. Am J Cardiol 83:237-240
17. Ramdat Misier AR, Opthof T, Hemel NM et al (1992) Increased dispersion of "refractoriness" in patients with idiopathic paroxysmal atrial fibrillation. J Am Coll Cardiol 19:1531-1535
18. Prakash A, Delfaut Ph, Krol RB et al (1998) Regional right and left atrial activation patterns during single- and dual-site atrial pacing in patients with atrial fibrillation. Am J Cardiol 82:1197-1204
19. Spurrell P, Sulke N (2000) Pacing and defibrillation for the prevention and termination of atrial fibrillation. In: Ovsyshcher IE (ed) Cardiac arrhythmias and device therapy: results and perspectives for the new century. Futura, Armonk, PA, pp 181-188

20. Chirife R (1983) Left heart function during right heart pacing. Pacing Clin Electrophysiol 17:1451-1455

21. Luna ABL, Cladellas M, Oter R (1988) Interatrial conduction block and retrograde activation of the left atrium and paroxysmal supraventricular tachyarrhythmia. Eur Heart J 9:112-1118

22. Sopher SM, Murgatroyd FD, Slade AK et al (1995) Dual site atrial pacing promotes sinus rhythm in paroxysmal atrial fibrillation. Circulation 92:532

23. Allessie MA, Bonke FIM, Schopman FJG (1976) Circus movement in rabbit atrial muscle as a mechanism of tachycardia, II: the role of nonuniform recovery of excitability in the occurence of unidirectional block, as studied with multiple microelectrodes. Circ Res 39:168-177

24. Tsuji H, Fujiki A, Tani M et al (1992) Quantitative relationship between atrial refractoriness and the dispersion of refractoriness in atrial vulnerability. Pacing Clin Electrophysiol 15:403-410

25. Wood MA, Mangano RA, Schieken RM et al (1996) Modulation of atrial repolarization by site of pacing in the isolated rabbit heart. Circulation 94:1465-1470

26. Kopecky SL, Gersh BJ, McGoon MD et al (1987) The natural history of lone atrial fibrillation. A population–based study over three decades. N Engl J Med 317:669-674

27. Van Gelder IC, Crijns HJ, Blanksma PK et al (1993) Time course of hemodynamic changes and improvement of exercise tolerance after cardioversion of chronic atrial fibrillation unassociated with cardiac valve disease. Am J Cardiol 72:560-566

28. Wiffels M, Kirchhof C, Dorland R et al (1995) Atrial fibrillation begets atrial fibrillation. Circulation 92:1954-1968

29. Schoels W, Becker R (1998) Mechanism of pacing interventions in atrial fibrillation. J Cardiovertes Electrophys 8(suppl):13-17

30. Revishvili A SH, Thong T, Schadach M (2000) A new dual chamber cardioverter-defibrillator with left atrial pacing support. Progr Biomed Res 5:100-106

31. Van Gelder IC, Crijns HJ (1997) Cardioversion of atrial fibrillation and subsequent maintenance of sinus rhythm. Pacing Clin Electrophysiol 20:2675-2683

32. Timmermans C, Wellens H (1998) Effect of device-mediated therapy on symptomatic episodes of atrial fibrillation. J Am Coll Cardiol 31:331A

33. Cazeau S, Ritter P, Lazarius A et al (1996) Multisite pacing for end-stage heart failure: early experience. Pacing Clin Electrophysiol 19:1748-1757

34. Wilensky RL, Yudelman P, Cohen AI et al (1988) Serial electrocardiographic changes in idiopathic dilated cardiomyopathy confirmed at necropsy. Am J Cardiol 62:276-283

35. Xiao HB, Roy C, Fujimoto S et al (1996) Natural history of abnormal conduction and its relation to prognosis in patients with dilated cardiomyopathy. Int Cardiol 53:163-170

36. Xiao HB, Roy C, Gibson DG (1994) Nature of ventricular activation in patients with dilated cardiomyopathy: evidence for bilateral bundle branch block. Br Heart J 72:167-174

37. Alonso C, Leclercq C, Victor F et al (1999) Electrocardiographic predictive factors of long-term clinical improvement with multisite biventricular pacing in advanced heart failure. Am J Cardiol 84:1417-1421

38. Cazeau S, Leclercq C, Lavergne T et al (2001) Effects of multisite biventricular pacing in patients with heart failure and intraventricular conduction delay. N Engl J Med 344:873-880

39. Bordachar P, Garrigue S, Reuter S et al (2000) Importance of QRS duration during multisite ventricular stimulation in heart failure: a hemodynamic noninvasive study using peak endocardial acceleration measurements. Pacing Clin Electrophysiol 23:636

40. Walker S, Levy T, Rex S et al (2000) Does biventricular pacing decrease ventricular arrhythmogenesis? Eur Heart J 21:1124
41. Goldman S, Johnson G, Cohn JN et al (1993) Mechanism of death in heart failure. The vasodilator-heart failure trials. Circulation 87:124-131
42. Toubol P (1999) A decade of clinical trials: CAST to AVID. Eur Heart J C2-C10
43. Moss AJ, Hall WJ, Cannom DS et al (1996) Improved survival with an implanted defibrillator in patients with coronary disease at high risk of ventricular arrhythmia. N Engl J Med 335:1933-1940
44. Merkely B (1999) Possible advantages of dual-chamber implantable cardioverter defibrillator therapy. Progr Biomed Res 4:415-421
45. Dracup K, Walden JA, Stevenson LW et al (1992) Quality of life in patients with advanced heart failure. J Heart Lung Transplant 11:273-279
46. Vogt J, Hansky B, Lamp B (2000) Biventricular stimulation in heart failure patients with ICD-indication – first experience with a new implantable cardioverter/defibrillator. Pacing Clin Electrophysiol 23:657
47. Walker S, Levy T, Rex S et al (2000) Preliminary results with the simultaneous use of implantable cardioverter defibrillators and permanent biventricular pacemakers: implications for device interaction and development. Pacing Clin Electrophysiol 23:365-372
48. Siemon G, Schwacke H, Droegemueller A et al (2000) Biventricular pacing in patients with life-threatening tachyarrhythmias: how many patients are possible candidates? Eur Heart J 21:1112
49. Vogt J, Hansky B, Lamp B et al (2000) Biventricular stimulation in heart failure patients with ICD-indication: first experience with a new implantable cardioverter/defibrillator. Eur Heart J 21:2537
50. Higgins SL, Yong P, Sheck D et al (2000) Biventricular pacing diminishes the need for implantable cardioverter defibrillator therapy. Ventak CHF investigators. J Am Coll Cardiol 36:828-831
51. Merkely B, Vágó H, Zima E, Gellér L (2001) Multichamber pacing in patients with an implantable cardioverter defibrillator. Progr Biomed Res 6:17-24
52. Gaita F, Bocchiardo M, Porciani MC et al (2000) Should stimulation therapy for congestive heart failure be combined with defibrillation backup? Am J Cardiol 86:165K-168K

Ventricular Resynchronization: What May We Expect from Technological Advances?

M. Lunati, G. Magenta, G. Cattafi, R. Vecchi, M. Paolucci and T. Di Camillo

Introduction

Cardiac resynchronization therapy (CRT) with biventricular pacing has been recently explored as an adjunctive support to drugs to treat symptoms in patients with advanced heart failure (HF) (NYHA class III-IV), dilated cardiomyopathy (left ventricular end-diastolic diameter ≥ 60 mm), ventricular conduction disturbances (left bundle branch block with QRS duration $\geq$ 120-150 ms). Improvements in functional capacity and quality of life have been proven in two randomized trials (PATH-CHF, MUSTIC) and in some observational studies (Insync Study, Insync Italian Registry) [1-5].

In the past few years we have seen a dramatic improvement in the technology of CRT [6-8]. While at the beginning the technological platform was derived from the conventional implantable device, recently some devices designed specifically for HF have been introduced. The experience accumulated so far allows devices and tools to be designed that respond better to requirements related to the implant and to the management of HF patients.

Nevertheless, particular attention still needs to be paid to both simplification and improvement of the entire process involved in CRT delivery:
- Specifically designed HF devices
- Specifically designed left ventricular (LV) leads and delivery system

Specifically Designed HF Devices

One of the most desiderable features in a device for the treatment of HF is the possibility of activating the heart chambers (right atrium, right ventricle, and left ventricle) completely independently, i.e., the possibility of programming timing, output, and sensing separately for each chamber. This would allow electric, mechanical, and hemodynamic activation of the left ventricle in the most effec-

Unità Operativa di Elettrofisiologia e Elettrostimolazione, Dipartimento Cardio-Toraco-Vascolare "A. De Gasperis", Ospedale Cà Granda, Niguarda, Milan, Italy

tive way, optimizing the A-V interval and V-V timing for example with the echo test. Moreover, since many HF patients have atrial fibrillation (AF), an HF device should have an atrial arrhythmia detection algorithm to maintain cardiac resynchronization even during AF episodes and stabilize the ventricular rate.

In the clinical management of HF patients, HF diagnostic information is also relevant. First of all, the prognostic value of heart rate variability in HF patients is known. Thus, the device must record relevant information on heart rate variability to guide treatment strategy for each patient. It would be also valuable to monitor the effectiveness of the therapeutic approach, recording all the information relevant to better management of the tailored therapeutic approach, i.e., detailed histograms of daily heart rate, or a log of the patient's activity during the day.

The Medtronic Insync III Model 8042, which is in clinical evaluation for market release, is an atrial synchronous biventricular pacing device for CRT. The device has the following cardiac resynchronization capabilities and diagnostic features in addition to the functionality provided by the Medtronic Insync Model 8040:

- Sequential biventricular pacing. Either ventricle may be paced first, with up to 80 ms delay from the first ventricular pace to the second.
- Three independent pacing outputs. The device delivers pacing and resynchronization therapy via the right atrial (RA), right ventricular (RV), and LV leads. All pacing outputs and polarities are independently programmable. LV pacing can be programmed to use the RV ring as anode.
- Configurable sensing. The device senses cardiac activity via the RA lead and either the RV or LV lead, or a combination of both (RV tip to LV tip). Double sensing of ventricular activity can be avoided through the use of the interventricular refractory period.
- Ventricular sense response. The device can be programmed to pace the programmed ventricle(s) immediately after a ventricular sense in order to provide resynchronization in the presence of ventricular senses during the A-V interval (or at any time in single chamber ventricular pacing modes) up to a programmable maximum response rate. Ventricular safety pacing behaves similarly, pacing immediately in response to ventricular senses occurring within 110 ms after an atrial pace.
- Medtronic Kappa series features, including mode switch and auto-adjusting postventricular atrial refractory period (PVARP).
- Arrhythmia, heart failure, and cardiac resynchronization diagnostics, including: patient activity, night heart rate variability, atrial high rate, ventricular pacing, number and percentage of pacing episodes, and marker channel.

Specifically Designed LV Leads and Delivery Systems

Each patient's anatomy is unique: cardiac veins bend and turn, vein diameters vary, side branches leave at irregular angles. Moreover, in HF patients the distortion and enlargement of the heart make the coronary sinus (CS) cannulation and lead delivery more challenging. CRT is accomplished via biventricular pacing and epicardial pacing of the left ventricle is obtained by placing a lead in a cardiac vein.

Lead and delivery system options are necessary in order to make a left heart lead implantation successful. In an attempt to enable positioning at various venous sites and to select the part of the left ventricle whose pacing is associated with the best hemodynamic changes (probably the mid lateral portion), many options have been developed and/or will be shortly released.

To improve the rate of LV implantation (the failure rate can be as high as 10%), decrease implantation time (mean fluoroscopy time at present is 30 min more or less), and increase safety for patients and clinicians (time reduction reduces infection risk), it seems necessary to have at our disposal specific guiding catheters, different leads, other specific tools.

In the method of left-heart lead implantation the steps are as follows:
1. Engage the CS. Sheaths that combine a flexible body with a soft tip seem necessary for quick and safe CS cannulation, supporting the venography balloon, delivering the lead for the LV. Steerable electrophysiologic catheters can probably help in this step.
2. Visualize and select the appropriate vein. An occlusive balloon catheter is mandatory to obtain the best images of the venous tree with a CS venogram. Choosing the right lead for each patient requires looking closely at the cardiac anatomy in regard to diameters, angulation, and tortuousness of the veins.
3. Place the left-heart lead. The goal is a stable position, quickly attained, that could provide anatomical and electrical separation for the RV and LV leads, low pacing thresholds, good sensing characteristics, and no phrenic nerve stimulation. Experience obtained so far highlights the need to provide new tools dedicated to the procedure. Manufacturers give us various solutions. Medtronic provides a family of lead and delivery system choices that span the different anatomies: small-bodied leads with or without guide wire delivery ("side wire") for small to medium-sized veins, particularly those which depart from the CS at a sharp angle; larger leads with greater pushability and flexibility for medium-sized to large veins. Guidant provides the Easy Track leads, an "over the wire" system that enhances trackability and ability to reach smaller vein branches. St. Jude Medical, in order to guarantee stable wedging of the lead, provides a lead with a tip preshaped into an S-curve.
4. Remove the implantation tools. To simplify removal of the delivery system, after lead placement, a peel-away design of the sheath is probably the best.

Conclusions

In a selected population with advanced HF, CRT can achieve a significant and persistent benefit in up to 80% of patients. Improvement and facilitation of LV pacing, which is a reality, will allow us to improve and facilitate our success rate and offers the hope of further enhancing the hemodynamic response.

References

1. Auricchio A, Stellbrink C, Sack S et al (1999) The pacing therapies for congestive heart failure (PATH-CHF) study: rationale, design and endpoints of a prospective randomized multicenter study. Am J Cardiol 83:130D-135D
2. Cazeau S, Leclercq C, Lavergne T et al for the Multisite Stimulation in Cardiomyopathies (MUSTIC) Study Investigators (2001) Effects of multisite biventricular pacing in patients with heart failure and intraventricular conduction delay. N Engl J Med 344:873-880
3. Gras D, Mabo PH, Tang T et al (1998) Multisite pacing as a supplemental treatment of congestive heart failure: preliminary results of the Medtronic Inc. InSync study. Pacing Clin Electrophysiol 21:2249-2255
4. Ricci R, Ansalone G, Toscano S et al (2000) Cardiac resynchronization: materials, technique and results. The InSync Italian Registry. Eur Heart J 2[Suppl J]:J6-J15
5. Zardini M, Tritto M, Bargiggia G et al (2000) The InSync Italian Registry: analysis of clinical outcome and considerations on the selection of candidates to left ventricular resynchronization. Eur Heart J 2[Suppl J]:J16-J22
6. Curnis A, Neri R, Mascioli G, Cesario AS (2000) Left ventricular pacing lead choice based on coronary sinus venous anatomy. Eur Heart J 2[Suppl J]:J31-J35
7. Puglisi A, Bianchi S, Sgreccia F et al (2000) New materials to facilitate coronary sinus lead positioning. In: M Santini (ed) Progress in Clinical pacing, Cepi, Rome, pp 440-446
8. Leclerq C (2000) Which coronary lead for which patient? Does one design fit all patients? Europace [Suppl 97/3]:D112

VENTRICULAR ARRHYTHMIAS AND SUDDEN DEATH: RISK STRATIFICATION AND PREVENTION

Catecholaminergic Polymorphic Ventricular Tachycardia: Another Inherited Arrhythmia?

C. NAPOLITANO AND S.G. PRIORI

Introduction

The term "inherited arrhythmogenic disorders" identifies a group of cardiac diseases characterized by genetically determined cardiacion channel defects which create an electrically unstable substrate that may easily cause malignant ventricular tachyarrhythmias and sudden death. The lack of demonstrable cardiac structural abnormality is a landmark feature of these disorders, namely the long QT syndrome (LQTS), Brugada syndrome (BS), catecholaminergic polymorphic ventricular tachycardia (CPVT), and the short-coupled torsades de pointes (SCTdP) [1-4].

In recent years, mostly thanks to extensive use of molecular biological techniques, remarkable advancements have been achieved in our understanding of the pathophysiological basis of inherited arrhythmogenic diseases. Among these diseases, CPVT is the most recent clinical entity brought to light and its pathogenetical mechanisms elucidated by molecular genetics. In this review we will summarize the clinical features and the current knowledge concerning this newly identified genetic arrhythmogenic disease.

Clinical Features of CPVT

Catecholaminergic ventricular tachycardia (VT) occurring in the structurally intact heart was described by Reid et al. in 1975 [5] and Coumel et al. in 1978 [3]. The first extensive description of this disease was provided by Leenhardt et al. in 1995 [6].

The clinical picture of the disease reported by Leenhardt et al. [6] showed a remarkably uniform pattern of bidirectional polymorphic VT that could be easily and reproducibly induced during exercise or catecholamine infusion (Fig. 1). Approximately one-third of cases had a family history of juvenile sudden death and/or stress-related syncope. Although the presence of bidirectional tachycar-

Molecular Cardiology Laboratories, IRCCS Fondazione Salvatore Maugeri, Pavia, Italy

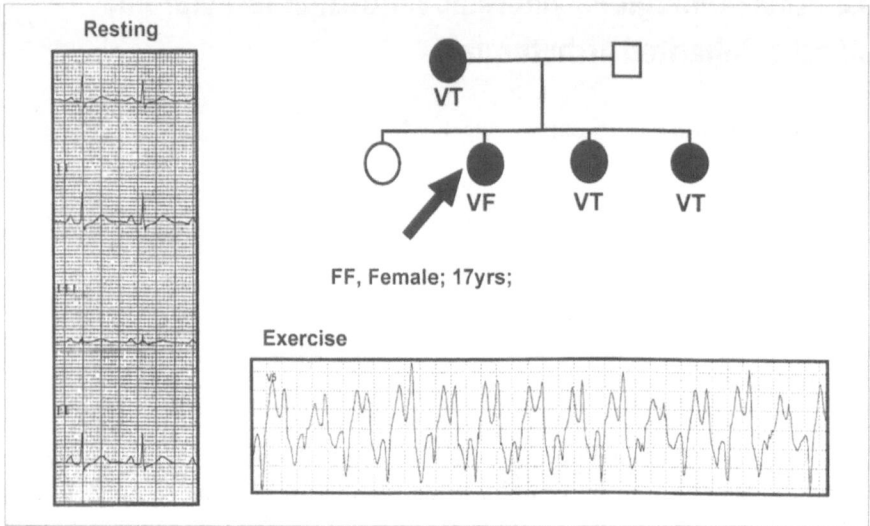

Fig. 1. Example of bidirectional VT in a patient affected with familial CPVT. The *upper right* panel shows the pedigree of the family and the *arrow* indicates the patient whose ECG are depicted (*filled circle* represent affected females). The *left panel* shows normal ECG at rest while typical bidirectional VT develops during exercise stress test (*lower panel*)

dia was described as a distinctive feature of CPVT, adrenergically mediated polymorphic VT in the absence of the typical bidirectional pattern was also shown [6]. Syncope, usually triggered by exercise or acute emotion, was the typical manifestation of the disease described in the earlier reports, but sudden cardiac death may also be the first manifestation of the disease in some families. The reported mean age at onset of symptoms is 8 years. However, other evidence shows that symptoms may also present for the first time at an older age [7, 8].

Additional landmark features of CPVT, as they emerge in the original description of the disease, are normal baseline ECG (with normal QT interval duration) and absence of myocardial abnormalities. No detectable cardiac structural alterations have been reported [3, 5-7, 9], nor have they become evident at follow-up [6].

In summary, CPVT is a distinct clinical entity that may cause the onset of repetitive VT and may lead to sudden cardiac death in a significant percentage of affected patients. At the present time little information is available concerning the natural history and the more effective therapeutic options. β-blockers have been empirically used in the majority of affected patients on the basis of the primary role of the adrenergic nervous system as the trigger for arrhythmias. β-blockers do indeed appear to reduce the incidence of arrhythmias during exercise, but prospective clinical evaluations are still needed in order to assess their effectiveness in the prevention of recurrences, as well as to define the role of implantable cardioverter-defibrillators for the prevention of fatal events in high-risk patients.

Genetic Basis of CPVT

Pathogenetic Hypothesis

The two distinctive features of CPVT are the bidirectional pattern of VT and the clearly identifiable triggering role of the adrenergic nervous system.

Bidirectional ventricular tachycardia is the typical arrhythmia developing during digitalis intoxication and intracellular Ca^{2+} overload [10]. On the other hand, intracellular Ca^{2+} overload is a condition that greatly facilitates the arrhythmogenic effect of β-adrenergic stimulation through delayed afterdepolarizations (DADs) and triggered activity [11, 12]. These two observations point to a genetically determined abnormality in the Ca^{2+} handling as a likely pathogenetic substrate for CPVT. Moreover, the evidence that DADs are increased by fast pacing and suppressed by administration of ryanodine [11], a specific blocker of the sarcoplasmic reticulum Ca^{2+} releasing channel, point to the ryanodine receptor as a possible candidate gene for CPVT.

The Identification of the CPVT Gene

Based on distribution of the CPVT phenotype in the affected families, an autosomal dominant pattern of inheritance was suggested [6]. Subsequently, Swan et al. reported two families with exercise-induced arrhythmias and found a statistically significant linkage between the CPVT phenotype and a set of microsatellite markers located in the region 1q42-43 (on the long arm of chromosome 1) [13]. On the other hand it was known that the region 1q42-43 contains the gene encoding for the human cardiac ryanodine receptor (*hRyR2*) [14, 15], a key protein involved in Ca^{2+} release from the sarcoplasmic reticulum [16].

Taken together, this evidence along with the hypothesized pathophysiological mechanisms of CPVT provided strong indications for a direct role of the *hRyR2* gene in the genesis of CPVT. In December 2000 Priori and co-workers identified *hRyR2* mutations in four families with the typical pattern of CPVT and history of sudden cardiac death, thus demonstrating that *hRyR2* is the gene for CPVT [7]. The fact that not all the probands screened carry *hRyR2* mutations suggests that, like the other inherited arrhythmogenic diseases so far identified, CPVT is a genetically heterogeneous disease.

Conclusions

CPVT has been described as a rare condition associated with VT and sudden death. Only recently has genetic analysis of affected individuals allowed at least some of the genetic defects underlying this disease to be revealed. Thanks to this, it has been shown that, unlike other known primary electrical diseases (e.g., LQTS), which are due to mutations of plasmalemmal ion channel proteins,

CPVT is linked to abnormalities in an intracellular ion channel devoted to the control of calcium handling and excitation-contraction coupling. In the near future, the availability of larger groups of genotyped patients will allow the prevalence of the disease, genotype-phenotype correlations, the natural history of the disease, and, ultimately, the optimal treatment options to be defined.

References

1. Brugada P, Brugada J (1992) Right bundle branch block, persistent ST segment elevation and sudden cardiac death: a distinct clinical and electrocardiographic syndrome. A multicenter report. J Am Coll Cardiol 20:1391-1396
2. Schwartz PJ, Priori SG, Napolitano C (2000) The long QT syndrome. In: Zipes DP, Jalife J (eds) Cardiac electrophysiology: from cell to bedside. Saunders, Philadelphia, pp 597-615
3. Coumel P, Fidelle J, Lucet V et al (1978) Catecholaminergic-induced severe ventricular arrhythmias with Adams-Stokes syndrome in children: report of four cases. Br Heart J 40:28-37
4. Leenhardt A, Glaser E, Burguera M et al (1994) Short-coupled variant of torsade de pointes. A new electrocardiographic entity in the spectrum of idiopathic ventricular tachyarrhythmias. Circulation 89:206-215
5. Reid DS, Tynan M, Braidwood L, Fitzgerald GR (1975) Bidirectional tachycardia in a child. A study using His bundle electrography. Br Heart J 37:339-344
6. Leenhardt A, Lucet V, Denjoy I et al (1995) Catecholaminergic polymorphic ventricular tachycardia in children. A 7-year follow-up of 21 patients. Circulation 91:1512-1519
7. Priori SG, Napolitano C, Tiso N et al (2000) Mutations in the cardiac ryanodine receptor gene (hRyR2) underlie catecholaminergic polymorphic ventricular tachycardia. Circulation 102:r49-r53
8. Martini B, Buja GF, Canciani B, Nava A (1988) Bidirectional tachycardia. A sustained form, not related to digitalis intoxication, in an adult without apparent cardiac disease. Jpn Heart J 29:381-387
9. Glikson M, Constantini N, Grafstein Y et al (1991) Familial bidirectional ventricular tachycardia. Eur Heart J 12:741-745
10. Rosen MR, Danilo P Jr (1980) Effects of tetrodotoxin, lidocaine, verapamil, and AHR-2666 on ouabain-induced delayed afterdepolarizations in canine Purkinje fibers. Circ Res 46:117-124
11. Priori SG, Corr PB (1990) Mechanisms underlying early and delayed afterdepolarizations induced by catecholamines. Am J Physiol 258:H1796-H1805
12. Priori SG, Mantica M, Schwartz PJ (1988) Delayed afterdepolarizations elicited in vivo by left stellate ganglion stimulation. Circulation 78:178-185
13. Swan H, Piippo K, Viitasalo M et al (1999) Arrhythmic disorder mapped to chromosome 1q42-q43 causes malignant polymorphic ventricular tachycardia in structurally normal hearts. J Am Coll Cardiol 34:2035-2042
14. Otsu K, Fujii J, Periasamy M et al (1993) Chromosome mapping of five human cardiac and skeletal muscle sarcoplasmic reticulum protein genes. Genomics 17:507-509
15. Otsu K, Willard HF, Khanna VK et al (1990) Molecular cloning of cDNA encoding the Ca2+ release channel (ryanodine receptor) of rabbit cardiac muscle sarcoplasmic reticulum. J Biol Chem 265:13472-13483
16. Sorrentino V, Barone V, Rossi D (2000) Intracellular Ca(2+) release channels in evolution. Curr Opin Genet Dev 10:662-667

The Link Between SIDS and Long QT Syndrome: from Theory to Evidence

P.J. Schwartz

Introduction

For reasons not immediately obvious, the suggestions made over the years that cardiac mechanisms and, specifically, life-threatening arrhythmias [1, 2] might account for a significant portion of cases of sudden infant death syndrome (SIDS) were always received in the pediatric world with a mixture of skepticism and irritation. Against this background, it is not surprising that these proposals – irrespective of whether they are supported by solid data – have consistently ended up in controversy.

I will describe the rationale and origin of the hypothesis linking part of SIDS to a fatal arrhythmia, ventricular fibrillation, associated with prolongation of the QT interval on the electrocardiogram (ECG). I will then summarize the results of our prospective study carried out recording an ECG in 34 000 infants over a period of almost 20 years [3], and I will conclude by presenting our new findings [4, 5], which provide for the first time the molecular evidence linking SIDS to the long QT syndrome (LQTS).

The QT Hypothesis

Many hypotheses have been proposed to explain SIDS but none has yet been proven. There is a consensus that SIDS is multifactorial [2, 6], a concept implying that a sudden and unexpected death in infancy may stem from different causes. A logical corollary is that the validity of one mechanism is not negated by validity of another.

Most SIDS cases probably result from an abnormality in either respiratory or cardiac function [7], or in their neural control, which may be transient in nature but sufficient to initiate a fatal sequence of events.

Department of Cardiology, Policlinico S. Matteo IRCCS and University of Pavia, Italy

In 1974, in a funded NIH grant application [8], and in 1976, in a peer-reviewed journal [1], I proposed that some cases of SIDS might have been due to a mechanism similar to that responsible for the sudden death of patients affected by the LQTS, the leading cause of sudden death below age 20 [9]. One such mechanism might have been a developmental abnormality in cardiac sympathetic innervation predisposing some infants to fatal arrhythmias in the first year of life [1]. Another likely mechanism might have been the same genetic alterations that only very recently have been shown to cause LQTS [9, 10]. The only clinically detectable marker for these mechanisms is a QT interval prolongation on the ECG.

Neonatal Electrocardiography and SIDS

To test the hypothesis of a relationship between QT interval prolongation and SIDS, in 1976 we designed a prospective study based on the recording of a standard ECG in 3- to 4-day-old infants. Given the low incidence of SIDS (0.5-1.0 per 1000 live births), we had to prospectively collect neonatal ECGs in a very large population and to subsequently follow these infants for 1 year to assess the occurrence of SIDS or deaths for other causes. The results of this study were published in 1998 [3] and, partly because of the accompanying editorial [11] and partly because of the media attention, were widely publicized. For this reason, I will simply summarize the main facts and findings here.

Twelve-lead ECGs were recorded in 34 442 neonates born in nine maternity hospitals. The QT interval was measured on the ECGs of all infants that died and on the ECGs of a random sample of 9725 infants taken from the entire study population. All measurements were performed by investigators blind to the survival status of the infant. The study lasted 19 years.

Of the 34 442 infants enrolled, 33 034 (96%) completed the 1-year follow-up. The losses to follow-up were due to change of residence. The mean QT_c (QT interval corrected for heart rate) was 400 ± 20 ms and did not differ between males and females (401 ± 19 vs 400 ± 20 ms). The normal and symmetrical distribution of the QT_c in our population made the 97.5th percentile value of QT_c correspond to 440 ms, 2 standard deviations above the mean. Consequently, we considered a value greater than 440 ms as a prolonged QTc.

During the 1-year follow-up there have been 34 deaths: 24 due to SIDS and 10 due to other causes. All post-mortem examinations of SIDS victims were negative and failed to document an adequate cause of death. No SIDS victim had a family history of LQTS or sudden death.

The mean QT_c was 435 ± 45 ms in the SIDS group, significantly longer than that of the non-SIDS victims (392 ± 26 ms, $p < 0.05$) and that of healthy controls (400 ± 20 ms, $p < 0.01$, Fig. 1). More importantly, the analysis of the individual values of QT_c in the two groups of victims (Fig. 1) showed that 12/24 (50%) infants who died of SIDS had a QT_c greater than 440 ms, whereas all the infants who died of other causes had a QT_c shorter than 440 ms.

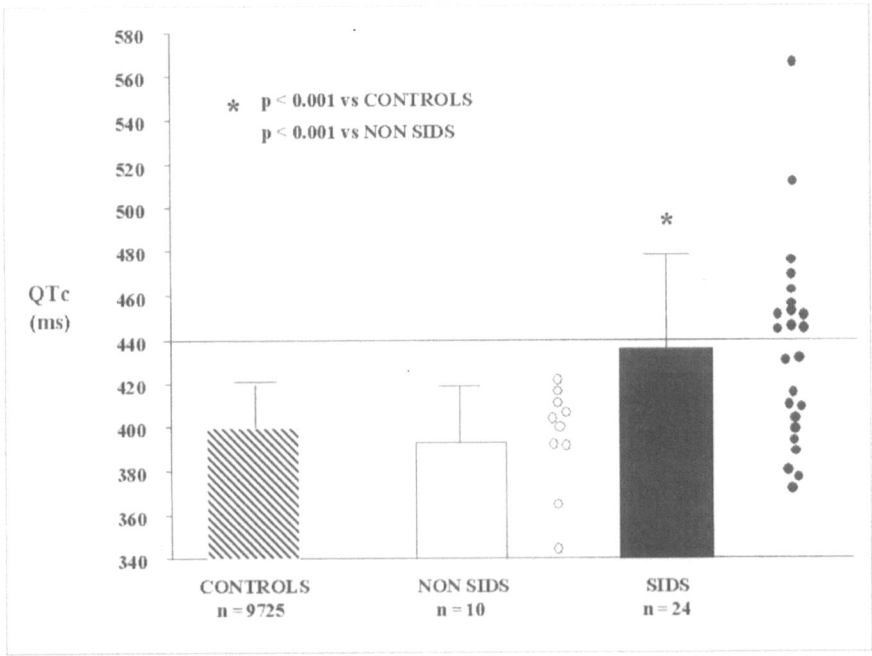

Fig. 1. Mean QT interval corrected for heart rate (QT_c) in control infants, in victims of sudden infant death syndrome (*SIDS*), and in victims of death from other causes (*NON SIDS*). The *line* represents the 97.5th percentile value of QT_c in the whole population and corresponds to 440 ms, 2 standard deviations above the mean. The *filled* and the *open* circles represent the individual values of QT_c of the SIDS victims and of the non-SIDS victims, respectively. (From [3], by permission)

Since heart rate in the neonatal period is relatively high, Bazett's formula might not be appropriate to correct QT interval for short cycle lengths. Accordingly, we also divided the RR intervals in 17 classes with progressively increasing values (20 ms stepwise), and for each class we calculated the percentile distribution of the corresponding absolute values of QT interval (from the 2.5th to the 97.5th). Figure 2 shows that the individual values of 12/24 (50%) SIDS victims were located above the 97.5th percentile, whereas all the values of the non-SIDS victims were below the 90th percentile.

On the basis of our results, the absolute risk of SIDS in infants with a normal QT_c is 0.37 per thousand, while that of infants with a $QT_c \geq 440$ ms is 15 per thousand. The odds ratio for SIDS associated with a prolonged QT_c (> 440 ms) is 41.3 (95% CI 17.3-98.4), significantly greater than that of infants with a normal QT_c.

This large prospective study based on more than 33 000 infants provided the demonstration that QT interval prolongation on the standard ECG recorded on the 3rd-4th day of life is a major risk factor for SIDS.

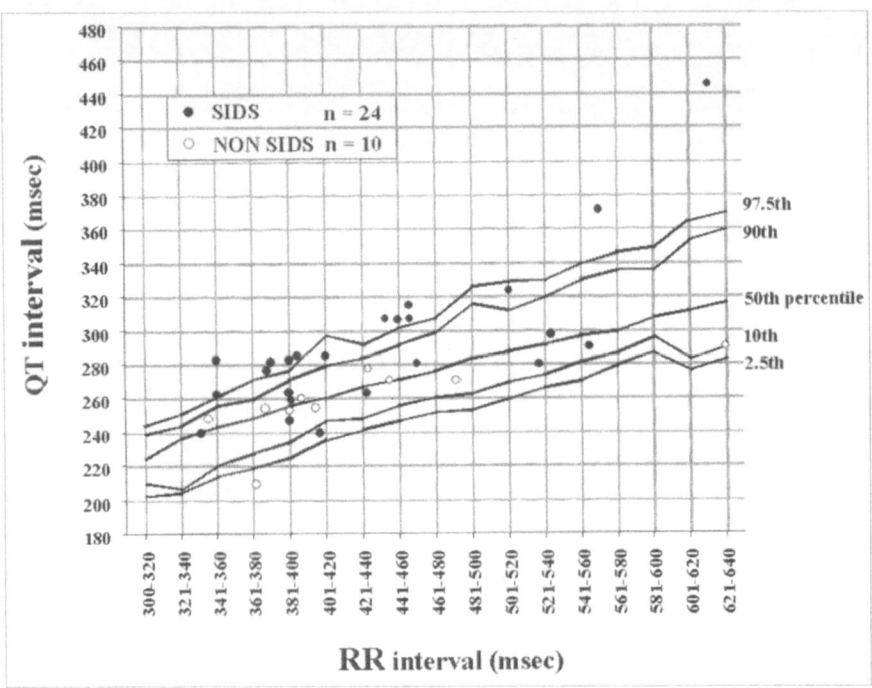

Fig. 2. Relation between QT interval and cardiac cycle length. Each *line* represents the percentile values of uncorrected QT intervals at the corresponding range of RR intervals. The *filled* and the *open* circles represent the individual values of QT_c of the SIDS victims and of the non-SIDS victims, respectively. (From [3], by permission)

Clinical Implications

Our article [3] ended by mentioning two rather obvious, but nonetheless potentially troublesome, clinical implications.

One was that the highly significant association between QT prolongation and occurrence of SIDS unavoidably raises the issue of the potential value of a routine neonatal ECG screening. The low incidence of SIDS in the general population (< 0.1%) forces a low predictive value for any factor associated with the event, and QT prolongation (1.5%) is no exception even though its relative risk of 41 is strikingly higher than any previously reported. Despite this limitation, a simple ECG screening might contribute to identify a portion of the infants at high risk for SIDS.

The second big issue is the management of the infants found to have a prolonged QT_c. Our study contained no data to justify new therapeutic recommendations; however, the association between prolonged QT interval and SIDS should allow some cautious speculation. The lethal arrhythmias favored by QT prolongation are usually triggered by sudden increases in sympathetic activity [12]. In the 1st year of life this may be often elicited by multiple conditions [2] including sudden noise, exposure to cold, REM sleep, apnea leading to a chemoceptive reflex, arousals, and, probably, the prone position. In LQTS, antiadrenergic interventions are quite successful [9, 13]. Data from almost 1000 LQTS families indicate that treatment with β-blockers has reduced mortality below 3% [9, 14]. This information is relevant to the prevention of SIDS in newborns with a prolonged QT interval. It also provides a ready therapy for those infants serendipitously identified by neonatal ECG screening as definitely affected by LQTS, and offers a valid option for the yet unproven but reasonable possibility of reducing risk in all neonates with a markedly prolonged QT interval.

The Molecular Link

Potential Causes for QT Prolongation in Infants

We established [3] that a prolonged QT interval increases the risk of SIDS. A major question, however, remained. Why should an infant have a QT prolongation? Which mechanisms would be involved? We have proposed three different mechanisms that might be involved in the genesis of QT interval prolongation in some newborns. The first is a developmental abnormality in cardiac sympathetic innervation [1]. The second is a de novo mutation in one of the LQTS genes. The third involves cases of LQTS with low penetrance [15].

The latter two possibilities, more easily testable, involve LQTS and some related concepts of genetics. LQTS is a familial disease, which may nonetheless present also "sporadic" cases (with no apparent familial involvement) and is characterized by QT prolongation and high risk of sudden death, usually under stressful conditions but also during sleep [9, 16]. LQTS has genetic heterogeneity, and LQTS genes located on chromosomes 3, 7, 11 and 21 have been identified [10]. A potential difficulty for linking LQTS to SIDS is that the latter is not a familial disease. Two important concepts are highly relevant here. The first is that among "sporadic" cases of LQTS, de novo (spontaneous) mutations have been found in the two genes, *HERG* and *KvLQT1*, which encode the potassium channels for I_{Kr} and I_{Ks}, two of the major repolarizing currents [10]. A de novo mutation, by definition, is not found among the parents. The second is represented by the demonstration of "low penetrance" in LQTS [15]. Penetrance is defined as the ratio between gene carriers and individuals showing the full phenotype of the disease. A low penetrance implies that clinical diagnosis is often inadequate and that many affected individuals may appear completely normal at clinical examination.

We have just obtained the evidence that the second of these three possibilities may indeed account for some cases of SIDS and thus explain prolongation of the QT interval in some SIDS victims with parents who have a completely normal QT interval.

Molecular Evidence

We recently reported a case which demonstrates that de novo mutations in LQTS genes may manifest as, and be indistinguishable from, classic cases of "near miss" for SIDS or as SIDS itself [4]. A 7-week old infant was found by his parents cyanotic, apneic, and pulseless. He was rushed to a nearby hospital while his father was attempting cardiopulmonary resuscitation; in the emergency room an ECG showed ventricular fibrillation. Thus, this infant presented as a typical "near-miss" for SIDS. After defibrillation, the ECG revealed a major QT prolongation (QT$_c$ 648 ms), LQTS was diagnosed and effective therapy was instituted by combining β-blockade and the sodium channel blocker mexiletine. A critical point is that the QT interval of both parents was normal, paternity being confirmed. Molecular screening of the infant identified a mutation on *SCN5A*, the cardiac sodium channel gene responsible for the LQT3 subtype of LQTS [10]. This disease-carrying mutation was not present in the mother nor in the father, thus establishing that this is a de novo mutation.

The documentation of ventricular fibrillation at arrival in the emergency room is quite important given the frequency of statements such as "*no one has recorded ventricular arrhythmias in infants at risk for SIDS*" [17]. Had the infant died – a certainty without cardioversion – the absence of an ECG and the normal QT interval of both parents would have ruled out any suspicions of LQTS and would have prompted the classic diagnosis of SIDS. Thus, infants who have similar de novo mutations involving one of the ionic channels controlling ventricular repolarization may have a prolonged QT interval at birth. Some of them may die from ventricular fibrillation already in utero, and thus become stillbirths, or during the first few months of life, when without an available ECG they would be labeled as SIDS victims. Others would probably begin to have syncopal episodes or nonfatal cardiac arrests during their childhood and would then be diagnosed as sporadic cases of LQTS.

The significance of this finding exceeds by far that commonly associated with a single case report because it represents "proof of concept" for the link between LQTS and SIDS. It does indeed provide the first unequivocal demonstration that a life-threatening event in infancy, with all the characteristics of SIDS or of a "near miss" for SIDS, can depend on a de novo mutation in one of LQTS genes, thus escaping recognition in the parents, and lead to sudden death due to ventricular fibrillation.

More recently, we obtained additional and perhaps even more important evidence of the link between SIDS and LQTS [5]. A 4-month old baby was found dead in her crib. After a negative autopsy, the diagnosis of SIDS was made. No ECG was available. Post-mortem molecular diagnosis identified a de novo mutation on *KCNQ1*, the gene responsible for LQT1 which is the most common genetic variant of LQTS. Importantly, the same mutation is present in one of the LQTS families followed at our center in Pavia. With normal parents and lack of an ECG of the victim no one could have suspected the presence of LQTS. Molecular screening has allowed us to provide the first evidence that an infant thought to have died of SIDS actually had LQTS.

These two cases should put to rest a controversy which has lasted more than 20 years. They provide definitive evidence for one of the mechanisms involved in SIDS, they support the concept of widespread neonatal ECG screening, and they indicate that at least this subset of infants at high risk of sudden infant death can be diagnosed early on and that their impending death probably be prevented.

References

1. Schwartz PJ (1976) Cardiac sympathetic innervation and the sudden infant death syndrome. A possible pathogenetic link. Am J Med 60:167-172
2. Schwartz PJ (1987) The quest for the mechanism of the sudden infant death syndrome. Doubts and progress. Circulation 75:677-683
3. Schwartz PJ, Stramba-Badiale M, Segantini A et al (1998) Prolongation of the QT interval and the sudden infant death syndrome. N Engl J Med 338:1709-1714
4. Schwartz PJ, Priori SG, Dumaine R et al (2000) A molecular link between the sudden infant death syndrome and the long QT syndrome. N Engl J Med 43:262-267
5. Schwartz PJ, Priori SG, Bloise R et al (2001) Molecular diagnosis in victims of sudden infant death syndrome. Medical and legal implications. Lancet (in press)
6. Schwartz PJ (1981) The sudden infant death syndrome. In: Scarpelli EM, Cosmi EV (eds) Reviews in perinatal medicine, vol 4. Raven Press, New York, pp 475-524
7. Schwartz PJ, Southall DP, Valdes-Dapena M (eds) (1988) The sudden infant death syndrome: cardiac and respiratory mechanisms and interventions. Ann NY Acad Sci, 533:474
8. NIH Grant HDO8796 1975/1978: Experimental reproduction of long QT syndrome and SIDS
9. Schwartz PJ, Priori SG, Napolitano C (2000) Long QT syndrome. In: Zipes DP, Jalife J, (eds) Cardiac electrophysiology: from cell to bedside, 3rd edn. Saunders, Philadelphia, pp 597-615
10. Priori SG, Barhanin J, Hauer RNW et al (1999) Genetic and molecular basis of cardiac arrhythmias: impact on clinical management. Parts I and II: Circulation 99:518-528, and Part III: Circulation 99:674-681; and Eur Heart J 20:174-195
11. Towbin JA, Friedman RA (1998) Prolongation of the QT interval and the sudden infant death syndrome. N Engl J Med 338:1760-1761
12. Schwartz PJ, Priori SG (1990) Sympathetic nervous system and cardiac arrhythmias. In: Zipes DP, Jalife J (eds) Cardiac electrophysiology: from cell to bedside. Saunders, Philadelphia, pp 330-343
13. Schwartz PJ, Locati EH, Moss AJ et al (1991) Left cardiac sympathetic denervation in the therapy of congenital long QT syndrome: a worldwide report. Circulation 84:503-511
14. Moss AJ, Zareba W, Hall WJ et al (2000) Effectiveness and limitations of β-blocker therapy in congenital long QT syndrome. Circulation 101:616-623
15. Priori SG, Napolitano C, Schwartz PJ (1999) Low penetrance in the long QT syndrome. Clinical impact. Circulation 99:529-533
16. Schwartz PJ, Priori SG, Spazzolini C et al (2001) Genotype-phenotype correlation in the long QT syndrome. Gene-specific triggers for life-threatening arrhythmias. Circulation 103:89-95
17. Guntheroth WG, Spiers PS (1999) Prolongation of the QT interval and the sudden infant death syndrome. Pediatrics 103:813-814

Brugada Sign: What Is the Prevalence in an Apparently Healthy Population?

A. Nava[1], B. Bauce[1], S. Cannas[2], A. Rampazzo[3] and B. Martini[2]

Introduction

The syndrome of right bundle branch block, ST elevation and sudden death, described in more than 350 international papers, was first reported in 1988-1989 by Italian scientists in the *Giornale Italiano di Cardiologia* [1, 2], in *Mises a Jour Cardiologiques* [3] and in the *American Heart Journal* [4] and by Aihara [5] in 1990. This syndrome was lately called world-wide, "Brugada syndrome" by the name of those who reported the same entity in 1992 [6].

The most fascinating feature of the syndrome is the ECG pattern, which is characterized by:

1. Different degrees of right bundle branch block and sometime left axis deviation and prolonged PR interval.
   The most popular ECG, published by Nava (Fig. 1), and now called Brugada's sign, shows a r' pattern in V1, quite similar to an incomplete right bundle branch block, followed by a coved ST elevation, initially called "early repolarization". Differently from a right bundle branch delay, there is not a late and slurred S wave in V6, and the vectorcardiographic terminal loop does not reach the beginning of QRS [3]. Late potentials often characterize this atypical conduction disturbance, where are absent in pure incomplete right bundle branch block. Late QRS depolarizations are recordable at the right ventricular outflow tract, coincident with r' wave and initial ST elevation [3]. This r' pattern is often incorrectly called a J wave [7], while the true J wave is that recorded in left lateral and inferior leads in vagotonia, which shows a notch in the descending portion of the QRS, often associated with a saddle-like ST elevation, so-called "early repolarization". A similar wave can be recorded, always in left lateral leads in severe hypothermia, brain damage and radical neck surgery.
2. ST segment elevation in V1-V3 (which can be an isolated pattern, according to some experience, not always confirmed), can be coved, saddle-like or

[1]Cattedra di Cardiologia, Università di Padova; [2]Unità Operativa di Cardiologia, Ospedale Boldrini, Thiene; [3]Dipartimento di Biologia, Università di Padova, Italy

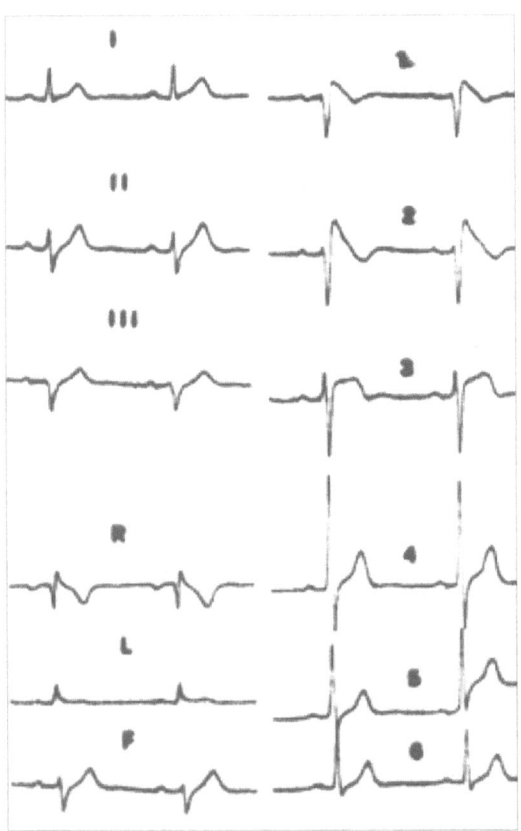

Fig. 1. The syndrome is a clinico-electrocardiographic association between sudden death, ventricular fibrillation and an ECG pattern of different degrees of RBBB and different-shaped ST segment elevation. This ECG is the typical ECG of the syndrome, and was published 4 years before the article of Brugada [3]. It shows an r' pattern in V1, and a coved ST elevation in the precordial leads. The patient is still alive, without an AICD, after an episode of resuscitated cardiac arrest 18 years ago

dome-shaped. In the first Brugada series, the ST elevation was described as persistent [6]. After the paper from Sumiyoshi [8], it was realised that in approximately 30% of patients this pattern may vary in different observations, and may be elicited by the Class 1C drugs flecainide, ajmaline, propaphenon, and pilsicainide.

The ECG discussed above may occasionally be recorded at the third intercostal space [9]. The ST elevation may, incidentally, occur only during arrhythmic events.

While the recording of isolated right bundle branch disturbance or of ST segment elevation is not especially rare, their association is quite unusual, according to 0.01-0.63% of the ECG traces in the normal population. The pathophysiologic mechanism underlying the ECG, as well as the pathologic substrate of the syndrome, have been extensively debated. A few authors insist on an organic substrate inducing a conduction disturbance and a depolarization abnormality [10-18], while the vast majority accept the theory of a functional disorder of repolarization not associated with any organic heart disease.

Recent Personal Experience

The first complete description that related ventricular fibrillation (VF) and juvenile sudden death in the presence of a peculiar ECG aspect characterized by right bundle branch block (RBBB) and ST segment elevation in the right precordial lead was published in 1989 [4]. Among patients described in this series, one was a male who died suddenly at the age of 32; 6 years before he had presented an episode of VF. After the sudden death of this patient, in whom right ventricular cardiomyopathy and major conduction disturbances were detected [4, 10, 11], the whole family was investigated and some asymptomatic members were found to show the same ECG features [19]. A genetic study is still in progress, searching for the presence of associated mutations in SCN5A, previously described in some patients presenting the same ECG pattern but without a cardiac pathology [20].

At the present time, the prevalence of the SCN5A mutation in patients with the syndrome is no more than 15%, despite initial enthusiasm [16, 20, 21]. These data could be explained by assuming that this syndrome is characterized by genetic heterogeneity or that the ECG criteria for the Brugada syndrome lead to overestimating the incidence of the disease.

We report additional data of a family, already published in 1996 [10], that has the longest follow-up in the literature (18 years) and that could lead to a better understanding of different features of the syndrome characterized by RBBB and ST segment elevation. The family comprises 47 subjects (27 males, 20 females, mean age 39 ± 17 years). All family members underwent the following study protocol: 12 lead ECG, signal-averaged ECG (SAECG), 24-h Holter ECG, 2D-echocardiogram.

Twelve patients presented an abnormal ECG: RBBB + ST segment elevation in V1-V2 in three and RBBB in nine. Seventeen showed the presence of late potentials at SAECG, four at all filters setting, 12 at 40-80 Hz, one at 80 Hz. Late potentials were present in all patients with ECG alterations. With regard to echocardiographic examination, 14 subjects presented right ventricular alterations (ventricular dilatation, kinetics alterations, trabecular thickening, high reflectability of the moderator band) consistent with the diagnosis of arrhythmogenic right ventricular cardiomyopathy. Holter ECG showed the presence of isolated ventricular premature beats (Lown 3), in two patients. Thus, our clinical study revealed pathologic findings in 17 patients (13 males, four females, mean age 42 ± 16 years), who were considered to be affected. Additional two subjects without clinical signs of the disease but able to transmit it to their progeny were considered healthy carriers. Anti-arrhythmic drug treatment was not undertaken in any of them.

Follow-up: the study began in 1982 (maximum follow-up 18 years, minimum 1 year, mean 8 years). In this period no subject had symptoms such as palpitations, dizziness or syncopal episodes, or died suddenly.

The lack of symptoms in all family members, except the one who had a ventricular fibrillation and later died suddenly, demonstrates that the clinical manifestation of this syndrome is different in each subject in the presence of the same cardiac disease.

The entire phenotype of the syndrome could be expressed by the presence of additional precipitating factors that could trigger the onset of a lethal arrhythmia. This assumption should stimulate many cautions when dealing with subjects in whom the isolated presence of a typical or similar ECG cannot be ascribed as the typical feature of the syndrome.

Discussion

It must be pointed out that there is no typical ECG of this syndrome, although the trace presented in Fig. 1 is the most popular. However, much confusion exists in the literature, with several papers discussing a "typical ECG", which is quite different from the syndrome [22-24]. An ECG pattern of RBBB + ST segment elevation has been detected by Namiki in 0.64% of 10 420 adults, by Hata in 0.2-0.005 of Japanese people, by Michaud in 0.02% of 32 641 ECGs, by Miyasaka in 0.7% of 12 929 ECGs, by Kan-Ichi in 0.41% of 34 520 ECGs, and by Hermida in 0.1-6% of 1000 ECGs (only 0.1% had a coved ST) [25-31].

The fortuitous discovery of the ECG pattern in a healthy individual does not fit with the diagnosis of the syndrome, as this includes a typical ECG (RBBB + ST elevation) pattern and a significant clinical event (sudden death), both with familial distribution.

This assumption has significant medico-legal implications. After excluding a familial involvement, a significant clinical history, an organic heart disease, and a normal non-invasive arrhythmologic study, at the present time it seems controversial to classify a healthy subject as affected by the syndrome, even in the occasional presence of a SCN5A abnormality or after Class 1C drugs challenge.

Brugada reported an 8% (total number not available) occurrence of major events in subjects with the ECG (but he did not specify which type of ECG) [32]. In a previous report [33] this percentage was 22%. Takenada, however, has recently described 12 individuals with a long benign follow-up [34]. This benign pattern was also described by Atarashi [27] in 34 asymptomatic individuals.

This benign behaviour is particularly relevant when an isolated ST elevation (usually saddle-like or dome-shaped), without right conduction disturbance, is detected in a young individual, particularly a sportsperson. A recent report [21] described an 89% prevalence of ST elevation > 1 mm in top-ranking male athletes and 72% in controls. No-one in this series, however, had the typical ECG pattern (Fig. 1), despite the author's misleading assumption that the trace 1B was similar.

Thus, it is demonstrated that many people have a normal ECG that shows some degree of RBB, or minor ST abnormality, and that a small percentage of healthy people (0.1%) can have the same standard ECG pattern as patients affected with the syndrome. Apart from the clinical background, from an electrical point of view, this last group might be differentiated by more frequently recordable late potentials at both signal-averaged ECG and intracavitary mapping, and prolonged HV interval. In this last group, in our opinion, an organic heart disease, which is not impossible to detect by careful investigation, must be excluded.

Autopsy data of patients with the syndrome have not been available until now; on the contrary, an accurate necropsy study and direct heart examination in the operating room have documented that a right ventricular cardiomyopathy underlies the syndrome [4, 10-18, 35]. Moreover, at least 30% of the patients reported in the medical literature had angiographic NMR, endomyocardial biopsy, and echocardiographic evidence of right heart disease [11, 12, 16, 36].

The histologic study of the conduction system in the first patient had demonstrated a fibrotic His and right bundle, and marked myocardial atrophy at the right ventricular outflow tract, consistent with a right ventricular cardiomyopathy [4, 10, 11, 17]. A genetic concordance between patients with the syndrome and the typical chromosome abnormalities of right ventricular cardiomyopathy has not been yet demonstrated, apart from one incidental report [34]. This would lead to the assumption that right ventricular cardiomyopathy and the right heart disease underlying the syndrome are not the same entity, but a gap in our present knowledge cannot be excluded. Other chromosomes, not yet identified, may be involved, and patients with the syndrome, due to demonstrated right ventricular cardiomyopathy, might have other associated genetic disorders, as reported in this paper.

According to histology [4, 10, 11], the ECG pattern might represent a double conduction defect: a septal defect, responsible for RBBB and HV prolongation, and a peripheral defect at the right ventricular outflow tract level, responsible for the ST elevation and for intracavitary or signal-averaged late potentials. So, in this theory, the ST elevation wave is an atypical late infundibular depolarization abnormality [16].

The evidence of a conduction defect underlying the syndrome is well documented in literature. A number of patients in the Brugada series [6, 18] also show prolonged PR interval, left axis deviation and prolonged HV interval. All these abnormalities are well consistent with a His-fascicular heart disease, which cannot be assumed as functional.

Going to the ST elevation, there is evidence that it represents a "strange" conduction disturbance at the infundibular level, possibly responsible for micro-re-entry arrhythmias. This ST wave can be detected, or is more pronounced, by recording the precordial leads at the third right intercostal space [10], with the exploring electrode just over the right ventricular outflow tract. Intracavitary recordings at the same level have clearly demonstrated late depolarization waves coincident with the ST elevation [3]. Body surface mapping has also confirmed a conduction disturbance in this structure [12, 16]. A demonstration of a late depolarization abnormality comes more easily from a study of late potentials [16, 20], which is so often positive in these patients, indicating again a conduction heart disease.

It must be remembered that in patients with ST elevation due to a true repolarization abnormality, such as early repolarization, myocardial infarction or pulmonary embolism, late potentials are always negative [16], because in these patients the ECG feature is linked to disturbed ionic currents and not to conduction delays.

Conclusions

This fascinating new syndrome needs more scientific studies and fewer journal speculations. In the nearly 350 published papers (according to the Brugada website), most of the conclusions derive from an incomplete analysis of the available data, with uncritical acceptance and repetition of only the most popular theory on the subject [11, 16].

Two syndromes, identical but different, have been reported, but recent papers give credit only to the functional base of the disease, while the papers documenting an organic origin are hardly accepted and can only be presented as abstracts [15, 20]. Wang, the co-discoverer of the SCN5A gene anomaly, recently wrote, "*Sometimes politics does penetrates basic sciences*", and this may be a sufficient explanation for what is happening. At the present time there is anatomical evidence only of organic heart disease underlying the syndrome, and electrocardiographic documentation of a conduction abnormalities both at His-fascicular and right ventricular outflow tract level, underlying the RBBB + ST elevation pattern. A genetically-based repolarization abnormality is a fascinating theory that lacks clinical and experimental demonstrations. The organic and sodium channel theories are not mutually exclusive, as evidentiated in our case, and this is what the scientist should demonstrate in the future.

We very much appreciate, however, all the different and contrasting opinions on this topic, and will give all our requested contribution to the knowledge of this disease without any mental limitation. We will welcome any new contribution to the study of the syndrome and will be glad if somebody in the future will discover, and correctly document, new theories. A third or a fourth true syndrome would be appreciated, but science fiction will not be encouraged. At the present time nobody knows the truth about this fatal disease, and the whole scientific community must humbly recognize this and work fairly only for the patient's health. As wisely said recently by Farré [24], the syndrome of sudden death, RBBB + ST elevation is a clinical-ECG association, and not a typical ECG abnormality, especially if it is induced by drugs like flecainide, which are not specific for any disease. We are not ethically allowed to investigate, treat or threaten asymptomatic subjects who have the ECG but not the syndrome, and who may occasionally present important symptoms like syncope, but of vagal origin.

"*We need other diagnostic tools rather than the ECG to make a correct diagnosis*" [22].

References

1. Nava A, Canciani B, Martini B et al (1988) La ripolarizzazione precoce nelle precordiali destre. Correlazioni ECG-VCG-elettrofisiologia. G Ital Cardiol (abstr) (Suppl 1)18:118
2. Martini B, Nava A, Buja GF et al (1988) Fibrillazione ventricolare in apparente assenza di cardiopatia. Descrizione di 6 casi. G Ital Cardiol (abstr) (Suppl 1)18:136

3. Nava A, Canciani B, Schiavinato ML, Martini B (1988) La repolarisation precoce dans le precordiales droites: trouble de la conduction intraventriculaire droite? Correlations de l'electrocardiographie-vectorcardiographie avec l'electro-physiologie. Mises J Cardiol 17:157-159

4. Martini B, Nava A, Thiene G et al (1989) Ventricular fibrillation without apparent heart disease: description of six case. Am Heart J 18:1203-1209

5. Aihara N, Ohe T, Kamakura S et al (1990) Clinical and electrophysiologic characteristics of idiopathic ventricular fibrillation. Shinzo 22 (Suppl 2):80

6. Brugada P, Brugada J (1992) Right bundle branch block, persistent ST segment elevation and sudden cardiac death: a distinct clinical and electrocardiographic syndrome. J Am Coll Cardiol 20:1391-1396

7. Yan GX, Antzelevitch C (1996) Cellular basis for the electrocardiographic J wave. Circulation 93:372-379

8. Sumiyoshi M, Nakata Y, Hisaoka T et al (1993) A case of idiopathic ventricular fibrillation with incomplete right bundle branch block and persistent ST segment elevation. Japan Heart J 34:661-666

9. Naccarella F, Coluccini M, Gatti M et al (1999) Familial distribution of the Brugada-Martini syndrome. Personal observations of nine families who underwent clinical evaluation and genetic screening. Mediterr J Pacing Electrophysiol 1:31-38

10. Corrado D, Nava A, Buja GF, Martini B (1996) Familial cardiomyopathy underlies syndrome of right bundle branch block, ST segment elevation and sudden death. J Am Coll Cardiol 27:443-448

11. Martini B, Corrado D, Nava A, Thiene G (1997) Syndrome of right bundle branch block, ST segment elevation and sudden death. Evidence of an organic substrate. In: Nava A, Rossi L, Thiene G (eds) Arrhythmogenic right ventricular cardiomyopathy/dysplasia. Elsevier, Amsterdam, pp 438-453

12. Martini B, Nava A, Ruzza L et al (1999) La sindrome "Morte improvvisa giovanile, blocco di branca destra e sopraslivellamento del tratto ST". G Ital Aritmol Cardiostim 2:157-77

13. Tada HT, Aihara N, Ohe T et al (1998) Arrhythmogenic right ventricular cardiomyopathy underlies syndrome of right bundle branch block, ST-segment elevation, and sudden death. Am J Cardiol 81:519-522

14. Kirschner RH, Echner FAO, Baron RC (1986) The cardiac pathology of sudden unexplained nocturnal death in southeast Asian refugees. J Am Med Assoc 256:2700-2705

15. Martini B, Nava A, Thiene G, Corrado D (2000) Right bundle branch block, ST-segment elevation, and sudden death. Circulation 101:176

16. Martini B, Cannas S, Ruzza L (2000) The syndrome of right bundle branch block, ST segment elevation and sudden death: Nava-Martini and/or Brugada syndrome. In: Adornato E. (ed) Cardiac arrhythmias: how to improve the reality in the third millennium? Luigi Pozzi, Rome, pp 206-219

17. Corrado D, Basso C, Buja GF et al (2001) Right bundle branch block, right precordial ST-segment elevation, and sudden death in young people. Circulation 103:710-717

18. Aligns M, Wilde A (1999) Brugada syndrome: clinical data and suggested pathophysiological mechanisms. Circulation 99:666-673

19. Nava A, Bauce B, Rampazzo A (1999) Further evidence that "Brugada syndrome" can be due to arrhythmogenic right ventricular cardiomyopathy with disease locus in chromosome 14q24.4. G Ital Cardiol 29 (Suppl 5):366-369

20. Chen Q, Kirsch GE, Zhang D et al (1998) Genetic basis and molecular mechanisms for idiopathic ventricular fibrillation. Nature 392:293-296

21. Priori SG, Napolitano C, Gasparini M et al (2000) Clinical heterogeneity of right bundle branch block and ST-segment elevation syndrome. Circulation 102:2509-2515

22. Martini B, Nava A, Cannas S (2000) There is not a typical ECG pattern for the syndrome of sudden death, RBBB and ST elevation. (rapid response) Heart, August. Electronic pages

23. Bianco M, Bria A, Gianfelici A et al (2001) Does early repolarization in the athlete have analogies with the Brugada syndrome? Eur Heart J 22:504-510

24. Farré J (2000) The Brugada syndrome: do we need more than 12-lead ECG? Eur Heart J 21:264-265

25. Namiki T, Ogura T, Kuwabara Y et al (1995) Five-year mortality and clinical characteristics of adult subjects with right bundle branch block with ST elevation. Circulation 92(abstr):159

26. Hata Y, Chiba N, Hotta K et al (1997) Incidence and clinical significance of right bundle branch block and ST segment elevation in V1-V3 in 6-18 year-old school children in Japan. Pacing Clin Electrophysiol 20(abstr):2310

27. Atarashi H, Ogawa S, Harumi K et al (1996) Characteristic of patients with right bundle branch block and ST-segment elevation in right precordial leads. Am J Cardiol 78:581-583

28. Michaud G (2000) Incidence of electrocardiographic finding of right bundle branch block and ST elevation in asymptomatic patients. Circulation 102 (Suppl II):584

29. Miyasaka Y (2000) Prevalence and mortality of right bundle branch block and right precordial ST-Segment elevation (Brugada type ECG) in a general population. Circulation 102 (Suppl II):676

30. Kan-Ichi F (2000) Incidence of asymptomatic Brugada syndrome among middle to high-aged subjects: an exhaustive investigation of local residents in Japan. Circulation 102 (Suppl II):676

31. Hermida JS, Lemoine JL, Anoun FB et al (2000) Prevalence of the Brugada syndrome in apparently healthy population. Am J Cardiol 86:91-94

32. Brugada J, Brugada R, Brugada P (2001) Asymptomatic patients with a Brugada electrocardiogram: are they at risk? J Cardiovasc Electrophysiol 12:7-8

33. Brugada J, Brugada R, Brugada P (1998) Right bundle branch block and ST-segment elevation in leads V1-V3. A marker for sudden death in patients without demonstrable heart disease. Circulation 97:457-460

34. Takenada S, Fukushima K, Hisamatsu K et al (2001) Relatively benign clinical course in asymptomatic patients with Brugada-type electrocardiogram without family history of sudden death. J Cardiovasc Electrophysiol 12:2-6

35. Nava Martini Syndrome:
http://www.angelfire.com/mb/bortolomartini/STSegmentElevation.html

36. Yan GX, Antzelevitch C (1999) Cellular basis for the Brugada syndrome and other mechanism of arrhythmogenesis associated with ST segment elevation. Circulation 100:1660-1666

Asymptomatic Patients with Brugada Syndrome: Does the Risk of Sudden Death Justify ICD Implantation?

S. FAVALE AND F. NACCI

Brugada syndrome is an arrhythmogenic clinical and electrocardiographic entity consisting of syncope and/or sudden death associated with a typical electrocardiographic pattern in sinus rhythm, characterized by aspects of QRS such as a right bundle-branch block and ST elevation at V1 and V3, but with no structural heart disease. Arrhythmias include polymorphous ventricular tachycardia or ventricular fibrillation, which may cease spontaneously [1].

Nademanee et al. demonstrated a recurrence of potentially lethal tachyarrhythmic events in 62% of symptomatic patients with typical ECG after a mean follow-up period of 11.8 ± 7 months [2]. In similar groups of subjects 34% incidence was reported at a mean follow-up of 37 ± 31 months [3], 33% at a follow-up of 81 ± 53 months [4], and 16% at a follow-up of 34 ± 36 months [5]. These data, although varied, leave no doubt as to the therapeutic choice of automatic defibrillator implantation for secondary prevention in this group of subjects.

Moreover, there are subjects with a typical ECG who are totally asymptomatic and identified only by chance during familial screening following a sudden death event at a young age. In 1996 a prospective study of 63 subjects with a typical baseline ECG, 34 of whom were asymptomatic (32 male, mean age 52 ± 10 years) was published [6]. Of these, one patient (3%) had had a sudden death in the family, and none underwent intracavitary electrophysiological study. Thirty-three subjects (97%) were not treated and one (3%) was treated with dysopiramide. No patient presented symptoms at a mean follow-up of 452 ± 75 days.

Eleven asymptomatic patients (11 male, mean age 40.5 ± 9.6 years) with typical ECG and without a previous family history of sudden death, eight of whom underwent intracavitary electrophysiological study (one had ventricular fibrillation induced) did not present symptoms during follow-up (42.5 ± 21.6 months) [7].

In another prospective analysis of 63 subjects (56 male, mean age 38 ± 17 years) with typical baseline ECG, 22 of whom were asymptomatic, 9 subjects (41%) reported familial sudden death [3]. Fourteen subjects underwent intra-

Interventional Arrhythmology Unit, Cardiosurgery Section, Department of Emergency and Organ Transplant, University of Bari, Italy

cavitary electrophysiological study following a nonuniform stimulation protocol, with a maximum of 3 extrastimuli in at least one site on the right ventricle. In 12 subjects (86%) polymorphous, nonsustained ventricular tachycardia of more than 10 s or ventricular fibrillation was induced. Eleven subjects (50%) had no further treatment, 3 (14%) were given drug therapy (β-blockers and/or amiodarone), and 8 (36%) underwent automatic defibrillator implantation. At a follow-up of 27 ± 32 months, 6 subjects (27%) reported a sudden death event (aborted), 4 of whom had a family history of sudden death [8]. In this study, familial sudden death and inducibility of ventricular tachyarrhythmias were not identified as predictive factors for sudden death in the pooled symptomatic and asymptomatic groups. Moreover, the authors proposed automatic defibrillator implantation in asymptomatic subjects with familial sudden death and/or inducibility of ventricular tachyarrhythmias, and close clinical follow-up for asymptomatic subjects with no familial history of sudden death or inducibility of ventricular tachyarrhythmias.

Recently, a prospective study [5] of 60 subjects from 52 families with a typical ECG either at baseline or after drug testing identified 30 asymptomatic subjects (25 male, mean age 42 ± 14 years). Eleven families (21%) reported episodes of sudden death. The distribution of familial sudden death between symptomatic and asymptomatic patients was not reported. Nineteen asymptomatic subjects underwent intracavitary electrophysiological studies, following a nonuniform stimulation protocol. In 13 subjects (68%) polymorphous sustained ventricular tachycardia or ventricular fibrillation was induced, with a single extrastimulus in 2 cases, double extrastimulus in 8, and triple extrastimulus in 3 cases. Twenty-six subjects (86%) were not treated, 2 subjects (7%) were treated with sotalol, and 2 had automatic defibrillator implantation. At a mean follow-up of 30 ± 43 months no patient presented potentially lethal ventricular tachyarrhythmias. In the two automatic defibrillator recipients the device reported episodes of nonsustained ventricular tachycardias. The authors proposed automatic defibrillator implantation in asymptomatic subjects with a history of familial sudden death and loop-recorder implantation in nonfamilial subjects. For this latter group, training of family members in cardiopulmonary resuscitation and the use of an external defibrillator was also proposed.

In subjects with other genetically determined heart diseases which also include sudden death as a possible first clinical event, a family history of sudden death was identified as a predictive risk factor. This simple clinical datum, as a possible predictive factor of sudden death events, merits more detailed study.

More recently, 25 families with Brugada syndrome, consisting of 334 family members (192 male, aged between 6 months and 92 years, mean age 52 ± 27 years), were evaluated [9]. Brugada syndrome patients were identified on the basis of the typical ECG present at baseline or after administration of flecainide, ajmaline, or procainamide, in the absence of other heart diseases. Genetic analysis was not available and the authors presumed a 100% correlation between the typical ECG and the disease genotype. Eighteen families were found to be symptomatic as one or more members affected by the disease had had an aborted sudden death event (of these 7 families also had a previous history of sudden death). Seven families, however, were asymptomatic as no member affected by the disease had had a sudden death event (of these only 1 family had a previous history of sudden death). The study evaluated the incidence of sudden death linked and sudden death not linked to Brugada syndrome, and sudden death due to unclear causes but unlikely to be linked to the syndrome. Sudden death was considered as linked to the disease if caused by polymorphous ventricular tachycardia or occurring during sleep. Fifty of the 334 subjects studied were identified as having the syndrome. During the follow-up period (of an unknown length), 42 subjects had a sudden death event, 24 (57%) of which were linked to Brugada syndrome. In 7 of the 8 families who had a history of sudden death, both symptomatic and asymptomatic, at least 1 death linked to the syndrome was observed. On the other hand, in 5 of the 17 families without a history of sudden death, whether they were symptomatic or not, at least 1 death was linked to the syndrome. Therefore, in this study no statistically significant difference was observed in the incidence of sudden death linked to Brugada syndrome between families with a history of sudden death and those without.

A subgroup of asymptomatic patients is that of gene carriers. In a prospective study [10], testing of flecainide was negative in 80% of asymptomatic subjects with normal baseline ECG and who were carriers of an anomaly of the SCN5A gene [11, 12]. In this subgroup the risk of sudden death is unknown. Genetic analysis is not generally used to define the prognosis and treatment of subjects with Brugada syndrome. However, understanding of the genetic aspect of the disease is progressing rapidly. Various mutations of the SCN5A gene have already been identified; moreover, there are asymptomatic subjects with a typical Brugada syndrome ECG in whom no mutation of this gene has been identified. It is, therefore, probable that mutation of other genes can be a substrate of the disease [13]. It is also possible that specific genetic mutations are associated with a particularly high risk of potentially lethal arrhythmic events. The discovery of the whole spectrum of mutations underlying the syndrome and each individual association between a specific alteration of the function of the Na^+ channel and a specific clinical phenotype will probably permit future identification of which asymptomatic subjects to treat as well as the use of more specific drug or genetic therapy.

The therapeutic approach to asymptomatic patients with a typical ECG at baseline or after drug testing cannot be based on any reassuring evidence as in these cases no single clinical or electrophysiological predictive factor for future occurrence of sudden death has been identified. There are, however, well-known data on which to base any treatment decision, although these are not supported by large, randomized, prospective studies.

In subjects with Brugada syndrome an arrhythmic first event usually occurs at an age between 2 and 77 years, peaking around 40 years of age [2-5]. Therefore, the patients are usually young, disease-free, and at the prime of their personal and professional life. Moreover, sudden death resulted the first clinical event in 62% [3] and 18% [5] of subjects evaluated for aborted sudden death.

Arrhythmic events are more common at night and during sleep. In 12 subjects with Brugada syndrome who were symptomatic for aborted sudden death and underwent automatic defibrillator implantation [14], the recording of the intracavitary electrograms permitted the identification of the circadian rhythm of the recurring ventricular tachyarrhythmias; 93.3% of potentially lethal events occurred at night (between 6 p.m. and 6 a.m.) and 86.7% during sleep.

In the affected subjects the ECG varies with time, as, probably, does the degree of electrical stability of the myocardium, since both are expressions of the same cellular and ionic mechanisms, only partially understood to date [15]. For example, sympathetic stimulation reduces the ST elevation; conversely, vagal stimulation and administration of class Ia, Ic, and III antiarrhythmic drugs increases it. Effort has a variable effect on the entity of the ST elevation: in some subjects it produces a decrease, in others an increase. This is probably the reason why induction of sustained ventricular tachyarrhythmias has a low positive and negative predictive power. It follows that the administration of cardiac and noncardiac drugs, electrolytic imbalances, and myocardial ischemia can alter an initially stable equilibrium.

The prognosis totally depends on efficient prevention of recurring, potentially lethal arrhythmias. In this case amiodarone is not effective [3] and class Ic drugs and β-blockers [16] may even increase the risk.

Experimental evidence shows that I_{to} current is not only responsible for the typical ECG pattern of patients with Brugada syndrome, but also for the phase 2 re-entry which causes ventricular tachyarrhythmias in these subjects [17]. These experimental data and limited clinical data [18] suggest that, due to its $I(to)$ current blocking effect, quinidine may be a more effective drug in protecting these subjects from sudden death.

The automatic defibrillator is considered a totally safe and efficient therapy for the prevention of ventricular tachyarrhythmias and sudden death, given the absence of mortality reported in patients with Brugada syndrome implanted with one [2, 3, 5]. However, in subjects with asymptomatic Brugada syndrome, automatic defibrillator implantation may be a costly procedure for an as yet unclearly defined risk. The problem of cost is even more important in regions such as South-East Asia, where the highest incidence of the syndrome is observed and health spending is greatly below that of Western countries.

Given the economic analysis of subjects enrolled in the CIDS study [19], the use of less expensive prophylactic implantable cardioverter-defibrillator with a battery capacity which would guarantee sufficient recording of data could be a reasonable solution until future large-scale trials define the risk of sudden death in asymptomatic subjects.

In conclusion, subjects who are asymptomatic with a typical Brugada syndrome ECG are usually young (mean age 40 years) and have a relatively high incidence of sudden death (up to 10% a year) – which may be the first clinical event. A circadian pattern with events usually occurring at night leads to a poor survival rate.

Moreover, the automatic defibrillator has completely eradicated sudden death while antiarrhythmic drugs have proved to be ineffective, and therefore research into efficacious drugs without the back-up of an automatic defibrillator is no longer ethically possible. The automatic defibrillator has become so small as to allow a very low risk of adverse events. Moreover, due to the more recent discriminatory algorithms which avoid inappropriate interventions, a good quality of life is also possible. The high cost of automatic defibrillators is not an insurmontable limitation given the small population suitable to receive them, and in this phase of the research the ability to record arrhythmic events as they occur is mandatory: it is the only means by which to achieve prospective evaluation for better clarification of the natural history of asymptomatic subjects with a typical ECG of Brugada syndrome, thus avoiding young victims. However, ethical reasons, the low rate of prevalence of the disease in the general population, and the relatively low rate of event occurrence make it difficult to perform a prospective and randomized study to compare the therapeutic efficacy of the implantable cardioverter-defibrillator and drugs.

References

1. Brugada P, Brugada J (1992) Right bundle branch block, persistent ST segment elevation and sudden cardiac death. J Am Coll Cardiol 20:1391-1396
2. Nademanee K, Veerakul G, Nimmannit S et al (1997) Arrhythmogenic marker for the sudden unexplained death syndrome in Thai men. Circulation 96:2595-2600
3. Brugada J, Brugada R, Brugada P (1998) Right bundle branch block, persistent ST segment elevation and sudden cardiac death. Circulation 97:457-460
4. Remme CA, Wever EFD, Wilde AAM et al (2001) Diagnosis and long term follow up of the Brugada syndrome in patients with idiopathic ventricular fibrillation. Eur Heart J 22:400-409
5. Priori SG, Napolitano C, Gasparini M et al (2000) Clinical and genetic heterogeneity of right bundle branch block and ST-segment elevation syndrome. A prospective evaluation of 52 families. Circulation 102:2509-2515
6. Atarashi H, Ogawa S, Harumi K (1996) Characteristics of patients with right bundle branch block and ST-segment elevation in right precordial leads. Am J Cardiol 78:581-583
7. Takenaka S, Kusano KF, Hisamatsu K et al (2001) Relatively benign clinical course in asymptomatic patients with Brugada-syndrome without family history of sudden death. J Cardiovasc Electrophysiol 12:108-111
8. Brugada J, Brugada P, Brugada R (1999) The syndrome of right bundle branch block, ST segment elevation in V1 to V3 and sudden death – the Brugada syndrome. Europace 1:156-166
9. Brugada P, Brugada R, Brugada J (2000) Sudden death in patients and relatives with the syndrome of right bundle branch block, persistent, ST segment elevation in the precordial leads V1 to V3 and sudden death. Eur Heart J 21:321-326
10. Priori SG, Napolitano C, Terrini L et al (1999) Incomplete penetrance and variable response to sodium channel blockade in Brugada syndrome. Eur Heart J 20[Suppl]:465 (abstr)
11. Chen Q, Kirsch GE, Zhang D et al (1998) Genetic basis and molecular mechanism for idiopathic ventricular fibrillation. Nature 392:293-296
12. Alshinawi C, Mannens M, Wilde A (1998) Mutations in the human cardiac sodium channel gene (SCN5A) in patients with Brugada syndrome. Eur Heart J 19:78 (abstr)

13. Guicheney P, Descheces I, Nicolas L et al (1999) Novel mutations in the cardiac Na$^+$ channel alpha subunit gene (SCN 5A) in patients with Brugada syndrome. Eur Heart J 20[Suppl]:465 (abstr)
14. Matsuo K, KuritaT, Inagaki M et al (1999) The circadian pattern of the development of ventricular fibrillation in patients with Brugada syndrome. Eur Heart J 20:465-470
15. Miyazaki T, Mitamura H, Miyoshi S et al (1996) Autonomic and antiarrhythmic drug modulation of ST segment elevation in patients with Brugada syndrome. J Am Coll Cardiol 27:1061-1070
16. Kasanuki H, Ohnishi S, Ohtuka M et al (1997) Idiopathic ventricular fibrillation induced with vagal activity in patients without obvious heart disease. Circulation 95:2277-2285
17. Antzelevitch C (1998) The Brugada syndrome. J Cardiovasc Electrophysiol 9:513-516
18. Belhassen B, Viskin S, Fish R et al (1999) Effects of electrophysiologic-guided therapy with class IA antiarrhythmic drugs on the long term outcome of patients with idiopathic ventricular fibrillation with or without the Brugada syndrome. J Cardiovasc Electrophysiol 10:1301-1312
19. Zipes DP (2001) Implantable cardioverter defibrillator: a Volkswagen or a Rolls Royce. How much will we pay to save a life? Circulation 103:1372-1374

Will the Spectrum of Ion Channel Diseases Increase Further in the Near Future?

C. Napolitano and S.G. Priori

Ten years ago Keating and co-workers [1] paved the way to an understanding of the genetic defects causing inherited arrhythmogenic disorders in the structurally normal heart. Since then, our knowledge has grown remarkably and cardiologists have become progressively more interested in molecular genetics. They have rapidly realized that genetic analysis, gene-specific treatments, and gene-based risk stratification algorithms are entering clinical cardiology and will influence clinical practice in the next years. In the pregenetic era, clinical conditions such as long QT syndrome, Brugada syndrome, progressive cardiac conduction defect, and catecholaminergic polymorphic ventricular tachycardia were quite extensively characterized at the clinical level, but until recently only speculation was possible concerning their pathophysiologic background. In the present paper we will briefly summarize current knowledge and the likely future developments relating to the inherited arrhythmogenic disorders and in particular the ion channel diseases.

Primary Electrical Disorders Associated with Ventricular Arrhythmias

Long QT Syndrome

In the early 1960s Romano and Ward [2, 3] independently described a disease characterized by QT prolongation, abnormal T wave morphology, and fatal cardiac arrhythmias transmitted as an autosomal dominant trait (Romano-Ward syndrome, RWS). A similar phenotype associated with neurosensorial deafness and autosomal recessive inheritance had been described few years earlier by Jervell and Lange-Nielsen (Jervell and Lange-Nielsen syndrome, JLNS) [4]. Syncope is the typical symptom of long QT syndrome, and its occurrence is very often associated with conditions of physical or emotional stress, although in a smaller subset of individuals cardiac events occur at rest [5].

Molecular Cardiology Laboratories, IRCCS Fondazione Salvatore Maugeri, Pavia, Italy

As of today five genes and six loci have been implicated in the genesis of long QT syndrome. Linkage analysis applied to large kindred allowed the mapping of four long QT syndrome loci on chromosomes 11 [1], 3 and 7 [6], and 4 [7]. The gene on chromosome 11 (LQT1) is *KCNQ1* [8], on chromosome 7 (LQT2) it is *HERG*, and on chromosome 3 (LQT3) it is *SCN5A* [9, 10]. Two additional genes have been more recently identified on chromosome 22, *KCNE1* and *KCNE2* [11, 12], but they appear to account for only a small percentage of patients [13]. All these genes encode for ionic channel subunits critical for the physiological excitability of cardiac myocytes.

Genotype-Phenotype correlation

In the last few years a number of genotype-phenotype correlation studies have been performed in the attempt to provide novel indicators for risk stratification. The analysis of the electrocardiographic patterns revealed gene-specific alterations of the ST-T segment [14], and different behavior of QT interval adaptation to changes in heart rate, with increased shortening at high frequency among LQT3 patients [15] and reduced adaptation among LQT1 patients [16]. Schwartz et al. [17] have recently provided evidence that *KCNQ1* mutations increase the risk of cardiac events during physical or emotional stress. Analysis of event-free survival by genotype shows that LQT3 patients have fewer events but with higher fatality [18].

Prediction of the severity of clinical manifestation from in vitro studies is not possible [19] since even the same mutation may cause variable severity of clinical manifestations [20]; however, it has been suggested that the position of a mutation may allow some level of prediction of the phenotype. For example, mutations located in the carboxy terminus of *KCNQ1* [21] are mostly benign and associated with a mild clinical phenotype.

Finally, the variable penetrance of long QT syndrome mutations [22] and the evidence that up to 6% of genotyped long QT syndrome probands may in fact carry two independently inherited genetic defects [23, 24] introduce additional complexity and limit the possibility of predicting prognosis in the individual patient.

Brugada Syndrome

In 1992 Brugada et al. [25] described a novel clinical entity characterized by ST segment elevation in right precordial leads (V1 to V3), incomplete or complete right bundle branch block, and susceptibility to develop ventricular tachyarrhythmias. This disease is now frequently called "Brugada syndrome". Familial occurrence has been described with an autosomal dominant pattern of inheritance. The age at onset of clinical manifestations is the third or fourth decade of life, and the cardiac events typically occur during sleep or at rest [25]. Malignant forms with earlier onset and even with neonatal manifestations have been reported [26].

The diagnostic electrocardiographic pattern is intermittently present in affected individuals. Pharmacological challenge with class I antiarrhythmic drugs, namely, ajmaline, flecainide, and procainamide, may unmask the typical ECG pattern in affected patients and has been proposed as a diagnostic test in patients with borderline ECGs [27].

In 1998 the molecular basis of Brugada syndrome was identified and the disease demonstrated to be allelic to the long QT syndrome (LQT3) [28]. However, data from our laboratory as well as others suggest that no more than 20%-25% of patients with Brugada syndrome carry *SCN5A* mutations, indicating that the disease is genetically heterogeneous.

The overlapping phenotypes of long QT syndrome 3 (LQT3) and Brugada syndrome were reported by Bezzina et al. [29], who described the simultaneous presence of QT prolongation and ST segment elevation in a family where a *SCN5A* mutation (InsD1795) was present. Subsequently we demonstrated that ST segment elevation may be induced in LQT3 patients by administration of intravenous flecainide [30], suggesting that the response to this drug is similar in the two diseases, which further supports the existence of clinical overlapping.

Catecholaminergic Polymorphic Ventricular Tachycardia

Coumel et al. [31] and Leenhardt et al. [32] described a typical pattern of ventricular arrhythmias manifesting in children and young adults, characterized by polymorphic tachyarrhythmias often showing a typical bidirectional pattern. In these patients arrhythmias are precipitated by stress or emotion: patients have a normal ECG, a normal QT interval, and no structural abnormalities of the right and the left ventricle. Familial occurrence of the disease was noted in approximately 30% of cases described by Leenhardt et al. [32] and an autosomal dominant pattern of inheritance was suggested. The condition has since been referred to as "catecholaminergic polymorphic ventricular tachycardia" (CPVT). Based on the typical pattern of arrhythmias and the primary pathogenetic role of the adrenergic nervous system, we hypothesized that genes encoding proteins responsible for intracellular calcium handling were likely candidates for this genetic disorder. In 1999 Swan et al. mapped the locus of CPVT to the chromosomal locus 1q42-q43 in two families [33]. This region contains the gene encoding for the human cardiac ryanodine receptor (hRyR2) [34], the key protein involved in calcium release from the sarcoplasmic reticulum. We therefore decided to perform molecular screening on the conding region of the hRyR2 gene after having determined its genomic structure. This genetic analysis allowed the identification of four different hRyR2 mutations in families presenting with a clinical diagnosis of CPVT, thus demonstrating that hRyR2 is the gene for catecholaminergic ventricular tachycardia [35].

Progressive Cardiac Conduction Defect

Progressive cardiac conduction defect (PCCD), also called Lenegre-Lev disease [36, 37], is a cardiac conduction defect characterized by progressive impairment of intracardiac conduction. In the early stages the diagnosis of the disease is mainly electrocardiographic; when complete atrioventricular (AV) block develops, patients manifest syncope and even sudden death. PCCD is considered a degenerative disorder of the conduction system histologically characterized by focal sclerosis and is one of the major reasons for pacemaker implantation.

Familial occurrence of conduction disturbances of the heart leading to complete AV block have been described [38, 39]. Because of the heterogeneous clinical manifestation and the variable penetrance, it is difficult to assess whether the families reported by different authors have a single disease (caused by a single genetic abnormality) or represent a heterogeneous group of conduction disturbances.

In 1999, Schott et al. [40] described two families with conduction defects and identified in both an *SCN5A* gene mutation. This gene has been previously implicated in long QT syndrome (LQT3) and Brugada syndrome (see above). Thus, according to Schott et al., PCCD is allelic to LQT3 and Brugada syndrome. This finding is supported by a more recent study by the same group reporting an *SCN5A* mutation (G514C) associated with "conduction defect in five families" [41]. Biophysical analysis of the in vitro effects of this mutation and computational evaluation in an action potential computer simulation model were consistent with selective slowing of myocardial conduction without the typical abnormalities observed in the "classical" long QT syndrome and Brugada syndrome *SCN5A* mutations. Overall, these findings are puzzling and stimulating at the same time. Particularly, the phenotypic characterization of PCCD families is still incomplete since only few cases associated with *SCN5A* mutations have been reported. Moreover, it has to be pointed out that Brugada syndrome is frequently associated with prolonged HV interval at electrophysiologic evaluation. It is intriguing to speculate that these families may carry a form of Brugada syndrome.

Will the Spectrum of Ion Channel Diseases Increase Further in the Future Near?

Despite the remarkable advance achieved in the last few years by the application of molecular genetics to the field of inherited ion channel diseases, many unresolved issues still remain. All the diseases so far identified are characterized by a high degree of genetic heterogeneity, and it is common experience of all the centers that perform mutational screening that only a fraction (from 20%-25% for Brugada syndrome to 55%-60% for long QT syndrome) of the clinically affected patients may be successfully genotyped. Therefore, one of the primary endpoints will be identification of the remaining genes for these diseases. Research in this field will focus primarily on the identification and screening of candidate genes, which will presumably be represented by other ion channel coding genes.

The gene hunting process will also have to pursue identification of the molecular bases of diseases that are still of unknown origin, such as the short-coupled variant of torsade de pointes [42] or to finding the gene for diseases where so far only a chromosomal locus has been identified. This latter is the case of familial atrial fibrillation [43] and of familial AV block locus on chromosome 19 [44].

An additional important point which deserves extensive evaluation is the study of the so-called "modifier factors", i.e. those genetic or epigenetic variables that, given a specific genetic substrate, may play a role in the modulation of the clinical phenotype. It is a common experience for the clinical cardiologist that the manifestation of these diseases may be extremely different even among patients carrying the same genetic defect. The identification of such modulating factors will give crucial information for the identification of the patient at higher risk of life-threatening events.

In summary, several pieces of information are still needed before it will be possible to reach a comprehensive understanding of the whole picture of ion channel diseases and to derive the full clinical benefit from the genetic knowledge. Only through active collaboration between clinical cardiologists and basic scientists will it be possible to acquire and achieve these targets, and ultimately to improve the quality of our daily clinical practice.

References

1. Keating MT, Atkinson D, Dunn C et al (1991) Linkage of a cardiac arrhythmia, the long QT syndrome, and the Harvey ras-1 gene. Science 252:704-706
2. Romano C, Gemme G, Pongiglione R (1963) Aritmie cardiache rare in età pediatrica. Clin Pediatr 45:656-657
3. Ward DC (1964) New familial cardiac syndrome in children. J Irish Med Assoc 54:103
4. Jervell A, Lange-Nielsen F (1957) Congenital deaf mutism, functional heart disease with prolongation of the QT interval and sudden death. Am Heart J 54:59-61
5. Schwartz PJ, Priori SG, Napolitano C (2000) The Long QT Syndrome. In: Zipes DP, Jalife J (eds) Cardiac electrophysiology: From cell to bedside. Saunders, Philadelphia pp 597-615
6. Jiang C, Atkinson D, Towbin JA et al (1994) Two long QT syndrome loci map to chromosomes 3 and 7 with evidence for further heterogeneity. Nat Genet 8:141-147
7. Schott JJ, Charpentier F, Peltier S et al (1995) Mapping of a gene for long QT syndrome to chromosome 4q25-27. Am J Hum Genet 57:1114-1122
8. Wang Q, Curran ME, Splawski I et al (1996) Positional cloning of a novel potassium channel gene: KVLQT1 mutations cause cardiac arrhythmias. Nat Genet 12:17-23
9. Curran ME, Splawski I, Timothy KW et al (1995) A molecular basis for cardiac arrhythmia: HERG mutations cause long QT syndrome. Cell 80:795-803
10. Wang Q, Shen J, Splawski I et al (1995) SCN5A mutations associated with an inherited cardiac arrhythmia, long QT syndrome. Cell 80:805-811
11. Splawski I, Tristani-Firouzi M, Lehmann MH et al (1997) Mutations in the hminK gene cause long QT syndrome and suppress IKs function. Nat Genet 17:338-340
12. Abbott GW, Sesti F, Splawski I et al (1999) MiRP1 forms IKr potassium channels with HERG and is associated with cardiac arrhythmia. Cell 97:175-187
13. Napolitano C, Ronchetti E, Memmi M et al (2001) Molecular epidemiology of the long QT Syndrome in a cohort of 267 probands. J Am Coll Cardiol 37[Suppl A]:87A
14. Moss AJ, Zareba W, Benhorin J et al (1995) ECG T-wave patterns in genetically distinct forms of the hereditary long QT syndrome. Circulation 92:2929-2934

15. Schwartz PJ, Priori SG, Locati EH et al (1995) Long QT syndrome patients with mutations of the SCN5A and HERG genes have differential responses to Na+ channel blockade and to increases in heart rate. Implications for gene-specific therapy. Circulation 92:3381-3386

16. Moretti P, Calcaterra G, Napolitano C et al (2001) High prevalence of concealed long QT syndrome among carriers of KVLQT1 defects. Circulation 102[Suppl]:II-584 (abstr)

17. Schwartz PJ, Priori SG, Spazzolini C et al (2001) Genotype-phenotype correlation in the long-QT syndrome: gene-specific triggers for life-threatening arrhythmias. Circulation 103:89-95

18. Zareba W, Moss AJ, Schwartz PJ et al (1998) Influence of genotype on the clinical course of the long-QT syndrome. International Long-QT Syndrome Registry Research Group. N Engl J Med 339:960-965

19. Priori SG, Napolitano C, Brown AM et al (1998) The loss of function induced by HERG and KVLQT1 mutations does not correlate with the clinical severity of the long QT syndrome. Circulation 98[Suppl 1]:I-457 (abstr)

20. Priori SG, Napolitano C, Schwartz PJ et al (1998) Variable phenotype of long QT syndrome patients with the same genetic defect. Circulation 30[Suppl]:82 (abstr)

21. Donger C, Denjoy I, Berthet M et al (1997) KVLQT1 C-terminal missense mutation causes a forme fruste long-QT syndrome. Circulation 96:2778-2781

22. Priori SG, Napolitano C, Schwartz PJ (1999) Low penetrance in the long-QT syndrome: clinical impact. Circulation 99:529-533

23. Napolitano C, Memmi M, Ronchetti E et al (1999) Silent mutation on cardiac ion channel genes and sudden death: a lesson from the long QT syndrome. Circulation 100[Suppl I]:I495

24. Berthet M, Denjoy I, Donger C et al (1999) C-terminal HERG mutations: the role of hypokalemia and a KCNQ1-associated mutation in cardiac event occurrence. Circulation 99:1464-1470

25. Brugada P, Brugada J (1992) Right bundle branch block, persistent ST segment elevation and sudden cardiac death: a distinct clinical and electrocardiographic syndrome. A multicenter report. J Am Coll Cardiol 20:1391-1396

26. Priori SG, Napolitano C, Giordano U et al (2000) Brugada syndrome and sudden cardiac death in children. Lancet 355:808-809

27. Brugada R, Brugada J, Antzelevitch C et al (2000) Sodium channel blockers identify risk for sudden death in patients with ST-segment elevation and right bundle branch block but structurally normal hearts. Circulation 101:510-515

28. Chen Q, Kirsch GE, Zhang D et al (1998) Genetic basis and molecular mechanism for idiopathic ventricular fibrillation. Nature 392:293-296

29. Bezzina C, Veldkamp MW, van Den Berg MP et al (1999) A single Na(+) channel mutation causing both long-QT and Brugada syndromes. Circ Res 85:1206-1213

30. Priori SG, Napolitano C, Schwartz PJ et al (2000) The elusive link between LQT3 and Brugada syndrome: the role of flecainide challenge. Circulation 102:945-947

31. Coumel P, Fidelle J, Lucet V et al (1978) Catecholaminergic-induced severe ventricular arrhythmias with Adams-Stokes syndrome in children: report of four cases. Br Heart J 40:28-37

32. Leenhardt A, Lucet V, Denjoy I et al (1995) Catecholaminergic polymorphic ventricular tachycardia in children. A 7-year follow-up of 21 patients. Circulation 91:1512-1519

33. Swan H, Piippo K, Viitasalo M et al (1999) Arrhythmic disorder mapped to chromosome 1q42-q43 causes malignant polymorphic ventricular tachycardia in structurally normal hearts. J Am Coll Cardiol 34:2035-2042

34. Otsu K, Fujii J, Periasamy M et al (1993) Chromosome mapping of five human cardiac and skeletal muscle sarcoplasmic reticulum protein genes. Genomics 17:507-509
35. Priori SG, Napolitano C, Tiso N et al (2000) Mutations in the cardiac ryanodine receptor gene (hRyR2) underlie catecholaminergic polymorphic ventricular tachycardia. Circulation 102:r49-r53
36. Lenegre J (1964) Etiology and pathology of bilateral bundle branch block in relation to complete heart block. Prog Cardiovasc Dis 6:409-444
37. Lev M, Kinare SG, Pick A (1970) The pathogenesis of atrioventricular block in coronary disease. Circulation 42:409-425
38. De Meeus A, Stephan E, Debrus S et al (1995) An isolated cardiac conduction disease maps to chromosome 19q. Circ Res 77:735-740
39. Stephan E, de Meeus A, Bouvagnet P (1997) Hereditary bundle branch defect: right bundle branch blocks of different causes have different morphologic characteristics. Am Heart J 133:249-256
40. Schott JJ, Alshinawi C, Kyndt F et al (1999) Cardiac conduction defects associate with mutations in SCN5A. Nat Genet 23:20-21
41. Tan HL, Bink-Boelkens MT, Bezzina CR et al (2001) A sodium-channel mutation causes isolated cardiac conduction disease. Nature 409:1043-1047
42. Leenhardt A, Glaser E, Burguera M et al (1994) Short-coupled variant of torsade de pointes. A new electrocardiographic entity in the spectrum of idiopathic ventricular tachyarrhythmias. Circulation 89:206-215
43. Brugada R, Tapscott T, Czernuszewicz GZ et al (1997) Identification of a genetic locus for familial atrial fibrillation. N Engl J Med 336:905-911
44. Brink PA, Ferreira A, Moolman JC et al (1995) Gene for progressive familial heart block type I maps to chromosome 19q13. Circulation 91:1633-1640

Left Ventricular Hypertrophy: A Neglected Risk Factor for Sudden Cardiac Death?

G. Turitto, R.P. Pedalino, S. Soliman, V. Togay and N. El-Sherif

Sudden Cardiac Death and Left Ventricular Hypertrophy: Magnitude of the Problem

Despite recent declines in mortality from coronary artery disease (CAD), this entity remains the major cause of death in the United States for blacks and whites [1]. A majority of deaths from CAD are classified as sudden cardiac deaths (SCDs). A significant body of evidence from epidemiology and pathology studies has emerged showing that the presence of left ventricular hypertrophy (LVH) is an important predictor for SCD, and that the mortality risk associated with LVH may be particularly high when underlying CAD is present. Conventional risk stratification algorithms have not taken into account the adverse effects of LVH on prognosis and its interaction with other indices of increased risk.

Epidemiological Data on the Prognostic Significance of LVH

Studies on the underlying morphologic substrate for SCD in black and white Americans have resulted in an appreciation of the role of LVH in promoting SCD [2]. In particular, two major anatomic differences have emerged from autopsy studies of victims of SCD: (1) blacks seem to have less extensive CAD, and (2) they have heavier hearts compared to whites. Thus, an increased tendency to SCD is associated with increased LV mass.

Data derived from large epidemiological studies also support the proposition that LVH may be associated with electrical instability and an increased incidence of SCD. In the Framingham Study, ECG LVH carried an eight-fold increase in cardiovascular mortality [3]. Increased LV mass on echocardiogram was also associated with an increased incidence of cardiovascular death (relative risk: 1.73 in

Cardiac Electrophysiology Section, Department of Medicine, State University of New York, Downstate Medical Center, Brooklyn, New York, USA

men and 2.12 in women) [4]. Furthermore, this large community-based study clearly demonstrated that LVH and increased LV mass are associated specifically with increased risk of SCD [5]. The adverse prognostic value of LVH has been confirmed in other settings and holds true in patients with or without obstructive CAD, and with or without a history of previous myocardial infarction (MI) [6-14]. The effects on survival of echocardiographic LVH in comparison to the number of stenosed vessels and LV systolic dysfunction has been assessed by several studies [11, 14]. In a cohort of 1089 patients undergoing both echocardiogram and coronary angiography and followed for a mean of 5 years, LVH was detected in 50% of the study patients, while no obstructive CAD, single-vessel disease, or multi-vessel disease was present in 48%, 16%, and 36% of patients, respectively [14]. Among patients with CAD, 36% had history of previous MI. There were no differences in the prevalence of LVH between patients with and without CAD. When LVH, number of diseased vessels, and LV dysfunction were subjected to multivariate analysis, LVH conferred a relative risk of death of 2.4. Calculation of the attributable risk fraction showed that for every 100 deaths in this cohort, LVH independently accounted for 37. This study concluded that LVH is associated with a greater relative risk and attributable risk than the traditional measures of CAD [14].

Mechanisms for Increased Incidence of SCD in the Presence of LVH

The risk associated with LVH is real and severe. Nevertheless, the mechanism(s) by which cardiac hypertrophy may increase the risk of SCD are inadequately understood [15, 16]. LVH reduces coronary flow reserve while increasing myocardial oxygen consumption [16]. This imbalance may predispose to ischemia and/or fatal ventricular tachyarrhythmias (VT) [16-18]. Studies in laboratory animals with hypertensive LVH have demonstrated a three-fold risk of SCD as well as increased myocardial infarct size after coronary occlusion [19, 20].

A prominent mechanism for the poor prognostic significance of LVH is that ischemia/infarction superimposed on LVH may result in increased early and late post-MI mortality. Early MI mortality can result from (1) the development of a more extensive ischemic zone with failure of the hypertrophied LV to compensate for loss of myocardial function, resulting in pump failure, and (2) an increased susceptibility to early malignant VT. A possible mechanism of the latter is the development of a greater degree of dispersion of repolarization, recognized as a critical substrate for development of malignant VT. Late post-MI mortality could be related to differences in post-MI remodeling of the hypertrophied heart. This could result in an early onset and/or an enhanced degree of (1) diastolic/systolic dysfunction, leading to early onset of heart failure, and (2) alterations in the active and passive electrophysiological properties of the myocardium, leading to enhanced susceptibility to malignant VT. One possible mechanism for enhanced arrhythmogenesis that is supported by preliminary observations in Dr. El-Sherif's laboratory is that ischemia results in a greater degree of shortening of the action potential duration (APD) of hypertrophied myocytes. This could result in the development of a greater degree of dispersion of repolarization at the border between the ischemic and nonischemic regions and would accentuate the already present increased dispersion of repolarization associated with hypertrophy per se. Additionally, early onset and/or enhanced degree of alterations of the transient outward potassium channel gene expression and current density as well as the expression of connexin 43 in the post-MI noninfarcted remodeled myocardium in hearts with LVH may play a major role in the enhanced propensity for ventricular arrhythmias shown by these hearts [21]. Differential regional alterations in transient outword current (I_{to}) and connexin 43 can increase the spatial heterogeneity of both active and passive electrical properties of the post-MI heart and contribute to enhanced arrhythmogenesis.

Identification and Modulation of Indices of Sudden Cardiac Death in Survivors of MI With or Without LVH

A currently held position in the clinical electrophysiology community is that, other than a low left ventricular ejection function (LVEF), no other risk stratifier for arrhythmic death is powerful enough to be included in a risk stratification strategy for primary prevention of SCD. However, although LVEF is an excellent predictor of total cardiac mortality, it is not specific enough for arrhythmic death. This would result in redundancy in management strategy if, for example, an implantable cardioverter-defibrillator (ICD) is prescribed for primary prevention in a subject with low LVEF who would eventually succumb to terminal pump failure rather than to a lethal arrhythmic event. The problem of risk stratification for SCD is also magnified by the fact that conventional risk stratification algorithms do not take into account the adverse prognostic effects of LVH and its interaction with other risk stratifiers. Commonly utilized markers for risk stratification include: LVEF, ventricular arrhythmias on ambulatory Holter recording, signal-averaged electrocardiography (SAECG), and heart rate variability (HRV). In addition, there are a number of more recently described or less commonly utilized markers of arrhythmic death, such as QT dispersion, baroreflex sensitivity (BRS), and T wave alternans (TWA). However, with the exception of LVEF, none of the other tests, at present, has proven to be solely adequate as a powerful risk stratifier. An optimal algorithm that combines more than one index of high risk has not yet been identified or agreed upon.

Left Ventricular Ejection Fraction

LV function is one of the best predictors of total cardiac mortality and morbidity in patients with CAD, especially after MI [22]. However, LV systolic dysfunction is not a very specific marker of sudden or arrhythmic death [23, 24].

Ambulatory Holter Recording

In post-MI patients, the presence of complex ventricular arrhythmias (frequent ventricular premature complexes or nonsustained ventricular tachycardia) on Holter ECG is associated with an increased incidence of SCD, but is also characterized by a low predictive accuracy. In patients with hypertension, there is a statistically significant relationship between LVH and complex ventricular arrhythmias [18, 25-28]. However, the prognostic value of this marker is also poor in this setting [29]. In the Framingham Study, the presence of asymptomatic ventricular arrhythmias on 1-h recordings obtained in subjects with LVH was associated with a statistically significant increase in mortality, which became marginally significant after adjusting for covariates [30].

Signal-Averaged Electrocardiography

Several prospective studies have confirmed the increased likelihood of malignant VT and SCD in post-MI patients with an abnormal SAECG [31]. LVH does not seem to correlate with an increased incidence of abnormal SAECG [32], even though in one report a relationship was found between the occurrence of ventricular tachycardia during Holter recording and the presence of abnormal SAECG parameters in hypertensive subjects with LVH [33]. No studies have evaluated the effects of LVH on measures of spectral turbulence, a technique for frequency-domain analysis of the SAECG.

QT Dispersion

Dispersion of ventricular repolarization is a well-recognized electrophysiologic substrate for malignant VT. The QT interval has been the index of choice for assessing repolarization abnormalities. However, the role of QT dispersion for risk stratification of SCD remains controversial, in large measure due to methodological issues [34]. Patients with LVH have been found to have increased QT dispersion on 12-lead ECG. In these reports, the degree of QT dispersion, defined as the difference between maximum and minimum QT interval on a 12-lead ECG, directly correlated with echocardiographic LV mass [35-37]. The prognostic significance of QT dispersion in patients with LVH is presently unknown.

T Wave Alternans

Alternation of the configuration and/or duration of the repolarization wave of the ECG, usually referred to as "TWA", is seen under diverse experimental and clinical conditions. Interest in repolarization alternans is attributed to the hypothesis that it may reflect underlying dispersion of repolarization in the ventricle, i.e., an arrhythmogenic substrate [38]. Although overt TWA in the

ECG is not common, in recent years digital signal-processing techniques capable of detecting subtle degrees of TWA have suggested that the phenomenon may be more prevalent than previously recognized and could represent an important marker of vulnerability to SCD. Several studies have shown that microvolt TWA elicited with heart rate elevation with bicycle exercise is a strong predictor of arrhythmia inducibility and arrhythmia-free survival [39-41]. A preliminary report from our group has specifically addressed the relationship between LVH, TWA, and SCD [42]. The aim of our study was to investigate the relationship between TWA and LVH, as defined by echocardiographically measured LV mass. The study population included 30 patients with organic heart disease who had technically adequate echocardiograms for LV mass measurement and TWA recordings during a symptom-limited bicycle exercise test. Sixteen patients had a history of malignant VT. Out of 30 patients, 13 developed exercise-induced TWA, while 17 did not. LV mass was significantly greater in patients with TWA, as compared to those without TWA ($p < 0.04$). This preliminary report suggested that LVH may be a risk factor for the development of exercise-induced TWA.

HRV and BRS

Several studies have revealed an association between the autonomic nervous system and SCD [43]. In post-MI patients, a shift of sympathovagal balance towards a predominance of sympathetic activity and a reduction in parasympathetic tone has been demonstrated. It is the enhanced sympathetic activation that predisposes to malignant VT and SCD, while increased vagal tone has been shown to have protective effects [24, 43]. Both HRV and BRS are measures of the sympathovagal balance [44]. Methods to analyze HRV employ both time- and frequency-domain measurements that quantify periodicity in the data [43]. Depressed HRV is a powerful predictor of mortality and arrhythmic events in survivors of MI, as well as in unselected patient populations, and in cohorts of apparently healthy middle-aged and elderly subjects [43, 45, 46]. The predictive value of HRV is independent of other factors established for post-MI risk stratification, such as LV dysfunction, abnormal SAECG, and complex ventricular arrhythmias on Holter monitoring [45, 46]. For prediction of total cardiac mortality, the value of HRV is similar to that of LVEF. However, HRV is superior to LVEF in predicting serious arrhythmic events (SCD and ventricular tachycardia) [45, 46]. A continuous inverse relationship between LV mass and HRV has been reported in patients with hypertension and LVH [47, 48]. Thus, it is possible that disturbances in cardiac autonomic function may contribute to the increased risk of SCD associated with LVH. BRS assessed with phenylephrine injection is an alternative noninvasive test to evaluate sympathovagal balance [44]. Overall, BRS decreases whenever the autonomic balance shifts towards sympathetic dominance and increases whenever the autonomic balance shifts towards parasympathetic dominance. There are no investigations comparing BRS in patients with and without LVH.

Metaiodobenzylguanidine Imaging

[123]I-labeled metaiodobenzylguanidine (MIBG) scintigraphic imaging reflects the relative distribution of adrenergic neurodensity and function in the myocardium. Impaired sympathetic innervation as assessed by MIBG activity has been proposed as a powerful risk factor (independent of LVEF) for cardiac mortality and SCD in patients with heart failure due to ischemic or nonischemic dilated cardiomyopathy [49-51]. MIBG myocardial imaging has been shown to be abnormal in patients with LVH, and the degree of abnormality had a positive correlation with LV mass [52, 53]. The exact pathogenesis of these abnormalities and their relationship with physiologic markers of cardiac autonomic nervous system activity is currently unknown.

Conclusions

A comprehensive risk stratification strategy that assesses how LVH modulates the predictive value of traditional risk factors for cardiac death and SCD is currently lacking. Such a strategy should take into account the potential effects of LVH on the arrhythmogenic substrate, and could result in the identification of a subset of patients at high risk of SCD, who may become candidates for interventions aimed at reducing this risk. Planning and carrying out such studies seems to be of paramount importance in view of the data summarized in this review.

References

1. Sytkowski PA, D'Agostino RB, Belanger AJ, Kannel WB (1996) Secular trends in long-term sustained hypertension, long-term treatment, and cardiovascular mortality: the Framingham Heart Study 1950 to 1990. Circulation 93:697-703
2. Kuller LH, Cooper M, Perper J, Fisher R (1973) Myocardial infarction and sudden death in an urban community. Bull NY Acad Med 49:532-543
3. Kannel WB, Gordon T, Castelli WP, Margolis JR (1970) Electrocardiographic left ventricular hypertrophy and risk of coronary heart disease. The Framingham Study. Ann Intern Med 72:813-822
4. Levy D, Garrison RJ, Savage DD et al (1990) Prognostic implications of echocardiographically determined left ventricular mass in the Framingham Heart Study. N Engl J Med 322:1561-1566
5. Haider AW, Larson MG, Benjamin EJ, Levy D (1998) Increased left ventricular mass and hypertrophy are associated with increased risk for sudden death. J Am Coll Cardiol 32:1454-1459
6. Boden WE, Kleiger RE, Schechtman KB et al and the Diltiazem Reinfarction Study Research Group (1988) Clinical significance and prognostic importance of left ventricular hypertrophy in non-Q-wave acute myocardial infarction. Am J Cardiol 62:1000-1004

7. Knutsen R, Knutsen SF, Curb JD et al (1988) The predictive value of resting electro-cardiograms for 12-year incidence of coronary heart disease in the Honolulu Heart Program. J Clin Epidemiol 41:293-302

8. Wong ND, Levy D, Kannel WB (1990) Prognostic significance of the electrocardiogram after Q wave myocardial infarction. The Framingham Study. Circulation 81:780-789

9. Koren MJ, Devereux RB, Casale PN et al (1991) Relation of left ventricular mass and geometry to morbidity and mortality in uncomplicated essential hypertension. Ann Intern Med 114:345-352

10. Behar B, Reicher-Reis H, Abinader E et al (1992) Long-term prognosis after acute myocardial infarction in patients with left ventricular hypertrophy on the electrocar-diogram. Am J Cardiol 69:985-990

11. Ghali JK, Liao Y, Simmons B et al (1992) The prognostic role of left ventricular hyper-trophy in patients with or without coronary artery disease. Ann Intern Med 117:831-836

12. Sullivan JM, Vander Zwaag R, El-Zeky F et al (1993) Left ventricular hypertrophy: effect on survival. J Am Coll Cardiol 22:508-513

13. Levy D, Salomon M, D'Agostino RB et al (1994) Prognostic implications of baseline electrocardiographic features and their serial changes in subjects with left ventricu-lar hypertrophy. Circulation 90:1786-1793

14. Liao Y, Cooper RS, McGee DL et al (1995) The relative effects of left ventricular hypertrophy, coronary artery disease, and ventricular dysfunction on survival among black adults. JAMA 273:1592-1597

15. Burke AP, Farb A, Liang Y et al (1996) Effect of hypertension and cardiac hyper-trophy on coronary artery morphology in sudden cardiac death. Circulation 94:3138-3145

16. Zehender M, Faber T, Koscheck U et al (1995) Ventricular tachyarrhythmias, myocar-dial ischemia, and sudden cardiac death in patients with hypertensive heart disease. Clin Cardiol 18:377-383

17. Szlachcic J, Tubau JF, O' Kelly B et al (1992) What is the role of silent coronary artery disease and left ventricular hypertrophy in the genesis of ventricular arrhythmias in men with essential hypertension? J Am Coll Cardiol 19:803-808

18. Zehender M, Meinertz T, Hohnloser S et al (1992) Prevalence of circadian variations and spontaneous variability of cardiac disorders and ECG changes suggestive of myocardial ischemia in systemic arterial hypertension. Circulation 85:1808-1815

19. Dellsperger KC, Clothier JL, Hartnett JA et al (1988) Acceleration of the wavefront of myocardial necrosis by chronic hypertension and left ventricular hypertrophy in dogs. Circ Res 63:87-96

20. Dellsperger KC, Martins JB, Clothier JL, Marcus ML (1990) Incidence of sudden car-diac death associated with coronary artery occlusion in dogs with hypertension and left ventricular hypertrophy is reduced by chronic beta-adrenergic blockade. Circulation 82:941-950

21. Peters NS (1996) New insights into myocardial arrhythmogenesis: distribution of gap-junctional coupling in normal, ischaemic and hypertrophied human hearts. Clin Sci 90:447-452

22. Rouleau JL, Talajic M, Sussex B et al (1996) Myocardial infarction patients in the 1990s – their risk factors, stratification and survival in Canada: the Canadian Assessment of Myocardial Infarction (CAMI) Study. J Am Coll Cardiol 27:1119-1127

23. Kober L, Torp-Pedersen C, Elming H, Burchardt H, on behalf of the TRACE Study Group (1997) Use of left ventricular ejection fraction or wall-motion score index in predicting arrhythmic death in patients following an acute myocardial infarction. Pacing Clin Electrophysiol 20:2553-2559

24. Hohnloser SH, Klingenheben T, Zabel M, Li YG (1997) Heart rate variability used as an arrhythmia risk stratifier after myocardial infarction. Pacing Clin Electrophysiol 20:2594-2601

25. McLenachan JM, Henderson E, Morris KI, Dargie HJ (1987) Ventricular arrhythmias in patients with hypertensive left ventricular hypertrophy. N Engl J Med 317:787-792

26. Siegel D, Cheitlin MD, Black DM et al (1990) Risk of ventricular arrhythmias in hypertensive men with left ventricular hypertrophy. Am J Cardiol 65:742-747

27. Ghali JK, Kadakia S, Cooper RS, Liao YL (1991) Impact of left ventricular hypertrophy on ventricular arrhythmias in the absence of coronary artery disease. J Am Coll Cardiol 17:1277-1282

28. Bayes-Genis A, Guindo J, Vinolas X et al (1995) Cardiac arrhythmias and left ventricular hypertrophy in systemic hypertension and their influences on prognosis. Am J Cardiol 76:54D-59D

29. Galinier M, Balanescu S, Fourcade J et al (1997) Prognostic value of arrhythmogenic markers in systemic hypertension. Eur Heart J 9:1484-1491

30. Bikkina M, Larson MG, Levy D (1993) Asymptomatic left ventricular arrhythmias and mortality risk in subjects with left ventricular hypertrophy. J Am Coll Cardiol 22:1111-1116

31. Turitto G, Sorgato A, Alakhras M, El-Sherif N (2001) QRS averaging. In: Zareba W, Maison-Blanche P, Locati EH (eds) Noninvasive electrocardiology in clinical practice, Futura, Armonk, NY, pp 49-69

32. Fragola PV, De Nardo D, Calo' L, Cannata D (1994) Use of the signal-averaged QRS duration for diagnosing left ventricular hypertrophy in hypertensive patients. Int J Cardiol 44:261-270

33. Palatini P, Maraglino G, Accurso V et al (1995) Impaired left ventricular filling in hypertensive left ventricular hypertrophy as a marker of the presence of an arrhythmogenic substrate. Br Heart J 73:258-262

34. Lux RL, Fuller MS, MacLeod RS et al (1998) QT interval dispersion: dispersion of ventricular repolarization or dispersion of QT interval? J Electrocardiol 30 (Suppl):176-180

35. Perkiomaki JS, Ikaheimo MJ, Pikkujamsa SM et al (1996) Dispersion of QT interval and autonomic modulation of heart rate in hypertensive men with and without left ventricular hypertrophy. Hypertension 28:16-21

36. Ichkhan K, Molnar J, Somberg J (1997) Relation of left ventricular mass and QT dispersion in patients with systematic hypertension. Am J Cardiol 79:508-511

37. Mayet J, Shahi M, McGrath K et al (1996) Left ventricular hypertrophy and QT dispersion in hypertension. Hypertension 28:791-796

38. Chinushi M, Restivo M, Caref EB, El-Sherif N (1998) Electrophysiological basis of the arrhythmogenicity of QT/T alternans in the long QT syndrome. Tridimensional analysis of the kinetics of cardiac repolarization. Circ Res 83:614-628

39. Rosenbaum DS, Jackson LE, Smith JM et al (1994) Electrical alternans and vulnerability to ventricular arrhythmias. N Engl J Med 330:235-241

40. Estes NAM 3rd, Michaud G, Zipes DP et al (1997) Electrical alternans during rest and exercise as a predictor of vulnerability to ventricular arrhythmias. Am J Cardiol 80:1314-1318

41. Gold MR, Bloomfield DM, Anderson KP et al (2000) A comparison of T-wave alternans, signal averaged electrocardiography and programmed ventricular stimulation for arrhythmia risk stratification. J Am Coll Cardiol 36:2247-2253

42. Pedalino R, Graham S, Obeidou B et al (2000) Left ventricular hypertrophy as a major determinant of exercise-induced T-wave alternans. Europace I (Suppl D):D62

43. Task Force of the European Society of Cardiology and the North American Society of Pacing and Electrophysiology (1996) Heart rate variability. Standards of measurement, physiological interpretation, and clinical use. Circulation 93:1143-1165

44. La Rovere MT, Schwartz PJ (1997) Baroreflex sensitivity as cardiac and arrhythmia mortality risk stratifier. Pacing Clin Electrophysiol 20:2602-2613

45. Odemuyiwa O, Malik M, Farrell T et al (1991) Comparison of the predictive characteristics of heart rate variability index and left ventricular ejection fraction for all-cause mortality, arrhythmic events and sudden death after acute myocardial infarction. Am J Cardiol 68:434-439

46. Farrell TG, Bashir Y, Cripps T et al (1991) Risk stratification for arrhythmic events in postinfarction patients based on heart rate variability, ambulatory electrocardiographic variables and the signal-averaged electrocardiogram. J Am Coll Cardiol 18:687-697

47. Mandawat MK, Wallbridge DR, Pringle SD et al (1995) Heart rate variability in left ventricular hypertrophy. Br Heart J 73:139-144

48. Petretta M, Bianchi V, Marciano F et al (1995) Influence of left ventricular hypertrophy on heart period variability in patients with essential hypertension. J Hypertens 13:1299-1306

49. Nakata T, Miyamoto K, Doi A et al (1998) Cardiac death prediction and impaired cardiac sympathetic innervation assessed by MIBG in patients with failing and nonfailing hearts. J Nucl Cardiol 5:579-590

50. Cohen-Solal A, Esanu Y, Logeart D et al (1999) Cardiac metaiodobenzylguanidine uptake in patients with moderate chronic heart failure: relationship with peak oxygen uptake and prognosis. J Am Coll Cardiol 33:759-766

51. Merlet P, Benvenuti C, Moyse D et al (1999) Prognostic value of MIBG imaging in idiopathic dilated cardiomyopathy. J Nucl Med 40:917-923

52. Kuwahara T, Hamada M, Hiwada K (1998) Direct evidence of impaired cardiac sympathetic innervation in essential hypertensive patients with left ventricular hypertrophy. J Nucl Med 39:1486-1491

53. Sakata K, Shirotani M, Yoshida H, Kurata C (1999) Cardiac sympathetic nervous system in early essential hypertension assessed by ^{123}I-MIBG. J Nucl Med 40:6-11

Post-Extrasystolic Heart Rate Turbulence as a Risk Predictor: What are the Perspectives and Limitations?

E. Sade and A. Oto

Introduction

Sudden cardiac death (SCD) is one of the leading causes of mortality, and early identification of patients at high risk is of critical importance for its prevention. There is a need for precise, reliable, and, preferably, noninvasive diagnostic tools for accurate selection of the patients at high risk and targeting of preventive and therapeutic strategies. Several parameters have been studied over the years. To date, various noninvasive studies such as measurement of the left ventricular ejection fraction (LVEF) [1, 2], signal-averaged electrocardiography (SAECG) [3, 4], ventricular ectopic activity on Holter monitoring, heart rate variability (HRV), baroreflex sensitivity (BRS) [5], and tests to evaluate ventricular repolarization abnormalities [6] have been proposed as useful tools for identification of patients at high risk of SCD. However, the predictive value of each of these tests alone is low. Assessment of mortality risk and prevention of SCD are not yet ideal.

Two distinct mechanisms may be responsible for the majority of lethal arrhythmic episodes. Coronary artery disease is the most frequent cause of SCD in these patients. Acute ischemia may trigger ventricular arrhythmias by creating abnormalities in impulse propagation, conduction velocity, changes in refractoriness, areas of block and enhanced automaticity. Secondly, reentrant circuits created within and around the infarct scar may be the causative mechanism [7]. In the absence of an ischemic trigger, arrhythmic events probably occur on the basis of a combination of conditions including the substrate properties of myocardium, inhomogeneous repolarization, premature depolarization, and neurohormonal factors [8]. The different underlying mechanisms of SCD may explain the inconclusive results in terms of survival benefit from arrhythmia suppression by medical treatment or ICD implantation based upon noninvasive SCD markers. Due to the low positive predictive accuracy and high false positive results obtained with present methods, it seems unlikely that any of them will be sufficient to assess the risk of the individual patient. For this

Department of Cardiology, Hacettepe University School of Medicine, Ankara, Turkey

reason it is a common approach to use a combination of several of these parameters to increase the accuracy of prediction of high-risk patients. Even by combining different risk indicators, the positive predictive accuracy barely exceeds 30% [9, 10].

In addition, there are difficulties in the practical application of some of these methods. For instance, the conventional way of assessing baroreflex sensitivity is based on phenylephrine administration and on measurement of the relationship between blood pressure and cardiac cycle length. Although it is stated that this method could be used safely after recent acute myocardial infarction (AMI) deleterious effects could emerge in the very early phase of AMI [11]. Recently T wave alternans (TWA), which reflects specific fluctuations in the morphology of the T wave during alternating beats, has been shown to be associated with ventricular arrhythmias and has been investigated as a clinical tool by which to identify patients at high risk of developing SCD [12-14]. However, the need for exercise or atrial pacing to accelerate the heart rate in order to detect microvoltage TWA is an important limitation of its application in AMI patients.

There is therefore still a need for reliable noninvasive markers for assessment. This paper focuses on heart rate turbulence (HRT), which has emerged as a new method by which to predict high-risk patients.

Heart Rate Turbulence

HRT is defined as the fluctuations of sinus rhythm cycle length after a single ventricular premature beat (VPB). It is basically related to the ventriculophasic mechanism of sinus arrhythmia [15-17]. Schmidt et al. [18] showed that after a VPB, sinus rhythm shows a characteristic pattern of early acceleration and subsequent deceleration in low-risk patients, while this fluctuation pattern of the sinus cycle does not occur in high-risk patients. After developing and optimizing the method in a training sample of 100 patients with coronary artery disease with more than 10 VPBs per hour, Schmidt and colleagues validated this new risk predictor in two large independent populations of myocardial infarction survivors, namely the population of the Multicenter Post-Infarction Program (MPIP) study and the placebo group of the European Myocardial Infarction Amiodarone Trial (EMIAT) [10, 19, 20].

Mechanism

It is recognized that VPBs can alter sinus node discharge rate even in the absence of retrograde conduction to atria. The main concept relies upon the ventriculophasic arrhythmia to explain the mechanism of HRT. Changes in autonomic tone, tractions of the atrial wall as well as atrial appendages, atrioventricular junction, and the sinus node region, and transient improvement of the blood supply to the sinus node have all been discussed as possible patho-physiological mechanisms underlying the ventriculophasic arrhythmia [15, 17, 21-24]. HRT is thought to be triggered by a baroreflex mechanism [25]. A single VPB causes inefficient contraction of the ventricle, which produces a slight drop in arterial blood pressure. However, a higher blood pressure amplitude follows, with the ensuing normal beat after the post-extrasystolic pause. This slight fluctuation in blood pressure is recorded by the sinus node and triggers the HRT response. Thus, the RR interval changes in a similar manner to the fluctuation of blood pressure [26]. The hemodynamically inefficient contrac-tion transiently inhibits the afferent vagal activity which causes the first phase of HRT, early abrupt acceleration of heart rate, termed "turbulence onset" (TO). Then the powerful contraction ensuing after the compensatory pause together with unopposed sympathetic activity causes an increase in blood pressure which is responsible for the second phase of HRT. This counter-reaction is called "turbulence slope" (TS), which is late deceleration of the heart rate. Current opinion states that both autonomic tone and the mechanistic proper-ties of the myocardium should be intact for this reaction to occur in response to a trigger as minor as a single premature beat. Indeed, although there is correla-tion between TO, TS, and BRS, the low correlation coefficients suggest that other intrinsic modulators may also be important in regulating the pathophysi-ology of HRT [27].

Measurement of HRT

TO, which is the immediate initial acceleration, is the percentage difference between the heart rate immediately following VPB and the heart rate immedi-ately preceding VPB. It is calculated using the equation

$$TO = [(RR1 + RR2) - (RR\text{-}2 + RR\text{-}1)] / (RR\text{-}2 + RR\text{-}1) \times 100$$

where RR-2 and RR-1 are the first two normal intervals preceding the VPB and RR1 and RR2 are the first two normal intervals following the VPB. Positive val-ues for TO indicate deceleration, negative values indicate acceleration of the sinus rhythm. These measurements are first performed for each individual VPB and then averaged to obtain the value characterizing the patient [18].

TS, the subsequent deceleration after VPB, is quantified by the steepest regression line between the RR interval count and duration assessed over any sequence of five consecutive sinus-rhythm RR intervals within the first 20 sinus beats following the VPB. The value of the TS is expressed in milliseconds per RR interval. It is easily made out from the tachogram of the RR intervals following the VPB. The present algorithm dedicated to HRT calculations uses an appropriate filter to ensure that the sinus rhythm preceding and following the VPB is free from arrhythmia, artefacts, and false classification as VPB. RR intervals shorter than 300 ms and longer than 2000 ms, and those showing more than 200 ms difference from the preceding sinus interval and more than 20% difference from the reference interval (mean of the five last sinus intervals) are excluded by the filter. Furthermore, HRT calculations are limited to VPBs with a minimum prematurity of 20% and a post-extrasystolic pause which is at least 10% longer than the normal interval (for quantification of HRT, see www.h-r-t.com).

It is also possible to quantify HRT by means of frequency domain analysis. The dominant frequency (TF) and the related amplitude (TA) of the dominant peak describing the strength of the HRT are calculated from the power spectrum of HRT tachogram. TA but not TF discriminated survivors from nonsurvivors and TA provided similar information to TS and appeared to be as strong as TS [28].

Clinical Relevance of HRT

The fact that HRT is a consistent phenomenon in low-risk patients and that it is absent in high-risk patients suffering from ischemic heart disease has been proven in the MPIP population and the placebo arm of the EMIAT population [10, 20]. On the basis of the data obtained from these large validation populations TO was dichotomized at 0% and TS at 2.5 ms/RR interval. In EMIAT TS was the strongest univariate predictor of mortality; however, in the MPIP study it was the second most powerful univariate predictor of mortality after low LVEF [18]. TS and TO in combination provided more powerful risk prediction for mortality, relative risk being 5.0 in the MPIP population and 4.4 in the EMIAT population. In the multivariate regression analysis too, the combination of abnormal TS and TO was the most powerful mortality predictor. The combination of TS and TO and low LVEF were the only independent mortality predictors in the MPIP population. In EMIAT four variables emerged as independent risk predictors in the multivariate analysis. However, the combination of TS and TO was more powerful than other significant predictors, namely, previous MI, mean RR interval shorter than 800 ms, and LVEF less than 30%. TO and TS are both predictors of mortality containing information additional to each other [18]. Later, the predictive value of HRT was studied in the ATRAMI (Autonomic Tone and Reflexes after Myocardial Infarction) population in whom, besides BRS, TS and the combination of TS and TO were potent predictors of mortality. Furthermore, in the ATRAMI population HRT was found to be additive to other mortality predictors, namely BRS, LVEF, HRV, and mean heart rate. At 40% sensitivity, TS best combined with HRV and with LVEF [29]. Interestingly enough, in the MPIP population Holter recordings were done in the second week after the index infarction, while in the EMIAT population the recordings were obtained in the second or third week after the infarction.

In a prospective study we evaluated HRT in 107 AMI patients. Quantification of HRT was from Holter recordings obtained during the first 24 h of the index MI to explore changes of HRT in the acute phase of MI and to assess the predictive value for long-term prognostication in these patients. In our study, median follow-up period was 10 (mean 19 ± 5) months. A cut-off value of 1.5 for TS and a cut-off value of -0.2% for TO were determined. We found that only TS along with low LVEF were independent predictors of total mortality, among many other univariate risk predictors, namely, TO, SDNN (defined below), LF/HF, QTe/RR slope (defined below), QTa/RR slope (defined below), frequency of VPBs, mean RR interval [for LVEF < 30% relative hazard = 5.9 (1.4-24) 95% CI, $p = 0.015$; and for TS relative hazard = 13 (2.5-69) 95% CI, $p = 0.002$]. We also investigated the additive role of HRT (TO and TS combined) to HRV and LVEF for mortality prediction (Table 1).

Table 1. Additive value of HRT to HRV and LVEF in long-term prediction of mortality in patients with AMI

	Mortality					
	Relative hazard (95% CI)	p value	Sensitivity (%)	Specificity (%)	PPV (%)	NPV (%)
LVEF < 30%	15.9 (4.5-57)	< 0.0001	60	94	50	96
HRT (TO and TS)	20 (5.2-79)	< 0.0001	70	92	47	97
HRV (SDNN)	20 (2.5-160)	= 0.004	90	71	98	25
LVEF + HRV	28.4 (7.6-105)	< 0.0001	60	97	67	97
LVEF + HRT	22 (5.8-84)	< 0.0001	40	98	67	94
HRT + HRV	23 (5.8-91)	< 0.0001	70	93	50	97
LVEF + HRV +HRT	22 (5.8-84)	< 0.0001	40	98	67	94

HRT, heart rate turbulence; *HRV*, heart rate variability; *LVEF*, left ventricular ejection fraction; *AMI*, acute myocardial infarction; *PPV*, positive predictive value; *NPV*, negative predictive value; *SDNN*, standard deviation of RR intervals of all normal beats

As shown in the table, when HRT is combined with HRV the specificity and negative predictive value of the latter increase from 71% to 93% and from 25% to 97% respectively, and the sensitivity, although reduced from 90% to 70%, still remains good enough. When HRT is added to low LVEF, the sensitivity of the latter decreases from 60% to 40% and the positive predictive value increases from 50% to 67%, while the specificity and negative predictive value do not change.

Another important finding is that HRT predicted arrhythmic deaths in post-MI patients with left ventricular dysfunction in the EMIAT population [30]. This finding may have important implications in selecting post-MI patients who are likely to benefit from prophylactic intervention such as ICD implantation.

HRT has also been investigated in patients with congestive heart failure. In a study comprising 199 patients where HRT was compared with previously validated prognostic markers such as age, LVEF, NYHA class, peak VO_2, BRS, triangular index, nonsustained VT, and QT dispersion, HRT has been found to hold promise as a new prognostic marker in congestive heart failure [31]. It is particularly helpful when HRV cannot be assessed due to frequent ectopy.

Various aspects of HRT have been investigated so far. The correlation between HRT and HRV studied in the EMIAT population suggests that HRT is at least partly mediated by sympathovagal activity [32]. TO and TS correlated significantly with almost all time-domain HRV parameters in such a manner that reduced HRV was associated with reduced TO and TS. We have also shown that both TS and TO correlated with HRV. The best correlates of TS and TO were SDNN (standard deviation of normal RR intervals) among time-domain variables and TP (total frequency power) and (logarithm of total power) among frequency domain variables. We have also investigated the correlation between HRT and QT dynamicity in AMI patients and found that QTa/RR (the regression line relating QT and RR intervals where QTa is the QT measured to the apex of the T wave) slope is the best correlate of both TS and TO. However QTe/RR (QTe is the QT interval measured to the end of T wave) correlated only with TO. HRT spectra determined from 24-h Holter recordings obtained 2 weeks after an index MI were compared in patients with and without diabetes who were included in the placebo arm of the EMIAT study [33]. TA was significantly reduced in patients with diabetes as compared to patients without diabetes. Again, this finding favors the suggestion that HRT is caused by an intact autonomic baroreflex.

Recent data suggest that HRT is influenced by heart rate, age, LVEF, NYHA class, diabetes, frequency of VPBs, thrombolysis, β-blockers, and ACE inhibitors, but not amiodarone or angiotensin receptor antagonists [34, 35]. Our study conducted in AMI patients parallels the recent finding related to thrombolysis. We found that 88% of patients with a normal TS value had TIMI III (Thrombolysis in Myocardial Infarction, where grade III represents prompt and complete opacification of the vascular bed by contrast material) flow grade, whereas only 12% of patients with abnormal TS had a TIMI III flow grade. Furthermore, TS > 1.5 ms/RR interval was predictive of successful reperfusion ($p = 0.03$; relative hazard 3.6 and 95% CI 1.2-12). On the other hand it has also been reported that amiodarone therapy, by improving abnormal TO, provides survival benefit in post-MI patients who are already on β-blockers [36]. This latter finding appears to be inconsistent with the former. Also, in 1999 it was reported that HRT was an equally strong predictor of mortality in post-MI patients with and without β-blockers, while mean RR interval, previous MI, and LVEF, although good prognosticators in patients without β-blockers, lost their predictive power in post-MI patients with β-blockers [37]. These conflicting findings should be further investigated in prospective large trials.

Limitations and Future Perspectives

The available data so far are convincing that HRT is one of the most powerful risk predictors for mortality. However, some points still remain unclear, and the method still has limitations. The exact mechanism of HRT is not yet completely understood. The relative contributions of the autonomic nervous system, mechanistic properties of the myocardium, and environmental conditions in the modulation of HRT remain to be explored. HRT has the advantage of being a practical and reliable noninvasive method when there are frequent premature beats, the situation which limits the usefulness of HRV as a predictor. However, the practice of this method is also limited by the presence of atrial fibrillation, which is common in both post-MI and congestive heart failure patients, the main population of interest for risk stratification. This method necessitates the presence of VPBs, and it is not clear how long the recordings should last to obtain a sensible average value for all individual measurements of each VPB. The discrimination of VPBs with and without retrograde conduction should also be recognized and the retrogradely conducted beats should be extracted from calculations with further sophisticated methods. Large groups of patients are needed to clarify the effect of different therapeutic interventions on TS and TO. It is of paramount importance to explore the predictive power of HRT in discriminating those patients who are likely to benefit in terms of survival from preventive interventions, including both medical approaches and ICD implantation. The value of adding HRT to other risk stratification methods such as measurement HRV, TWA, SAECG, BRS, and QT dynamicity should also be investigated in order to increase the positive predictive accuracy in identifying high-risk patients.

References

1. Copie X, Hnatkova K, Staunton A et al (1996) Predictive power of increased heart rate versus depressed left ventricular ejection fraction and heart rate variability for risk stratification after myocardial infarction: results of a two-year follow-up study. J Am Coll Cardiol 27:270-276
2. Bigger JT Jr, Fleiss JL, Kleiger R et al (1984) The relationships among ventricular arrhythmias, left ventricular dysfunction, and mortality in the 2 years after myocardial infarction. Circulation 69:250-258
3. Gomes JA, Winters SL, Stewart D et al (1987) A new non-invasive index to predict sustained ventricular tachycardia and sudden death in the first year after myocardial infarction: based on signal-averaged electrocardiogram, radionuclide ejection fraction, and Holter monitoring. J Am Coll Cardiol 10:349-357
4. Kuchar DL, Thornburn CW, Sammel NL (1987) Prediction of serious arrhythmic events after myocardial infarction: signal-averaged electrocardiogram, Holter monitoring and radionuclide ventriculography. J Am Coll Cardiol 9:531-538
5. Barron HV, Viskin S (1998) Autonomic markers and prediction of cardiac death after myocardial infarction. Lancet 351:461-462
6. Barr CS, Naas A, Freeman M et al (1994) QT dispersion and sudden unexpected death in chronic heart failure. Lancet 343:327-329
7. Mehta D, Curwin J, Gomes JA, Fuster V (1997) Sudden death in coronary artery disease: acute ischemias versus myocardial substrate. Circulation 96:3215-3223
8. Santoni-Rugiu F, Gomes JA (1999) Methods for identifying patients at high risk of subsequent arrhythmic death after myocardial infarction. Curr Probl Cardiol 24:121-154

9. McCallister BD, Christian TF, Gersh BJ, Gibbons RJ (1993) Prognosis of myocardial infarction involving more than 40% of the left ventricle after acute reperfusion therapy. Circulation 88:1470-1475

10. The Multicenter Post-infarction Research Group (1983) Risk stratification and survival after myocardial infarction. N Engl J Med 309:331-336

11. La Rovere MT, Specchia G, Mortara A, Schwartz PJ (1988) Baroreflex sensitivity clinical correlates and cardiovascular mortality among patients with a first myocardial infarction. Circulation 78:816-824

12. Rosenbaum DS, Jackson LE, Smith JM et al (1994) Electrical alternans and vulnerability to ventricular arrhythmias. N Engl J Med 330:235-241

13. Ikeda T, Sakata T, Takami M et al (2000) Combined assessment of T-wave alternans and late potentials used to predict arrhythmic events after myocardial infarction: a prospective study. J Am Coll Cardiol 35:722-730

14. Gold MR, Bloomfield DM, Anderson KP et al (2000) A comparison of T wave alternans, signal averaged ECG and programmed ventricular stimulation for arrhythmia risk stratification. J Am Coll Cardiol 36:2247-2253

15. Parsonnet AE, Miller R (1944) Heart block. Influence on ventricular systole upon the auricular rhythm in complete and incomplete heart block. Am Heart J 27:676-687

16. Jedlicka J, Martin P (1987) Time course of vagal effects studies in clinical electrocardiograms. Eur Heart J 8:762-772

17. Skanes AC, Tang ASL (1998) Ventriculophasic modulation of atrioventricular nodal conduction in humans. Circulation 97:2245-2251

18. Schmidt G, Malik M, Barthel P et al (1999) Heart rate turbulence after ventricular premature beats as a predictor of mortality after acute myocardial infarction. Lancet 353:1390-1396

19. Schneider R, Barthel P, Schmidt G (1999) Methods for assessment of heart rate turbulence in Holter-ECGs. J Am Coll Cardiol 33[Suppl A]:351A

20. Julian DG, Camm AJ, Frangin G et al (1997) Randomised trial of effect of amiodarone on mortality in patients with left ventricular dysfunction after recent myocardial infarction: EMIAT. Lancet 349:667-674

21. Chung EK, Jewson DV (1970) Ventriculophasic sinus arrhythmia in the presence of artificial pacemaker induced ventricular rhythm. Cardiology 55:65-68

22. Rosenbaum M, Lepeschkin E (1995) The effect of ventricular systole on auricular rhythm in atrioventricular block. Circulation 11:240-261

23. Hashimoto K, Tanaka S, Hirata M, Chiba S (1967) Responses of the sinoatrial node to change in pressure in the sinus node artery. Circ Res 21:297-304

24. Kappagoda CT, Linden RJ, Saunders DA (1972) The effect off heart rate on distending the atrial appendages in the dog. J Physiol Lond 225:705-719

25. Barthel P, Schmidt G, Schneider R et al (1999) Heart rate turbulence in patients with and without autonomic dysfunction. J Am Coll Cardiol:136A

26. Malik M, Wichterle D, Schmidt G (1999) Heart-rate turbulence. G Ital Cardiol 29[Suppl 5]:65-69

27. Ghuran A, Schmidt G, La Rovere et al (2000) Pathophysiologic correlate of heart rate turbulence and baroreceptor reflex sensitivity from the ATRAMI Study. Eur Heart J 21[Suppl]:333

28. Schneider R, Schmidt G, Röck et al (2000) Heart rate turbulence: analysis in the frequency domain. J Am Coll Cardiol 35[2 Suppl A]:159A

29. Malik M, Schmidt G, Barthel P et al (1999) Heart rate turbulence is a post-infarction mortality predictor which is independent of and additive to other recognised risk factors. Pacing Clin Electrophysiol 22:741

30. Yap G, Camm AJ, Schmidt G, Malik M (2000) Heart rate turbulence predicts arrhythmic mortality in post myocardial infarction patients with left ventricular dysfunction – EMIAT substudy. Eur Heart J 21:332

31. Morley-Davies A, Dargie HJ, Cobbe SM et al (2000) Heart rate turbulence: a novel holter derived measure and mortality in chronic heart failure. Eur Heart J 21[Suppl]:408

32. Yap YG, Camm AJ, Schmidt G, Malik M (2000) Heart rate turbulence is influenced by sympathovagal balance in patients after myocardial infarction – EMIAT substudy. Eur Heart J 21[Suppl]:474

33. Barthel P, Schmidt G, Röck A et al (2000) Decreased heart rate turbulence in patients with diabetes mellitus. Eur Heart J 21[Suppl]:551

34. Yap GY, Camm J, Schmidt G, Malik M (2001) Heart rate turbulence is influenced by heart rate, age, left ventricular ejection fraction, NYHA class, diabetes, drugs and frequency of ventricular ectopics in patients after acute myocardial infarction – EMIAT substudy. J Am Coll Cardiol 37[Suppl A]:1A-648A

35. Chowdhary S, Ozman F, Ng GA et al (2000) Effects of quinapril and candesartan on heart rate turbulence in heart failure. Pacing Clin Electrophysiol 23:643

36. Schmidt G, Barthel P, Schneider R et al (2001) EMIAT substudy: prediction of the efficacy of amiodarone by heart rate turbulence. J Am Coll Cardiol 37[Suppl A]:1A-648A

37. Schmidt G, Malik M, Barthel P et al (2000) Heart rate turbulence in post myocardial infarction patients on and off betablockers. Pacing Clin Electrophysiol 23:619

T-Wave Alternans, a Powerful Index for Malignant Ventricular Arrhythmias – Fact or Fiction?

N. El-Sherif, G. Turitto, R.P. Pedalino, D. Robotis, V. Togay and S. Soliman

Introduction

In spite of recent improvement in overall cardiovascular mortality, sudden cardiac death (SCD) remains a formidable clinical challenge. Given the magnitude of the problem of SCD – representing up to 50% of all cardiac deaths – cardiologists have long struggled to identify individuals at specific risk for SCD [1]. Traditional strategies have focused on the very-high-risk subgroups in which SCD rates are high. These include survivors of acute myocardial infarction (AMI), and populations such as those studied in MADIT [2] and AVID [3] trials. This strategy has limited population impact, however, because it addresses only a small part of the spectrum of SCD risk. For example, 20%-30% of the population with known or unsuspected coronary artery disease experience SCD as the first clinically recognized manifestation of the disease [1].

Management strategies of SCD – which in the majority of cases is due to malignant ventricular tachyarrhythmias (VT), defined as hypotensive ventricular tachycardia and ventricular fibrillation – have centered over the years on two closely related aspects [4]: (1) how to identify those at risk of SCD, and (2) what the best management modalities, are - pharmacotherapy or the implantable cardioverter - defibrillator (ICD). Recent publications of the results of several multicenter studies have not so far proven pharmacotherapy, mainly antiarrhythmic drugs, to be an effective management modality for those at risk of SCD. This has cleared the way for more widespread use of the ICD as the sole, or main, management modality. Primarily because of the high cost of the ICD and the invasive nature of this therapeutic modality, the prophylactic use of the device for primary prevention of SCD did not gain momentum until recently. This aspect of management strategy for SCD is still in the clinical research domain, with several primary ICD prevention trials currently underway. However, this trend has highlighted the urgent need for more powerful risk stratification algorithms for SCD. Further, the recent results of

Cardiology Division, Department of Medicine, State University of New York, Downstate Medical Center and New York Harbor VA Health Care Center, Brooklyn, New York, USA

the MADIT [2] and AVID [3] trials on one hand and the CABG-PATCH trial [5] on the other hand underscored the point that the ICD works only when implanted in patients at high risk of arrhythmic death.

In order to provide impact on a significant proportion of the total population at risk, methods that allow increased resolution of SCD risk within more general populations will be required. Besides the invasive electrophysiology study (EPS), noninvasive risk stratifiers that have been commonly utilized include: left ventricular ejection fraction (LVEF), ventricular arrhythmias on ambulatory Holter recording, signal-averaged electrocardiography (SAECG), heart rate variability (HRV), baroreflex sensitivity (BRS), and QT dispersion. In addition, there are a number of other less commonly utilized markers of arrhythmic death, e.g., the recently introduced heart rate turbulence [6]. However, with the exception of LVEF, none of the other indicators, at present, has proven to be solely adequate as a powerful risk stratifier [4]. An optimal algorithm that combines more than one index of high risk has not yet been identified or agreed upon.

A new noninvasive technique that detects microvolt levels of T-wave alternans (TWA) has attracted increased interest in recent years [7]. Although overt TWA in the electrocardiogram (ECG) is not common [8], digital signal processing techniques capable of detecting subtle degrees of TWA have suggested that TWA is more prevalent than previously recognized and may represent an important marker of vulnerability to VT [9]. This review will examine the electrophysiologic basis that links TWA to electrical vulnerability and the recent clinical data that investigated TWA as a risk stratifier of VT.

Electrophysiologic Mechanisms of the Arrhythmogenicity of TWA

Interest in repolarization alternans is attributed to the hypothesis that it may reflect underlying dispersion of repolarization in the ventricle, a well-recognized electrophysiologic substrate for reentrant VT [10]. Investigations of the arrhythmogenicity of QT/T wave alternans in experimental models of the long QT syndrome (LQTS) have provided significant insight into the role of dispersion of ventricular repolarization in the generation of reentrant VT. Chinushi et al. studied an in vivo canine surrogate model of LQTS utilizing the neurotoxin anthopleurin-A (AP-A) and analyzed tridimensional repolarization and activation patterns during tachycardia-induced QT/T alternans [11]. The arrhythmogenicity of QT/T alternans was primarily due to the greater degree of spatial dispersion of repolarization during alternans than during slower rates not associated with alternans. The dispersion of repolarization was most marked between mid-myocardial (M) and epicardial zones in the LV free wall. In the presence of a critical degree of dispersion of repolarization, propagation of the activation wavefront could be blocked between these zones to initiate reentrant excitation and polymorphic VT. Two factors contributed to the modulation of repolarization during QT/T alternans, resulting in greater magnitude of dispersion of repolarization between M and epicardial zones at critical short cycle lengths: (1) differences in restitution kinetics at M sites, characterized by larger differences of the activation recovery interval (ARI), an accurate in vivo marker of the duration of repolarization, and a slower time constant as compared with epicardial sites; and (2) differences in the diastolic interval that would result in different input to the restitution curve at the same constant cycle length. The longer ARI of M sites resulted in shorter diastolic interval during the first short cycle, and thus a greater degree of ARI shortening.

An important observation was that marked repolarization alternans could be present in local electrograms without manifest alternation of the QT/T segment in the surface ECG. The latter was seen at critically short cycle lengths associated with reversal of the gradient of repolarization between epicardial and M sites, with a consequent reversal of polarity of the intramyocardial QT wave in alternate cycles. This observation provides the rationale for the digital processing techniques that attempt to detect subtle degrees of TWA.

The association of TWA with a greater degree of dispersion of repolarization was later confirmed in two other experimental models. Shimizu et al. [12] studied an in vitro surrogate model of LQTS utilizing the neurotoxin ATX-II and a perfused wedge preparation of canine LV wall. Simultaneous transmembrane action potentials were recorded from epicardial, M, and endocardial cells together with a simulated unipolar ECG. When the preparation was paced at a critical fast rate there was pronounced alternation of action potential duration (APD) of M cells, resulting in a reversal of repolarizing sequence across ventricular wall leading to alternation in the polarity of the T wave in the unipolar ECG. The authors concluded that TWA observed at rapid rates under long QT conditions is largely the result of alternation of the M-cell APD, leading to exaggeration of transmural dispersion of repolarization during alternate beats, and thus the potential for development of torsade de pointes. The data also suggested that, unlike transient forms of TWA which damp out quickly and depend on electrical restitution factors, the steady-state electrical and mechanical alternans demonstrated in their study appears to be largely the result of beat-to-beat alternans of I_{Ca}. Pastore et al. [13] investigated TWA in a Langendorff-perfused guinea pig heart using optical mapping of epicardial action potentials and showed that repolarization alternans at the level of the single cell accounts for TWA on the surface ECG. They also showed that discordant alternans produces spatial gradients of repolarization of sufficient magnitude to cause unidirectional block and reentrant VT.

Optimal Target Heart Rate for Exercise-Induced TWA

TWA is a threshold phenomenon, tending to appear abruptly when the heart rate exceeds a patient-specific onset heart rate threshold. Sustained TWA is defined as TWA that is present continuously while the patient's heart rate is above his/her onset heart rate. The occurrence of sustained TWA is the clinically predictive phenomenon. Because experimental evidence suggests that TWA is dependent on both heart rate and the sympathetic nervous system [14], the difference in the electrophysiologic mechanisms of rate-dependent TWA when heart rate is increased by exercise versus atrial pacing was investigated. The prevalence and heart rate threshold for TWA were compared in the same group of patients during exercise and atrial pacing [15]. This study showed that, during both exercise and atrial pacing, TWA developed when the heart rate reached a patient-specific threshold, and that the average threshold for TWA was similar whether the heart rate was increased by exercise or with pacing. This would suggest that the increase in heart rate rather than autonomic changes is primarily responsible for TWA. However, in this study a submaximal exercise was utilized that may not have been associated with significant activation of the sympathetic nervous system [16].

TWA is a rate-dependent phenomenon and microvolt TWA could develop in normal subjects at sufficiently high heart rate. The onset heart rate for sustained TWA in patients susceptible to VT tends to be relatively low. In clinical studies of TWA, a voltage > 1.9 μV and an alternans ratio higher than 3 at a heart rate below 110 beats/min was empirically utilized as the criterion of a positive test (Fig. 1). Recently, the optimal heart rate for the use of TWA as an index of ventricular vulnerability was systematically investigated [17]. Two groups of age-matched elderly subjects were studied: group I, 50 patients with malignant VT who received an ICD and constituted a "true positive" high-risk group, and group II, 55 normal subjects considered "true negative" for arrhythmic risk. The best sensitivity and specificity could be achieved at a target heart rate of 115 beats/min (100% and 96%, respectively) (Fig. 2). A target heart rate of 110 beats/min had a similar specificity (98%) but a lower sensitivity (82%). Lower target heart rates were associated with rapid decline of the sensitivity of the test, while maintaining a relatively high specificity.

This study was not designed to investigate the predictive value of exercise-induced TWA for malignant VT at large or to compare it with other indices of arrhythmic risk, such as programmed stimulation or the SAECG. However, in group I, which comprised patients at very high risk for arrhythmic death in whom the ICD was indicated according to currently approved guidelines, a TWA utilizing a target heart rate of 115 beats/min had only a 61% positivity. On the other hand, 11% of these patients had false negative results, while in the remaining 28% the test was indeterminate, because the patients could not exercise up to a target heart rate of 115 beats/min. In this group, it could be argued that the use of a pharmacological agent, e.g., isoproterenol, to increase heart rate to the target level may be advised and could conceivably enhance the sensitivity of the test. However, a comparison of the sensitivity/specificity of TWA induced by exercise versus pharmacological means is yet to be reported. It should be emphasized, however, that the two study groups with markedly contrasting arrhythmic risk are not appropriate for evaluating the predictive value of TWA for malignant VT, nor for comparing TWA with other potential risk stratifiers. Further, the study utilized an analysis algorithm for defining TWA that has been previously reported [18]. It is possible that a different algorithm would have resulted in a different optimal target heart rate. For example, a recent study has shown that the use of individual orthogonal leads plus a vector

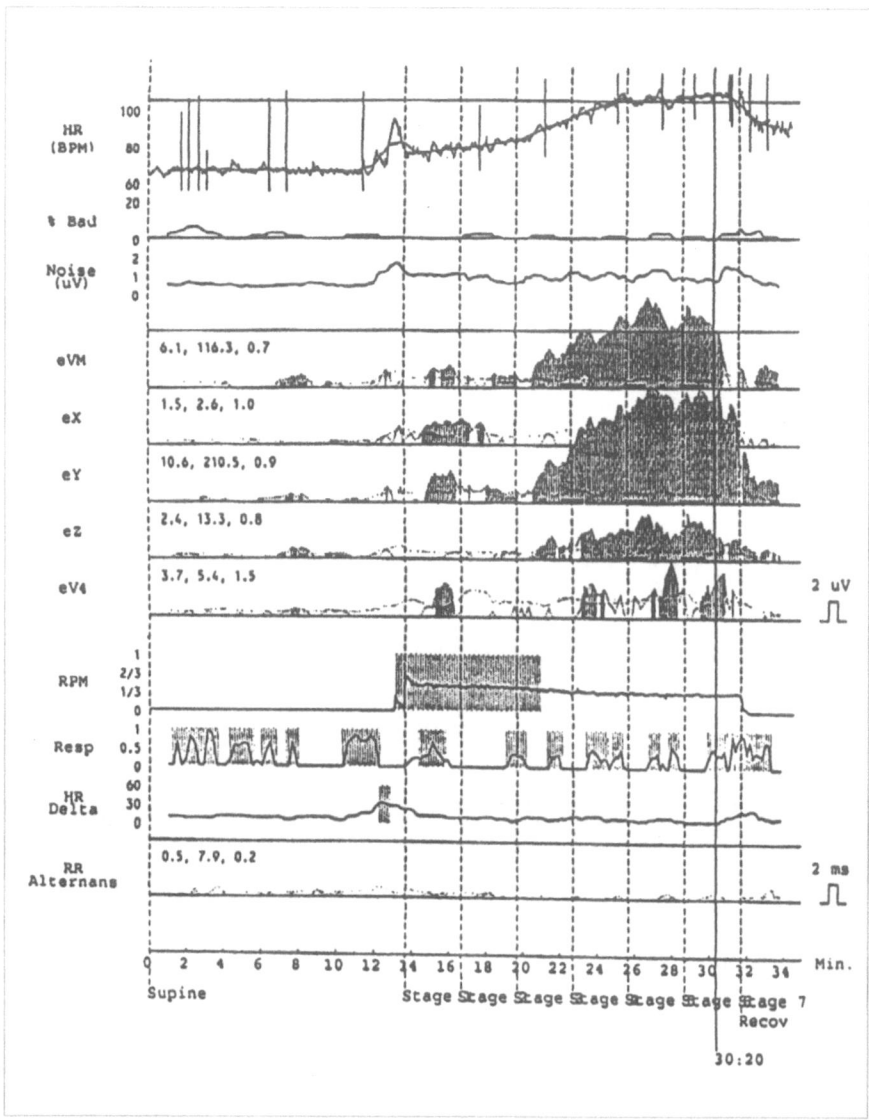

Fig. 1. A representative trend graph of TWA during bicycle exercise test in a 62-year-old male patient with coronary artery disease, prior myocardial infarction, and spontaneous and inducible sustained monomorphic ventricular tachycardia. Marked TWA (voltage > 1.9 mV with alternans ratio > 3) developed when the patient's heart rate reached 85 beats/min during stage I of exercise, increased until peak exercise, and gradually decreased during the recovery phase (shaded area in X,Y, Z leads and the vector magnitude eVM). (Reproduced by permission from [17])

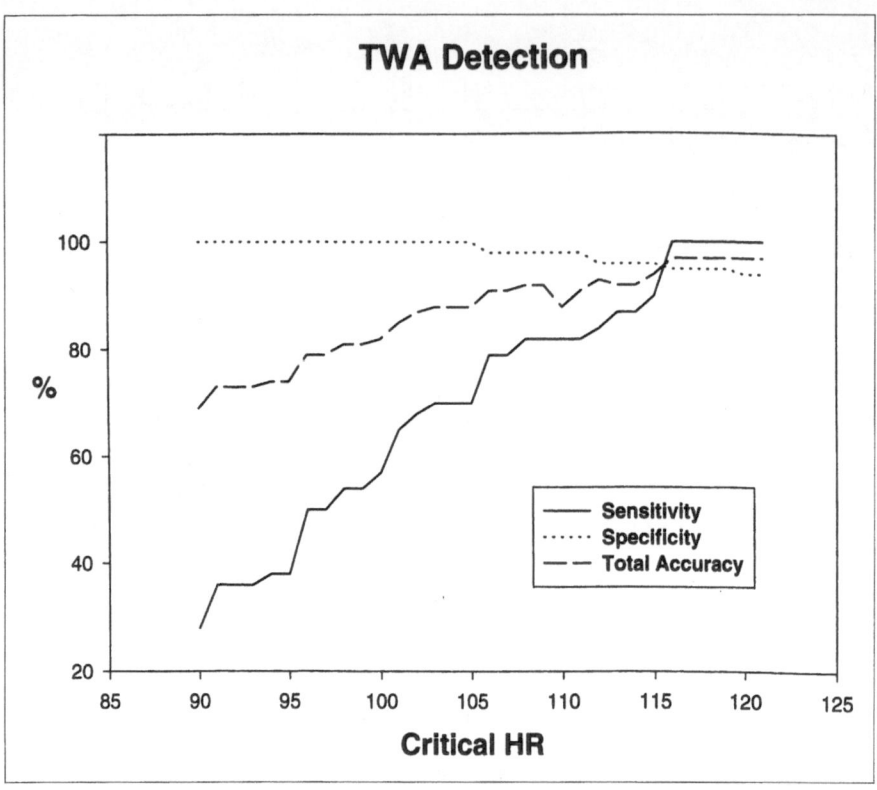

Fig. 2. Sensitivity, specificity, and total accuracy curves plotted to identify the optimal target heart rate for TWA detection. HR; heart rate (in beats/min). (Reproduced by permission from [17])

magnitude lead (as was utilized in the above study) results in increased sensitivity of the test as a predictor of VT inducibility [19]. On the other hand, the study raises the important issue of the sensitivity versus specificity of a diagnostic test in relation to the degree and severity of the risk investigated in a given population. For example, if TWA is to be used as a screening test for malignant VT in a population with low-to-moderate risk, it is comforting to know that the specificity of the test remains high up to a heart rate of 115 beats/min. However, in a high-risk population, e.g., those with coronary artery disease and LV dysfunction, to achieve a high degree of sensitivity for identification of those at risk (and who could, for example, receive a prophylactic ICD) it may be necessary to reach a high target heart rate.

Clinical Studies of TWA for Risk Stratification

The first study to demonstrate the value of TWA for arrhythmic risk stratification was published in 1994. Rosenbaum et al. [20] showed that microvolt-level TWA measured during atrial pacing prior to EPS identified patients at high risk of VT events (defined as sustained ventricular tachycardia, ventricular fibrillation, or SCD). Patients who did not have significant levels of TWA had only a 6% event rate over the following 20 months, while those with significant levels of TWA had an 81% rate of VT events. TWA performed equivalently to EPS as a predictor of VT events.

In subsequent studies of TWA, the increased heart rate was achieved by bicycle exercise test. In a pilot study of 27 patients who presented with sustained VT and underwent EPS, the TWA measured at rest and during exercise had a sensitivity of 89% and a specificity of 75%, and an overall clinical accuracy of 80% in predicting inducibility during EPS [18]. Based on the results of this study, a multicenter trial of 313 patients in sinus rhythm who were undergoing EPS was conducted [21]. TWA, assessed with bicycle ergometry, and the SAECG were measured before EPS. The primary endpoint was SCD, sustained VT, or appropriate ICD therapy, and the secondary endpoint was any of these arrhythmias or all-cause mortality. All follow-up data were censored at 400 days. Kaplan-Meyer survival analysis of the primary endpoint showed that TWA predicted events with a relative risk of 10.9, EPS with a relative risk of 7.1, and SAECG with a relative risk of 4.5. The relative risks for the secondary endpoint were 13.9, 4.7, and 3.3, respectively ($p < 0.05$). Multivariate analysis of 11 clinical parameters identified only TWA and EPS as independent predictors of events. In the prespecified subgroup with known or suspected VT, TWA predicted primary endpoints with a relative risk of 6.1 and secondary endpoints with a relative risk of 8.0. The study concluded that TWA is a strong independent predictor of spontaneous VT or death. It performed as well as programmed stimulation and better than the SAECG in risk stratifying patients for life-threatening VT.

Several other clinical studies of TWA were published in the last few years [22-29]. One study focused on patients receiving ICDs [22]. At the time of implantation of the ICD, 95 patients underwent a battery of diagnostic tests involving essentially all the arrhythmic risk stratifiers currently in use. These tests included TWA and invasive EPS, as well as measurement of LVEF, BRS, 24-h HRV, the presence of nonsustained ventricular tachycardia during 24-h ECG monitoring, and QT dispersion. The endpoint of the study was the first appropriate discharge of the ICD as documented by review of stored ECGs. Of all the diagnostic tests, only TWA and LVEF were statistically significant predictors of appropriate ICD therapy. Other studies investigated the predictive value of TWA for arrhythmic risk in patients with organic heart disease other than coronary artery disease. Murda'h et al. [23] measured TWA noninvasively in 64 patients with hypertrophic cardiomyopathy in an attempt to predict arrhythmic events in this high-risk patient population. A positive TWA was found in 34 out of 64 patients. TWA was the only significant marker with respect to identification of patients who survived a VT event. The predictive power could be increased by combining TWA with the clinical history (sensitivity: 86%; specificity: 79%). Adachi et al. [24] investigated the value of TWA in 58 patients with nonischemic dilated cardiomyopathy. EPS as well as many other noninvasive markers of arrhythmic risk are known to have less predictive accuracy in this group of patients compared to patients with ischemic heart disease. In this study, the sensitivity, specificity, and predictive accuracy of TWA for

VT were 88%, 72%, and 77%, respectively. Multivariate analysis showed that the presence of VT was a major independent determinant of TWA in patients with nonischemic dilated cardiomyopathy. The study concluded that TWA is a useful noninvasive test for identifying high-risk patients with dilated cardiomyopathy who have VT. Hennersdorf et al. [25] investigated the correlation of TWA and resuscitated SCD in patients with nonischemic cardiomyopathy, including dilated cardiomyopathy, chronic myocarditis, and LV hypertrophy. The study found a significant correlation between a positive TWA and a history of resuscitated arrhythmic event, with a sensitivity of 65% and a specificity of 98%.

There are currently a number of ongoing multicenter SCD primary prevention trials in patients with ischemic or nonischemic cardiomyopathy [30]. In some of the trials the only requirements for entering the study are LVEF < 35% and NYHA class II/III symptoms. The annual cardiac mortality in this group of patients is high and it is generally considered that approximately half of the deaths are sudden and presumably due to malignant VT, while the rest of the deaths are due to terminal pump failure [26]. It is obvious that a strategy that requires a prophylactic ICD in all of these patients represents significant redundancy, since at least half of the patients would not have benefited from such a highly expensive therapeutic modality. It stands to reason that better risk stratification in these patients is an important requirement before the ICD can be recommended as primary prophylaxis for SCD in this population. With this goal in mind, a recent report from Klingenheben et al. [27] investigated the predictive value of TWA for arrhythmic events in 107 patients with congestive heart failure and no history of sustained VT. The patients were followed up for arrhythmic events during the next 18 months. Of the patients with events, 11 had positive and 2 indeterminate TWA results; there were no arrhythmic events among patients with negative TWA results. Of 7 different noninvasive risk stratifiers, only TWA was a significant ($p = 0.0036$) and independent predictor of arrhythmic events.

TWA and the SAECG

The concept of combining more than one risk index for serious arrhythmic events in order to increase their combined predictive accuracy is a valid one. However, the combination of more than one risk index should be based on thorough understanding of their relationship to the underlying electrophysiologic mechanism(s) of malignant VT. In this regard, the combined application of the SAECG and TWA for risk stratification of malignant VT makes the most sense. The SAECG can provide evidence of ventricular conduction disorders while TWA detects underlying inhomogeneity of ventricular repolarization. These two electrophysiologic parameters contribute to a varying degree to the development of reentrant VT. A number of recent studies that examined the predictive value of these two techniques in the same group of patients reported inconsistent results [21, 28, 29]. For example, in the report by Gold et al. [21], both TWA and SAECG predicted arrhythmic events in univariate analysis with a relative risk of 10.9 and 4.5, respectively. However, in a multivariate analysis only TWA (and EPS) were independent predictors of events. On the other hand, Ikeda et al. [30] examined the combined predictive power of TWA and the SAECG in post-AMI patients. In this study, the event rate was significantly higher in patients with TWA, late potentials in the SAECG, and low LVEF. The negative predictive accuracy of TWA was very high whereas the positive value was lower than those of late potentials and LVEF. The study concluded that the combined indices of positive TWA and late potentials were associated with a high positive predictive value for arrhythmic events in the post-AMI patient. It is also important to emphasize that all the studies that examined both SAECG and TWA in the same group of patients utilized time-domain analysis of the SAECG. Several studies have shown that combined time-domain and frequency-domain analysis of the SAECG can significantly increase its positive predictive accuracy [31].

Some limitations of TWA

There are several technical and electrophysiologic limitations of the TWA that should be considered in the design of the best strategy for risk stratification of serious arrhythmic events. The two most obvious technical limitations are: (1) TWA could not be measured in patients with atrial fibrillation, a relatively common arrhythmia in patients with organic heart disease, and (2) the presence of frequent ectopic beats, motion artifacts, and in particular the inability of patients to achieve the target heart rate would render the results "indeterminate". Unfortunately, indeterminate results approach 20%-25% in most of the published studies. Some of these technical limitations could be reduced by refinement of the technique and by investigating, for example, exercise-induced versus pharmacologically induced increase in heart rate. On the electrophysiological aspect, there is evidence that the test may lose much of its predictive power when applied in the first few weeks after-AMI, a period of time known to be associated with a relatively high incidence of SCD [32].

Conclusions

The detection of rate-dependent microvolt TWA seems to be a powerful marker for the risk of malignant VT. This concept has a solid electrophysiological basis. The combination of this technique with other established risk indices such as SAECG (with combined time- and frequency-domain analysis) may provide a strong algorithm for risk stratification, especially in patients with organic heart disease. More importantly, the noninvasive nature and the relative low cost of both techniques make them ideal as screening tests in the much larger group of patients with only moderate risk for arrhythmic events. However, the real chal-

lenge is to prove the validity of the test in a prospective multicenter ICD primary prevention trial of SCD. Such a trial (Alternans Before Cardioverter
Defibrillator, ABCD) is currently underway.

Acknowledgements. This work was supported in part by VA MERIT and REAP grants to Nabil El-Sherif.

References

1. Myerburg RJ, Kessler KM, Castellanos A (1993) Sudden cardiac death: epidemiology, transient risk, and intervention assessment. Ann Intern Med 119:1187-1197
2. Moss AJ, Hall WJ, Cannom DS et al for the Multicenter Automatic Defibrillator Implantation Trial Investigators (1996) Improved survival with an implanted defibrillator in patients with coronary artery disease at high risk for ventricular arrhythmias. N Engl J Med 335:1933-1940
3. The Antiarrhythmics Versus Implantable Defibrillator (AVID) Investigators (1997) A comparison of antiarrhythmic-drug therapy with implantable defibrillators in patients resuscitated from near-fatal ventricular arrhythmias. N Engl J Med 337:1576-1583
4. El-Sherif N, Turitto G (1999) In search of the optimal algorithm for risk stratification of sudden cardiac death in the era of prophylactic ICD. MESPE 1:65-70
5. Bigger JT, for the Coronary Artery Bypass Graft (CABG) Patch Trial Investigators (1997) Prophylactic use of implanted cardiac defibrillators in patients at high risk for ventricular arrhythmias after coronary-artery bypass graft surgery. N Engl J Med 337:1569-1573
6. Schmidt G, Schneider R, Barthel P (1999) Heart rate turbulence. Cardiac Electrophysiol Rev 3:297-301
7. Smith JM, Clancy EA, Vereri CR et al (1988) Electrical alternans and clinical electrical instability. Circulation 77:110-121
8. Habbab MA, El-Sherif N (1992) TU alternans, long QTU, and torsade de pointes: clinical and experimental observations. Pacing Clin Electrophysiol 15:916-931
9. El-Sherif N (1999) T-wave alternans: a marker of vulnerability to ventricular tachyarrhythmias. In: Raviele A (ed) Cardiac arrhythmias. Springer-Verlag Italia, Milan, pp 12-16
10. Han J, Moe GK (1964) Nonuniform recovery of excitability in ventricular muscle. Circ Res 14:44-60
11. Chinushi M, Restivo M, Caref EB, El-Sherif N (1998) Electrophysiological basis of the arrhythmogenicity of QT/T alternans in the long QT syndrome. Tridimensional analysis of the kinetics of cardiac repolarization. Circ Res 83:614-628
12. Shimizu W, Antzelevitch C (1999) Cellular and ionic basis for T-wave alternans under long QT conditions. Circulation 99:1499-1507
13. Pastore JM, Girouard SD, Laurita KR et al (1999) Mechanism linking T-wave alternans to the genesis of cardiac fibrillation. Circulation 99:1385-1394
14. Verrier RL, Nearing BD (1999) Electrophysiologic basis for T-wave alternans as an index of vulnerability to ventricular fibrillation. J Cardiovasc Electrophysiol 5:445-461
15. Hohnloser SH, Klingenheben T, Zabel M et al (1997) T wave alternans during exercise and atrial pacing in humans. J Cardiovasc Electrophysiol 8:987-993
16. Verrier RL, Stone PH (1997) Exercise stress testing for T-wave alternans to expose latent electrical instability. J Cardiovasc Electrophysiol 8:994-996

17. Turitto G, Caref EB, El-Attar G, et al (2001) Optimal target heart rate for exercise-induced T-wave alternans. Ann Noninv Electrocardiol 6:123-128
18. Estes III NAM, Michaud G, Zipes DP, et al (1997) Electrical alternans during rest and exercise as predictors of vulnerability to ventricular arrhythmias. Am J Cardiol 80:1314-1318
19. Kavesh NG, Shorofsky SR, Sarang SE, Gold MR (1998) Effect of heart rate on T wave alternans. J Cardiovasc Electrophysiol 9:703-708
20. Rosenbaum D, Jackson LE, Smith JM et al (1994) Electrical alternans and vulnerability to ventricular arrhythmias. N Engl J Med 330:235-241
21. Gold MR, Bloomfield DM, Anderson KP et al (2000) A comparison of T-wave alternans, signal averaged electrocardiography and programmed ventricular stimulation for arrhythmia risk stratification. J Am Coll Cardiol 36:2248-2253
22. Hohnloser SH, Klingenheben T, Li YG et al (1998) T wave alternans as a predictor of recurrent ventricular tachyarrhythmias in ICD recipients. J Cardiovasc Electrophysiol 9:1258-1268
23. Murda'h M, McKenna W, Camm J (1997) Repolarization alternans: techniques, mechanisms, and cardiac vulnerability. Pacing Clin Electrophysiol 20(part II):2641-2657
24. Adachi K, Ohnishi Y, Shima T et al (1999) Determinants of microvolt-level T wave alternans in patients with dilated cardiomyopathy. J Am Coll Cardiol 34:374-380
25. Hennersdorf MG, Perings C, Niebch V et al (2000) T wave alternans as a risk predictor in patients with cardiomyopathy and mild-to-moderate heart failure. Pacing Clin Electrophysiol 23:1386-1391
26. Goldman S, Johnson G, Cohn JN et al (1993) Mechanisms of death in heart failure. The vasodilator-heart failure trials. The V-HeFT VA Cooperative Studies Group. Circulation 87:124-131
27. Klingenheben T, Zabel M, D'Agostino RB et al (2000) Predictive value of T-wave alternans for arrhythmic events in patients with congestive heart failure. Lancet 356:651-652
28. Armoundas AA, Rosenbaum DS, Ruskin JN et al (1998) Prognostic significance of electrical alternans versus signal averaged electrocardiography in predicting the outcome of electrophysiologic testing and arrhythmia free survival. Heart 80:251-256
29. Ikeda T, Sakata T, Takami M et al (2000) Combined assessment of T-wave alternans and late potentials used to predict arrhythmic events after myocardial infarction. J Am Coll Cardiol 35:722-730
30. El-Sherif N, Turitto G (2000) The need for powerful risk stratification of sudden cardiac death in the era of prophylactic ICD. In: Ovsyschcher IE (ed) Cardiac arrhythmias and devise therapy: results and perspective for the new century. Futura, Armonk, NY, pp 273-284
31. Vazquez R, Caref EB, Torres F et al (1999) Improved diagnostic value of the combined time- and frequency-domain analysis of the signal-averaged electrocardiogram after myocardial infarction. J Am Coll Cardiol 33:385-394
32. Tapainen JM, Still A-M, Airaksinen J, Huikuri HV (2001) Prognostic significance of risk stratifiers of mortality following an acute myocardial infarction including T-wave alternans. Results of a prospective follow-up study. J Cardiovasc Electrophysiol 12:645-652

Prevention of Sudden Death in Different Realities: Can We Reach a Consensus?

D.S. Cannom

Sudden death presents a challenge to the North American electrophysiology community which is unmet at many levels. Innovations in medical care over the past two decades have decreased the numbers and perhaps the characteristics of those who suffer sudden death. However, current data suggests that patients who survive a malignant cardiac arrhythmia are being undertreated in most areas of the world including North America. More importantly, survivors of malignant arrhythmias and candidates for prophylactic implantable cardioverter-defibrillators (ICDs) constitute only a small percentage of those patients who will die in the United States.

The magnitude of the sudden death problem has been widely publicized, and the accepted number is that some 300 000 patients die suddenly in the United States each year. This figure is based on calculations rather than actual counts and assumes that 50% of all cardiac deaths are sudden [1]. While there has been a sharp reduction in age-adjusted risk of cardiovascular death over the past 30 years, the percentage of these patients who die suddenly is unchanged. The widespread use of thrombolysis and angioplasty reduces the number of patients who die due to myocardial infarction, and patients live longer due to the post-procedure use of β-blockers, statins, and aspirin. We are probably converting the short-term mortality from myocardial infarction (which approached 30% 35 years ago) to a group of chronic coronary patients who remain at risk of sudden death because of their associated congestive failure. These epidemiologic considerations, plus greater awareness in the United States of less common causes of sudden death in the young (e.g., long QT and ARVD), strongly suggest that we need an accurate count of the victims of sudden death. A national registry of sudden death victims would be helpful, although this, too, would be hampered by inadequate definitions and documentation.

The 1990s were a golden age of clinical trials which focused primarily on patients who had already experienced an episode of out-of-hospital cardiac arrest or symptomatic ventricular tachycardia (VT). The results of the

Division of Cardiology, Good Samaritan Hospital, Los Angeles, California, USA

Antiarrhythmics Versus Implantable Defibrillators (AVID) study, Canadian Implantable Defibrillator Study (CIDS), and Cardiac Arrest Study Hamburg (CASH) are widely known and accepted. These trials all showed, in carefully designed randomized prospective trials, that the ICD improved survival in a statistically significant way compared to amiodarone, especially among patients with an ejection fraction (EF) under 36% [2-4]. Thus, for the patient with a higher EF (> 36%), either drugs or an ICD was adequate therapy. The ICD did not show a benefit in this population because the overall mortality was so low (< 20%) at the termination of the study. The benefit of the ICD in patients with lower EF was confirmed in CIDS and CASH as well. While trial data are not available in other populations of interest (e.g., sudden cardiac death either due to reversible causes, after coronary artery bypass graft, or in high EF patients), there are usually enough clinical data to make well-informed decisions in most patients.

The North American electrophysiology community has enthusiastically accepted these trial results. While there was much debate about the design and even the ethics of the AVID trial during its enrollment, there is now no organized professional resistance to the published results. Both the American Heart Association and the American College of Cardiology accepted the AVID data as class I indications for the ICD after the AVID results were published [5, 6]. This endorsement has made it relatively easy to assure that payors will accept the published device indications and not provide barriers to payment to the hospital and physician.

In the 1990s there was a steady increase in the number of newly implanted ICDs on a per annum basis, with the number going from 22 000 in 1995 to 49 000 in 1999 (Equity Research Bank of America Securities, April 30, 2000). This dramatic increase in the number of ICDs came at a time when the results of studies such as AVID, CIDS, and CASH were widely disseminated in North America. However, in the past year or two, the rate of new ICD implantations has leveled. The growth between 1999 and 2000 was only 8000 units. This stabilization of ICD implantation numbers has concerning implications for both device manufacturers and potential patients.

One major device company has done an extensive analysis of potential patient populations based on available data (M. McGrory, Medtronic Inc., personal communication). They analyzed both Medicare and managed care claims data representing the experiences of some 2.6 million managed care lives and 2.0 million Medicare patients during the year 1997. Based on appropriate diagnosis codes, including all patients with ventricular tachycardia or ventricular fibrillation as a primary or secondary diagnosis, they found some potential 334 000 ICD candidates in the US. By excluding patients with comorbidities (15%) and those with a left ventricular ejection fraction above 35% (40%), the number was reduced to 200 000 potential ICD candidates, or 763 potential ICD candidates per million population.

This number (763/million) of potential implantations contrasts dramatically with the actual ICD implantation numbers in North America. The current figure for ICD implantation in the US is only 185 per million population. If these calculations are correct, it means that only a small fraction of the eligible patients in the US are actually receiving an ICD. Yet, the US implantation rate is high compared to countries in Europe and the Far East. These data are both surprising and concerning. One conclusion might be that more physician education about ICD indications is necessary, perhaps at the level of the primary care physician, including internists and family practitioners. Another strategy might be to begin direct patient education about cardiac arrhythmias and their appropriate treatment. Pharmaceutical companies have done a good job of educating the American public about statin therapy using sports figures as spokesmen in newspaper sports pages.

Another interpretation of these data is that we do not have enough trained electrophysiologists to implant these devices, or that available electrophysiologists are too involved in ablation therapy and pacing therapies to implant devices. This theory implies that the rate-limiting step in device implantation growth is the availability of adequately trained physicians. The US has roughly three times as many implanting physicians per million as Western Europe. With industrial support, the North American Society of Pacing and Electrophysiology (NASPE) recently awarded US$ 5 million to fund 20 additional advanced electrophysiology fellowships at 20 major university training programs funded over 5 years. An exhaustive manpower study of the electrophysiology community in North America, intended to assess actual capacity, is underway and should be complete by January, 2002.

The use of the ICD as a prophylactic tool for the prevention of sudden death is much less well developed. Virtually every electrophysiologist is well aware of the surprisingly effective role of the ICD in the so-called MADIT I trial. Mortality was reduced by 54% in coronary patients with an ejection fraction below 35% who were inducible and nonsuppressed in the electrophysiology laboratory and treated with an ICD [7]. A further analysis of these data showed that the ICD benefit in the MADIT population was limited to patients with an ejection fraction under 26%, patients with left bundle branch block, and patients with recently treated congestive heart failure [8]. While MADIT I was heavily criticized after its publication, subsequent data from the MUSTT trial, while using a completely different design and a large (2200) population, indirectly confirmed the MADIT I data by identifying the ICD as the reason for survival benefit in the antiarrhythmic drug arm of the trial [9].

The surprising data from the MUSTT trial in high-risk patients have made the primary prevention field one of the most interesting in electrophysiology. Not only do patients in primary prevention ICD trials have dramatic reductions in mortality compared to secondary prevention patients (approximately 50% reduction in mortality versus 30%), but also the numbers of patients are large enough that the widespread application of the ICD might begin to have a favorable impact on the US sudden death figures. The primary prevention trials underway, MADIT II and SCD-HEFT, are both studying patients with cardiomyopathy with a low ejection fraction (30% in MADIT and 35% in SCD-HEFT) and using no other risk stratifier [10, 11]. ICD therapy is being compared to either best medical therapy (MADIT II) or amiodarone versus placebo (SCD-HEFT), and trial data should be available for MADIT II in 2001 and SCD-HEFT in 2002-3 (Fig. 1).

However, all of the potential survival benefit offered by the ICD in primary and secondary populations only accounts for some 15%-25% of the patients who will have an episode of sudden death in a given year. As Myerburg has pointed out, if we aggressively treat cardiac arrest survivors and patients with sustained ventricular tachycardia with an ICD, we will have treated only 5%-10% of the population of sudden cardiac death victims. If we expand attention to patients with left ventricular dysfunction and congestive failure, as in SCD-HEFT and MADIT II, we may prevent another 10%-15% of potential sudden deaths (Fig. 2). Only if we successfully treat *all* categories of coronary ischemia in addition to attenuating traditional risk factors for coronary artery disease will we have a statistically significant impact on sudden deaths due to coronary artery disease.

The real solution to the sudden death problem lies in improved medical and possibly even genetic therapy to prevent coronary disease and at the same time successfully risk stratifying the small numbers of patients with congenital diseases. The ultimate assault on the sudden death problem will be a medical one through the aggressive use of a variety of medications including β-blockers, statins, and aspirin. The impressive and relatively cheap promise of such treatments is becoming an everyday reality as the medical community prescribes

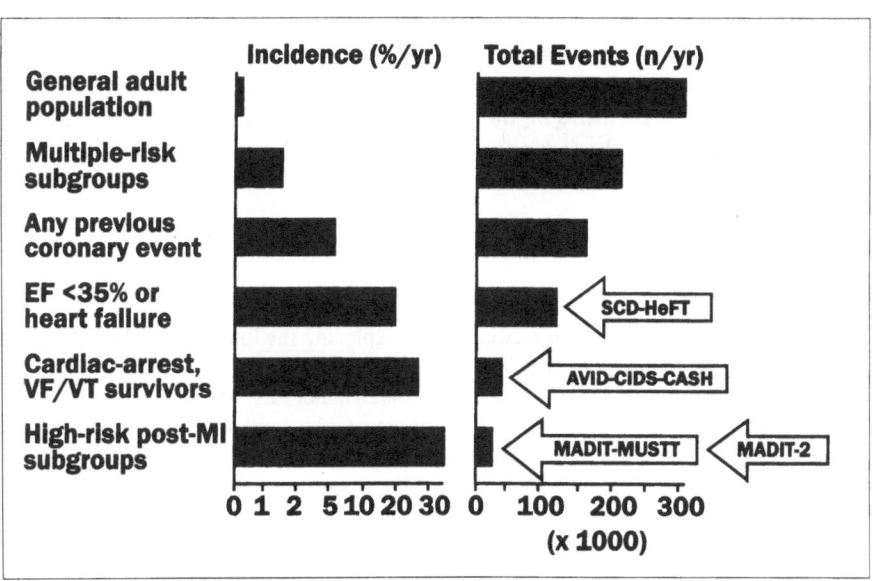

Fig. 1. Relationship between population subsets, incidence of sudden cardiac death, and total population burden for each group. With increasing incidence, based on subgroup profiling, there is a decreasing proportion of the total sudden death burden. The population groups under study in the major ICD trials are shown for each subgroup: note that the total events per year represented in these trials is small in relation to the total sudden death population. (Used with permission from [1], p. 371)

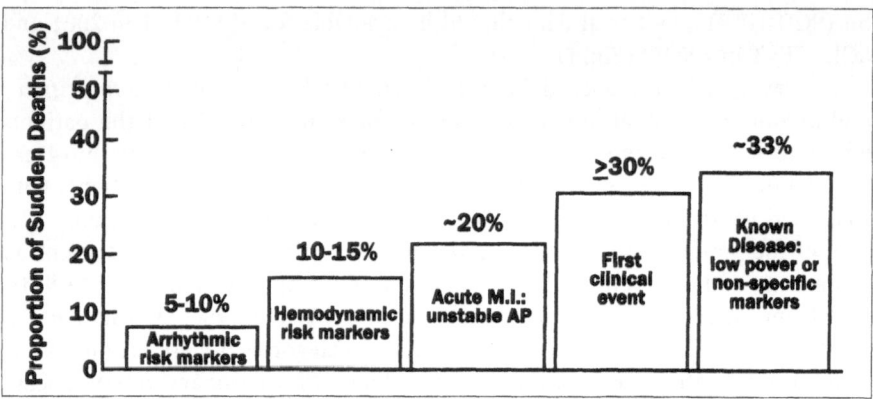

Fig. 2. Subgroups at risk of sudden cardiac death within the category of ischemic heart disease. The population subset with high-risk arrhythmia markers constitute less than 10% of the total sudden death burden attributable to coronary artery disease. A somewhat larger group is associated with hemodynamic risk markers and congestive heart failure. More than 50% of the total sudden death burden is accounted for by those victims among whom sudden cardiac death is the first clinical event or those who have known coronary heart disease but a low power of risk. (Used with permission from [1], p. 372)

more of these drugs in an increasingly aggressive manner. This hope is realistic to a certain level but not beyond. In most clinics, the patients presenting for treatment after a cardiac arrhythmia are those who developed their heart disease in the late 1980s and early 1990s. The number of patients available for device implantation as primary prophylactic therapy is also large, but may diminish as fewer patients present with low ejection fraction. For the next few years, however, the immediate need seems to be that of appropriately treating high-risk patients based on the data from the secondary and primary ICD trials of the 1990s.

References

1. Myerburg RJ (2001) Sudden cardiac death: exploring the limits of our knowledge. J Cardiovasc Electrophysiol 12:369-381
2. The Antiarrhythmics Versus Implantable Defibrillators (AVID) Investigators (1997) A comparison of antiarrhythmic drug therapy with implantable defibrillators in patients resuscitated from near-fatal ventricular arrhythmias. N Engl J Med 337:1576-1583
3. Connolly SJ, Gent M, Roberts RS et al, on behalf of the CIDS investigators (2000) Canadian Implantable Defibrillator Study (CIDS): a randomized trial of the implantable cardioverter defibrillator against amiodarone. Circulation 101:1297-1302
4. Kuck KH, Cappato R, Siebels J et al (2000) Randomized comparison of antiarrhythmic drug therapy with implantable defibrillators in patients resuscitated from cardiac arrest. The Cardiac Arrest Study Hamburg (CASH). Circulation 102:748-754
5. Gregoratos G, Cheitlin MD, Conill A et al (1998) ACC/AHA guidelines for implantation of cardiac pacemakers and antiarrhythmic devices: a report of the ACC/AHA Task Force on practice guidelines. J Am Coll Cardiol 31:1175-1209

6. Lerman RD, Cannom DS (2001) Indications for implantable cardioverter defibrillator therapy in year 2000. Card Electrophysiol Rev 5:6-14
7. Moss AJ, Hall WJ, Cannom DS et al (1996) Improved survival with an implanted defibrillator in patients with coronary disease at high risk for ventricular arrhythmia. N Engl J Med 335:1933-1940
8. Moss AJ, Fadi Y, Zareba W et al for the Multicenter Automatic Defibrillator Implantation Trial Research Group (2001) Survival benefit with an implanted defibrillator in relation to mortality risk in chronic coronary heart disease. Am J Cardiol, (in press)
9. Buxton AE, Lee KL, Fisher JD et al (1999) A randomized study of the prevention of sudden death in patients with coronary artery disease. Multicenter Unsustained Tachycardia Trial (MUSTT) Investigators. N Engl J Med 341:1882-1890
10. Moss AJ, Cannom DS, Daubert JP et al for the MADIT II investigators (1999) Multicenter Automatic Defibrillator Implantation Trial II (MADIT II): design and clinical protocol. Ann Noninvas Electrocard 4:83-91
11. Klein H, Auricchio A, Reek S, Geller C (1999) New primary prevention trials of sudden cardiac death in patients with left ventricular dysfunction: SCD-HEFT and MADIT II. Am J Cardiol 83:91D-97D

Drug Prevention of Sudden Death after Myocardial Infarction: Role of Angiotensin Converting Enzyme Inhibitors

G.V. Naccarelli, D.L. Wolbrette, J.C. Luck and J.P. Boehmer

After a patient survives a myocardial infarction (MI), his or her risk of death from nonarrhythmic and arrhythmic cardiac causes averages 5%-10% per year. Sudden cardiac death accounts for about half of these deaths. The highest risk is in patients with the largest infarction (lowest ejection fractions) and is increased further in patients with concomitant ventricular arrhythmias, latent ischemia, and other noninvasive risk stratifiers such as an abnormal signal average electrocardiogram (SAECG), decreased heart rate variability, abnormal reflex baroreceptor sensitivity, or the presence of repolarization alternans [1]. Although a single positive test may predict future events in 15%-30% of patients, even the addition of several positive tests is only predictive in 30%-40% of patients. Given this group's enhanced risk of reinfarction and sudden death, with less than a 20% survival probability if an out-of-hospital cardiac arrest should occur, prophylactic therapies have been studied as a primary preventative strategy in post-MI patients.

ACE Inhibitors After MI

Several prospective clinical trials have demonstrated that angiotensin converting enzyme (ACE) inhibitors improve survival and decrease morbidity in patients with a depressed ejection fraction after a recent MI [1-14]. The HOPE trial demonstrated a benefit of ramipril in patients at high cardiovascular risk including patients whose MI was remote [15]. Although ACE inhibitors have no known direct electrophysiologic effects, they may be antiarrhythmic by enhancing left ventricular remodeling, decreasing maladaptive hypertrophy, improving endothelial dysfunction, preventing left ventricular dilatation, and possibly by reducing stretch receptors [16]. Although a small study demonstrated a decrease in ventricular ectopic activity in patients treated with ACE inhibitors [17], this antiarrhythmic effect was not seen in the larger SOLVD

Division of Cardiology, Cardiovascular Center, Penn State University College of Medicine, Hershey, Pennsylvania, USA

prevention study. A consideration is that ACE inhibitors may decrease the sudden cardiac death rate by a nonarrhythmic mechanism such as reducing reinfarction or stroke.

Multiple studies [1-10] have studied the beneficial effects of various ACE inhibitors on post-MI survival. Meta-analyses of randomized trials of early ACE inhibitor used in MI patients have demonstrated a 6.5% statistical ($p = 0.006$) reduction in mortality [11-14].

In ISIS-4 [2], 58 050 post-MI patients were randomly assigned to receive captopril (up to 50 mg b.i.d.) or placebo at any time up to 7 days after infarction. By 35 days of therapy, mortality was reduced by 7% in the captopril group ($p = 0.02$) and the benefit persisted for a year. Greater benefit was noted in patients with previous MI or congestive heart failure (CHF).

In GISSI-3 [3], there was a 12% reduction ($p = 0.03$) in mortality in 19 934 patients treated with lisinopril (within 24 h of MI) when compared to the usual care group. Most of the benefit occurred in patients with CHF.

In contrast to studies demonstrating benefit, CONSENSUS II [4] did not reveal any benefit of an ACE inhibitor. In this study, 6090 patients presenting within 24 h of acute MI were treated with 1 mg i.v. enalaprilat followed by oral enalapril (≤ 20 mg/day) or placebo for 6 months. This trial was prematurely terminated due to early hypotensive reactions in high-risk elderly patients as well as absence of benefit in the enalapril-treated patients. Six-month mortality was 10.2% in the placebo versus 11% in the enalapril group ($p = 0.26$).

In the Survival and Ventricular Enlargement (SAVE) trial [5], patients with asymptomatic left ventricular dysfunction (ejection fraction ≤ 40%) 3-16 days after MI were treated with captopril (≤ 50 mg t.i.d.) or placebo. After 42 months of follow-up, captopril reduced mortality by 19% ($p = 0.019$), cardiovascular events by 21% ($p = 0.01$), and severe heart failure by 37% ($p < 0.001$). There was no statistical difference in the 5.6% sudden death rate in the captopril compared to the 6.7% rate in the placebo group ($p > 0.25$). Benefits were noted even in patients treated with thrombolytics, aspirin, and β-blockers.

The Acute Infarction Ramipril Efficacy (AIRE) study [6] evaluated the effects of ramipril (≤ 5 mg b.i.d.) in 2206 patients with heart failure within 3-10 days of an MI. Ramipril reduced mortality by 27% ($p = 0.002$) and a combined endpoint of death, severe heart failure, MI, and stroke by 19%.

In the Trandolapril Cardiac Evaluation (TRACE) study [7] trandolapril (≤ 4 mg q.d.) reduced mortality by 22% ($p = 0.001$) in patients who had echocardiographic evidence of left ventricular dysfunction 3-7 days after MI. Trandolapril also significantly reduced sudden death by 24% ($p = 0.03$) and severe heart failure by 29% ($p = 0.003$).

Zofenopril administered during the first 24 h of an anterior MI tended to reduce total mortality by 22% ($p = 0.17$) and sudden cardiac death (from 1.4% to 0.5%, $p = 0.17$) in high risk post-MI patients in the Survival of Myocardial Infarction in Long-Term Evaluation (SMILE) study [8].

Recently the HOPE trial [15] demonstrated a beneficial effect of ramipril which included a large number (52%) of patients with a prior MI, although their infarction was remote and not recent. Ramipril produced a large decrease in the combined endpoint of MI, stroke, and cardiovascular death (relative risk 0.78, 95% CI 0.70-0.86). All-cause mortality was also reduced (relative risk 0.84, 95% CI 0.75-0.95).

Although individual trials, except for TRACE, have not demonstrated that ACE inhibitors reduce sudden cardiac death, meta-analyses have demonstrated that these drugs reduce sudden death by 20% (odds ratio 0.80; 95% CI 0.70-0.92) consistent with positive trends of individual trials [18].

Clinical Perspective on ACE Inhibitors After MI

ACE inhibitor treatment should be routinely started to improve survival and promote left ventricular remodeling within 24 h of the onset of an MI if there is no contraindication to therapy [14, 19]. Except for hypotension, drug-induced cough, or azotemia, there appears to be little downside risk with the use of these drugs. The ACC/AHA class I indications [20] include: (1) patients within the first 24 h of a suspected MI with ST-segment elevation in two or more anterior precordial leads or with CHF; and (2) patients with MI and left ventricular ejection fraction < 40% or CHF during or after an MI. The reduction in mortality using several different agents suggests this benefit may be secondary to a class effect. This finding is consistent with meta-analytic studies reporting the benefit of ACE inhibitors on prolonging survival in CHF patients [21]. In addition, one should keep in mind that this effect is additive to other drugs that prolong survival after MI such as β-blockers [22].

References

1. Naccarelli GV, Wolbrette DW, Dell'Orfano JT et al (1999) A decade of clinical trial developments in postmyocardial infarction, congestive heart failure, and sustained ventricular tachyarrhythmia patients: From CAST to AVID and beyond. J Cardiovasc Electrophysiol 9:864-891
2. ISIS-4 (Fourth International Study of Infarct Survival) Collaborative Group (1995) ISIS-4: a randomised factorial trial assessing early oral captopril, oral mononitrate, and intravenous magnesium sulphate in 58,050 patients with suspected acute myocardial infarction. Lancet 345:669-685
3. Gruppo Italiano per lo Studio della Sopravvivenza nell'Infarto Miocardico (1994) GISSI-3: effects of lisinopril and transdermal glyceryl trinitrate singly and together on 6-week mortality and ventricular function after acute myocardial infarction. Lancet 343:1115-1122
4. Swedberg K, Held P, Kjekshus J et al (1992) Effects of early administration of enalapril on mortality in patients with acute myocardial infarction: results of the Cooperative New Scandinavian Enalapril Survival Study II (CONSENSUS II). N Engl J Med 327:678-684
5. Pfeffer MA, Braunwald E, Moye LA et al on behalf of the SAVE Investigators (1992) Effect of captopril on mortality and morbidity in patients with left ventricular dysfunction after myocardial infarction. N Engl J Med 327:669-677

6. The Acute Infarction Ramipril Efficacy (AIRE) Study Investigators (1993) Effect of ramipril on mortality and morbidity of survivors of acute myocardial infarction with clinical evidence of heart failure. Lancet 342:821-828

7. Kober L, Torp-Pedersen C, Carlsen JE et al (1995) A clinical trial of the angiotensin-converting-enzyme inhibitor trandolapril in patients with left ventricular dysfunction after myocardial infarction. N Engl J Med 333:1670-1676

8. Ambrosini E, Booghi C, Magnani B, for the Survival of Myocardial Infarction Long-Term Evaluation (SMILE) Study Investigators (1995) The effect of the angiotensin-converting enzyme inhibitor zofenopril on mortality and morbidity after anterior myocardial infarction. N Engl J Med 332:80-85

9. Chinese Cardiac Study Collaborative Group (1995) Oral captopril versus placebo among 13,634 patients with suspected acute myocardial infarction: interim report from the Chinese Cardiac Study (CCS-1). Lancet 345:686-688

10. Kingma JH, VanGilst WH, Peels CH et al (1994) Acute intervention with captopril during thrombolysis in patients with first anterior myocardial infarction: results from the Captopril and Thrombolysis Study (CATS). Eur Heart J 15:898-907

11. Lau J, Antman EM, Jimenez-Silva J et al (1992) Cumulative meta-analysis of therapeutic trials for myocardial infarction. N Engl J Med 327:248-254

12. Hennekens CH, Albert CM, Godfried SL et al (1996) Adjunctive drug therapy of acute myocardial infarction – evidence from clinical trials. N Engl J Med 335:1660-1667

13. Latini R, Maggioni AP, Flather M et al (1995) ACE inhibitor use in patients with myocardial infarction. Summary of evidence from clinical trials. Circulation 92:3132-3137

14. Ball SG, Hall AS, Murray GD (1995) Angiotensin-converting enzyme inhibitors after myocardial infarction: Indications and timing. J Am Coll Cardiol 25:42S-46S

15. The Heart Outcomes Prevention Evaluation Study Investigators (2000) Effects of an angiotensin-converting enzyme inhibitor, ramipril, on cardiovascular events in high risk patients. N Engl J Med 342:145-153

16. Pratt C, Gardner M, Pepine C et al (1995) Lack of long-term ventricular arrhythmia reduction by enalapril in heart failure. Am J Cardiol 75:1244-1249

17. Sogaard P, Gotzsche CO, Ravkilde J et al (1994) Ventricular arrhythmias in acute and chronic phases after acute myocardial infarction. Effect of intervention with captopril. Circulation 90:101-107

18. Domanski MJ, Exner DV, Borkowf CB et al (1999) Effect of angiotensin converting enzyme inhibition on sudden cardiac death in patients following acute myocardial infarction. J Am Coll Cardiol 33:598-604

19. Brunner F, Kukovetz WR (1995) Postischemic antiarrhythmic effects of angiotensin enzyme inhibitors. Role of suppression of endogenous endothelin secretion. Circulation 94:1752-1761

20. Ryan TJ, Anderson JL, Antman EM et al (1996) ACC/AHA guidelines for the management of patients with acute myocardial infarction: a report of the American College of Cardiology/American Heart Association Task Force on Practice Guidelines (Committee on Management of Acute Myocardial Infarction). J Am Coll Cardiol 28:1328-1428

21. Garg R, Yusuf S, for the Collaborative Group on ACE Inhibitor Trials (1995) Overview of randomized trials of angiotensin-converting enzyme inhibitors on mortality and morbidity in patients with heart failure. JAMA 273:1450-1456

22. Vantrimpont P, Rouleau JL, Wun CC et al, for the SAVE Investigators (1997) Additive beneficial effects of beta-blockers to angiotensin-converting enzyme inhibitors in the Survival and Ventricular Enlargement (SAVE) study. J Am Coll Cardiol 29:229-236

Post-Infarction: When and How to Use Amiodarone

P. J. Schwartz

The choice of an antiarrhythmic drug to reduce the risk for sudden cardiac death after an acute myocardial infarction should be left to neither chance nor personal preference. This concept, not mindboggling but certainly sound, has been over the years a consistent theme of the Sicilian Gambit [1-4].

A presentation aimed at discussing when and how to use, after a myocardial infarction (MI), a highly specific and unique antiarrhythmic drug, such as amiodarone [5], should follow a certain logical process. It will refrain, for example, from giving excessive weight to a meta-analysis based on patients suffering from different types of cardiac disorders [6]. It will recognize the meaningful point of a relatively small but significant reduction in all-cause mortality, and will then move on.

It will consider, briefly again, a meta-analysis [7] based on two large clinical trials, such as EMIAT and CAMIAT [8, 9], and will acknowledge the value of relatively similar sizes of the populations under study and particularly the fact that the two trials were carried out simultaneously. It will consider also the very similar outcomes in terms of all-cause mortality and of arrhythmic mortality. It will, however, give proper weight to the fact that one of these trials, CAMIAT, was performed without information on the left ventricular ejection fraction of the patients – not a small point, given the general consensus that a depressed ejection fraction remains the single most important predictor of post-MI mortality. The fact that an unknown percentage of patients in CAMIAT might have had a well-preserved ejection fraction will be taken into account when examining nonidentical observations, for example the interaction with β-blockers.

It should, thus, not be surprising if this presentation would eventually focus on the results of one adequately large randomized study, such as EMIAT [8]. Moreover, as the audience will be represented not only by trialists but also, and more importantly, by practicing cardiologists used to deal with an "n of 1" (because such should be the patient-physician relationship), this presentation could give careful consideration also to subgroup analyses, and more than one has been performed on the EMIAT database [10, 11]. This would mean looking at subgroups, probably not pre-specified in the study protocol, which, according to the books, should at best serve to produce hypothesis-generating observa-

Department of Cardiology, Policlinico S. Matteo IRCCS and University of Pavia, Italy

tions. These subgroups analyses could nonetheless stimulate unconventional approaches when we are doing all we can to save a patient's life while remaining mindful of the quality of the same life, which we try to prolong.

Finally, such an unorthodox presentation might even flirt with anathema and approach the forbidden area of the "on-treatment" analysis. And this could happen because it might be considered that, while the "intention-to-treat" analysis remains and should remain the gold standard for randomized clinical trials, the "on-treatment" analysis becomes the most informative about the efficacy of a single intervention when there is a high number of patients who, for whatever reason, discontinue the study medication. In EMIAT, this happened for 38.5% of patients assigned to amiodarone treatment.

As Bernard Lown wrote, more than 20 years ago [12], "*The physician is not unmindful of the ultimate futility, but although there is no cure for sudden death there is a high art in its deferment*". Art requires creativity and physicians, in the era of megatrials and of evidence-based medicine, should not give up the privilege of their freedom to combine "hard statistical significance" with "interesting and biologically meaningful trends" and chose management strategies tailored to their individual patients.

References

1. Task Force of the Working Group on Arrhythmias of the European Society of Cardiology (Bigger JT Jr, Breithardt G, Brown AM et al) (1991) The Sicilian Gambit. A new approach to the classification of antiarrhythmic drugs based on their actions on arrhythmogenic mechanisms. Eur Heart J 12:1112-1131, and Circulation 84:1831-1851
2. Members of the Sicilian Gambit (1998) The search for novel antiarrhythmic strategies. Eur Heart J 19:1178-1196, and Jpn Circ J 62:633-648
3. Allessie MA, Boyden PA, Camm AJ et al (2001) Pathophysiology and prevention of atrial fibrillation. Circulation 103:769-777
4. Members of the Sicilian Gambit. New approaches to antiarrhythmic therapy: emerging therapeutic applications of the cell biology of cardiac arrhythmias (submitted for publication)
5. Schwartz PJ (2001) (ed) Focus on amiodarone. Ital Heart J [Suppl]: in press
6. Amiodarone Trials Meta-Analysis Investigators (1997) Effect of prophylactic amiodarone on mortality after acute myocardial infarction and in congestive heart failure: meta-analysis of individual data from 6500 patients in randomised trials. Lancet 350:1417-1424
7. Boutitie F, Boissel JP, Connolly SJ et al (1999) Amiodarone interaction with β-blockers. Analysis of the merged EMIAT (European Myocardial Infarct Amiodarone Trial) and CAMIAT (Canadian Amiodarone Myocardial Infarction Trial) databases. Circulation 99:2268-2275
8. Julian DG, Camm AJ, Frangin G et al for the European Myocardial Infarct Amiodarone Trial Investigators (1997) Randomised trial of effect of amiodarone on mortality in patients with left-ventricular dysfunction after recent myocardial infarction: EMIAT. Lancet 349:667-674

9.   Cairns JA, Connolly SJ, Roberts R, Gent M for the Canadian Amiodarone Myocardial
     Infarction Arrhythmia Trial Investigators (1997) Randomised trial of outcome after
     myocardial infarction in patients with frequent or repetitive ventricular premature
     depolarisations: CAMIAT. Lancet 349:675-682
10. Janse MJ, Malik M, Camm AJ et al on behalf of the EMIAT investigators (1998)
     Identification of post-acute myocardial infarction patients with potential benefit
     from prophylactic treatment with amiodarone. A substudy of EMIAT (the European
     Myocardial Infarct Amiodarone Trial). Eur Heart J 19:85-95
11. Malik M, Camm AJ, Janse MJ et al (2000) Depressed heart rate variability identifies
     postinfarction patients who might benefit from prophylactic treatment with amioda-
     rone: a substudy of EMIAT (The European Myocardial Infarct Amiodarone Trial). J
     Am Coll Cardiol 35:1263-1275
12. Lown B (1979) Sudden cardiac death: the major challenge confronting contemporary
     cardiology. Am J Cardiol 43:313-328

Amiodarone and β-Blockers: Why This Combination?

P. ALBONI, L. GIANFRANCHI, G. FUCÀ AND S. SCARFÒ

Survivors of cardiac arrest, patients with sustained ventricular tachyarrhythmias and those with systolic left ventricular dysfunction, above all when associated with frequent premature ventricular beats (PVB), are considered at high risk of sudden death.

The CAST trial [1] showed an increase in cardiac death in patients with previous acute myocardial infarction (AMI) and frequent PVB, treated with Class I antiarrhythmic agents (AAs). The same agents facilitate the appearance of heart failure in patients with systolic left ventricular dysfunction [2]. In survivors of cardiac arrest, amiodarone is superior to Class I AAs; in fact, the CASCADE trial [3] showed a lower mortality at 2 years in patients treated with amiodarone than in those treated with Class I AAs (18% vs 31%, $p = 0.007$). Moreover, the incidence of ventricular tachycardia (VT) recurrences was lower in the amiodarone group. On the basis of these results, Class III AAs, amiodarone and sotalol, appear to be the only antiarrhythmic drugs proposable to patients at high risk of sudden death. However, it must be considered that the automatic implantable cardioverter defibrillator (ICD) has been used in clinical practice for more than 10 years; this device represents important progress in the prevention of sudden death and, therefore, all the treatments prescribed to this purpose should be compared with the ICD.

Patients with Sustained Ventricular Tachyarrhythmias or with Cardiac Arrest

Up to now there have been no placebo-controlled trials of amiodarone against sustained VT and ventricular fibrillation.

Three randomized trials, AVID [4], CIDS [5] and CASH [6], of ICD therapy vs AA treatment for the prevention of death in survivors of cardiac arrest and in patients with sustained VT causing severe hemodynamic compromise, have

Division of Cardiology, Ospedale Civile, Cento, Ferrara, Italy been reported. The AVID study reported a statistically significant reduction in total mortality, whereas in the other two studies the reduction was not statistically significant. In these three trials, patients > 80 years or with haemodynamically well-tolerated VT were excluded. Recently a meta-analysis of these three trials was performed and only patients treated with amiodarone were included in the medical arm [7]. ICD therapy appeared superior to amiodarone, since the device significantly reduced total mortality (absolute risk, –3.5%, relative risk, –27%, $p < 0.001$) during a mean follow-up of 2.3 years. However, in a post hoc analysis it emerged that only patients with a left ventricular ejection fraction (LVEF) ≤ 35% derived significant benefit from ICD therapy, whereas in patients with LVEF > 35% the survival curves were superimposible. This behavior was well evident in all the three trials analysed.

Patients with Previous AMI and Systolic Left Ventricular Dysfunction or Frequent PVB

A number of small trials, published over the decade from 1985 to 1995, explored the effect of amiodarone on mortality in patients with previous AMI or with systolic left ventricular dysfunction; the results were contrasting. Recently, four placebo-controlled or no treatment-controlled trials were carried out. In two, GESICA [8] and CHF-STAT [9], the effect of amiodarone on mortality was investigated in patients with heart failure and in the other two, EMIAT [10] and CAMIAT [11], in patients with previous AMI. In the GESICA, amiodarone reduced both total mortality (–28%, $p = 0.02$) and sudden death, but not in the CHF-STAT. The divergent findings of these two trials have led to the suggestion that the underlying cause of heart failure may affect the efficacy of amiodarone. The two studies carried out in patients with previous AMI and left ventricular systolic dysfunction [10] or frequent PVB [11] showed that the use of amiodarone had no benefit on total mortality. In fact, they suggested only a significant antiarrhythmic benefit: survival from sudden death or cardiac arrest was significantly improved by amiodarone.

To understand the effect of this drug better, a meta-analysis of all reported randomized controlled trials of amiodarone against placebo was carried out [12]. There were eight trials conducted using post-AMI patients and five trials performed in patients with heart failure, giving rise to 6553 patients enrolled in the meta-analysis. A total of 89% of patients had suffered previous AMI; the mean LVEF was 31%. With amiodarone, total mortality was slightly reduced by 13% ($p = 0.03$); sudden death was reduced by 29% ($p = 0.003$). There was a slight non-significant increase in noncardiac death with amiodarone, but the effect on all nonsudden deaths was neutral.

The slight effect of amiodarone on total mortality does not suggest the use of this drug alone for the prevention of cardiac death; however, it has a relevant role in the treatment of symptomatic nonsustained ventricular arrhythmias in order to improve quality of life.

In patients with systolic left ventricular dysfunction, who are at risk of sudden death, the effect of ICD on mortality has been investigated in three randomized trials, CABG [13], MADIT [14] and MUSTT [15]. In the CABG trial, patients undergoing surgery who had a LVEF < 35% were screened by means of a signal-averaged electrocardiogram. Patients with abnormal tests were randomized at the time of surgery to receive either a thoracotomy ICD or conventional therapy. This trial enrolled 900 patients and was terminated early because these was no discernible benefit of ICD therapy. On the contrary, in the MADIT and MUSTT trials a significant reduction of total mortality has been reported. However, in the MUSTT trial total mortality was not a primary endpoint. Both the MADIT and the MUSTT trials present several methodological limitations; moreover, we do not know whether the results obtained in a few hundred highly selected patients are translatable in a large patient population at risk of sudden death.

Combination of Amiodarone and β-blockers

In a nonrandomized study by Tonet et al. [16], it was suggested that a combination of amiodarone and low dose β-blockers inhibited VT inducibility.

In both the EMIAT [10] and that CAMIAT [11] trials an interaction between amiodarone and β-blockers was suggested, and to explore this interaction in that, the data of the two trials were pooled in a common file (ECMA study) [17]. The number of patients with and without β-blockers at entry was well balanced: 1314 and 1373, respectively. The patients were subdivided into four groups: placebo, amiodarone, β-blockers, and amiodarone plus β-blockers. Both adjusted and unadjusted relative risks for the five outcomes (all-cause mortality, cardiac death, arrhythmic cardiac death, nonarrhythmic cardiac death, arrhythmic death or resuscitated cardiac arrest) were lower in patients receiving β-blockers at entry and randomized to amiodarone than for those receiving amiodarone alone, indicating a tendency for a more favourable effect of amiodarone in the patients treated with β-blockers. The interaction was statistically significant for cardiac death and arrhythmic death or resuscitated cardiac arrest ($p = 0.05$ and $p = 0.03$, respectively), although formal statistical analysis was limited by the small number of subgroups. More specifically, the results showed a reinforced antiarrhythmic effect of amiodarone in patients receiving β-blockers compared with those in any of the other three groups, leaving a slight excess of noncardiac death in the subgroups of patients without β-blockers.

In the placebo group, the mortality rate was about 10% per year and half of these deaths were sudden (about 5%), whereas in the amiodarone plus β-blockers group the mortality rate was about 5% per year and the rate of sudden death was only 1% per year. This reduction of sudden death obtained with the combination of amiodarone and β-blockers is similar to that obtained with ICD therapy [5-7, 14, 15]. At present there is no obvious explanation for the amiodarone-β-blockers interaction.

The heart rate variable was stratified into three classes; heart rate at entry, when introduced into the model, did not make the correlation disappear. To explore more precisely the role of heart rate at entry, the adjusted relative risks for three classes of heart rate were computed. No trend emerged for an interaction between the effect of amiodarone and heart rate in any of the death categories. This means that the antiarrhythmic effect of amiodarone appears to be similar whatever the level of the patient's heart rate. The same analysis was performed on the average heart rate from the entry 24 h Holter recordings, available for 81% of the patients, and similar results were found.

The discontinuation survival curves were analysed and the combination of amiodarone with β-blockers did not seem to alter the withdrawal rate from amiodarone. Discontinuation of amiodarone because of excessive bradycardia was no more frequent in the amiodarone plus β-blockers group than in the amiodarone alone group: 1.2% and 1%, respectively. Regarding the discontinuation of β-blockers, there were more patients withdrawn who were receiving the combination group than receiving β-blockers alone.

These results are provisional because they are based on a post hoc analysis and a prospective trial is needed to confirm them. However, in the clinical setting we often have to take a decision in the absence of strong data and, at present, the combination of amiodarone and β-blockers can be proposed to patients at risk of sudden death in whom there is no clear evidence of the beneficial effects of ICD. The indications could be:

- Patients with sustained VT causing severe haemodynamic compromise and LVEF > 35%
- Patients with haemodynamically well-tolerated sustained VT
- Patients with sustained VT and age > 80 years
- Patients with sustained VT and severe comorbidities
- Patients with syncope of unknown cause and induction of ventricular tachyarrhythmias during electrophysiologic study
- Patients with systolic left ventricular dysfunction and "symptomatic" nonsustained ventricular arrhythmias
- Patients with previous AMI and "symptomatic" nonsustained ventricular arrhythmias

References

1. Echt DS, Liebson PR, Mitchell LB et al (1991) Mortality and morbidity in patients receiving encainide, flecainide, or placebo: the Cardiac Arrhythmia Suppression Trial. N Engl J Med 324:781-788
2. Myerburg RJ, Kessler KM, Kmura S (1992) Sudden cardiac death: future approaches based on identification and control of transient risk factors. J Cardiovasc Electrophysiol 3:626-640

3. The CASCADE investigators (1993) Randomized antiarrhythmic drug therapy in survivors of cardiac arrest (the CASCADE study). Am J Cardiol 72:280-287

4. The Antiarrhythmics versus Implantable Defibrillators (AVID) Investigators (1997) A comparison of antiarrhythmic-drug therapy with implantable defibrillators in patients resuscitated from near-fatal ventricular arrhythmias. N Engl J Med 337:1576-1583

5. Connolly SJ, Gent M, Roberts RS et al (2000) Canadian implantable defibrillator study (CIDS). A randomised trial of the implantable cardioverter defibrillator against amiodarone. Circulation 101:1297-1302

6. Kuck KH, Cappato R, Siebels J, Ruppel R (2000) Randomized comparison of antiarrhythmic drug therapy with implantable defibrillators in patients resuscitated from cardiac arrest. The Cardiac Arrest Study Hamburg (CASH). Circulation 102:748-754

7. Connolly SJ, Hallstrom AP, Cappato R et al (2000) Meta-analysis of the implantable cardioverter defibrillator secondary prevention trials. Eur Heart J 21:2071-2078

8. Doval HC, Nul DR, Grancelli HO et al (1994) Randomized trial of low-dose amiodarone in severe congestive heart failure. Lancet 344:493-498

9. Singh SN, Fletcher RD, Fisher SG et al (1995) Amiodarone in patients with congestive heart failure and asymptomatic ventricular arrhythmia. Survival Trial of Antiarrhythmic Therapy in Congestive Heart Failure. N Engl J Med 333:77-82

10. Julian DG, Camm AJ, Frangin G et al (1997) Randomised trial of effect of amiodarone on mortality in patients with left ventricular dysfunction after recent myocardial infarction: EMIAT. Lancet 349:667-674

11. Cairns JA, Connolly SJ, Roberts R, Gent M (1997) Randomised trial of outcome after myocardial infarction in patients with frequent or repetitive ventricular premature depolarisations: CAMIAT. Lancet 349:675-682

12. Amiodarone Trials Meta-Analysis Investigators (1997) Effect of prophylactic amiodarone on mortality after acute myocardial infarction and in congestive heart failure: meta-analysis of individual data from 6500 patients in randomised trial. Lancet 350:1417-1424

13. Bigger JT Jr, for the Coronary Artery Bypass Graft (CABG) Patch Trial Investigators (1997) Prophylactic use of implanted cardiac defibrillators in patients at high risk for ventricular arrhythmias after coronary artery bypass graft surgery. N Engl J Med 337:1569-1575

14. Moss AJ, Hall WJ, Cannom DS et al (1996) Improved survival with an implanted defibrillator in patients with coronary disease at high risk for ventricular arrhythmia. N Engl J Med 335:1933-1940

15. Buxton AE, Lee KL, Fisher JD et al (1999) A randomised study of the prevention of sudden death in patients with coronary artery disease. N Engl J Med 341:1882-1890

16. Tonet J, Frank R, Fontaine G, Grosgogeat Y (1988) Efficacy and safety of low doses of beta-blockers agents combined with amiodarone in refractory ventricular tachycardia. Pacing Clin Electrophysiol 11:1984-1989

17. Boutitie F, Boissel JP, Connolly SJ (1999) Amiodarone interactions with β-blockers. Analysis of the merged EMIAT and CAMIAT databases. Circulation 99:2268-2275

Impact of MADIT and MUSTT on Clinical Practice

S. NISAM

Introduction

The very first trial aiming at evaluating the role of the implantable cardioverter defibrillator (ICD) as *prophylaxis* was the Multicenter Automatic Defibrillator Trial (MADIT), initiated by Moss and co-workers in 1990 [1]. MADIT demonstrated that ICD therapy dramatically reduced all-cause mortality in high-risk chronic coronary artery disease patients *without* previous sustained ventricular tachyarrhythmias. This trial, now recognized as a landmark study, was met by some skepticism [2, 3], but five further positive ICD trials have reinforced the conclusions from the MADIT trial [4]. The most important of these with respect to establishing the role of ICDs in *primary* prevention of sudden death was the Multicenter UnSustained Tachycardia Trial (MUSTT) [5]. Some authors have contended that these studies would have little clinical impact [6] (D. Andresen, responsible for German EURID registry, personal communication, 1999), and the purpose of our paper here is to investigate precisely that question: what impact have MADIT and MUSTT had on clinical practice?

MADIT and MUSTT: What Did They Really Prove?

To avoid possible misinterpretations emanating from the many other studies involving other patient populations, we will begin by describing the patients in MADIT and MUSTT and summarizing the main findings from these two studies. By definition, patients with any history of sustained ventricular tachyarrhythmias were excluded. Table 1 shows that the patient cohorts were nearly identical: patients enrolled *late* after myocardial infarction (on average over 2 years in MADIT and over 3 years in MUSTT), having depressed left ventricular function, with nonsustained ventricular tachycardia (NSVT), and inducible via programmed ventricular stimulation into sustained VT. The

Guidant Corporation, Diegem, Belgium

Table 1. Patient characteristics in MUSTT and MADIT (from [7], by permission)

Patient characteristics	MUSTT	MADIT
Mean age (years)	66	63
Sex (M/F, %)	90/10	92/8
LVEF (mean %)	30	26
Mean time post-MI (months)	39	27
Prior CABG/ PTCA (% patients)	66	71
NSVT (mean number of beats)	5	9
CHF class II-III (% patients)	64	65
Active therapy	AARx (45%)/ICD (46%)	ICD
	No AARx (7%)	
Control limb therapy (discharge)	No AARx (96%)	75% Amiodarone
Patients on ACE-inhibitors (%)	75	58
Patients on β-blockers (%)		
ICD limb	34	26
Control limb	51	15*

LVEF, left ventricular ejection fraction; *MI*, myocardial infarction; *CABG*, coronary artery bypass graft; *NSVT*, nonsustained ventricular tachycardia; *CHF*, congestive heart failure; *AARx*, antiarrhythmic drug therapy; *ICD*, implantable cardioverter defibrillator
* Includes 7% receiving sotalol

patients were certainly a high-risk group, as evidenced by the fact that approximately three-quarters were being treated for heart failure at the time of enrolment. Great attention was taken in both studies to assure optimal revascularization before patients were permitted into the trials. The study designs have been reported in detail [1, 5]. The most important outcome of the two studies was the demonstration of over 50% reduction in all-cause mortality for patients treated by ICDs compared to controls (MADIT: hazard ratio 0.46, $p < 0.009$; MUSTT: hazard ratio 0.49, $p < 0.001$). MUSTT responded to essentially all the criticisms leveled at the MADIT study [7]. For example, the so-called "β-blocker imbalance" strongly *disfavored* ICD therapy in MUSTT [8]; and MUSTT included a true "natural history" arm (no antiarrhythmic drugs). So, what MADIT and MUSTT proved for this patient population can be summarized quite succinctly:

1. The patients as described are truly at high risk, with all-cause mortality in the absence of ICD therapy of approximately 30% at 2 years.
2. The screening cascade as used in both studies is remarkably specific in identifying patients with high arrhythmic risk.
3. Such patients receive a huge (> 50%) life-saving benefit when treated by ICD therapy compared to amiodarone therapy (MADIT), or electrophysiologically guided drug therapy or no antiarrhythmic drug therapy (MUSTT).

How Have MADIT/MUSTT Impacted Clinical Practice?

In the era of "evidence-based medicine", the MADIT and MUSTT results *should* have a dramatic impact on clinical practice, but have they in fact? There are several pieces of evidence we can use to answer this – the essential question we are responding to in this article. In early 1999, prior to the publication of MUSTT and 3 years after MADIT had been announced, we conducted a survey of centers highly experienced with ICD implantation in Europe and the United States, and found out that 9% (6% in Europe, 15% in the US) of all first implants at those centers had been carried out for "MADIT" indications [9] (Fig. 1). One year later, we repeated the survey in order to determine the impact of an additional year and of the MUSTT study on this practice, and the 133 responding centers (86 Europe, 47 US) indicated that this rate had increased significantly, reaching 18% of implants worldwide, ranging from 10% for the European centers to 24% for the American centers [10]. Data from the German EURID Registry (data from European countries on pacemaker and ICD implantations) on the rate of "prophylactic indications" in Germany from 1994 to 1999 are shown in Fig. 2. The 9% for 1998 coincides precisely with the survey results from the 14 German responders. What is clear from the figure and from our two surveys is that rate of implants for MADIT/MUSTT indications is increasing: 9% in 1998, 18% in 1999, and an unknown figure currently.

The surveys also attempted to establish how patients were being identified and screened for MADIT and MUSTT. The results showed that most of the patients screened were already in hospital – either for routine follow-up or receiving treatment. There was relatively little systematic screening or looking at patient charts for potential candidates.

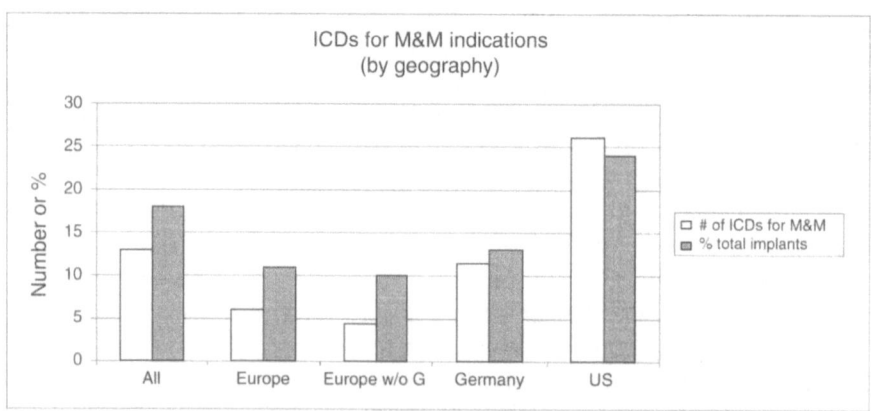

Fig. 1. ICD implantation for MADIT and MUSTT indications in 1999 by geographical area. The *light bars* indicate the average number of implants per center for MADIT and MUSTT indications, and the *dark bars* the percentage of total *initial* implants per center that were for these indications

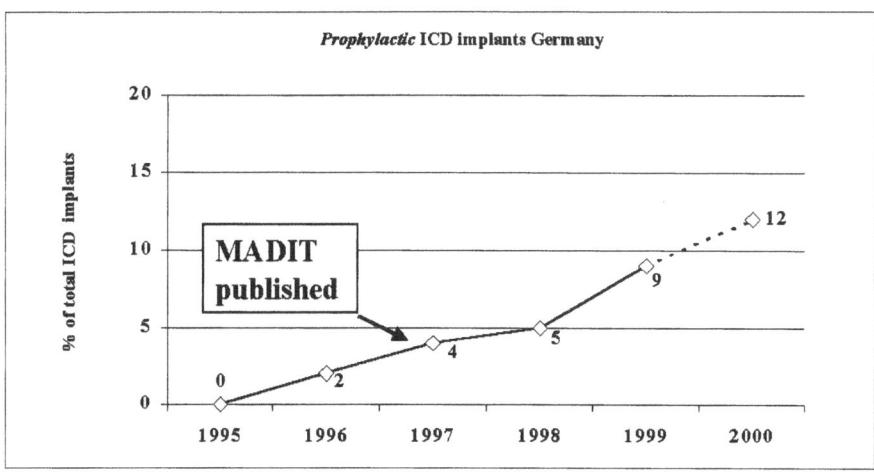

Fig. 2. The rate of "prophylactic indications" in Germany, from 1994 to 1998, as recorded in the German EURID registry (data provided from European countries on pacemaker and ICD implantations) (D. Andresen, responsible for German EURID registry, personal communication, 1999)

Impact of MADIT and MUSTT on ICD Guidelines

Inasmuch as guidelines reflect the consensus of thought leaders in cardiology, they also reflect the extent to which these leaders believe that medical practice should adhere to such guidelines. So, a good test of whether MADIT and MUSTT were considered of sufficient validity and clinical importance to be integrated into medical practice is to examine whether they have been included in the most recent guidelines for the use of the ICD. The US Food and Drug Administration gave its OK for the "MADIT strategy" within a few weeks of the announcement of the results [11]. Within 2 years, the joint American College of Cardiology/American Heart Association Taskforce made MADIT a class I indication for ICD therapy [12]. In short order, the national guidelines for ICD implantation in most European countries all integrated the MADIT indication as a class I indication, with only slight variations in the precise conditions [13].

To summarize: MADIT and MUSTT have been integrated into clinical practice, and accounted for nearly one-fifth of initial ICD implants during 1999, double the rate from 1 year earlier. The rate varies significantly between various countries, reaching 24% in the US and 10% in Europe. Nevertheless, all geographies showed significant increases from 1998 to 1999, indicating that the rate world-wide is now likely well over 20%. The prophylactic indications for ICD implantation, as established by these studies, have now been integrated into most national guidelines.

Most patients being identified by the MADIT and MUSTT screening were already in the hospital, either for routine follow-up or receiving treatment.

Relatively few were being identified by checking patient charts to look prospectively for patients who might fit the criteria. Thus, as long as systematic screening remains infrequent, many potential patients who could be protected will not be identified in time.

References

1. MADIT Executive Committee (1991) Multicenter Automatic Defibrillator Implantation Trial (MADIT): design and clinical protocol. Pacing Clin Electrophysiol 14:920-927
2. Friedman P, Stevenson W (1996) Unsustained ventricular tachycardia – to treat or not to treat (editorial). N Engl J Med 335:1984-1985
3. Coumel P (1998) The MADIT trial: what was wrong? In: Vardas PE (ed) Cardiac arrhythmias, pacing and electrophysiology. Kluwer Academic Publishers, Dordrecht, pp 121-124
4. Prystowsky E, Nisam S (2000) Prophylactic implantable cardioverter defibrillator trials (ICD): MUSTT, MADIT, and beyond. Am J Cardiol 86:1214-1215
5. Buxton A, Lee K, Fisher J et al for the Multicenter UnSustained Tachycardia Trial (MUSTT) Investigators (1999) A randomized study of the prevention of sudden death in patients with coronary artery disease. N Engl J Med 341:1882-1890
6. Hohnloser S, Andresen D, Block M, et al (2000) Guidelines for implantation of automatic cardioverter/defibrillator. Z Kardiol 89:126-135 (German), 136-143 (English)
7. Gold M, Nisam S (2000) Primary prevention of sudden cardiac death with implantable cardioverter-defibrillators: lessons learned from MADIT and MUSTT. Pacing Clin Electrophysiol 23:1981-1985
8. Gold M, Rottman J, Wood M et al (1999) The effect of clinical factors on the benefit of implantable defibrillators in the MUSTT trial (abstract). Circulation 100:I-642
9. Wilber D, Nisam S (2000) Survey of prophylactic defibrillator implantation following MADIT. Ann Noninvasive Electrocardiol 248-254
10. Nisam S, Wilber D, Henry S (2001) Evolution of practice patterns related to prophylactic defibrillator implantation: results of an international survey (Abstract). PACE
11. FDA Talk Paper T96-33 (1996) FDA speeds approval of wider use of heart attack device. Food and Drug Administration, Rockville, MD, 16 May 1996
12. Gregoratos G, Cheitlin M, Conill A et al (1998) ACC/AHA guidelines for implantation of cardiac pacemakers and antiarrhythmia devices: a report of the ACC/AHA task force on practice guidelines (committee on pacemaker implantation). J Am Coll Cardiol 31:1175-1209
13. Camm J, Nisam S (2000) The utilization of the implantable defibrillator – a *European* Enigma. Eur Heart J 21:1998-2004

How Many ICD Recipients Really Need Dual-Chamber Pacing?

A. Proclemer, D. Facchin and M. Trentin

Introduction

Dual-chamber pacing showed a mortality decrease in comparison to ventricular pacing, and a lower incidence of atrial fibrillation and thromboembolic complications, especially in patients with congestive heart failure [1, 2]. The dual-chamber implantable cardioverter-defibrillator (DDD-ICD) became available in July 1997; this device enables atrioventricular pacing and sensing in case of bradycardia, as well as sensing of atrial events in case of atrial tachyarrhythmias. The proportion of patients in whom DDD-ICD is indicated is still a subject of debate, and so far no prospective data about the clinical indications and possible advantages of the DDD-ICD in comparison to the single-chamber DDD-ICD are available [3]. However, accurate identification of candidates for the DDD-ICD is essential because of the higher technological complexity and cost of this device in comparison to the single-chamber ICD.

Clinically, the main indications for DDD-ICD are based on (1) the need for physiologic pacing due to the occurrence of bradyarrhythmias, (2) the possibility of better discriminating supraventricular tachyarrhythmias from ventricular tachycardia on the basis of atrial sensing, (3) improved diagnostic function if arrhythmia recurs, (4) a possible hemodynamic benefit in patients with heart failure or low left ventricular ejection fraction, and (5) prevention and treatment of atrial tachyarrhythmias in selected cases.

The purpose of this review was to consider the real need for DDD-ICD in an unselected population of ICD recipients.

Dual-Chamber Sensing and Pacing Indications

In a recent retrospective multicenter study [4], the clinical and electrocardiographic indications for dual-chamber ICD were examined at the time of implantation, and during a medium-term follow-up period. The study population presented the classical clinical and arrhythmological characteristics of ICD recipi-

Istituto di Cardiologia, Ospedale S. Maria della Misericordia, Fondazione IRCAB, Udine, Italy

ents. All patients were treated with a single-chamber ICD and no patient was concomitantly treated with a pacemaker during the study period. *Definite indications* such as sinus node dysfunction and second- or third-degree AV block was found at the time of ICD placement in 10.5% of cases, and this value remained stable during the follow-up time (11%). Consistent with this figure, Geelen et al. [5] found that 21 of 139 patients (15%) required dual-chamber antibradycardia pacing for high-degree AV block or sick sinus syndrome. To Best et al. [6] and Higgins et al. [7] as well, dual-chamber ICD placement appeared definitely indicated for NASPE class 1 pacing indications [8] in 28 of 253 patients (11%) and 26 of 122 patients (21.3%), respectively. By contrast, dual-chamber pacing was needed in only 6% of 200 consecutive patients who received an ICD with VVI capability in the series of Andrews et al. [9]. This discrepancy may be related to the different clinical characteristics of the study populations or to differing uses of antiarrhythmics. Unfortunately, only the first of the five studies cited evaluated modifications of NASPE class 1 indications during the follow-up period.

Possible indications such has minor AV conduction defects and history of paroxysmal atrial fibrillation accounted for respectively 11% and 6.5% of the cases in one series [4]. During the follow-up period these figures remained stable (11% and 8.5%, respectively). However, the authors hypothesized that the number of atrial fibrillation episodes was underestimated, due to the possibility of asymptomatic atrial fibrillation and to the lack of atrial diagnostic memory function in the single-chamber ICD used. The study did not evaluate the possibility of a hemodynamic benefit of dual-chamber pacing and sensing in patients with severe left ventricular dysfunction and/or history of congestive heart failure in the absence of classical pacing indications. In the series of Best et al. [6], dual-chamber ICD usage was considered probably indicated in 72 patients (28%), who met the NASPE class 2 pacing indications and who were in NYHA functional class III or IV. Dual-chamber ICD therapy was regarded as possibly indicated in another 35 patients (14%), on the basis of the presence of a less than 20% left ventricular ejection fraction or a history of paroxysmal atrial fibrillation. During the follow-up period, 0.8% of the patients developed chronic atrial fibrillation and 2.4% of the patients had a first episode of paroxysmal atrial fibrillation. In the study by Higgins et al. [7], "other or ICD-specific indications" including conduction defects, inappropriate shocks, and heart failure were documented in 32 patients (26.3%). In the Andrews et al. study [9], supraventricular tachycardia – mostly atrial fibrillation – occurred in 63 of 200 patients (32%). The differing definitions of "possible" and "probable" dual-chamber ICD indications make it difficult to compare the cited studies.

Arrhythmia Discrimination and Diagnostic Function

A theoretically important advantage of the DDD-ICD is its better discrimination between supraventricular arrhythmias with fast ventricular response and ventricular arrhythmias, thus avoiding inappropriate ICD therapy (30%-40% in single-chamber ICD era). The detection algorithms of single-chamber ICDs traditionally have been based on analysis of rate stability, sudden change of ventricular rate, and/or different morphology of the QRS complex during ventricular tachycardia (VT). These algorithms allowed 90%-100% sensitivity and 50%-98% specificity of the ventricular arrhythmia therapy.

Kühlkamp et al. [10], in an open-label, nonrandomized prospective study, compared the discrimination algorithms of the Ventak AV 1810 DDD-ICD (Guidant) and the Ventak Mini I-II single-chamber ICD. The two ICDs have similar device operation, but differ because the DDD-ICD Ventak AV provides two main arrhythmia discrimination enhancements to differentiate atrial arrhythmias from only VT. The first is the "atrial fibrillation rate threshold", which withholds ventricular treatment if the atrial rate is above 250 bpm. The second detection parameter is defined as "ventricular rate > atrial rate" and guarantees ventricular therapy when the ventricular rate is at least 10 bpm greater than the atrial rate. Both parameters can be programmed in conjunction with sudden onset and rate stability criteria. The *Ventak AV* group included 39 patients with a high percentage of sick sinus syndrome (23%), conduction defects (54%), and history of paroxysmal atrial fibrillation (21%). Twelve patients (31%) suffered a total number of 199 episodes of supraventricular tachycardias (17% sinus tachycardia, 83% atrial fibrillation or flutter). Mean RR cycle length stability during atrial fibrillation was 50 ms and mean detected atrial rate 249 bpm. Of the supraventricular episodes in the VT detection zone, 41% were inappropriately treated by antitachycardia pacing or shock therapy. All the 8 of 166 atrial fibrillation episodes in the ventricular fibrillation (VF) zone were treated by shock. The *Ventak Mini* group consisted of 55 patients, with a history of paroxysmal atrial fibrillation in 18% of them. During the follow-up period 218 episodes of atrial fibrillation or flutter were documented in 10 patients. Mean ventricular rate was 173 bpm and mean RR stability 54 ms. All episodes were in the VT zone and 24% of them were treated by overdrive ventricular pacing or shock. Detection and treatment of sustained VT or VF were similarly efficient in the two groups of patients. Despite the presence of the new dual-chamber discrimination algorithm, significantly more episodes of atrial fibrillation underwent inappropriated therapy in the Ventak AV group than in the Ventak Mini group ($p < 0.001$). One explanation was the high incidence of atrial undersensing due to atrial blanking period of 86 ms and to absence of atrial rate detection when the ventricular rate activated the ICD before the atrial rate could be determined (51% of all atrial fibrillation episodes). The other explanation is the high cutoff value (250 bpm) of the atrial fibrillation threshold criterion in the Ventak AV 1810; this parameter has been modified in the new series of Ventak AV.

A more recent observational multicenter study [11] reported the clinical results of the arrhythmia detection obtained by another dual-chamber discrimination algorithm (PR Logic) in a group of 933 patients receiving the Medtronic GEM DR 7271 ICD. The PR Logic has three independently programmable criteria to discriminate between supraventricular tachycardias such as sinus tachycardia, atrial fibrillation-flutter, other 1:1 supraventricular arrhythmia and VT or VF, with the aim of reducing the possibility of inappropriate VT/VF therapy.

The algorithm analyzes the following aspects: atrial and ventricular rate, pattern of atrial and ventricular events, ventricular cycle length regularity, atrioventricular dissociation, evidence of atrial fibrillation-flutter, and far-field R-wave sensing on the atrial lead. If supraventricular tachycardia without coexistence of VT/VF is confirmed, then antitachycardia therapy is withheld. A total of 4856 sustained arrhythmia episodes with stored electrogram and marker channel were documented; 3488 episodes in 232 patients were classified as VT or VF, 1368 episodes in 149 patients as supraventricular tachycardia. The relative sensitivity for detection of sustained VT and/or VF was 100%, the VT/VF positive predictivity 88.4%, and the supraventricular tachycardia positive predictivity 100%. There were 457 true atrial episodes in 86 patients for which the PR Logic algorithm did not withhold VT/VF detection. Main causes of all inaccurate diagnoses were intermittent far-field R-wave oversensing (84 of 457, 17%), rapidly conducted atrial fibrillation in the VF detection zone despite supraventricular tachycardia limit (44 episodes, 9.6%), sinus or atrial tachycardia episodes with long PR intervals (> 50% RR interval) interpreted for VT with 1:1 VA conduction (174, 38%), PR Logic not correctly applied (68, 14.8%), and atrial fibrillation with regular ventricular cycle length (26, 5.6%). The majority of these pitfalls could be modified by correction of ICD detection characteristic and programming (e.g., ventricular rate during atrial fibrillation in the VT or fast VT zone and not in the VF zone) or atrial lead sensing or placement.

Similar results were obtained in other two studies [12, 13] that reported a 15%-20% incidence of inappropriate therapy despite the presence of the PR Logic algorithm. Stored electrograms in the majority of pitfall cases showed sinus tachycardia with first-degree AV block interpreted as VT with 1:1 VA conduction, atrial fibrillation with fast ventricular rate within the VF zone, atrial tachycardia with ventricular rate around the shortest programmable supraventricular tachycardia limit, and supraventricular tachycardia redetection following VT therapy. In particular, in the Dijkman et al. series [12] tachycardia classification was not corrected in 59 (19%) of 310 arrhythmia episodes, in which the rate criterion alone was not sufficient for diagnosis. Detection of true VT or VF, however, was never interrupted or delayed by the rhythm detected on the atrial channel either in "VT only" episodes or in "double tachycardia" episodes (VT+atrial arrhythmia).

Dual-chamber diagnostics consisting of simultaneous atrial and ventricular channel registrations in DDD-ICD are very important to allow better insight into the mechanisms of the onset and maintenance of sustained ventricular arrhythmias. The information from the atrial channel can also guide the ventricular electrical treatment. Dijkman and Wellens evaluated in 41 patients 724 spontaneous VT/VF episodes detected and treated by three types of dual-chamber ICD from two manufacturers [14]. All the patients had structural heart disease. The relation between atrial and ventricular rhythm was assessed from the onset until the interruption of VT/VF episodes. Sinus tachycardia was the most frequent supraventricular rhythm (23%) either before or after the onset of VT and VF, and was observed more often during hemodynamically stable VT then during fast VT. The simultaneous dual-chamber electrogram registration also showed that the majority of ventricular arrhythmias arising during atrial fibrillation or flutter were preceded by a high ventricular rate despite wide use of β-blocking drugs. Finally, dual-chamber diagnostics allowed better evaluation of arrhythmia-ICD interaction, thus providing useful information for programming the detection zones.

The Medtronic Jewel AF 7250 is the only commercially available DDD-ICD able to detect and treat specific atrial and ventricular arrhythmias. The device functions as a DDD pacemaker and has independently programmable therapy for VT, VF, and atrial tachycardia and fibrillation. The detection of atrial arrhythmias is based on the PR Logic algorithm. Other main functions include: mode switching to prevent inappropriate tracking of rapid atrial rhythms, withholding inappropriate ventricular therapy, delivery of atrial therapy by means of overdrive pacing, 50 Hz burst stimulation for few seconds, dual-chamber shock, and prevention of atrial premature beats and/or atrial arrhythmias by pacing algorithms such as "atrial rate stabilization", and "switchback delay". Swerdlow et al. [15] studied 80 patients with dual tachycardia treated with the Jewel AF 7250. During a mean follow-up of 6 months, supraventricular tachycardia detection was considered appropriate in 98% of 132 episodes of atrial fibrillation and 88% of 190 episodes of atrial tachycardia. During Holter monitoring, the sensitivity of the detection of both atrial arrhythmias was 100%; the specificity of the detection of other rhythms was 99.9%. Atrial tachycardia was terminated by overdrive pacing in 45% of cases. Intermittent sensing of far-field R waves caused 27 inappropriate detections of atrial tachycardia and fibrillation. The authors' conclusions are that atrial tachyarrhythmias can be detected successfully by a dual-chamber atrial ICD, and eventual shocks may be programmed for long-lasting atrial tachycardia or fibrillation. The detection interval of atrial tachycardia should be programmed to less than 300 ms to avoid oversensing of far-field R waves.

GEM II-III DR Registry

Correct identification of candidates for DDD-ICD may be achieved by randomizing new ICD recipients to a single-chamber or a DDD-ICD device. However, this type of study may have limited usefulness because new devices and algorithms are quickly available and results from large randomized trials are very difficult to obtain. Therefore, we planned a prospective registry to evaluate new-technology dual-chamber ICD.

This multicenter registry includes consecutive patients with 7273-7275 GEM II-III DR ICDs implanted in five Italian hospitals (see Appendix). The main technical characteristics of this atrio-ventricular ICD are the previously described PR Logic detection algorithm and the advanced diagnostic and therapeutic features of a dual-chamber rate-responsive pacemaker. The clinical indications for dual-chamber ICD in this registry are based on (1) the need for physiologic pacing, (2) the correct identification of supraventricular and ventricular arrhythmias, and (3) the possible hemodynamic benefit in patients with heart failure and/or left ventricular dysfunction. Main endpoints are (1) the incidence of atrial arrhythmias detected in the VT zone due to rapid ventricular rate, (2) the incidence of atrial arrhythmias activating the mode switch due to a ventricular rate under the cutoff of the VT zone, (3) the correct identification of atrial and ventricular arrhythmias based on PR Logic, and (4) the relation between atrial arrhythmias and programmed pacing modality. Clinical follow-up and ICD control are planned at 3 and 6 months after device implantation, and every 6 months thereafter. The tachycardia episodes are documented with stored atrial and ventricular electrograms and classified as (1) VT, (2) VF, or (3) supraventricular tachycardia with or without a concomitant ventricular arrhythmia. This information is copied to disk for investigator evaluation and confirmation of correct arrhythmia classification (Figs. 1-3). Information about the number and duration of mode switch episodes is also obtained when this function is activated.

So far, the study population consists of 42 consecutive patients with a mean age of 66 years (Table 1). All the patients had classical indications for ICD implantation, including 3 MADIT type cases. Coronary artery disease was present in 32 patients (76.5%), left and right ventricular cardiomyopathy in 9 (21%). Seven patients had previously undergone coronary artery bypass graft, and 3 radiofrequency ablation of VT. Sick sinus syndrome was evident only in 1 case, while conduction defects were detected in 7 (first-degree AV block in 4, second- or third-degree AV block in 3). Eight patients (19%) had a history of paroxysmal atrial fibrillation or atrial flutter. At enrollment, DDD pacing mode was programmed in 27 patients, DDI in 6, DDDR in 4, and VVI in 3. Mode switch was activated in 20 cases. Amiodarone treatment was administered to 22 patients, sotalol to 5, and β-blockers to 19. At the moment the mean follow-up is 9 ± 6 months, and the first follow-up data will be available in the next few months.

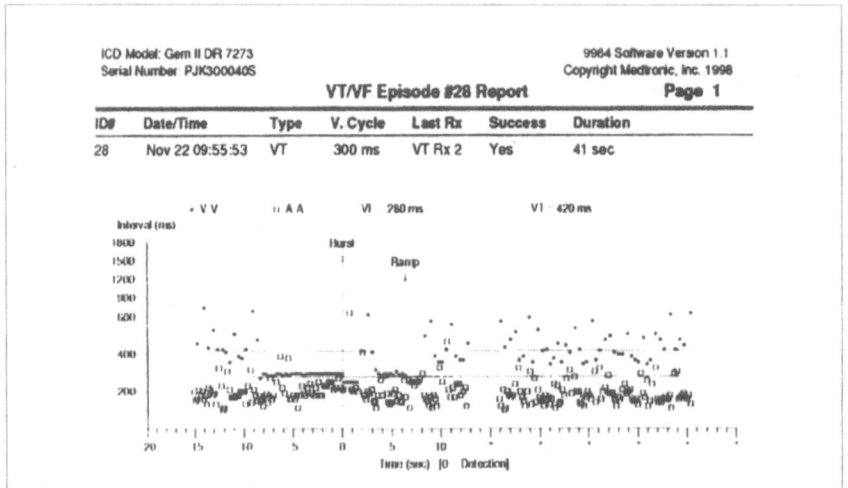

Fig. 1. Start of VT episode with a cycle length of 300 ms in a patient with persistent atrial fibrillation. Before VT onset, a clear irregularity of atrial (*open square*) and ventricular (*black circle*) cycle length is evident. Burst pacing is ineffective, whereas rump pacing clearly stops the VT episode. Irregularity of VV cycles reappears after VT interruption

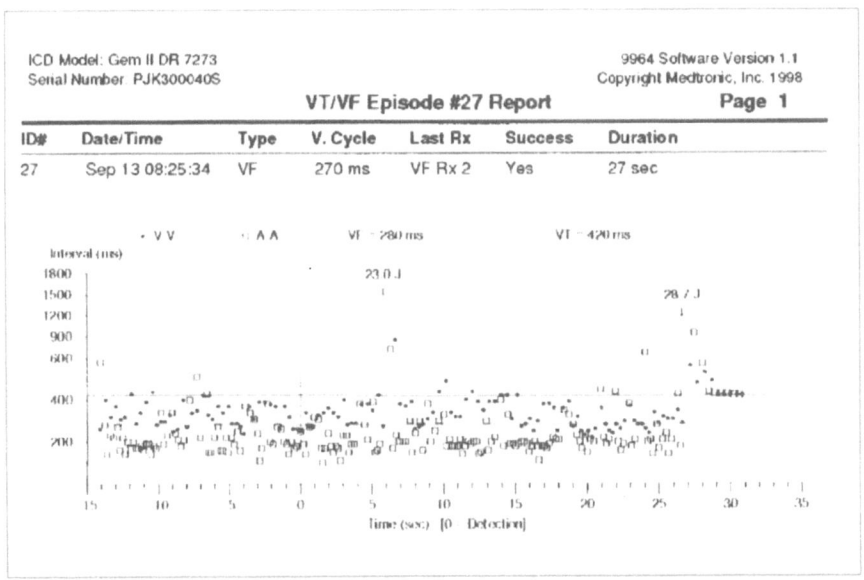

Fig. 2. Inappropriate ICD intervention during atrial fibrillation with fast ventricular response detected in the VF zone (VV cycle length 270 ms). The second shock (28.7 J) interrupted the atrial fibrillation; the atrial and ventricular cycle became regular and equal

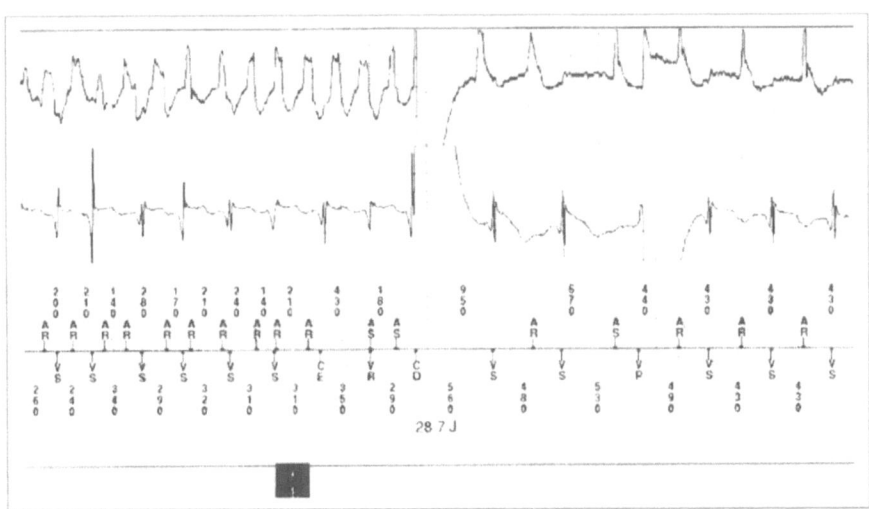

Fig. 3. Detail of the episode in Fig. 2. The interruption of atrial fibrillation by the 28.7-J shock succeeds in obtaining regular atrial and ventricular rhythm at a cycle length of 430 ms

Table 1. GEM II-III DR Registry. Characteristics at enrollment of 42 patients (preliminary data)

	n	%
Male sex	37	88
Mean age (years)	66 ± 11	
Index arrhythmia		
Sustained VT	28	67
Nonsustained VT (MADIT)	4	9
VF	7	17
VT + VF	3	7
Etiology		
CAD, post-MI	31	74
CAD, no MI	1	2.5
Cardiomyopathy–dilated	7	16
Cardiomyopathy–right ventricle	2	5
Valvular heart disease	1	2.5
NYHA class		
1	6	15
2	29	70
3	6	15
Mean left ventricular ejection fraction	35 ± 11	
Sick sinus syndrome – AV conduction defects	8	19
Atrial fibrillation or flutter	8	19

VT, ventricular tachycardia; *VF*, ventricular fibrillation; *CAD*, coronary artery disease; *MI*, myocardial infarction; *AV*, atrioventricular

Conclusions

The DDD-ICD provides dual-chamber pacing, therapy, and advance diagnostic features in the same device. On the basis of retrospective studies [4-7, 9] including unselected ICD recipients, dual-chamber pacing appeared definitely indicated in 10%-15% of cases owing to sinus node dysfunction and second- or third-degree AV block, and possibly indicated in an additional 25%-30% on the basis of minor AV conduction defects, paroxysmal atrial fibrillation, left ventricular dysfunction, and congestive heart failure. Other rare but "highly recommended" indications include long QT syndrome and hypertrophic cardiomyopathy [8, 16-18].

DDD-ICD of new technology seem to improve the sensitivity and specificity of both atrial and ventricular arrhythmia detection, reducing the incidence of inappropriate ICD intervention and allowing dual-chamber arrhythmia treatment. Refinements and programmability of DDD-ICD algorithms are needed to improve diagnostic accuracy in subgroups of difficult arrhythmias. Ongoing randomized trials and prospective observational registries will define more precisely the role of the DDD-ICD.

Appendix

GEM II-III DR Registry: Participating Investigators and Medical Centers:
A. Proclemer, D. Facchin, Az. Osp. Santa Maŕia della Misericordia Udine; A. Vincenti, Ospedale S. Gerardo di Monza, Milan; F. Zardo, M. Brieda, Az. Osp. S.M. degli Angelii Pordenone; T. Morgera, E. Barducci, P.O. di Monfalcone, Gorizia; E. Nicotra, Ospedale Vittorio Emanuele II, Gorizia.

Data Coordinators
M. Trentin, IRCAB Foundation, Udine; M. Maggi, M. Passardi, C. De Michele, Medtronic Italia.

References

1. Alpert MA, Curtis JJ, Sanfelippo JF et al (1987) Comparative survival following permanent ventricular and dual-chamber pacing for patients with chronic symptomatic sinus node dysfunction with and without congestive heart failure. Am Heart J 113:958-965
2. Rediker DE, Eagle KA, Homma S et al (1988) Clinical and hemodynamic comparison of VV vs DDD pacing in patients with DDD pacemaker. Am J Cardiol 61:323-329
3. Iskos D, Fahy GJ, Lurie KG et al (1998) Physiologic cardiac pacing in patients with contemporary implantable cardioverter-defibrillators. Am J Cardiol 82:66-71
4. Proclemer A, Della Bella P, Facchin D et al (2001) Indication for dual-chamber cardioverter defibrillator at implant and at 1 year follow-up: a retrospective analysis in the single-chamber defibrillator era. Europace 3:132-135
5. Geelen P, Lorga FA, Chauvin M et al (1997) The value of DDD pacing in patients with an implantable cardioverter defibrillator. Pacing Clin Electrophysiol 20:177-181
6. Best PJM, Hayes DL, Stanton MS (1999) The potential usage of dual chamber pacing in patients with implantable cardioverter defibrillators. Pacing Clin Electrophysiol 22:79-85
7. Higgins SL, Seth KW, Pak JP, Meyer DB (1998) Indications for implantation of dual-chamber pacemaker combined with an implantable cardioverter-defibrillator. Am J Cardiol 81:1360-1362
8. Gregoratos G, Cheitlin MD, Conill A et al (1998) ACC/AHA guidelines for implantation of cardiac pacemakers and antiarrhythmia devices: a report of the American College of Cardiology / American Heart Association Task Force on Practice Guidelines (Committee on Pacemaker Implantation). J Am Coll Cardiol 31:1175-1209
9. Andrews NP, Gudgel·R, Evans JJ et al (1997) How frequently is dual chamber pacing indicated in patients with implantable defibrillators? Pacing Clin Electrophysiol 20:1071

10. Kühlkamp V, Dörnberger V, Mewis C et al (1999) Clinical experience with the new detection algorithms for atrial fibrillation of a defibrillator with dual chamber sensing and pacing. J Cardiovasc Electrophysiol 10:905-915
11. Wilkoff BL, Kühlkamp V, Volosin K et al (2001) Critical analysis of dual-chamber implantable cardioverter-defibrillator arrhythmia detection. Results and technical considerations. Circulation 103:381-386
12. Dijkman B, Wellens HJJ (2000) Detection in the implantable cardioverter defibrillator. J Cardiovasc Electrophysiol 11:1105-1115
13. Fan K, Lee K, Pak Lau C (1999) Dual-chamber implantable cardioverter defibrillator benefit and limitations. J Interv Card Electrophysiol 3:239-245
14. Dijkman B, Wellens HJJ (2000) Importance of the atrial channel for a ventricular arrhythmia therapy in the dual chamber implantable cardioverter defibrillator. J Cardiovasc Electrophysiol 11:1309-1319
15. Swerdlow CD, Schsls W, Dijkman B et al (2000) Detection of atrial fibrillation and flutter by a dual-chamber implantable cardioverter-defibrillator. Circulation 101:878-885
16. Hayes DL (1996) Evolving indication for permanent pacing. New Engl J Med 334:89-97
17. Hesselson AB, Parsonnet V, Berstein AD, Bonavita GJ (1992) Deleterious effects of long-term single chamber pacing in patient with sick sinus syndrome: the hidden benefits of dual chamber pacing. J Am Coll Cardiol 17:1542-1549
18. Sutton R, Bourgeois I (1996) Cost benefit analysis of single and dual chamber pacing for sick sinus syndrome and atrioventricular block. An economic sensitivity analysis of literature. Eur Heart J 17:574-582

ATRIAL FLUTTER AND OTHER SUPRAVENTRICULAR TACHYARRHYTHMIAS

Acute Termination of Atrial Flutter: Are New Class Antiarrhythmic Drugs the Best Choice?

N. Baldi, V.A. Russo, V. Morrone, L. Di Gregorio, L. Liconso and G. Polimeni

Introduction

The expression "atrial flutter" (AFl) covers a series of arrhythmias which are related to different physiopathological mechanisms: typical AFl (common and uncommon, referring respectively to the anti-clockwise and clockwise routes through the anatomical substrate of right atrium, septum-lateral wall and isthmus inferior vena cava-tricuspid) and the atypical AFl, in which the circuit is located differently. In the population the prevalence of AFl is less than one in a thousand. Uncommon AFl is ten times less frequent than common AFl. The atypical form includes a heterogeneous series of arrhythmias whose electrogenetic mechanism is not exhaustively known and in which the absence of an excitable gap makes it very difficult to achieve entrainment or reset through the technique of pacing. Recently Cheng et al. [1] have shown that the site of the atypical flutter circuit is the lower part of the right atrium, while Jais et al. [2] have reported some cases of left AFl. As a consequence of this, we suggest that the arrhythmias generally referred to as typical and atypical flutter can be considered as electrophysiologically different entities. This element might influence the different actions of drugs on AFl "tout-court".

Theoretical-Experimental Physiopathological Assumptions Regarding the Action of Drugs in the Interruption of AFl

Concerning the typical flutter at least, in which the presence of an excitable gap is recognizable, a double modality of interruption of the arrhythmia has been experimentally defined: (1) abolition of the excitable gap through greater prolongation of the refractory period compared with a lesser slowing down of conduction; and (2) interruption of arrhythmia by suppressing conduction to a

Cardiovascular Department, Azienda Ospedaliera S.S.Annunziata, Taranto, Italy

crucial point beyond which propagation of conduction becomes impossible. When there is a greater slowing down of conduction relative to prolongation of the effective refractory period, reentry is not terminated.

Drugs prevalently acting on the refractory period belong to class III; those prevalently acting on conduction belong to class I. In some cases these theoretical assumptions have been experimentally verified [3]. We will see their impact in the clinical field. Concerning atypical flutter, especially if we consider it at a high frequency and without an excitable gap, the only vulnerable parameter is represented by prolonging the atrial refractory period, which can be obtained through class III drugs. To conclude this section, it must be remembered that it is commonly known that AFl into often changes atrial fibrillation (AF) and vice versa, both spontaneously and when caused by the action of some drugs. There are few systematic studies in which the incidence of this alternating process has been analyzed: they include the study by Murdock et al. [4] and the one by Tunick et al. [5].

Pharmacological Acute Treatment of AFl

Until the last generation of class III drugs were introduced onto the market, such as ibutilide and dofetilide (information concerning azimilide is still very poor), the available antiarrhythmic drugs were effective in AFl cardioversion in only a small percentage of cases. Most authors therefore preferred trans-esophageal or atrial overdrive suppression pacing, particularly in typical flutter, or DC shock in all forms of flutter. However, a big limitation in evaluating the effectiveness of drugs is the fact that AF and AFl have almost always been considered together, despite the considerable electrogenetic differences between them. In the few studies in which the two arrhythmias have been considered separately - although with very heterogeneous study populations - class I drugs were not very effective in restoring the sinus rhythm. As concerns propafenone, the success rates range between 33% (5 out of 15 patients) [6] and 40% (2 out of 5 patients) [7]; concerning flecainide the percentages of success rate ranges between 0% [8] and 33% [9].

An indubitable and decisive step forward in the acute treatment of AFl has been represented by the introduction into the market of some drugs, particularly ibutilide and dofetilide (the latter not yet available in Italy). So far few studies have focused on the action of such drugs on this arrhythmia which seemed to be poorly respondent to drugs; there are indications that these drugs have a beneficial effect, although the data are as yet sparse.

Ibutilide

Ibutilide is an intravenous class III antiarrhythmic drug that prolongs the atrial and ventricular action potential via two mechanisms: blockade of the delayed

rectifier potassium current and an increase in the slow inward sodium current. This drug is not associated with the reverse use-dependence phenomenon [10], has no significant effect on heart rate, PR interval, or QRS interval, and does not have any negative inotropic effect [11]. Two major placebo-controlled dose-ranging studies [12, 13] have been performed. Both were designed as double-blind, placebo-controlled, randomized dose-response trials. Other studies involved comparing ibutilide with other drugs or as an addition to other drugs, but really with rather low patient numbers. From the two major studies in which, as usually occurs, AFl and AF are considered together, we will try, where possible, to identify the results concerning AFl. In the study by Stambler et al. [12], 266 patients were enrolled, 133 of whom had AFl. Out of the total number of patients, 86 were randomized to receive placebo, 86 to a 1.0 mg + 0.5 mg dose of ibutilide, and 94 to 1.0 mg + 1.0 mg ibutilide. Importantly, the patient population was very similar to that commonly reported in cardiology departments. The mean age was 67 years; the average duration of arrhythmias was about 2 weeks; and 75% of patients had a history of heart disease other than AFl or AF. Eighty-three percent of patients had a depressed left ventricular ejection fraction and 71% had valvular heart disease. The greater conversion efficacy of ibutilide, compared with placebo, was significant in both the AFl and the AF group, but the conversion rate after two infusions of ibutilide was significantly ($p < 0.0001$) higher for AFl (63%) than for AF (31%). The mean termination time was 30 min in the flutter group. In the study by Ellenbogen et al. [13], the efficacy of ibutilide therapy was evaluated in 197 patients. There were 98 patients with AFl and 99 with AF. Of the patients with AFl, 78 were treated with increasing doses of ibutilide and 20 with placebo. Seventy-three percent of the patients with AFl had a history of heart disease other than their arrhythmias. The mean duration of the AFl was very significant: 93 ± 374 days. Overall, 72% had structural heart disease; 74% had significant left atrial enlargement and 50% had decreased left ventricular function. The overall success rate in ibutilide-treated patients was 38% among those with AFl and 29% among those with AF. The mean time of termination was 19 ± 15 min. In both studies the drug was significantly more effective than placebo.

In our opinion, some points must be emphasized. Although there were differences in the drug efficacy, as shown in both study populations - probably due to higher doses of the drug in the study of Stambler et al. [12] and to the greater duration of arrhythmia in the study of Ellenbogen et al. [13] – its efficacy was significantly higher than that of placebo, and it was effective in (1) patients with long-lasting arrhythmia and (2) patients with various types of heart disease and different levels of left ventricular dysfunction - characteristics which differentiate it from other drugs and make it extremely useful. In a randomized comparison study with procainamide [14] carried out in 127 patients (86 AF and 41 AFl), the ibutilide (2 mg intravenously) conversion rate was 76% for AFl and 51% for AF compared to 12% and 20% respectively for procainamide ($p < 0.003$). In another comparison study with another class III drug, dl-sotalol, ibutilide *was also more efficacious*. In a multicenter, double-blind randomized study, Vos et al. [15] compared 308 patients with each other (48% with heart disease), 251 of whom had AF and 57 AFl. Ibutilide was given at doses of 1 mg and 2 mg and dl-sotalol at a dosage of 1.5 mg/kg. Ibutilide was superior to dl-sotalol in terminating AFl (56% and 70% vs 19%) ($p < 0.005$).

We want to underline two further points about the action of the drug: the possibility of administering it even in patients treated with amiodarone, and the facilitation of overdrive suppression pacing. Glatter et al. [16] carried out the infusion of the drug (1 mg + 1 mg) in 70 patients undergoing long-term treatment with amiodarone, 57 of whom had AF and 13 AFl. Seven of the patients with AFl (54%) had sinus rhythm restoration, vs 22 (39%) of those with AF. The mean QT interval for the entire group increased from 371 ± 61 to 479 ± 92 ms after ibutilide treatment, and there was one episode of nonsustained torsade de pointes. The drug had already been tested in patients taking digoxin, calcium antagonists, or β-blockers. Although it must be further tested, the study by Glatter et al. [16] has emphasized that the two drugs do not have increased adverse effects, even thought they belong to the same class. Concerning the capacity of enhancing termination of AFl by atrial overdrive suppression pacing, in a study in which ibutilide and procainamide were compared with placebo [17], both drugs significantly enhanced pacing-induced termination of AFl compared with placebo. Of 59 episodes of AFl in 54 patients, pacing converted 2 of 11 patients (18%) who received placebo, 13 of 15 patients (87%) who received ibutilide, and 29 of 33 (88%) who received procainamide. Therefore, both drugs, despite their differing electrophysiologic effects, enhanced the termination of AFl by atrial pacing. The other class III drug tested in the treatment of AFl is dofetilide, which is not yet available in Italy.

Dofetilide

Dofetilide is a highly selective blocker of the inward potassium current and appears to specifically block the rapid component of the delayed rectifier current (I_{Kr}). As such, it leads to prolongation of the action potential duration with a resultant increase in myocardial refractoriness. Its further characteristics are: (1) the propriety of the reverse use-dependence phenomenon; (2) excellent bioavailability (> 90%), so it is well absorbed after oral administration. In addition, this drug does not have any effect on PR, QRS, or HV interval, and is excellently tolerated even by patients with functional class III or IV CHF [18]. Dofetilide has also been tested in hospital in populations including patients with AF or AFl. Extrapolating data concerning AFl, which are really very poor, the following results have been observed. For Suttorp et al. [19], in a series of 24 patients, 5 of them with AFl lasting less than 6 months, conversion to sinus rhythm was achieved in 4 of the 5 patients (80%) in a mean time of 40 ± 52 min. In a double-blind multicenter study, Falk et al. [20] randomized 91 patients – 75 with AF and 16 with AFl – to receive one or two doses of dofetilide (4 or 8 µg/kg) or placebo. A high percentage of patients also presented underlying heart disease, functional class III or IV. The mean duration

of arrhythmia was about 2 months. Pharmacological conversion within 4 h was observed in 31% of the high-dose group, 12.5% of the low-dose group, and 0% of the placebo group. Conversion was more frequent in the small group with AFl compared with those with AF (54% versus 12.5%) overall. In a similar study in 96 patients with AF ($n = 79$) or AFl ($n = 17$) with a median arrhythmia duration of 62 days, 66 of whom were treated with dofetilide and 30 with placebo, and in which a high percentage of patients had an underlying heart disease, Norgaard et al. [21] studied the efficacy of 8 µg/kg dofetilide. Pharmacological conversion to sinus rhythm was seen in 64% of those with AFl and in 39% of those with AF treated with dofetilide, in contrast with 0% and 4% respectively in the placebo group ($p<0.006$). In comparison studies with other class I and III drugs, dofetilide has also proved superior in restoring sinus rhythm in patients with AFl. Crijns et al. [22], in 21 patients with AFl, 11 of whom were treated with flecainide 2 mg/kg and 10 with dofetilide 8 µg/kg, obtained conversion to sinus rhythm in 1 patient in the flecainide group (10%) versus 7 (70%) in the dofetilide group. In an Italian multicenter randomized, double-blind, placebo-controlled study, dofetilide was compared with amiodarone and placebo in the acute treatment of 150 patients with AF or AFl [23]. Thirty-one of these had AFl: 12 were given dofetilide, 9 amiodarone, and 10 placebo. In the majority of patients the arrhythmia had lasted longer than 7 days. Overall the conversion rate to sinus rhythm was 35% (17 of 48) in patients treated with dofetilide, 4% (2 of 50) in patients treated with amiodarone, and 4% (2 of 52) in patients treated with placebo, within the 3-h study period (dofetilide vs placebo, $p < 0.001$; amiodarone vs placebo, n.s.). In this population, too, the efficacy of dofetilide was significantly higher in AFl than in AF ($p = 0.004$): conversion rate at 3 h were 75% and 22% respectively. Finally, it is interesting that even when given orally, dofetilide has proved significantly more efficacious than placebo in sinus rhythm restoration in AFl. In a double-blind, multicenter, placebo-controlled, dose-ranging study, Singh et al. [24] evaluated 325 patients, 277 of whom (85%) had AF and 48 (15%) AFl. A structural heart disease was present in more than 50% of patients. The analysis of pharmacological conversion by primary diagnosis for the 500 mg b.i.d. dofetilide group showed a 21.6% rate for the AF subgroup and 66.7% for the AFl subgroup. Both of these rates are statistically highly significant with respect to the conversion rate for placebo.

Side Effects

Undoubtedly the most relevant side effect for both ibutilide and dofetilide is polymorphic unsustained or sustained VT. Among the patients treated with ibutilide, polymorphic VT was observed in proportions ranging from 0.9% to 8.3%. In 0.5%-2% a DC shock was required for termination. There were three predictive factors: low body weight, history of a CHF, and presence of bradycardia. The episodes of polymorphic VT were independent of LVEF, total patient dose, patient sex, and basal duration of QT. In all studies, however, high-risk patients had been excluded, such as those with prolonged basal QT (QTc > 440 ms), hypopotassemia, and previous episodes of torsade de pointes.

Concerning dofetilide, polymorphic unsustained or sustained VT was observed in 0%-8.3% of patients, of whom 0%-2.2% required DC shock for termination; one sudden death in a patient treated with a drug per os was unwitnessed and presumed to be a sudden cardiac death. At the moment, there is no agreement about possible predictive factors of such adverse effects.

In conclusion, to answer the question of the organizers of this meeting, I think that the following certainties can be underlined: first of all, it is undoubted that the new class III drugs have provided a further possibility for the acute treatment of AFl, in addition to DC shock, to which arrhythmia responds well, and transesophageal atrial pacing, but with the undisputed advantage that pharmacological treatment has with respect to such techniques – provided, obviously, that it does not cause significant side effects. Secondarily, rather than the efficacy percentages (although for AFl these were quite good, generally above 50%), the advantages of these drugs are represented by the fact that they can be used even if arrhythmia is long-lasting, and this is particularly favorable if prophylactic anticoagulation treatment has to be undertaken in patients with an underlying heart disease (over 50% of patients in whom the drugs have been tested had a heart disease), with reduced systolic function or in functional classes III-IV or with intraventricular conduction disorders. These are the population groups usually referred to cardiology departments.

Unsolved Questions

In the introduction we said that the expression "atrial flutter" covers a series of supraventricular arrhythmias that are electrogenetically dissimilar. This is probably one of the reasons why drugs are efficacious in some types of flutter but not in others. In future studies, therefore it would be better to select the different types of flutter, in order to verify this hypothesis. Another unsolved question is identifying factors predictive of efficacy, on the one hand, and adverse effects - apart from well-known effects - on the other. Since the number of patients treated is relatively low, especially given the low prevalence of the arrhythmia, we hope (and this is really a necessity) that future studies will be carried out on a much more selected and homogeneous patient population, in order to take advantage of these drugs as much as possible and perhaps reduce adverse effects. At present, however we think that, since factors predictive of adverse effects are not yet completely known, these drugs must be used only in hospitals, where any serious event due to their administration can be dealt with.

References

1. Cheng J, Cabeen WR, Scheinman MM (1998) Mechanism and anatomic substrates of atypical atrial flutter in the right atrium. Pacing Clin Electrophysiol 21:795 (abstr)
2. Jais P, Haïssanguerre M, Shah DC et al (1998) A new electrophysiological substrate for spontaneous left atrial flutter (abstract). Pacing Clin Electrophysiol 21:794
3. Inoue H, Yamashita T, Nozaki A, Sugimoto T (1999) Effects of antiarrhythmic drugs on canine atrial flutter due to reentry: role of prolongation of refractory period and depression of conduction to excitable gap. J Am Coll Cardiol 18:1089-1104
4. Murdock CJ, Kyles AF, Yeung-Lai-Wah JA et al (1990) Atrial flutter in patients treated for atrial fibrillation with propafenone. Am J Cardiol 66:755-757
5. Tunick PA, Mc Elhinney L, Mitchell T, Kronzon J (1992) The alternation between atrial flutter and atrial fibrillation. Chest 101:34-36
6. Bianconi L, Boccadamo R, Pappalardo A et al (1989) Effectiveness of intravenous propafenone for conversion of atrial fibrillation and flutter of recent onset. Am J Cardiol 64:335-338
7. Suttorp MJ, Kingma JH, Jessuron ER et al (1990) The value of class IC antiarrhythmic drugs for acute conversion of paroxysmal atrial fibrillation or flutter to sinus rhythm. J Am Coll Cardiol 16:1722-1727
8. Suttorp MJ, Kingma JH, Lie-A-Huen L, Mast EG (1989) Intravenous flecainide versus verapamil for acute conversion of paroxysmal atrial fibrillation or flutter to sinus rhythm. Am J Cardiol 63:693-696
9. Goy JJ, Hurni M, Maendly R et al (1985) Conversion of supraventricular arrhythmias to sinus rhythm using flecainide. Eur Heart J 6:518-524
10. Murray KT (1998) Ibutilide. Circulation 97:493-497
11. Foster RH, Wilde MI, Markhan A (1997) Ibutilide. A review of its pharmacological properties and clinical in the acute management of atrial flutter and fibrillation. Drugs 54:1-17
12. Stambler BS, Wood MA, Ellenbogen KA et al (1996) Efficacy and safety of repeated intravenous doses of ibutilide for rapid conversion of atrial flutter or fibrillation. Circulation 94:1613-1621
13. Ellenbogen KA, Stambler BS, Wood MA et al (1996) Efficacy of intravenous ibutilide for rapid termination of atrial fibrillation and atrial flutter: a dose-response study. J Am Coll Cardiol 28:130-136
14. Volgman AS, Stambler BS, Kappagoda C et al (1996) Comparison of intravenous ibutilide versus procainamide for the rapid termination of atrial fibrillation or flutter (abstract). Pacing Clin Electrophysiol 19:169
15. Vos MA, Golitsyn SR, Stangl K et al (1998) Superiority of Ibutilide (a new class III agent) over dl-sotalol in converting atrial flutter and atrial fibrillation. Heart 79:568-575
16. Glatter K, Yang Y, Chatterjee K et al (2001) Chemical cardioversion of atrial fibrillation or flutter with ibutilide in patients receiving amiodarone therapy. Circulation 103:253-257
17. Stambler BS, Wood MA, Ellenbogen KA (1996) Comparative efficacy of intravenous ibutilide versus procainamide for enhancing termination of atrial flutter by atrial overdrive pacing. Am J Cardiol 77:960-966
18. Mounsey JP, Di Marco JP (2000) Dofetilide. Circulation 102:2665-2670
19. Suttorp MJ, Polak P, Van't Hof A et al (1992) Efficacy and safety of a new selective class III antiarrythmic agent dofetilide in paroxysmal atrial fibrillation or atrial flutter. Am J Cardiol 69:417-419

20. Falk RH, Pollak A, Singh SN, Friedrich T (1997) Intravenous dofetilide, a class III antiarrhythmic agent, for the termination of sustained atrial fibrillation or flutter. J Am Coll Cardiol 29:385-390

21. Norgaard BL, Wachtell K, Christensen PD et al (1999) Efficacy and safety of intravenously administered dofetilide in acute termination of atrial fibrillation and flutter: a multicenter, randomized, double-blind, placebo-controlled trial. Am Heart J 137:1062-1069

22. Crijns HJG, Van Gelder IC, Kingma JH et al (1994) Atrial flutter can be terminated by a class III antiarrhythmic drug but not by a class I C drug. Eur Heart J 15:1403-1408

23. Bianconi L, Castro A, Dinelli M et al (2000) Comparison of intravenously administered dofetilide versus amiodarone in the acute termination of atrial fibrillation and flutter. Eur Heart J 21:1265-1273

24. Singh S, Zoble RG, Yellen L et al (2000) Efficacy and safety of oral dofetilide in converting to and maintaining sinus rhythm in patients with chronic atrial fibrillation or atrial flutter. The symptomatic atrial fibrillation investigative research on dofetilide (SAFIRE-D) study. Circulation 102:2385-2390

Typical Atrial Flutter: Antiarrhythmic Drugs or Ablation as First-Line Therapy?

N.F. Marrouche and A. Natale

Since Lewis postulated in 1920 that atrial flutter is due to reentrant circuit, a large body of evidence has advanced our understanding of the electrophysiologic substrate of typical atrial flutter and has enhanced our ability to treat this arrhythmia. Rosenblueth and Garcia-Ramos [1] and Frame et al. [2, 3] first described in an animal model the critical role of the anatomical boundaries in maintaining the flutter circuit. By creating a lesion between the orifices of the venae cavae and extending the lesion to the appendage, a model of atrial flutter was developed. Interestingly, the tricuspid annulus served as the anterior barrier and the crush lesion or incision served as the posterior barrier of the macroreentrant flutter circuit. These models introduced the concept that atrial flutter is a macroreentrant circuit maintained by anatomical barriers including: (1) the tricuspid annulus; (2) the cavity of the right atrium; and (3) the induced surgical barrier that prevents short-circuiting of the macroreentrant circuit within the right atrial free wall. Boineau et al. demonstrated in a canine model that the crista terminalis could replace the crush incision as the posterior barrier of the flutter circuit [4].

Multiple mapping studies in humans with typical isthmus dependent atrial flutter defined the functional and anatomical boundaries of the flutter circuit. Kalman and colleagues elegantly showed using activation and entrainment mapping that the tricuspid annulus constitutes a continuous anterior anatomical barrier constraining the reentrant wavefront of human typical atrial flutter [5]. The eustachian ridge and the crista terminalis define the posterior barriers of the flutter circuit, as reported by Nakagawa and colleagues [6]. The typical atrial flutter wave propagates in a caudocranial direction from the coronary sinus along the right atrial septum towards the vena cava and comes back along the free wall towards the cavotricuspid isthmus bounded by the crista terminalis posteriorly and the tricuspid annulus anteriorly. The wavefront finally enters the narrow isthmus of atrial tissues *protected by the eustachian ridge posteriorly and the tricuspid annulus* anteriorly.

Division of Pacing and Electrophysiology, Department of Cardiology, The Cleveland Clinic Foundation, Cleveland, Ohio, USA

Electrophysiologic Characteristics of Atrial Flutter

Waldo and colleagues first demonstrated the classic criteria of concealed entrainment of typical atrial flutter by rapid atrial pacing from high right atrium in an animal model [7]. Concealed entrainment predicts that the pacing site is located within the critical flutter isthmus. In case of typical atrial flutter the critical isthmus is between the eustachian ridge and the tricuspid annulus. Applying the technique of transient entrainment, Kalman et al. showed that postpacing intervals at all sites of the tricuspid annulus were within the flutter circuit [5].

Nakagawa and colleagues reported double potentials with widely separated isoelectric intervals along the eustachian ridge that extended from the coronary sinus ostium to the inferior vena cava in patients with typical atrial flutter. Arenal et al. demonstrated the importance of the double potentials along the crista terminalis and the eustachian ridge, showing, by rapid pacing on both sides of the crista terminalis, that this structure serves as a functional barrier [8]. The inducibility of atrial flutter is dependent on both the site of pacing and the number of stimuli required to develop the functional block along the crista terminalis. For this reason burst pacing is more effective than atrial extrastimulus in inducing atrial flutter. With regard to the site of pacing, pacing from the coronary sinus or the low lateral right atrium is more likely to develop unidirectional block across the cavotricuspid isthmus, allowing the flutter circuit to propagate in one direction.

Ablation of Typical Atrial Flutter

The understanding of the reentrant circuit of typical atrial flutter has led to the present treatment strategy, which relies on the ability to create a lesion that transects the critical isthmus by connecting two anatomical barriers. Multiple reports have shown that dragging a radiofrequency lesion from the tricuspid annulus to the inferior vena cava and/or eustachian ridge and coronary sinus interrupts the typical flutter circuit [9-12]. The anatomical target for ablation of typical atrial flutter, although relatively complex, is surrounded by fixed anatomical landmarks, which facilitates placement of the linear lesion. Wang and Jorge examined the dimensions of this anatomical structure defining the flutter isthmus in 51 postmortem hearts [13]. They reported a wide variation in the distance between the tricuspid annulus and the eustachian ridge, ranging between 1.8 and 4.2 cm. Therefore in some cases a lesion many centimeters long is needed. These findings have important clinical implications and may explain the relatively high recurrence rates reported in some series.

Catheter ablation can be conducted either in atrial flutter or during pacing from the coronary sinus or the low right lateral atrium. Understanding the anatomical barriers involved in the substrate for typical atrial flutter led to the development of new endpoints to establish successful atrial flutter ablation. These include: (1) demonstration of bidirectional conduction block in the flutter isthmus during coronary sinus and low lateral atrial pacing; (2) change to upright P wave with low lateral right atrial pacing; (3) split potentials with wide and fixed timing between the two components along the linear lesion in the isthmus with coronary sinus ostium and/or low lateral right atrial pacing; and (4) change in circumannular activation sequence with low lateral right atrial and coronary sinus pacing after ablation [14-19].

Radiofrequency (RF) is the energy source generally used for treatment of atrial flutter. Monitoring of the catheter tip solidus tissue temperature interface is particularly important, with the goal of keeping the temperature between 55°C and 60°C. The long-term success rates of atrial flutter ablation using RF energy delivery by creating an isthmus line vary between 70% and 95% [11, 20-22].

In our preliminary experience and that of others [23], the use of cooled-tip catheters, or large-tip catheters (8-10 mm) with a high power generator, appeared to reduce greatly the recurrence rate and to facilitate acute procedural success (Table 1).

Table 1. Comparison between different catheter ablation technologies for typical atrial flutter

	8-mm-tip or 10-mm-tip or cooled-tip ablation catheter	Conventional ablation catheter (4- or 5-mm tip)	Overall p value
Patients (M/F)	50 (42/8)	38 (26/12)	NS
Mean age (years)	61.5 ± 13.8	60.0 ± 11.3	NS
Acute ablation success rate	100% (50/50)	71% (27/38)	< 0.01
Success rate after crossover	0%	29% (11/38)	< 0.005
Fluoroscopy time (min)	39 ± 19	54 ± 26	< 0.005
Recurrence rate after 8 ± 2 months	0%	18.4% (7/38)	< 0.005

NS, not significant

Management of Atrial Flutter

Due to the high success rates and low complication rates associated with typical flutter ablation, this therapy modality is becoming the preferred approach. At present, several antiarrhythmic drugs are available to treat typical atrial flutter. In the absence of heart disease the class IC drugs associated with atrioventricular (AV) node blocking agents are probably the best choice, because of the better toleration and the lower organ toxicity compared to class IA drugs, sotalol and amiodarone. Only one retrospective study by Wood and colleagues suggested that the stroke rate in patients with atrial flutter is comparable to that with atrial fibrillation [24]. Although at present there is no clear agreement on the use of anticoagulation in patients with atrial flutter, warfarin therapy should be considered in the same fashion as in atrial fibrillation.

Antiarrhythmic Therapy Versus First-Line Radiofrequency Ablation

Despite the high rate of cure achieved by RF catheter ablation, pharmacologic therapy is still considered the standard initial therapeutic approach for atrial flutter. We conducted a study to assess and compare the clinical efficacy of conventional drug therapy versus first-line catheter ablation to treat atrial flutter in a prospective randomized manner.

This was a multicenter prospective randomized study. Patients were considered eligible for the study if they had at least two symptomatic episodes of atrial flutter in the last 4 months. Exclusion criteria included the following: (1) prior evidence of atrial fibrillation; (2) the presence of significant left atrial enlargement (≥4.5 cm); and (3) previous treatment with antiarrhythmic medications (AAD). Sixty-one patients were included in the study (42 men; mean age 66 ± 10 years). Mean left ventricular ejection fraction was 49 ± 3%. After entering the study each patient was randomized to either AAD therapy or first-line RF catheter ablation. Drug therapy was given based on the physician's preference. An effort was made to keep each patient in the same treatment group for at least 1 year. Each investigator was required to attempt sinus rhythm maintenance with at least two drugs, including amiodarone, before resorting to rate control medications. Recurrence of atrial flutter during amiodarone therapy was not considered a failure during the initial 2 months of treatment with this drug. Following enrollment in the study, institution or change of AAD therapy was performed on an outpatient basis unless hospitalization was required by the patients' symptoms. Quality of life and symptoms questionnaires were administered before institution of therapy, and 6 and 12 months thereafter. The study endpoints were as follows: (1) recurrence of atrial flutter; (2) need for rehospitalization; and (3) quality of life and symptom scales.

RF catheter ablation was performed by creating a linear lesion from the tricuspid annulus to the inferior vena cava using 4- and/or 8-mm-tip electrode catheters advanced in the right atrium with a long 8F sheath (SRO, Daig Corp). The 8-mm tip was used if with the 4-mm tip catheter adequate RF energy could not be delivered due to immediate impedance rise even at low power setting. RF ablation was continued until either no electrogram or consistent reduction of the electrogram amplitude of at least 90% was present across the isthmus. We also assessed inducibility after ablation using extrastimulus testing and burst pacing. To prove bidirectional isthmus block, a 20-pole halo catheter (Cordis-

Webster, Inc.) was used in 11 patients, while a custom-made catheter with eight proximal and eight distal electrodes separated by a 9-cm gap (Cardiac Assist Device Inc., Cleveland) was used in 15 patients. In these 15 patients the distal electrodes were placed in the coronary sinus and the proximal electrodes were placed along the right lateral atrial wall anterior to the crista terminalis. In the remaining 3 patients isthmus conduction block was proven using the electroanatomical mapping system CARTO (Biosense-Webster).

An assessment of the patients' quality of life before and after the procedure was performed using a questionnaire that included 16 items to evaluate the physical, social, economic and psychological impairment (Endicott, Quality of Life Enjoyment and Satisfaction Questionnaire).

All patients were followed up in the outpatient clinic at regular intervals. In case of recurrence of atrial flutter after ablation, the procedure was repeated. In the case of recurrence of atrial flutter in patients treated with AAD therapy, a different AAD was initiated. If patients experienced atrial fibrillation after entering the study, the arrhythmia was treated with medical therapy.

The clinical characteristics of the two study groups are summarized in Table 2.

Table 2. First-time RF ablation versus drug therapy: baseline characteristics of the two patient groups

	RF ablation ($n = 31$)	Drug therapy ($n = 30$)	p value
Age (years)	67 ± 8	66 ± 11	NS
Male gender	20	22	NS
Mean ejection fraction (%)	49.4 ± 5.1	49.6 ±3 .1	NS
Structural heart disease			
Absent	16	17	
Coronary artery disease	12	11	
Valvular disease	2	1	
Other	1	-	
Paroxysmal atrial flutter (n)	-	1	NS
Persistent atrial flutter (n)	1	2	NS
Median episodes of atrial flutter per month	30 1 (0-3)	28 1 (0-2)	NS
Mean no. of cardioversions before entering the study	2.3 ± 0.5	2.2 ± 0.5	NS
Mean no. of cardioversions after entering the study	0.5 ± 1.2	4.4 ± 1.7	< 0.01
Atrial flutter recurrence	6% (2)	93% (28)	< 0.01
Atrial fibrillation after entering the study	29% (9)	60% (18)	< 0.05
Mean no. of arrhythmia episodes at follow-up	0.7 ± 1.4	5.1 ± 2.0	< 0.01
Percentage of patients requiring rehospitalization	22% (7)	63% (19)	< 0.01

Acute successful ablation was obtained in all 31 patients undergoing RF ablation. Twenty-six patients out of 31 had typical isthmus-dependent flutter. In the remaining five patients incisional atrial flutter was induced and documented as the only arrhythmia (3 patients) or in combination with typical flutter (2 patients). In all patients, the ablation was initiated with a 4-mm-tip electrode, and it was concluded with an 8-mm-tip electrode in five of them.

Among the 26 patients undergoing verification of bidirectional block along the ablation line we observed the following: (1) bidirectional block was present immediately following termination of atrial flutter by catheter ablation only in 11 patients (42%); (2) after demonstration of bidirectional block, additional lesions were required in four patients (15%) to satisfy the electrogram amplitude endpoint; and (3) uniform reduction of the electrogram amplitude across the isthmus was never associated with persistence of conduction throughout this region.

At the end of the 1-year follow-up two patients experienced recurrence of atrial flutter (6.4%) and both were successfully treated with ablation. Nine patients experienced atrial fibrillation after successful catheter ablation of atrial flutter (29%). Of these nine patients, five were treated with AAD with long-term persistence of sinus rhythm. Three patients had sporadic episodes of self-terminating atrial fibrillation and were treated with rate control drugs. One patient did not respond to AAD, and because rate control was difficult to achieve with medication, he underwent AV node ablation and implantation of a single-chamber permanent pacemaker 9 months after the initial ablation for atrial flutter.

The mean number of drugs initiated in the AAD group was 3.4 ± 1.1. The type of drugs administered in individual patients is shown in Table 3. At follow-up, 16 (53%) of these patients were treated with rate control drugs due to the inefficacy of active AAD in maintenance of sinus rhythm. Of these 16 patients, 15 had both recurrence of atrial flutter and development of atrial fibrillation. At the time of the first arrhythmia recurrence, atrial fibrillation was observed in one patient, whereas all the remaining patients had atrial flutter. Two patients crossed over to the atrial flutter ablation group before the end of the first year of follow-up and one patient required AV node ablation and pacemaker due to the inability to maintain sinus rhythm and achieve adequate rate control. Of the remaining 11 patients, 8 were treated with amiodarone, 1 with propafenone and atenolol, and 2 with procainamide and digoxin. Of the 16 patients receiving rate control drugs, 2 were treated with digoxin alone, 7 with diltiazem or verapamil combined with digoxin, 4 with β-adrenergic blocking agents alone, and 3 with a combination of β-blocker and digoxin.

In the patients randomized to drug therapy, with the exception of palpitations, there was no statistically significant change in all the quality of life variables (Table 4). In contrast to this, the patients treated with catheter ablation reported a significant improvement in their quality of life and symptoms scores (Table 5).

After a mean follow-up of 22 ± 11 months, 25 patients (80%) who underwent catheter ablation were in sinus rhythm without the need for active AAD,

Table 3. Types of drugs administered in the antiarrhythmic drug therapy group

Patient No.	Drug 1	Drug 2	Drug 3	Drug 4	Final therapy
1	Sotal	Prop + Ver	Amio		Amio
2	Flecain + Aten	Sotal	Amio	Aten	Aten
3	Dig + Prop	Amio			Amio
4	Sotal	Prop + Ver	Amio	Ver + Dig	Ver + Dig
5	Prop + Aten				Prop + Aten
6	Flecain + Dig	Procain + Dig	Sotal	Amio	Amio
7	Procain + Dig	Prop + Dig	Amio	Ver + Dig	Ver + Dig
8	Sotal	Amio			Amio
9	Flecain + Aten	Sotal	Amio	Aten + Dig	Aten + Dig
10	Flecain + Dig	Procain + Dig			Procain + Dig
11	Procain + Dig	Flecain + Dig	Sotal	Amio	RF Abl
12	Amio	Quinid + Dig	Prop + Aten	Aten + Dig	Aten + Dig
13	Procain + Dig	Prop + Aten	Amio	Dilt + Dig	Dilt + Dig
14	Sotal	Prop + Ver	Amio	Metop	Metop
15	Sotal	Amio	Dilt + Dig		Dilt + Dig
16	Procain + Dig	Prop + Dig	Sotal	Amio	AV node Abl + PPM
17	Sotal	Flecain + Aten	Amio	Ver + Dig	Ver + Dig
18	Dig + Prop	Sotal	Flecain + Aten	Amio	Amio
19	Flecain + Aten	Sotal	Amio	Procain + Dig	Aten + Dig
20	Sotal	Prop + Dig	Amio	Ver + Dig	Ver + Dig
21	Sotal	Prop + Dig	Amio	Dig	Dig
22	Amio	Sotal	Prop + Aten		RF Abl
23	Procain + Dig				Procain + Dig
24	Amio	Sotal	Prop + Dig	Metop	Metop
25	Sotal	Prop + Aten	Procain + Dig	Amio	Amio
26	Quinid + Dig	Prop + Ver	Amio	Aten	Aten
27	Flecain + Dig	Sotal	Amio	Dig + Dilt	Dig + Dilt
28	Sotal	Prop + Aten	Amio		Amio
29	Amio	Prop + Aten	Sotal	Dig	Dig
30	Amio				Amio

Amio, amiodarone; *Aten*, atenolol; *AV*, atrioventricular; *Dig*, digoxin; *Dilt*, diltiazem; *Flecain*, flecainide; *Metop*, metoprolol; *PPM*, permanent pacemaker; *Procain*, procainamide; *Prop*, propafenone; *Quinid*, quinidine; *RF Abl*, catheter ablation of atrial flutter; *Sotal*, sotalol; *Ver*, verapamil

whereas only 11 (36%, $p < 0.01$) of those receiving AAD remained in sinus rhythm. At follow-up, atrial fibrillation was seen in 9 patients undergoing catheter ablation (29%) versus 18 of those receiving AAD therapy (60%, $p < 0.05$). Eight of the nine patients (88%) experiencing atrial fibrillation following catheter ablation had this arrhythmia controlled by medical therapy. In contrast to this, in the drug therapy group only 1 of the 18 patients (6%) developing atrial fibrillation had this arrhythmia successfully managed with drugs. During the follow-up period, hospitalization was required for occurrence of severely symp-

Table 4. Quality of life and symptom scores in the drug therapy group

	Before treatment	After treatment 6 months	After treatment 12 months	Overall p value
Sense of well being	1.9 ± 0.4	2.0 ± 0.4	2.1 ± 0.3	NS
Function in daily life	2.1 ± 0.4	2.1 ± 0.3	2.3 ± 0.3	NS
Palpitation	3.2 ± 0.6*	2.0 ± 0.5	2.1 ± 0.7	< 0.05
SOB with exercise	3.4 ± 0.4	3.2 ± 0.4	3.0 ± 0.5	NS
Feeling weak	2.9 ± 0.3	3.0 ± 0.4	3.1 ± 0.4	NS
QOL total score	29 ± 3	28 ± 6	31 ± 5	NS

QOL, quality of life overall score; SOB, shortness of breath
*$p < 0.001$, pre-treatment versus post-treatment 6 months after post-treatment 12 months
Other comparisons did not show statistical significance

Table 5. Quality of life and symptom scores in the drug therapy group

	Preablation	Postablation 6 months	Postablation 12 months	Overall p value
Sense of well being	2.0 ± 0.3*	3.9 ± 0.3	3.8 ± 0.5	< 0.01
Function in daily life	2.3 ± 0.4	3.8 ± 0.5	3.6 ± 0.6	< 0.01
Palpitation	3.1 ± 0.6	1.0 ± 0.4	1.0 ± 0.5	< 0.01
SOB with exercise	3.0 ± 0.4	1.0 ± 0.5	1.2 ± 0.3	< 0.01
Feeling week	2.9 ± 0.5	0.8 ± 0.4	0.8 ± 0.5	< 0.01
QOL total score	30 ± 4**	59 ± 7	57 ± 6	< 0.001

QOL, quality of life overall score; SOB, shortness of breath
*$p < 0.001$, preablation versus postablation 6 months after postablation 12 months
**$p < 0.0001$, preablation versus postablation 6 months after postablation 12 months

tomatic arrhythmia in 7 patients (22%) undergoing catheter ablation and 19 (63%, $p < 0.01$) of those receiving medication. Among the patients treated with AAD, recurrence of atrial flutter was never associated with 1:1 AV conduction.

These data support the use of catheter ablation rather than AAD as the first-line therapy for treatment of atrial flutter. As shown in our study, atrial flutter ablation was not only more effective in the long-term management of this arrhythmia, but patients treated with this approach experienced fewer rehospitalizations and lower occurrence of atrial fibrillation during the follow-up. This clinical beneficial effect appeared to have a more positive impact on the quality of life.

Of interest is the lower rate of atrial fibrillation after cure of atrial flutter with ablation. This finding may suggest that ineffective prevention of atrial fibrillation by AAD therapy may potentiate an unfavorable electrical remodeling of the atrium which, in turn, could facilitate degeneration to atrial fibrillation at follow-up. On the other hand, pure atrial flutter could be the early manifestation of an atrial electrical disease, which may lead to atrial fibrillation over time. A longer-term follow-up is needed to exclude or confirm this hypothesis.

In conclusion, catheter-based treatment of atrial flutter appears superior to conventional drug therapy and should be considered the first-line approach. Whether cure of atrial flutter has a long-term effect in preventing development of atrial fibrillation remains unclear.

References

1. Rosenblueth A, Garcia-Ramos J (1947) Studies on flutter and fibrillation. Am Heart J 33:677-684
2. Frame LH, Page RL, Boyden PA et al (1987) Circus movement in the canine atrium around the tricuspid ring during experimental atrial flutter and during reentry in vitro. Circulation 76:1155-1175
3. Frame LH, Page RL, Hoffman BF (1986) Atrial reentry around an anatomic barrier with a partially refractory excitable gap. A canine model of atrial flutter. Circ Res 58:495-511
4. Boineau JP, Schuessler RB, Mooney CR et al(1980) Natural and evoked atrial flutter due to circus movement in dogs. Role of abnormal atrial pathways, slow conduction, nonuniform refractory period distribution and premature beats. Am J Cardiol 45:1167-1181
5. Kalman JM, Olgin JE, Saxon LA et al (1996) Activation and entrainment mapping defines the tricuspid annulus as the anterior barrier in typical atrial flutter [see comments]. Circulation 94:398-406
6. Nakagawa H, Lazzara R, Khastgir T et al (1996) Role of the tricuspid annulus and the eustachian valve/ridge on atrial flutter. Relevance to catheter ablation of the septal isthmus and a new technique for rapid'identification of ablation success [see comments]. Circulation 94:407-424
7. Waldo AL, MacLean WA, Karp RB et al (1977) Entrainment and interruption of atrial flutter with atrial pacing: studies in man following open heart surgery. Circulation 56:737-745
8. Arenal A, Almendral J, Alday JM et al (1999) Rate-dependent conduction block of the crista terminalis in patients with typical atrial flutter: influence on evaluation of cavotricuspid isthmus conduction block. Circulation 99:2771-2778
9. Olgin JE, Lesh MD (1997) The laboratory evaluation and role of catheter ablation for patients with atrial flutter. Cardiol Clin 15:677-688
10. Saoudi N, Atallah G, Kirkorian G, Touboul P (1990) Catheter ablation of the atrial myocardium in human type I atrial flutter [see comments]. Circulation 81:762-771
11. Cosio FG, Lopez-Gil M, Goicolea A et al (1993) Radiofrequency ablation of the inferior vena cava-tricuspid valve isthmus in common atrial flutter. Am J Cardiol 71:705-709
12. Cheng J, Cabeen WR Jr, Scheinman MM (1999) Right atrial flutter due to lower loop reentry: mechanism and anatomic substrates. Circulation 99:1700-1705
13. Wang Z, Wilber D, Jorge A (2001) Anatomic variability of the tricuspid annulus-inferior vena cava isthmus and the eustachian ridge (in press)
14. Shah D, Haïssaguerre M, Takahashi A et al (2000) Differential pacing for distinguishing block from persistent conduction through an ablation line. Circulation 102:1517-1522
15. Oral H, Sticherling C, Tada H et al (2001) Role of transisthmus conduction intervals in predicting bidirectional block after ablation of typical atrial flutter. J Cardiovasc Electrophysiol 12:169-174
16. Kottkamp H, Hindricks G (1999) Catheter ablation of atrial flutter. Thorac Cardiovasc Surg 47 (Suppl 3):357-361

17. Nakagawa H, Jackman WM (1998) Use of a three-dimensional, nonfluoroscopic map-
     ping system for catheter ablation of typical atrial flutter. Pacing Clin Electrophysiol
     21:1279-1286
18. Kalman JM, Vohra JK, Jayaprakash S, Sparks PB (1997) Radiofrequency ablation for
     cure of atrial flutter. Aust N Z J Med 27:653-657
19. Lesh MD, Van Hare GF, Fitzpatrick AP et al (1993) Curing reentrant atrial arrhythmias.
     Targeting protected zones of slow conduction by catheter ablation. J Electrocardiol
     26:194-203
20. Saxon LA, Kalman JM, Olgin JE et al (1996) Results of radiofrequency catheter ablation
     for atrial flutter. Am J Cardiol 77:1014-1016
21. Calkins H, Leon AR, Deam AG et al (1994) Catheter ablation of atrial flutter using
     radiofrequency energy. Am J Cardiol 73:353-356
22. Feld GK, Fleck RP, Chen PS et al (1992) Radiofrequency catheter ablation for the treat-
     ment of human type 1 atrial flutter. Identification of a critical zone in the reentrant cir-
     cuit by endocardial mapping techniques. Circulation 86:1233-1240
23. Schweikert R, Natale A, Chung M et al (2001) Use of different catheter ablation
     technologies for typical atrial flutter: acute results and follow-up. J Am Coll Cardiol
     3 (abstr)
24. Wood KA, Eisenberg SJ, Kalman JM et al (1997) Risk of thromboembolism in chronic
     atrial flutter. Am J Cardiol 79:1043-1047

What Is the Most Accurate and Simple Method to Assess Block Through the Cavotricuspid Isthmus?

D.C. SHAH, P. JAÏS, M. HOCINI, T. YAMANE, L. MACLE, K.-J. CHOI, M. HAÏSSAGUERRE AND J. CLÉMENTY

The determining factor in allowing the effective elimination of typical atrial flutter by catheter ablation has clearly been the progressive refinement of procedural endpoints (Table 1). In our own experience, three clear transitions, demarcated by progressive reductions in the recurrence rates for this arrhythmia, have been evident. Beginning with a high recurrence rate when flutter termination and noninducibility were considered sufficient endpoints, the demonstration of cavotricuspid isthmus block based on septal and lateral right atrial activation sequences reduced recurrence rates to about 12%. Further refinement with the routine use of local electrogram-based criteria [1], mapping double potentials supplemented with differential pacing [2], has led to an additional reduction in recurrence rates to < 5%.

The criteria for demonstrating the presence of complete isthmus conduction block may be classified into primary and secondary; the primary criteria are those observed within the right atrium alone or derived from it, and may be divided into right atrial and local electrogram criteria, while the secondary criteria (observed from outside of the right atrium or derived chiefly from the left atrium) include surface ECG changes [3, 4] as well as changes in the activation sequence of the coronary sinus (left atrial criteria) [5]. Modification of the sequence of lateral or septal right atrial activation is necessary, but not enough to indicate isthmus block and local criteria more directly evaluate the linear lesion with greater sensitivity and specificity [1]. While the sensitivity of local electrogram criteria derives from being assessed right on the linear lesion, their specificity relates to independence from catheter positioning as well as from posterior intercaval conduction. The presence of such conduction can shorten the timing to the second component of double potentials on the ablation line but cannot produce false-positive gap electrograms on the ablation line. The extent of reduction in timing of the second component would depend at least partly upon the level of posterior intercaval conduction. More than one technique can be used to demonstrate some of the above criteria of isthmus block, including multielectrode multicatheter techniques, basket catheters,

Hôpital Cardiologique du Haut-Lévêque, Pessac, France

Table 1. Endpoints of catheter ablation for atrial flutter

Endpoint	Evolution	Catheter hardware	Comments
Flutter Termination	Historically oldest endpoints	Ablation catheter	Nonspecific: only implies transient block
Noninducibility		Pacing catheter	Insensitive; Frequently induces AF
Block assessed by primary right atrial changes: Isthmus block demonstrated by sequential mapping of lat. RA and septum	First techniques demonstrating isthmus block	One pacing and another rove map catheter	Limited coverage and sensitivity: difficult to map septum with multielectrode catheter; False-positive induction shown despite block
Isthmus block demonstrated by simultaneous mapping of lat. RA and septum		Multielectrode catheters	Intra-atrial activation time a variable continuum
Block assessed by primary local changes: Local electrogram-based criteria of isthmus block	Recently described techniques	Two-catheter technique	Covers full isthmus width plus ablation line; Increased sensitivity for slow conduction and specificity for block
Differential pacing		One pacing and one stationary recording catheter	Adjunct to above; Different complex online potentials
Block assessed by secondary-surface ECG changes: Paced P change	Observed associated changes	Only pacing catheter required	Primary appeal simplicity; Pacing position crucial; No advantage in sensitivity and specificity; Useful surveillance for tracking conduction
Block assessed by secondary LA changes: CS activation		CS catheter	Limited coverage specificity and sensitivity: indirect and remote assessment of RA block

electroanatomic sequential mapping, as well as noncontact mapping [6]. Essentially, these technologically different forms present the same data, i.e. the right atrial and local electrogram criteria in one form or another and with some or other trade off. Sequential mapping is time-consuming and cannot be applied to single-beat analysis, while multielectrode multicatheter techniques are typically limited in their coverage and consistent positioning. It is also not clear whether noncontact mapping would be able to localize low voltage gaps based on (virtual) unipolar electrograms; this may be even more of a problem during flutter with 2:1 or 1:1 AV ratios because of prominent ventricular electrograms.

Notwithstanding the different criteria described above, a common feature instrumental in maximizing the sensitivity and specificity for complete isthmus block is the choice of pacing site. The chosen site must be as close as possible to the line of block in order to maximize the probability/sensitivity for detecting slow conduction through the line, and to avoid it being concealed/masked by the wavefront going around the lesion with a relatively shorter conduction time [2]. If the pacing site is positioned optimally close to the line, the choice of a low lateral RA pacing site vs a coronary sinus ostial pacing site is probably immaterial. With a coronary sinus catheter, however, frequently the most proximal stable pacing site is within the coronary sinus, and therefore tends to be at a significant distance from the line, although this can be easily assessed by the stimulus to first potential time (st-DP1) on the line. A st-DP1 of 30 ms or less is optimal [2]. On the other hand, the change in the surface ECG P wave produced by isthmus block is maximal when pacing from the low lateral right atrium, and is particularly sensitive to conduction recovery because of the location of the coronary sinus input to the LA, which is just adjacent to, but on the opposite side of, the lesion only when pacing from the low lateral right atrium. LA activation from the CS input [7] therefore acts as a surface ECG amplifier of P wave change, both for conduction block/delay and particularly for conduction recovery (see below).

Differential pacing involves assessing the response of local onsite electrograms to shifting the site of activation origin (pacing), by advancing or withdrawing it from its original position near the ablation line. If activation on both sides of the line (indicated by local double potentials) is linked directly by a conducting gap, withdrawing the pacing site will increase the activation time to both sides and by roughly the same magnitude. On the other hand, if there is no conducting gap across the line, withdrawing the pacing site will certainly increase the activation time upstream of the line, but will either shorten the activation time on the other side of the line or leave it unchanged, but will not increase it.

The demonstration of functional linking by changing pacing sites depends upon the relative conduction times to both flanks of the ablation line, and therefore may be affected by the selection of the pacing position, relative conduction velocities, length of the activation detour, as well as by intervening areas of slow conduction or block, which affect only one of the two pacing positions. The pacing catheter should therefore be positioned as close as possible to the lesion line and the magnitude of displacement of the pacing position limited (15 mm), so that the stimulus to the first potential time is about 40 ms during distal pacing and 60 ms during proximal pacing. To detect very slow conduction through the isthmus (e.g 0.05 m/s or less), both pacing sites may need to be even closer to the ablation line, i.e. with shorter stimulus to first potential times. As an example, assume that the impulse travels around a tricuspid annulus of 14 cm in circumference after isthmus block with a uniform conduction velocity of 0.7 m/s, and the isthmus lesion conducts with a velocity of 0.05 m/s over a width of 7 mm, then the distal pacing site must be within 1.75 cm of the ablation line – corresponding to a stimulus to first potential time of 30 ms – in order to distinguish block from slow conduction through the isthmus. A close pacing site is also important in order to avoid orthodromic capture by a single front during distal pacing and antidromic capture of the opposite flank during proximal pacing, in the presence of persistent but slow conduction. This may be suspected by a change in the morphology of the electrograms, in spite of an unchanged catheter position.

Similarly, although the same pacing maneuvre could be applied to assessing the functional linking of electrograms adjacent to, but some distance from, the line, this would limit the ability to detect slow penetrating conduction, which is maximized by assessment on the ablation line. The latter consideration means that the absence of any lengthening is strong support for the presence of block, which was borne out in our study, not only by comparison with accepted criteria for block but also by repeat assessment at another site on the ablation line, which demonstrated clear shortening of the timing of the second potential. Intervening areas of slow conduction or block may, however, impair accuracy if they selectively affect only one of the two pacing positions. These limitations also apply to other means of conduction assessment and are in fact common to all.

Very slow conduction through the isthmus, therefore, cannot be absolutely ruled out and, although we did not find any instances of false-positive diagnoses of persisting conduction, this is theoretically possible in the presence of a conduction delay affecting only activation from the second pacing position.

Another factor that has significant impact on the efficacy of curative ablation is the stability of the achieved conduction block. Although the achievement of block in the cavotricuspid isthmus is accepted to require an in-line and contiguous series of point lesions, by the same corollary, the probability of conduction recovery across this composite lesion can be estimated by the number of constituent lesions (mean of 6-10 point lesions) times their individual probability of recovery. If the latter is estimated to be 2%, based on data from WPW ablation (so called "point" ablation), this works out to 12%-20%. In accordance with this analysis, recent data from serial and continuous monitoring in patients undergoing ablation have indicated rather high rates of conduction recovery after the achievement of complete block (as also after the termination of flutter by RF delivery in the cavotricuspid isthmus). In practice, this mandates monitoring of the stability of isthmus conduction block after ablation: the exponential reduction in the incidence of recovery with time suggests an empirical cutoff for the duration of the monitoring period, keeping in mind that, since 97% of conduction recovery was found to occur within 15 min, this duration of monitoring is compatible with the present low recurrence rates observed in our laboratory [8]. As a corollary, an extended period of monitoring for recovery, followed by reablation, might reduce recurrence rates even further.

Clinical Implications

Differential pacing – a single site assessment technique – is best used as a complement to local electrogram assessment to provide an onsite evaluation of each double or triple fractionated potential, without having to move the recording ablation catheter from the recording site or perform supplemental mapping. This is an obvious additional advantage when a gap electrogram is validated to represent persistent conduction through the ablation lesion instead of bystander slow conduction, and permits prompt ablation, whereas recognizing conduction block in spite of triple or fractionated potentials prevented unnecessary ablation. It is also useful for confirming the achievement of block, particularly when limited mapping of the line is performed, or to rule out slow conduction when right atrial criteria are used to evaluate conduction.

The gold standard for complete (and stable) isthmus conduction block is ultimately only the absence of recurrence of typical atrial flutter – which, however, can only be evaluated at a distance from the ablation procedure.

References

1. Shah DC, Takahashi A, Jaïs P et al (1999) Local electrogram-based criteria of cavotricuspid isthmus block. J Cardiovasc Electrophysiol 10:662-669
2. Shah DC, Haïssaguerre M, Takahashi A et al (2000) Differential pacing for distinguishing block from persistent conduction through an ablation line. Circulation 102:1517-1522
3. Hamdan MH, Kalman JM, Barron HV, Lesh MD (1997) P wave morphology during right atrial pacing before and after atrial flutter ablation - a new marker for success. Am J Cardiol 79:1417-1420
4. Tsai CF, Chen SA, Tai CT et al (1998) A novel interval (OCS-DCS) is the only independent predictor of complete vs incomplete isthmus conduction block in ablation of common atrial flutter. J Am Coll Cardiol 31(2):254A (abstr)
5. Kottkamp H, Hügl B, Krauss B et al (2000) Electromagnetic versus fluoroscopic mapping of the inferior isthmus for ablation of typical atrial flutter: a prospective randomized study. Circulation 102:2082-2086
6. Shah DC, Haïssaguerre M, Jaïs P et al (1999) Dual input right to left atrial activation correlating with P wave morphology. Pacing Clin Electrophysiol 22(II):832 (abstr)
7. Shah DC, Takahashi A, Jaïs P et al (2000) Tracking dynamic conduction recovery across the cavotricuspid isthmus. J Am Coll Cardiol 35:1478-1484
8. Nabar A, Rodriguez LM, Timmermans C et al (1999) Isoproterenol to evaluate resumption of conduction after right atrial isthmus ablation in type I atrial flutter. Circulation 99:3286-3291

Class IC/Amiodarone Atrial Flutter: What Are the Long-Term Results of Radiofrequency Ablation?

A. Bonso, A. Rossillo, S. Themistoclakis, G. Gasparini, A. Corrado and A. Raviele

Atrial fibrillation is the most frequent arrhythmia in clinical practice. Its prevalence varies from 0.5% to 9% [1] of the general population between 50 and 80 years of age. It may appear in the clinical history of every patient with cardiopathy and even in appearently healthy persons or those with minor structural anomalies of the heart. Its presence causes a rise in morbidity and mortality rates due to the loss of atrial function and the consequent decrease in heart performance and increase in embolic risk. For this reason recovery and maintenance of sinus rhythm is one of the main objectives of treatment.

Antiarrhythmic drug therapy with class IC drugs has proved successful in preventing recurrences of atrial fibrillation in noncardiopathic subjects or those with minor cardiopathy, while amiodarone is widely used in treatment even in cardiopathic patients. However, antiarrhythmic treatment of atrial fibrillation is often unsatisfactory because recurrences frequently occur. It is well known that during treatment of atrial fibrillation with antiarrhythmic class IC or III drugs, the arrhythmias can spontaneously convert into typical atrial flutter. The percentages in different reports vary from 5% to 22% for class IC drugs [2-4]. This reported variability is probably due to the fact that in some studies only atrial flutter episodes with high ventricular response were recorded. With amiodarone a rate of 18.5% is reported [4]. Generally atrial flutter is a poorly tollerated arrhythmia, since impulses can be conducted to the ventricles at very high frequencies, particularly during effort. At all events, because of the occurrence of atrial flutter, the antiarrhythmic therapy is often considered ineffective or proarrhythmic and is therefore interrupted. Radiofrequency (RF) catheter ablation of typical atrial flutter is a well-established treatment, and its acute and long-term efficacy are high. For this reason several reports have evaluated the hypothesis that RF catheter ablation of atrial flutter combined with maintenance of the antiarrhythmic therapy which provoked the atrial flutter could prevent recurrence of both atrial flutter and atrial fibrillation.

Cardiovascular Department, Division of Cardiology, Umberto I Hospital, Mestre-Venice, Italy

Literature Review

The first report in 1997 [5] on 9 patients with atrial flutter after amiodarone therapy for paroxysmal atrial fibrillation showed 80% therapeutic success in preventing recurrences of atrial fibrillation in the relatively short follow-up time of 8 ± 2 months. Later, in a 1998 study of 11 patients – 4 with atrial flutter induced by class IC drugs (3 flecainide, 1 propafenone) and 7 with amiodarone-related atrial flutter – Huang et al. [6] reported 90% therapeutic success after flutter ablation, with a follow-up of 14 ± 7 months (range 1-28 months). In 1999 in a report on 16 patients with class IC drug atrial flutter, Nabar et al. [7] reported a 73% success rate in a short follow-up period of 4 ± 2 months; recently, in a longer follow-up period of 13 ± 6 months in a group of 24 patients – 13 with typical and 8 with atypical atrial flutter – the same authors [8] reported success rates of 85% and 50% respectively in the two groups.

Schumacher et al. [9] noted the occurrence of sustained, documented typical atrial flutter after therapy with class IC drugs in 24 patients (12.8%) out of a population of 187 patients whose paroxysmal atrial fibrillation was treated with flecainide (96) or propafenone (91). A control group was made up of 20 patients with atrial fibrillation treated with class IC drugs who did not have documented atrial flutter. After ablation of typical atrial flutter the patients were monitored for a mean follow-up period of 11 ± 4 months with the same antiarrhythmic therapy as they had received before ablation. The incidence of atrial fibrillation episodes was significantly higher in the control group (7.8 ± 9.2 per year) than in the group with combined therapy (2.7 ± 3.6 per year). Moreover, the yearly incidence of atrial fibrillation episodes was significantly lower after flutter ablation in the group with class IC drug atrial flutter (10.2 ± 5.4 compared to 2.7 ± 3.6). In 7 patients (37.8%) no arrhythmias were documented; they were completely asymptomatic. In another 8 (42.1%) patients there was a dramatic reduction of both symptoms and atrial fibrillation episodes. Generally, the combined therapy was effective in about 80% of cases. Only 4 (20%) patients had no improvement.

In our own early experience [10] we studied 9 patients (mean age 58 ± 11 years) with frequent recurrences of atrial fibrillation and without documented episodes of typical atrial flutter who were treated with class IC antiarrhythmic drugs (6 flecainide, 3 propafenone). In all of them, after the start of treatment only recurrent persistent episodes of typical atrial flutter were documented which required restoration with transesophageal overdrive or external DC shock. In a follow-up of 14 ± 9 months only one patient had recurrence of documented atrial fibrillation and another had episodes of focal atrial tachycardia.

Recently, Reithmann et al. [11] reported a success rate of 80% in 10 patients with recurrence of only atrial flutter after treatment with amiodarone for a short follow-up period of 8.3 ± 2.8 months.

Acute infusion of flecainide during atrial fibrillation [12] is able to detect, among patients developing atrial flutter, those who will benefit from drug therapy combined with cavo-tricuspid isthmus ablation. In a mean follow-up period of 24 ± 7.2 months only 42.3% of patients had documented atrial fibrillation recurrences, as compared to 78% of patients who continued only oral therapy with flecainide, 92% of patients who underwent ablation of the cavo-tricuspid isthmus, and 92% of patients who did not respond to flecainide treatment.

Present Personal Experience

Patients and Method

We studied 36 patients (28 male and 8 female, mean age 64 ± 10 years) with frequent recurrent episodes of paroxysmal and persistent atrial fibrillation alone [median 6 (range 4-30) during a median of 3 (range 2-9) years] without documented episodes of atrial flutter before treatment with class IC antiarrhythmic drugs and amiodarone. Twenty patients had no structural heart disease, 8 had moderate hypertension, 6 had mitral prolapse, and 2 had chronic ischemic heart disease. Atrial fibrillation was paroxysmal in 2 patients and paroxysmal/persistent in 34. Sixteen patients received flecainide at a dosage of 200 mg/day, 13 received propafenone at a dosage of 600 mg/da, and 7 received amiodarone 200 mg/day. In this population, at least two other antiarrhythmic drugs were ineffective in maintaining sinus rhythm. After the start of treatment with class IC antiarrhythmic drugs or amiodarone, 28 patients (group A), 22 of whom were receiving class IC drugs (11 flecainide, 11 propafenone) and 6 amiodarone, experienced only episodes of typical atrial flutter (mean 5 ± 1.5 episodes per patient during a mean of 12 ± 3 months), and 8 (group B), 7 of whom were receiving class IC drugs (5 flecainide, 2 propafenone) and 1 amiodarone, experienced recurrences of both typical atrial flutter and atrial fibrillation (mean 3 ± 1 and 4 ± 1 episodes per patient, respectively, during a mean period of 12 ± 3 months). There were no significant differences between the two groups in regard to age, gender, duration of history and episodes of atrial fibrillation, atrial flutter recurrences, drugs taken, left atrial diameter (4.2 ± 0.5 cm in group A vs 4.0 ± 0.7 cm in group B), and left ventricular ejection fraction (normal). All 36 patients underwent successful RF catheter ablation of the cavo-tricuspid isthmus, achieving bidirectional isthmus conduction block. After the ablation procedure, the first 18 patients on class IC antiarrhythmic drugs did not receive any therapy until the first recurrence of atrial fibrillation or atrial flutter. The patients were followed up by means of a monthly interview until the first recurrence of arrhythmia, and if they had experienced recurrences of atrial fibrillation, class IC antiarrhythmic drug treatment was restarted at the same dosage as before the ablation procedure. The next 18 patients were discharged with antiarrhythmic medication for a mean follow-up period of 21 ± 11 months (group A 21 ± 11 months, group B 20 ± 13 months). The patients underwent a medical examination every 3 months. If they reported palpitations, ECG and Holter monitoring were performed.

Results

During the washout period after the ablation procedure, at least one episode of sustained atrial fibrillation occurred in all of the first 18 patients within 3 months. During treatment in the follow-up period no patient in either group had recurrences of atrial flutter. Recurrences of documented atrial fibrillation in the two groups together amounted up to 38.8% (14/36): 21.4% of group A (6/28) vs 100% (8/8) of group B ($p < 0.001$). In group A these were 18.2% (4/22) of patients treated with class IC drugs and 33.3% (2/6) of patients treated with amiodarone. There were 61.2% (22/36) of patients who showed no recurrence of atrial fibrillation (78.6% in group A vs 0% in group B, $p < 0.001$); 44.4% (17/36) of patients remained completely asymptomatic during follow-up and 55.6% (19/36) were symptomatic for palpitations. Atrial fibrillation was documented in 73.6% (14/19) of symptomatic patients, paroxysmal in 64.3% (9/14) and persistent in 35.7% (5/14). In 26.3% (5/19) of symptomatic patients it was not possible to record episodes of atrial fibrillation.

Discussion

Experimental studies on animals showed that there is a strict relationship between atrial fibrillation and atrial flutter, since each of the two arrhythmias can transform into the other [13]. Studies in man found that the circuit run by typical atrial flutter is anatomically defined. It is formed anteriorly by the tricuspid anulus and posteriorly by the crista terminalis and eustachian ridge [14]. The circuit runs anticlockwise in common typical atrial flutter and clockwise in non-common typical atrial flutter. The mechanism and meaning of the transformation of one arrhythmia into the other is not well known. It seems that before the atrial flutter appears, a short period of atrial fibrillation is present and there is a critical slowdown of the atrial fibrillation cycles. In particular, Lesh [15] demonstrated how, before atrial fibrillation transforms into atrial flutter, a functional block appears along the trabeculated right atrium, and with the onset of typical atrial flutter a stable 1:1 relation between the activation sequence along the trabeculated right atrium and the atrial activation recorded in the coronary sinus is established. Mapping during atrial fibrillation often shows, next to fragmentation and slowdown areas, other very extended areas where the electrical activity is well organized. The mechanism of drug-related atrial flutter seems to involve depression of intra-atrial conduction velocity, followed by the transformation of conduction delay into conduction block. This prevents simultaneous occurrence of the multiple reentrant circuits necessary for the perpetuation of atrial fibrillation. However, in some cases the conduction slowdown can start the development of macrocircuits and thus the start of atrial flutter around the tricuspid valve. Recent studies [5-12, 16] have shown that in patients undergoing treatment for recurrent episodes of atrial fibrillation with class IC drugs and amiodarone, the onset of atrial flutter is not a reason to consider the treatment ineffective; on the contrary, the elimination of atrial flutter through RF ablation combined with antiarrhythmic therapy is able to prevent both arrhythmias in the follow-up period.

From data in the literature it emerges that this type of hybrid treatment can change the clinical course of patients, with a success rate in preventing atrial fibrillation recurrences ranging from 40% to 90% with class IC drugs and 80% with amiodarone. These data, however, relate to a very limited number of cases, ranging from 9 to 24 patients, with average follow-up periods of no longer than 2 years and often less than 1 year. The variability of results in patients treated with class IC drugs is probably due to both the small number of cases and to patient selection; and during antiarrhythmic therapy some patients had both flutter and atrial fibrillation recurrences. At all events, in all reports at least 40% of patients are completely free from atrial fibrillation recurrences and related symptoms such as palpitations (44.4% in our study). It is interesting to note how in the study by Shumacher et al. [9], another 40% of patients experienced great benefit from combined treatment, with a dramatic reduction in atrial fibrillation recurrences. Thus, there is a remarkable clinical improvement in nearly 80% of patients, with a rise in the quality of life in patients with palpitations as well [17]. In our experience, atrial fibrillation was documented in 74% of patients reporting palpitations, persistent in 35.7% and paroxysmal in 64.3%. Combined therapy transforms persistent atrial fibrillation into paroxysmal in many patients.

In the literature [18, 19], the most powerful predictor of atrial fibrillation recurrences in patients with spontaneous atrial flutter who have undergone RF ablation is the preexistence of atrial fibrillation recurrences. The greater their prevalence on atrial flutter, the lower the benefits of atrial flutter ablation, although there is a general improvement in the quality of life. Probably if patients with atrial flutter recurrences only (group A in our case report) undergo combined treatment, the success rate in preventing atrial fibrillation recurrences comes up to 80% (77% with amiodarone and 82% with class IC drugs). In this group of patients, however, about 26% reported palpitations with no documented atrial fibrillation. In these cases Holter monitoring recorded frequent supraventricular beats. In the cases where no atrial fibrillation episodes are documented, it is possible that the symptoms are caused by the persistence of triggers. Moreover, it is important to point out that in responder patients there is a complete adherence to the antiarrhythmic therapy, probably due to the fact that when it is interrupted, the atrial fibrillation recurrences start again, as shown in our patients and in the control group with only cavo-tricuspid isthmus ablation in the report by Stabile et al. [12].

The efficacy of combined treatment with amiodarone has not yet been adequately compared with the efficacy of class IC drug therapy [16]. From the data they seems to be equivalent. As for amiodarone, it must be pointed out that in two of our patients who were responders to combined therapy drug administration had to be interrupted because of the onset of hyperthyroidism in the follow-up, and this seems to be the major limitation of treatment with amiodarone, which, unlike class IC drugs, can be used in patients with severe cardiopathy.

References

1. Kannel W, Wolff P, Benjamin E, Levy D (1998) Prevalence, incidence, prognosis, and predisposing conditions for atrial fibrillation: population-based estimates. Am J Cardiol 82:2N-9N
2. Levy S, Breithard G, Campbell WF et al (1998) Atrial fibrillation: current knowledge and recommendations for management. Eur Heart J 19:1294-1320
3. Bianconi L, Mennuni M, Lukic V et al (1996) Effects of oral propafenone administration before electrical cardioversion of chronic atrial fibrillation: a placebo-controlled study. J Am Coll Cardiol 28:700-706
4. Riva S, Tondo C, Carbucicchio C et al (1999) Incidence and clinical significance of transformation of atrial fibrillation to atrial flutter in patients undergoing long-term antiarrhythmic drug treatment. Europace 1:242-247
5. Natale A, Tomassoni G, Fanelli R et al (1997) Occurrence of atrial flutter after initiation of amiodarone therapy of paroxysmal atrial fibrillation. Circulation 96:I-385 (abstr)
6. Huang DT, Monaham KM, Zimetbaum P et al (1998) Hybrid pharmacological and ablative therapy: a novel and effective approach for the management of atrial fibrillation. J Cardiovasc Electrophysiol 9:462-469
7. Nabar A, Rodriguez LM, Timmermans C et al (1999) Effect of right atrial isthmus ablation on the occurrence of atrial fibrillation. Circulation 99:1441-1445
8. Nabar A, Rodriguez LM, Timmermans C et al (2001) Class IC antiarrhythmic drug induced atrial flutter: electrocardiographic and electrophysiological findings and their importance for long term outcome after right atrial isthmus ablation. Heart 85:424-429
9. Schumacher B, Jung W, Lewalter T et al (1999) Radiofrequency ablation of atrial flutter due to administration of class IC antiarrhythmic drugs for atrial fibrillation. Am J Cardiol 83:710-713
10. Bonso A, Themistoclakis S, Gasparini G et al (1999) IC drug induced atrial flutter during treatment of atrial fibrillation: usefulness of a combined pharmacological and ablative therapy. Eur Heart J 20:634 (abstr)
11. Reithmann E, Hoffmann G, Spitzlberger U et al (2000) Catheter ablation of atrial flutter due to amiodarone therapy for paroxysmal atrial fibrillation. Eur Heart J 21:565-572
12. Stabile G, De Simone A, Turco P et al (2001) Response to flecainide infusion predicts long-term success of hybrid pharmacologic and ablation therapy in patients with atrial fibrillation. J Am Coll Cardiol 37:1639-1644
13. Waldo A, Cooper TB (1996) Spontaneous onset of type I atrial flutter in patients. J Am Coll Cardiol 28:700-706
14. Kalman J, Olgin J, Saxon L et al (1996) Activation and entrainment mapping defines the tricuspid annulus as the anterior barrier in typical atrial flutter. Circulation 94:398-406
15. Lesh M (1997) What is the relationship between atrial fibrillation and flutter in man? In: Raviele A (ed) Cardiac arrhythmias. Springer-Verlag Italia, Milan, pp 144-151
16. Tai CT, Chiang CE, Lee SH et al (1999) Persistent atrial flutter in patients treated for atrial fibrillation with amiodarone and propafenone: electrophysiologic characteristics, radiofrequency catheter ablation, and risk prediction. J Cardiovasc Electrophysiol 10:1180-1187
17. Anselme F, Saudi MD, Poty MD et al (1999) Radiofrequency catheter ablation of common atrial flutter. Significance of palpitations and quality-of-life evaluation in patients with proven isthmus block. Circulation 99:534-540

18. Philippon F, Plumb VJ, Epstein AE et al (1995) The risk of atrial fibrillation following radiofrequency catheter ablation of atrial flutter. Circulation 92:430-435

19. Paydak H, Kall JG, Burke MC et al (1998) Atrial fibrillation after radiofrequency ablation of type I atrial flutter. Time to onset, determinants, and clinical course. Circulation 98:315-322

Diagnosis and Treatment of Atrial Flutter Circuits

M.M. Scheinman[1], Y. Yang[1] AND J. Cheng[2]

Typical atrial flutter has a well-defined pattern in surface electrocardiography and is manifest by either negative initial forces in the inferior leads and positive forces in V1 (counterclockwise) or positive flutter waves in the inferior leads and negative flutter waves in V1 (clockwise) [1-10]. Isthmus-dependent flutter has been found to rotate around the tricuspid annulus [2-9, 11, 12]. A critical isthmus is defined as the region between the tricuspid valve annulus and the subeustachian muscle ridge. The designation "counterclockwise" or "clockwise" is used with the tricuspid annulus displayed in left anterior oblique projection. The typical patterns are isthmus-dependent and are readily ablated by producing bidirectional isthmus block.

More recently, a host of flutter circuits have been recognized which call for different diagnostic and therapeutic approaches [8, 13-22]. In this essay we shall consider only spontaneous flutter circuits (nonsurgical). Atrial flutter may be divided into right and left atrial flutter circuits.

Right Atrial Isthmus-Dependent Flutter

We initially described double wave reentry (DWR), a circuit where, basically, two separate wavefronts occupy a typical flutter circuit [17]. Double wave reentry may be initiated by an atrial premature beat which blocks in the isthmus and generates a new wavefront while the original wave is still active. DWR is a transient arrhythmia lasting only several beats before one of the waves blocks in the isthmus.

We next described an entity called lower loop reentry (LLR) [18]. LLR is characterized by a counterclockwise reentrant circuit with earlier than expected activation of a portion of the annulus with collision over the annulus with wavefront generated by the early break with the orthodromic wavefront (Figs. 1-3). It should be emphasized that LLR and its derivative arrhythmias are all isthmus-dependent and amenable to isthmus ablation (Fig. 3). Use of entrainment mapping is critical

[1]Cardiac Electrophysiology Section, Division of Cardiology, University of California, San Francisco, California; [2]Thoracic Cardiovascular Institute, Lansing, Michigan, USA

in determining whether the isthmus is part of the circuit. It was initially felt that LLR was characterized by conduction over the distal crista terminalis [14, 16, 23-27]. It is now appreciated that transcristal conduction may occur anywhere along the crista and result in early activation over any portion of the tricuspid annulus [28]. In addition, multiple annular breaks may occur. The early break may result in changes in the surface electrocardiogram depending on the site of early annular activation and conduction time to the atrial septum and left atrium (Fig. 4).

Upper Loop Reentry

Upper loop reentry (ULR) is a macroreentrant arrhythmia with a clockwise orientation with annular break resulting in collision of wavefronts over the isthmus. ULR is clearly independent of the subeustachian isthmus and is not isthmus-dependent (Fig. 5). Initial studies suggest that at least some ULR tachycar-

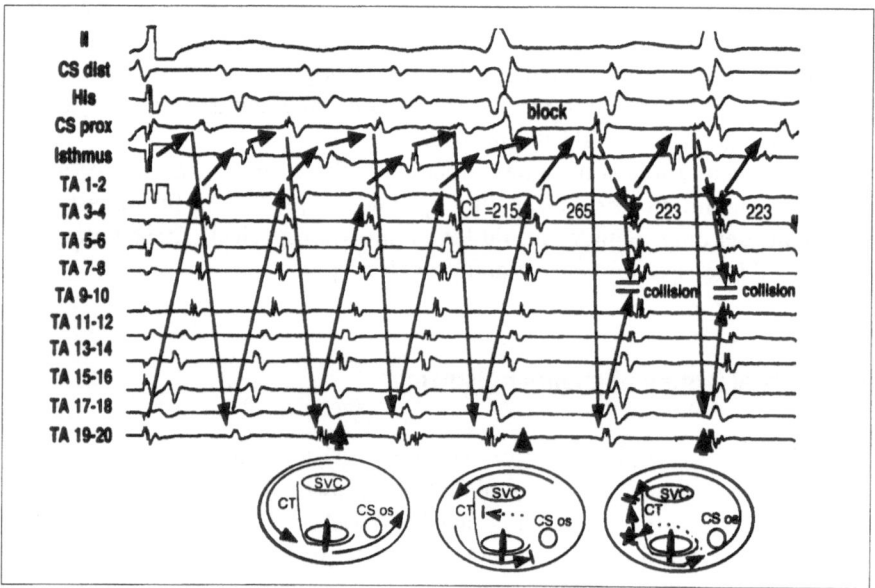

Fig. 1. An example of double wave reentry terminated by lower loop reentry. The figure shows simultaneous recordings from surface lead II and intracardiac electrogram from the coronary sinus (CS) His, isthmus and from a 20-pole catheter around the tricuspid annulus with poles TA1-2 at the low lateral annulus (7 o'clock position). The patient presented with counterclockwise lower loop reentry. A premature stimulus delivered at the isthmus (see pacing artifact) initiates a more rapid rhythm with identical electrogram morphology. The paced impulse initiates a new wave while the original wave is able to negotiate the flutter circuit allowing four beats of double wave reentry. One wavefront is blocked at the isthmus, allowing restoration of a single beat of counterclockwise flutter. This is followed by a sequence of two beats characterized by early activation of the low lateral tricuspid annulus (TA3-4) and results in collision at TA9-10 between the early eave break at TA3-4 and the original orthodromic counterclockwise wave (see cartoons at bottom of strip). These two beats are characteristic of lower loop reentry

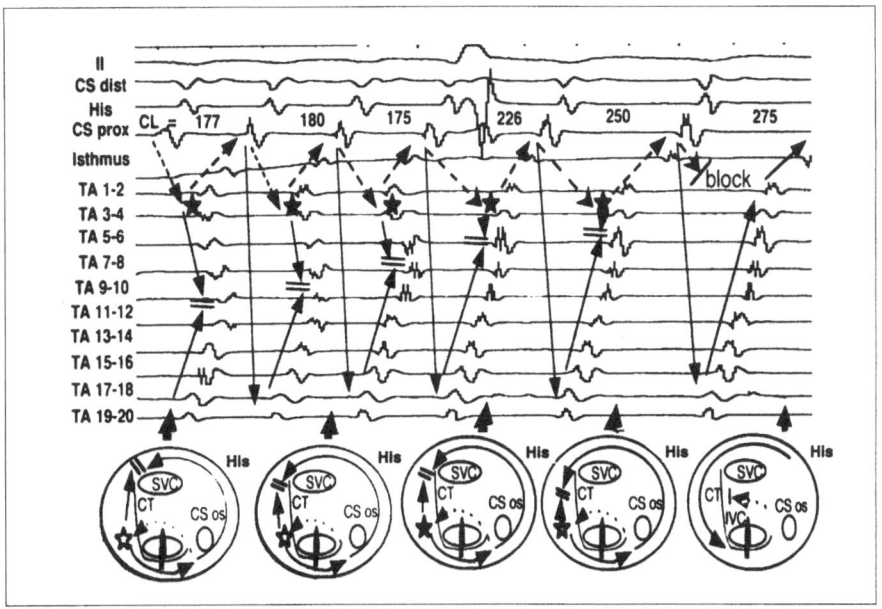

Fig. 2. Simultaneous surface and intracardiac recordings as in Fig. 1. The initial beats show a lower loop reentrant mechanism (see cartoon) with early break at TA3-4. The site of collision moves progressively higher and LLR is eventually terminated by block of the impulse from the coronary sinus (CS) to the low lateral RA. Typical counterclockwise flutter resumes

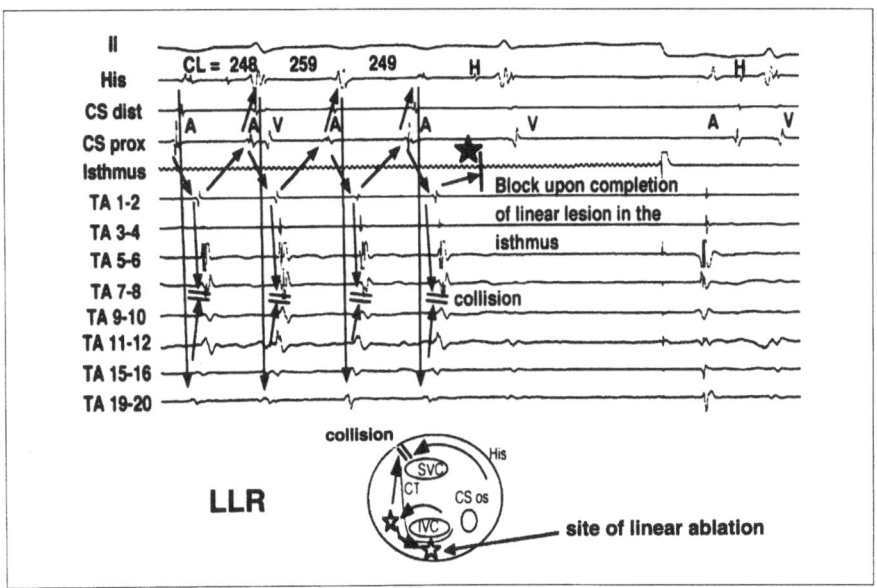

Fig. 3. Proof that LLR is isthmus-dependent. Typical LLR is present during application of RF to the subeustachian isthmus. LLR is terminated by block in the isthmus. After ablation tachycardia could no longer be induced

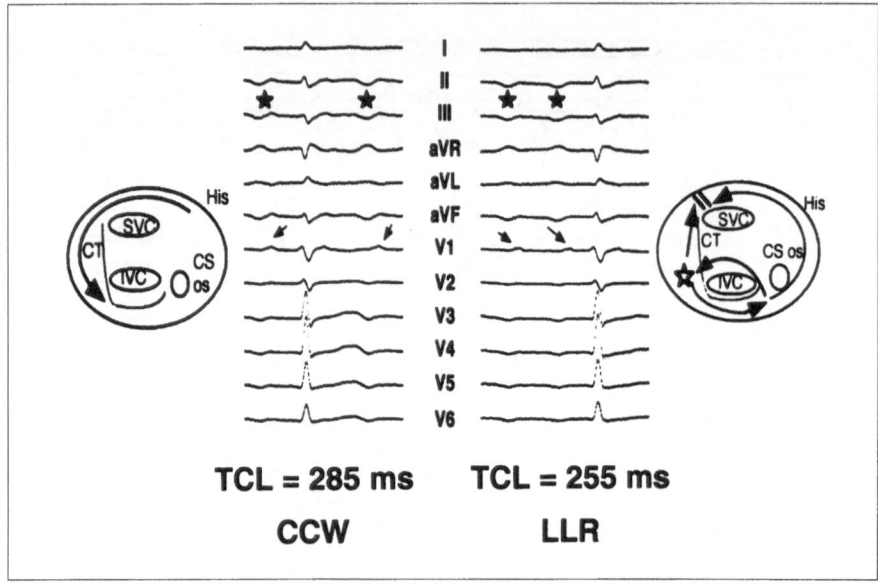

Fig. 4. Comparison of subtle morphological changes in the surface ECG of a patient who had typical counterclockwise (CCW) flutter (*left panel*) and LLR (*right panel*). The *right panel* shows the actual conversion from CCW to LLR. The changes are seen in lead III with loss of the terminal positive deflection. In addition, slight changes appear in lead V1

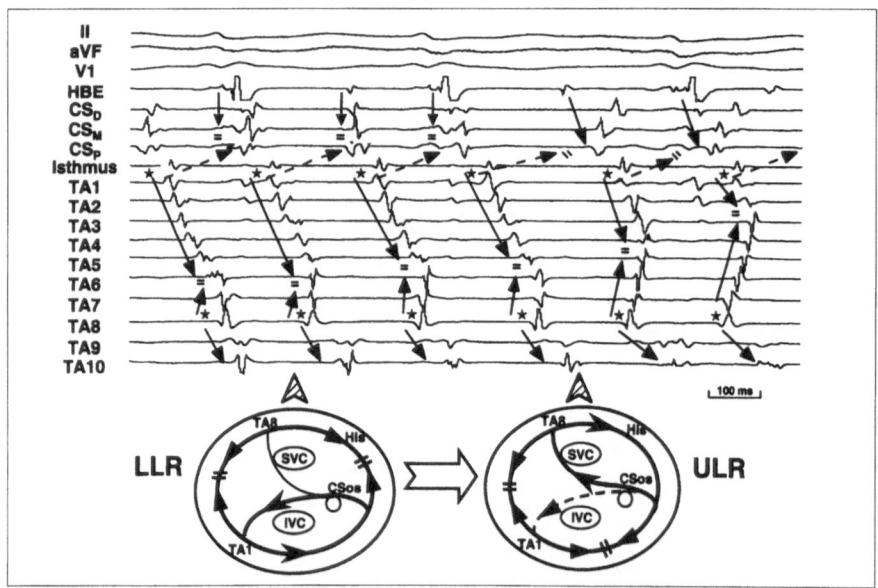

Fig. 5. Conversion of LLR to upper loop reentry (ULR). The figure shows a classic LLR flutter circuit initially (see cartoon at the *left* of the panel). The early break is over TA1 with collision at TA6. There is gradual increase in conduction over the isthmus (TA1 to CSP) until block occurs in the isthmus. With development of isthmus block, the tachycardia continues but is driven by the upper RA since there is repetitive collision in the isthmus. ULR is therefore non-isthmus-dependent

dias appear to rotate around an area of functional block over the right atrial septal region [28]. In one patient ablation from the zone of functional block to the tricuspid valve resulted in cure of tachycardia.

Macroreentrant Right Atrial Flutter

Others have described a variety of right atrial flutter circuits either around the crista terminalis or using wide areas of low voltage zones (scarred areas) as barriers [20, 28]. These zones may occur in the absence of prior surgery. Elucidation of these circuits is greatly augmented by use of three-dimensional imaging techniques. The Cartos Biosense system allows identification of both the activation sequence and areas of low voltage. Catheter ablation is performed in order to create bidirectional block over an isthmus found to be critical for maintenance of the tachycardia. It is important to remember that both isthmus-dependent and non-isthmus-dependent circuits may be found in the same patient. This is especially true for patients with surgical interatrial tachycardias.

Left Atrial Flutter Circuits

Olgin et al. were the first to describe a left atrial circuit involving the coronary sinus musculature [29]. Ablation of the musculature within the os of the coronary sinus resulted in cure. Subsequently, Shah et al. described a wide variety of left atrial circuits [30]. These circuits were associated with wide areas of low voltage recorded over the posterior left atrium. The described circuits included reentry around the mitral valve annulus as well as around and between the pulmonary veins. More recently, we described a left atrial flutter circuit that related around the left membranous septum [31]. This tachycardia could be successfully ablated by a lesion either from the left inferior pulmonary vein to the membranous septum or from the septum to the mitral annulus. Use of advanced imaging is particularly important in delineating the precise circuit for purposes of successful ablation of those circuits. It is very common for multiple macroreentrants to exist in a given patient.

Patients with left septal flutter circuits usually show large flutter waves (either positive or negative) in lead V1 associated with rather flat flutter waves in the limb leads. We hypothesize that this may be due to clockwise or counterclockwise rotation around the left membranous septum with cancellation of simultaneously generated right and left atrial activation wavefronts. Patients with other left atrial circuits may show a variety of surface electrocardiographic patterns.

Summary and Conclusions

Rapid growth in our understanding of the various flutter circuits highlights the inadequacies of current technologies for the flutter. It is probably time to abandon the well-worn terms "typical" and "atypical" flutter. It would appear preferable to have a terminology based on specific circuits. For example, right atrial flutter circuits are either isthmus-dependent or non-isthmus-dependent. The isthmus-dependent circuits would include DWR, LLR, and the various manifestations of LLR. ULR and right atrial macroreentrant arrhythmias are non-isthmus-dependent circuits. Left atrial circuits can now be divided into those that rotate around the mitral valve, those that rotate around and/or between the pulmonary veins, and those that rotate around the left septal isthmus. It is hoped that as knowledge accumulates in this area, it will lead to more effective catheter ablative techniques.

References

1. Okumura K, Plumb VJ, Page PL, Waldo AL (1991) Atrial activation sequence during atrial flutter in the canine pericarditis model and its effects on the polarity of the flutter wave in the electrocardiogram. J Am Coll Cardiol 17:509-518
2. Cosio FG, Goicolea A, Lopez-Gil M et al (1990) Atrial endocardial mapping in the rare form of atrial flutter. Am J Cardiol 66:715-720
3. Olshansky B, Okumura K, Hess PG, Waldo AL (1990) Demonstration of an area of slow conduction in human atrial flutter. J Am Coll Cardiol 16:1639-1648
4. Feld GK, Fleck PR, Chen PS et al (1992) Radiofrequency catheter ablation for the treatment of human type I atrial flutter. Identification of a critical zone in the reentrant circuit by endocardial mapping techniques. Circulation 86:1233-1240
5. Olgin JE, Kalman JM, Fitzpatrick AP, Lesh MD (1995) Role of right atrial endocardial structures as barriers to conduction during human type I atrial flutter. Circulation 92:1839-1848
6. Saoudi N, Nair M, Abdelazziz A et al (1996) Electrocardiographic patterns and results of radiofrequency catheter ablation of clockwise type I atrial flutter. J Cardiovasc Electrophysiol 7:931-942
7. Cosio FG, Arribas F, Lopez-Gil M, Nunez A (1996) Catheter mapping studies in atrial flutter. In: Waldo AL, Touboul P (eds) Atrial flutter: advances in mechanisms and management. Futura, Armonk, NY, pp 269-283
8. Kalman JM, Olgin JE, Saxon LA et al (1997) Electrocardiographic and electrophysiologic characterization of atypical flutter in man. Use of activation and entrainment mapping implications for catheter ablation. J Cardiovasc Electrophysiol 8:121-144
9. Cosio FG, Arribas F, Lopez-Gil M, Gonzalez HD (1996) Radiofrequency ablation of atrial flutter. J Cardiovasc Electrophysiol 7:60-70
10. SippensGroenewegen A, Lesh MD, Roithinger FX et al (2000) Body surface mapping of counterclockwise and clockwise typical atrial flutter: a comparative analysis with endocardial activation sequence mapping. J Am Coll Cardiol 35:1276-1287
11. Lesh MD, Van Hare GF, Epstein LM et al (1994) Radiofrequency ablation of atrial arrhythmias. Results and mechanisms. Circulation 89:1074-1089

12. Waldo AL, MacLean WAH, Karp RB et al (1977) Entrainment and interruption of atrial flutter with pacing. Studies in man following open heart surgery. Circulation 56:737-745

13. Gomes JA, Santoni-Rugiu F, Mehta D et al (1998) Uncommon atrial flutter: characteristics, mechanisms, and results of ablative therapy. Pacing Clin Electrophysiol 21:2029-2042

14. Zrenner B, Ndreppa G, Schneider M et al (1999) Computer-assisted animation of atrial tachyarrhythmias recorded with a 64-electrode basket catheter. J Am Coll Cardiol 34:2051-2060

15. Lai LP, Lin JL, Tseng CD et al (1999) Electrophysiologic study and radiofrequency catheter ablation of isthmus-independent atrial flutter. J Cardiovasc Electrophysiol 10:728-735

16. Chang KC, Lin YC, Chou HT et al (2000) Electrophysiologic characteristics and ablation of an atypical flutter in the right atrium. J Cardiovasc Electrophysiol 11:334-338

17. Cheng J, Scheinman MM (1998) Acceleration of typical atrial flutter due to double-wave reentry induced by programmed electrical stimulation. Circulation 97:1589-1596

18. Cheng J, Cabeen WR, Scheinman MM (1999) Right atrial flutter due to lower loop reentry: mechanism and anatomic substrates. Circulation 99:1700-1705

19. Kall JG, Rubinstein DS, Kopp DE et al (2000) Atypical atrial flutter originating in the right atrial free wall. Circulation 101:270-279

20. Nakagawa H, Matsudaira K, Monir G et al (1999) Macroreentrant atrial tachycardia not related to atriotomy. Circulation 100(Suppl I):I-652

21. Bogun F, Bender B, Li YG et al (2000) Ablation of atypical atrial flutter guided by the use of concealed entrainment in patients without prior cardiac surgery. J Cardiovasc Electrophysiol 11:136-145

22. Scheinman MM, Cheng J, Yang Y (1999) Mechanisms and implications of atypical atrial flutter. J Cardiovasc Electrophysiol 10:1153-1157

23. Shah DC, Jaïs P, Haïssaguerre M et al (1997) Three-dimensional mapping of the common atrial flutter circuit in the right atrium. Circulation 96:3904-3912

24. Tai CT, Chen SA, Chen YJ et al (1998) Conduction properties of crista terminalis in patients with typical atrial flutter: basis for a line of block in the reentrant circuit. J Cardiovasc Electrophysiol 9:811-819

25. Arenal A, Almendral J, Alday JM et al (1999) Rate-dependent conduction block of the crista terminalis in patients with typical atrial flutter: influence on evaluation of cavotricuspid isthmus conduction block. Circulation 99:2771-2778

26. Schumacher B, Jung W, Schmidt H et al (1999) Transverse conduction capabilities of the crista terminalis in patients with atrial flutter and atrial fibrillation. J Am Coll Cardiol 34:363-373

27. Friedman PA, Luria D, Fenton AM et al (2000) Global right atrial mapping of human atrial flutter: the presence of posteromedial (sinus venosa region) functional block and double potentials: a study in biplane fluoroscopy and intracardiac echocardiography. Circulation 101:1568-1577

28. Yang Y, Cheng J, Bochoeyer A et al (2001) Atypical right atrial flutter patterns. Circulation 103:3092-3098

29. Olgin JE, Jayachandran JV, Engesstein E et al (1998) Atrial macroreentry involving the myocardium of the coronary sinus: a unique mechanism for atypical flutter. J Cardiovasc Electrophysiol 9:1094-1099

30. Jaïs P, Shah DC, Haïssaguerre M et al (2000) Mapping and ablation of atrial flutters. Circulation 101:2928-2934

31. Cheng J, Steiner PR, Lee RJ, Scheinman MM (1999) Unusual form of atrial flutter utilizing the isthmus between the right pulmonary veins and fossa ovalis. Pacing Clin Electrophysiol 22:704

Is Inappropriate Sinus Tachycardia Really Inappropriate?

C.A. Morillo[1,2], H. León[1] and F. Pava[1]

Introduction

"Inappropriate sinus tachycardia" is a poorly defined clinical syndrome characterized by an increased resting sinus rate or an inappropriate and exaggerated acceleration of heart rate with minor physiological or emotional stress. Patients with inappropriate sinus tachycardia have a wide spectrum of clinical manifestations that range from mild palpitations to severely symptomatic incessant tachycardia [1]. Additionally, the clinical manifestation of orthostatic intolerance, primarily by severe tachycardia provoked by orthostatic changes, may also be associated with presyncope and syncope. These features have raised the possibility that inappropriate sinus tachycardia is more likely to be an alteration of autonomic response to orthostatic stress than a primary sinus node alteration.

The physiological effects of orthostatic stress on the heart rate response have been extensively studied [2]. Nonetheless, it is still unclear whether the heart rate response to orthostatic stress in patients with inappropriate sinus tachycardia is mediated by an abnormal response to orthostatic stress sensed by the arterial baroreceptors or a combination of increased β-adrenergic sensitivity and enhanced sinus node response [3]. We have recently evaluated both the spontaneous baroreceptor response to orthostatic stress and the response of the sinus node to incremental doses of isoproterenol and after complete autonomic blockade in a series of patients with inappropriate sinus tachycardia. We hypothesize that the exaggerated response in heart rate during orthostatic stress in patients with inappropriate sinus tachycardia is due to impaired baroreflex sensitivity mediated by increased sympathetic activity.

[1]Department of Cardiology and Cardiovascular Sciences, Laboratory of Autonomic Physiology, Instituto del Corazón, Fundación Cardiovascular del Oriente Colombiano, Floridablanca, Santander, Colombia; [2]Department of Medicine, Universidad Industrial de Santander, Bucaramanga, Santander, Colombia

Mechanisms

The mechanisms that lead to inappropriate sinus tachycardia remain a matter of controversy [1-3]. Nonetheless, from the different studies that have reported autonomic testing in patients with inappropriate sinus tachycardia some insight may be obtained regarding the mechanism of this rare disorder. Bauernfeind et al. [4] first described the effects of autonomic modulation in a series of seven patients with "idiopathic chronic sinus node tachycardia". These investigators described two different patterns of autonomic response, namely, augmented sympathetic activity caused by increased β-adrenergic sensitivity to isoproterenol, and impaired vagal control of resting heart rate. These investigators primarily studied patients with baseline sinus tachycardia in addition to sinus tachycardia triggered by orthostatic stress. These findings may be related to the chronic nature of the condition in the patients studied by Bauernfeind and may represent one spectrum of this disorder.

Morillo et al. [2] recently evaluated the result of a battery of autonomic tests in a group of patients with inappropriate sinus tachycardia that was defined by the following criteria: (1) atrial rate above > 100 beats per minute at rest or triggered by minimal physiological stress, (2) "normal" P wave axis and morphology during tachycardia documented electrocardiographically, and (3) absence of orthostatic hypotension, diabetes mellitus, hyperthyroidism, and drug abuse. Six patients were evaluated and all patients underwent analysis of heart rate variability with subsequent analysis of sympathovagal balance both at rest and during orthostatic stress. Similarly, tests assessing the cardiovagal reflexes were performed as well as an isoproterenol sensitivity test, and intrinsic heart rate after complete pharmacological denervation.

This study identified three potential mechanisms that may lead to inappropriate sinus tachycardia, namely increased β-adrenergic hypersensitivity, enhanced sinus node automaticity, and a depressed efferent cardiovagal reflex response. These findings suggest that two distinct mechanisms may be involved in the generation of inappropriate sinus tachycardia: (1) impaired autonomic response to either sympathetic stimulation or depressed vagal efferent reflex response and (2) an intrinsic alteration of the sinus node given by an increased firing rate. These two mechanisms are not mutually exclusive and usually interact to induce sustained inappropriate sinus tachycardia. Nonetheless, these findings do not answer the issue whether inappropriate sinus tachycardia really is inappropriate.

In an attempt to further understand the mechanisms that modulate heart rate response in individuals with inappropriate sinus tachycardia, we have recently assessed baroreflex function in a group of patients with this disorder [5].

Nine patients who fulfilled clinical diagnostic criteria for inappropriate sinus tachycardia were studied and their autonomic responses compared with those of nine age- and sex-matched controls with no previous cardiovascular or neurologic disease that could affect autonomic cardiac reflex response. Heart rate variability and spontaneous baroreflex gain were obtained by cross-spectral analysis of heart rate and systolic blood pressure recorded by noninvasive measurements. Similarly, intrinsic heart rate after complete denervation following intravenous propranolol and atropine administration was assessed. The isoproterenol chronotropic response test (CD_{25}) to determine β-adrenergic sensitivity was also performed. Response to orthostatic stress was assessed during 60° head-up tilt. All patients underwent a complete head-up tilt protocol with either nitrates or incremental low-dose isoproterenol [6, 7].

Baseline heart rate was significantly higher in patients with inappropriate sinus tachycardia. Similarly, these patients had a lower RMSSD, suggesting lower vagal tone at rest, possibly explaining the higher resting heart rate in patients with inappropriate sinus tachycardia. Baroreflex gain was also reduced in the supine position in the patients compared to the control group. Orthostatic stress induced a further reduction in baroreceptor gain particularly in patients with inappropriate sinus tachycardia. Two patients also had a neurally-mediated response induced during tilt. These same two subjects had an increased β-adrenergic sensitivity as shown by the isoproterenol CD_{25} response. These findings suggest that patients with β-adrenergic hypersensitivity who manifest inappropriate sinus tachycardia may be prone to neurally-mediated syncope triggered by head-up tilt probably related to the increased sympathetic drive potentiated by orthostatic stress. Intrinsic heart rate after complete pharmacological denervation was enhanced in eight of the nine patients.

Is inappropriate sinus tachycardia really inappropriate? Interpretation of the physiological response observed in the aforementioned patients poses the following hypothesis. Baseline impaired baroreceptor gain may be attributed to either a depressed baroreceptor response or an increased baseline sympathetic drive. The latter appears unlikely given the fact that increased β-adrenergic sensitivity was documented in only two patients. Of course, more sensitive measurements of sympathetic traffic such as catecholamine levels or sympathetic nerve traffic recordings are necessary to establish this issue. These findings suggest the possibility that the exaggerated heart rate response observed in patients with inappropriate sinus tachycardia triggered by orthostatic stress may be related to an inappropriate ability of the vagal baroreceptor reflex to be activated by positional changes. In this series, the majority of patients had an increased intrinsic heart rate. This finding suggests that the inappropriate heart rate response is due to enhanced sinus node automaticity that is not appropriately restrained at rest due to the decreased baseline vagal tone. In addition, orthostatic stress increases sympathetic activation and in combination with the enhanced sinus node automaticity leads to inappropriate sinus tachycardia. Returning to our initial question, "Is inappropriate sinus tachycardia really inappropriate?" – most likely it is. However, at least two different distinct autonomic patterns may be depicted in patients with so-called inappropriate sinus tachycardia. For this reason, detailed autonomic and pharmacological testing is necessary to define the mechanisms of inappropriate sinus tachycardia.

Rreferences

1. Krahn AD, Yee R, Klein GJ, Morillo CA (1995) Inappropriate sinus tachycardia: evaluation and therapy. J Cardiovasc Electrophysiol 6:1124-1128
2. Morillo CA, Klein GJ, Thakur RJ et al (1994) Mechanism of inappropriate sinus tachycardia: role of sympathovagal balance. Circulation 90:873-877
3. León H, Niño J, Tahvanainen K et al (2000) Comportamiento de la ganacia barorefleja durante el estrés ortostático en pacientes con taquicardia sinusal inapropiada. Acta Med Colombiana 25:253
4. Bauernfeind RA, Amat-Y-Leon F, Dhingra RC et al (1979) Chronic nonparoxysmal sinus tachycardia in otherwise healthy persons. Ann Intern Med 91:702-710
5. León H, Niño J, Tahvanainen K et al (2000) Is baroreflex gain impaired during orthostatic stress in patients with inappropriate sinus tachycardia? Clin Auton Res 10:234
6. Morillo CA, Klein GJ, Zandri S, Yee R (1995) Diagnostic accuracy of a low-dose isoproterenol head-up tilt protocol. Am Heart J 129:901-906
7. Raviele A, Menozzi C, Brignole M et al (1995) Value of head-up tilt testing potentiated with sublingual nitroglycerin to assess the origin of unexplained syncope. Am J Cardiol 76:267-272

"Pill in The Pocket" or Chronic Drug Prophylaxis for Patients with Paroxysmal Supraventricular Tachycardias without Indication for Catheter Ablation?

P. Alboni[1], C. Menozzi[2], C. Tomasi[2], N. Bottoni[2] and N. Paparella[1]

Paroxysmal supraventricular tachycardia (SVT) is commonly secondary to an atrioventricular (AV) nodal re-entry or to a re-entry involving an AV accessory pathway. Until 10 years ago, long-term antiarrhythmic prophylaxis represented the only therapeutic possibility. This treatment implies disadvantages, such as the daily intake of antiarrhythmic agents and the risk of drug-related adverse effects; moreover, despite optimal drug administration, relapses occur almost frequently [1]. The introduction of catheter ablation in clinical practice has deeply changed the therapeutic strategy of re-entrant SVT; in fact this procedure is effective in about 90% of the patients with this type of tachycardia. However, periprocedural death has been reported in 0.2%-0.3% and other major complications in about 3% of patients undergoing this therapy [2, 3]. These data suggest that catheter ablation should be recommended in those patients in whom paroxysmal SVTs induce a detrimental impact on their quality of life.

Some patients with SVT refer only rare and well-tolerated episodes, that are nevertheless long enough to require emergency room admission. In these patients, both long-term antiarrhythmic prophylaxis and catheter ablation do not seem to represent the most appropriate first-line treatment. In this group of patients, an appropriate approach appears to be an "episodic treatment", consisting of a single dose oral ingestion of an antiarrhythmic drug at the time and site of arrhythmia onset. This type of treatment has already been investigated in small groups of patients with frequent episodes of paroxysmal SVT [4, 5]. In a study by Yeh et al. [4], the combination of 120 mg diltiazem and 160 mg propranolol, administered as a single oral dose, was associated with termination within 3 h of drug intake of electrically induced SVT in 14 out of 15 patients (94%). However, at the dosage utilized by the investigators, two patients (13%) developed second degree AV block after SVT interruption. Musto et al. [5] tested the efficacy of a single oral dose of flecainide (about 3 mg/kg) to terminate electrically induced SVT in 25 children and young adults. Although this therapy was associated with SVT interruption within 3 h of drug

---

[1]Division of Cardiology, Ospedale Civile, Cento, Ferrara; [2]Department of Cardiology, Arcispedale S. Maria Nuova, Reggio Emilia, Italy

intake in 22 patients (88%), the true efficacy of flecainide could not be defined in the absence of a placebo group.

In this study we verified: (1) the efficacy of antiarrhythmic drugs as an acute oral dose to terminate SVT in patients with infrequent, long-lasting and well-tolerated episodes of this tachycardia; and (2) the out-of-hospital feasibility and safety of this treatment. To this purpose we have utilized, in a controlled design, oral flecainide and oral diltiazem plus propranolol because of the encouraging results reported in the literature.

Methods

All patients arriving at the emergency department of two hospitals with an episode of SVT were screened. Inclusion criteria were the following: (1) age 18-75 years; (2) infrequent (≤ 5 years), well-tolerated episodes of electrocardiographically documented paroxysmal SVT prompting for treatment in an emergency room at least once each year. The SVT episodes were defined as well-tolerated if they were not associated with severe symptoms and did not prevent normal activities, such as walking and driving. Exclusion criteria were the following: ventricular pre-excitation, ischaemic heart disease, resting sinus rate < 50 beats/min, left ventricular dysfunction or very severe general disease. The elegible patients underwent three electropharmacological studies on three different days in random order. The following treatments were tested in each patient: (1) placebo; (2) single oral dose of flecainide (about 3 mg/kg); and (3) single oral dose combination of 120 mg diltiazem and 80 mg propranolol. All drugs were administered 5 min after the induction of stable SVT. Electrical termination of SVT was attempted if no spontaneous conversion to sinus rhythm had occurred within 2 h from drug administration or arrhythmia-related severe symptoms were observed earlier on and treatment was considered ineffective.

Patients were discharged on the most effective treatment (showing the shortest conversion time; flecainide or diltiazem plus propranolol). If this treatment had induced severe adverse effects, the other treatment was prescribed. Before discharge, all patients were instructed to crush their tablet and to swallow it 5 min after the onset of the clinical arrhythmia.

Results

Out of 320 patients referred during a 3 year period for the treatment of SVT, 42 patients (13%) met the eligibility criteria. Of these, 37 (age 47 ± 11 years) gave written consent and were enrolled in the study. Two patients had hypertensive cardiovascular disease. In four patients (11%) SVT was not inducible during electrophysiological study or lasted < 5 min; these patients were excluded from analysis. Of the 33 patients with inducible SVT, conversion to sinus rhythm was achieved within 2 h in 17 (52%) after placebo, in 20 (61%) after flecainide and in 31 (94%) after diltiazem plus propranolol ($p < 0.001$). The conversion time to sinus rhythm was shorter after diltiazem plus propranolol (32 ± 22 min) than it was after placebo (77 ± 42 min, $p < 0.001$) or flecainide (74 ± 37 min, $p < 0.001$).

The treatment associated with the shortest conversion time was placebo in six patients (20%), flecainide in two (8%) and diltiazem plus propranolol in 21 (72%). The combination of diltiazem and propranolol was more effective than placebo ($p < 0.001$) and flecainide ($p < 0.001$), whereas the efficacy of flecainide did not significantly differ from that of placebo. Four patients (one placebo, one diltiazem plus propranolol, and two flecainide) had hypotension (systolic blood pressure ≤ 80 mmHg) and four (three diltiazem plus propranolol and one flecainide) a sinus rate < 50 beats/min after SVT interruption.

Twenty-six patients were discharged on diltiazem plus propranolol and five on flecainide. During a follow-up period of 17 ± 12 months, diltiazem plus propranolol was successful in 81% of the patients and flecainide in 80%, as all the arrhythmic episodes were interrupted out-of-hospital within 2 h. In the remaining patients a failure occurred during one or more episodes because of drug ineffectiveness or drug unavailability. The conversion time of the treated episodes was 41 ± 24 min and was similar to that observed during acute testing. One patient had syncope with trauma 15 min after ingestion of diltiazem plus propranolol, and drug treatment was discontinued.

During follow-up, the percentage of patients calling for emergency room assistance was significantly reduced as compared to the year before enrollment (9% vs 100%, $p < 0.0001$).

In seven patients (27%) the episodic treatment was discontinued after 13 ± 6 months of follow-up, in one patient because of syncope with trauma, in one because of concomitant atrial fibrillation requiring long-term prophylactic antiarrhythmic treatment, and in five patients because the arrhythmic episodes became more frequent and the patients underwent catheter ablation.

Discussion

Patients with the indication for "episodic treatment", i.e those with infrequent and well-tolerated episodes that were still long enough to call for emergency room assistance, account for 13% of all patients with paroxysmal re-entrant SVT, thus representing a small group. "Episodic treatment" is an appealing form of treatment for rarely symptomatic patients [6] because it prevents the disadvantages of long-term antiarrhythmic prophylaxis and the potential complications associated with catheter ablation. In the present study, selection of drug therapy based on the results of electropharmacological testing was associated with a satisfactory clinical outcome during the follow-up period. In fact, oral diltiazem plus propranolol interrupted within 2 h all out-of-hospital arrhythmic episodes in 81% of the patients and oral flecainide in 80%; in the remaining patients, a failure occurred during one or more episodes because of drug ineffectiveness or drug unavailability. An important impact of this treatment strategy was the dramatic reduction in emergency room admissions for medical care. These data have clinical implications, since emergency room admissions are often highly undesirable for SVT patients and represent the most important concern.

Although useful, the strategy we utilized to identify the most effective drug treatment in the individual patient appears to be of questionable practicability in clinical practice. In general, the combination of diltiazem plus propranolol proved efficacious in shortening the conversion time compared to placebo, whereas flecainide was not superior to placebo. For this reason, diltiazem plus propranolol could be tested as the first-choice treatment.

Based on the data of the present study, an acute success rate of about 70% would be expected (considering the possibility of SVT noninducibility and of severe side effects). Treatment of nonresponders remains to be investigated and, at this time, may include the testing of alternative drugs or other forms of therapy. Because "episodic treatment" with diltiazem plus propranolol was not tested in patients with ventricular pre-excitation, sinus bradycardia and left ventricular dysfunction, treatment with this drugs combination cannot be proposed in these patients. During follow-up, one patient had syncope with trauma 15 min after drug ingestion and, although paroxysmal SVT may cause syncope [7], it is likely that this symptom represents a drug-related adverse effect. Although rarely reported, the possibility of syncope should prompt physicians to recommend the patient to at least take a sitting position when using a self-administered single-dose oral treatment.

A not unexpected finding was that the clinical course of these patients may deteriorate with time. This was the case in five patients (16%) in this study, in whom the occurrence of more frequent episodes required discontinuation of the episodic treatment after 13 ± 6 months of follow-up; all five patients were referred for catheter ablation.

In conclusion, out-of-hospital "episodic treatment" with 120 mg diltiazem and 80 mg propranolol appears to be effective in patients with infrequent and well-tolerated episodes of paroxysmal SVT and the incidence of severe adverse events appears low. In particular, this treatment markedly reduces emergency room admissions. However, before being prescribed, diltiazem plus propranolol must be tested in hospital for assessment of efficacy and safety, possibly during a spontaneous SVT episode.

References

1. Mannino MM, Mehta D, Gomes A (1994) Current treatment options for paroxysmal supraventricular tachycardia. Am Heart J 127:475-480
2. Calkins H, Yong P, Miller JM et al (1999) Catheter ablation of accessory pathways,

atrioventricular nodal reentrant tachycardia, and the atrioventricular junction. Final results of a prospective, multicenter clinical trial. Circulation 99:262-270

3. Schaffer MS, Gow RM, Moak JP, Saul JP (2000) Mortality following radiofrequency catheter ablation (from the pediatric radiofrequency ablation registry). Am J Cardiol 86:639-643

4. Yeh SJ, Lin FC, Chou YY et al (1985) Termination of paroxysmal supraventricular tachycardia with a single oral dose of diltiazem and propranolol. Circulation 71:104-119

5. Musto B, Cavallaro C, Musto A et al (1992) Flecainide single oral dose for management of paroxysmal supraventricular tachycardia in children and young adults. Am Heart J 124:110-115

6. Wellens HJJ (1999) Catheter ablation of cardiac arrhythmias. Usually cure, but complications can occur. Circulation 99:195-197

7. Leitch JW, Klein GJ, Yee R et al (1992) Syncope associated with supraventricular tachycardia. An expression of tachycardia rate or vasomotor response? Circulation 85:1064-1071

Ablation of Fast and/or Slow Pathway for AV Nodal Reentrant Tachycardia: What Is the Risk of Late Block?

P. Delise[1], N. Sitta[1], F. Zoppo[2], L. Coro[1], R. Mantovan[3], L. Sciarra[1], P. Cannarozzo[1], R. Zecchel[3], A. Bonso[1], A. Raviele[4] and M. Fantinel[5]

Radiofrequency ablation of either the fast or the slow pathway in AV nodal re-entrant tachycardia was introduced in the early 1990s [1-4]. Both methods have a high success rate and low complications. As the procedures require the delivery of energy close to the AVN and the bundle of His, a possible complication is second or third degree AV block.

AV block can be acutely provoked by different mechanisms [5-15]: (a) an inadvertent damage of AVN or bundle of His; (b) a lesion of both fast and slow pathways during serial attemps at ablation of both pathways; (c) damage to the fast pathway during ablation of the slow pathway in cases in which the two pathways are abnormally close (about 8%, according to some authors) [12]; (d) simple damage of the slow pathway in cases in which the fast pathway does not have anterograde conduction and is only able to conduct retrogradely. The latter patients (about 3%) can be suspected when a long PR interval is present in the basal state [12-14]. In addition, second or third degree AV block can develop in the days after the procedure, owing to the edema induced by radiofrequency in the tissue surrounding the lesion [16, 17]. Finally, at least theoretically, AV block can develop during long-term follow-up owing to an anatomic evolution of the acute lesion.

Acute AV block requiring pacemaker implantation is more frequent during fast than during slow pathway ablation, according to some authors. E.g. the Multicenter European Radiofrequency Survey (MERFS) [5] reported an incidence of acute third degree AV block of 5.3% and 2% with the two techniques, respectively. In the same MERFS study, the incidence of block was lower in centers that had a greater experience (3.1% and 1.5% during fast and slow pathway ablation, respectively). An even smaller incidence of acute AV block (0-1%) has been reported in some recent studies with both techniques [16, 18].

The occurrence of a late block in the days after an uncomplicated procedure has been described by some authors. Perlagonio et al. [17], in a series of 418 patients treated with the slow pathway ablation, described two cases (0.4%) of AV block occurring 4 and 3 days, respectively, after a successful uncomplicated abla-

Divisions of Cardiology, Hospitals of [1]Conegliano, [2]Mirano, [3]Treviso, [4]Mestre, [5]Feltre, Italy

tion. In both cases AV conduction resumed after 10 and 8 days, respectively. Clague et al. [16], in a series of 379 patients treated with the slow pathway ablation, described six cases (1.5%) presenting with transient second or third degree AV block (< 1 h) following the procedure. In the same series they also observed one case (0.27%), who presented with presyncope and third degree AV block 1 month after a successful uncomplicated ablation requiring pacemaker implantation.

The long-term risk of AV block is not well established. Clague et al. [16], during a follow-up of 20.6 ± 10.8 months, did not observe any case of block. However, the incidence of block during a follow-up of many years is unknown.

Personal Experience

During February 1990-December 2000 we collected a total of 282 consecutive cases in four centers located in the Veneto Region of Italy (Conegliano, Mestre, Mirano, Feltre and Treviso).

The patients were divided into three groups according to the target of ablation (Table 1). In 25 patients (Group A), the only fast pathway was targeted in one or more sessions. In 250 patients (Group B) the only slow pathway was targeted in one or more sessions. In seven patients (Group C), the fast pathway was first targeted and the slow pathway was targeted subsequently in a different session. Multiple sessions were performed to deal with initial lack of success or arrhythmia relapse.

Table 1. In-hospital data

Targeted pathway	Group A (fast)	Group B (slow)	Group C (fast + slow)
n	25	250	7
Age (years)	56 ± 16	51 ± 15	52 ± 18
More than one procedure	7	16	7
n/pz	1.32	1.06	2.4
Acute second or third degree AV block			
· Transient	6	3	3*
· Persistent	0	3	0
Subcute second or third degree AV block			
· Transient	1	0	0
· Persistent	1	1 (+ 3**)	0
Pacemaker implantation for third degree AV block	1	2	0

*During fast pathway ablation (2/3 during first procedure)
** Three patients who had acute persistent AV block
n/pz, procedures/patient

In Group A, 7/25 (28%) had more than one session (mean, 1.32 sessions/patient). In Group B, 16/250 (2.4%) had more than one session (mean, 1.06 sessions/patient). In Group C, 7/7 patients had two or more sessions (mean, 2.4 sessions/patient). The final acute success rates were 92%, 99% and 100%, respectively, in the three groups. Electrophysiologic study and fast and slow pathway ablation were performed according to standard criteria, using previously described techniques [18].

All patients were followed up (Table 2) with clinical controls or by telephone interview when, for example, the patient lived far from the center where ablation was performed. The latter patients had electrocardiograms taken in another center and send it to us by fax.

Follow-up data were obtained in all patients of Groups A and C and in 235/250 (94%) of Group B. Follow-up was 8.7 ± 1.9 years in Group A, 3.8 ± 2.7 years in Group B and 7.9 ± 2.4 years in Group C. In Group B, 66 patients (Group B1) had a follow-up of at least 6 years (7.2 ± 0.8 years), 65 patients (Group B2) had a follow-up of 3-6 years (4.9 ± 7 years) and 104 patients (Group B3) had a follow-up of less than 3 years (1 ± 0.7 years).

Table 2. Follow-up data

Targeted pathway	Group A (fast)	Group B (slow)	Group C (fast + slow)
n	25	250	7
Follow-up (years)			
Drop-out	0	15 (6%)	0
Mean ± SD	8.6 ± 2	3.8 ± 2.8	7.3 ± 2.5
Range	1-11	0.15-8.7	2.2-10
Arrhythmia relapse	1	8	0
Second or third degree AV block	0 (+ 1*)	1 (+ 4*)	0
Pacemaker implantation for third degree AV block	0 (+ 1*)	1 (+ 2**)	0
Deaths [7 (2.4%)]			
· Sudden	1 (8.5) (FV post-dialysis)	0	0
· Accidental trauma	0	0	2
· Non-sudden cardiac deaths	2	0	0
· Noncardiac deaths	1	1	0

* patients who had the complications during hospital stay
** patients who had pacemaker implantation during hospital stay

Acute Complications

Transient acute second or third degree AV block was defined as a block disappearing before the end of the procedure. Persistent AV block was defined when it persisted at the end of the procedure.

Transient acute second or third degree AV block occurred during fast pathway ablation (Groups A and C) in 9/32 (28%; three second degree and six third degree AV blocks). Transient second or third degree AV block occurred during slow pathway ablation (Groups B and C) in 3/257 (1.2%). In all cases AV block disappeared after a mean of 18 seconds (range 1.8-120 seconds).

Persistent second or third degree AV block occurred in no case during fast pathway ablation and in 3/257 (1.2%; one second degree and two third degree AV blocks) during slow pathway ablation. No persistent block occurred in patients of Group C.

Subacute Complications (After the Procedure, During Hospital Stay)

Transient acute second or third degree AV block was defined as a block occurring during the days after the procedure and disappearing during the hospital stay. Persistent AV block was defined when it persisted during the hospital stay.

Second or third degree AV block persisted during hospital stay in all three cases of Group B, which consisted of patients having an acute persistent second or third degree AV block. Furthermore, one patient of Group A who had a transient acute third degree AV block developed a persistent third degree block 2 days after the procedure; and one patient of Group B who had a transient acute second degree AV block during slow pathway ablation showed a persistent second degree AV block the day after the procedure.

In summary, a persistent second or third degree AV block occurred in 1/32 cases (3%) during or after a fast pathway ablation and in 4/257 (1.5%) during or after slow pathway ablation. A pacemaker implantation for third degree AV block was required in 1/32 (3%) and 2/257 (0.7%) patients treated with fast and slow pathway ablations, respectively. Patients with second degree AV block were not implanted, owing to a good heart rate at rest and during effort.

As to transient acute second or third degree AV block, this was a frequent complication in fast pathway ablation, occurring in 9/32 (28%), but only in 1/9 (11%) was it followed by chronic AV block. In contrast, transient second or third degree AV block during slow pathway ablation was rare (3/257; 1.2%) but in one-third of patients it developed into persistent second degree AV block.

Finally, transient AV block in the days after an uncomplicated procedure was very rare, occurring in 1/32 (3%) in Group A, 0/250 in Group B and in 0/7 in Group C.

Long-term Follow-up

In all five patients who had a persistent second or third degree AV block during or after the procedure, it persisted during the follow-up. In addition, one further patient of Group B who had a slow pathway ablation developed a right bundle branch block with left axis deviation and 2:1 AV block 8 years after the procedure, which required a pacemaker implantation.

Conclusions

AV block is a possible complication of both fast and slow pathway ablation performed in patients suffering from AV nodal re-entrant tachycardia.

The acute incidence of persistent AV block, requiring pacemaker implantation, is rare with both techniques and it has been progressively reduced over time with the increasing experience of centers. The incidence of a permanent third degree AV block requiring pacemaker implantation is less during slow than fast pathway ablation. In our series it was 0.7% vs 3%. Some authors report a lower incidence of block during fast pathway ablation [16, 18]. The difference can be explained by the limited number of our series treated with fast pathway ablation (only 32 cases, with one block). According to most authors, the risk of persistent third degree AV block during slow pathway ablation is low (< 1%). Furthermore, its incidence could be reduced by guiding the ablation with the pacemapping of Koch's triangle [12]. In fact, with this technique it is possible to identify patients having close fast and slow pathways and also patients having anterograde conduction only via the slow pathway. In all these cases, slow pathway ablation, based only on an anatomical approach, has a high risk of inadvertent AV block.

Transient acute AV block is significantly more frequent during fast than slow pathway ablation (28% vs 1.2%, in our experience). However, with both methods the occurrence of late third degree AV block requiring pacemaker implantation is rare. In fact, only 1/9 patients who had a transient second or third degree AV block during fast pathway ablation required pacemaker implantation. On the other hand, 0/3 patients who had a transient second degree AV block during slow pathway ablation required a pacemaker, although one patient continued to present with episodes of second degree AV block.

Some authors [16, 17] suggest that after a successful uncomplicated procedure a transient late second or third degree AV block can occur. Perlagonio [17] and Clague [16] described this complication in 0.5% and 1.5% respectively. In both series the block resumed during 1 or 2 weeks, suggesting a transient edema involving the AV node. In our experience, this transient phenomenon occurred only in 1/32 (3%) cases who had a fast pathway ablation and in 0/257 of those who had a slow pathway ablation.

An unresolved issue is the long-term follow-up of patients treated with the fast or slow pathway ablation and in particular their risk to develop second or third degree AV block many years after the procedure, owing to an anatomic evolution of the acute lesion provoked by radiofrequency energy.

The incidence of AV block during a long-term follow-up was investigated by Clague et al. [16], who reported over a mean period of 20.6 months a single case (0.3%) of definite complete AV block requiring pacemaker implantation 1 month after an uncomplicated procedure.

In our study, we collected 282 consecutive patients during February 1990-December 2000 and we followed them for a maximum of 11 years, with a mean of 8.7, 3.8 and 7.9 years in Group A, B and C, respectively. Furthermore, in Group B 66 patients (28%) had a mean follow-up of 7.2 years.

During long-term follow-up we observed no case of AV block related to the procedure. One case from Group B, a 70 year-old man, developed a 2:1 AV block that was probably related to a progressive disease of the intraventricular conduction system. In particular, no case who had a transient second or third degree AV block during or soon after the procedure developed second or third degree AV block during long-term follow-up. Furthermore, during long-term follow-up we observed no syncope or sudden death possibly due to paroxysmal AV block. Only in the small series of Group C (fast + slow pathway ablation) did we find two deaths related to accidental traumas, which occurred in the first months after the procedure. In these cases we cannot exclude a paroxysmal AV block causing syncopal episodes.

In conclusion, the risk of late AV block in patients submitted to fast or slow pathway ablation is low and limited to the immediate days after the procedure. Frequently, late block is transient. Persistent late second or third degree block is rare and generally occurs in patients who had a transient AV block during the procedure. Patients submitted to fast or slow pathway ablation seem to have no risk of developing a second or third degree AV block during long-term follow-up.

The follow-up data are incertain in patients submitted to serial fast and slow pathway ablation. So, according to some authors [5], this latter method should be avoided whenever possible.

References

1. Haïssaguerre M, Warin JF, Lemetayer P et al (1989) Closed-chest ablation of retrograde conduction in patients with atrioventricular nodal re-entrant tachycardia. N Engl J Med 320:426-433
2. Delise P, Bonso A, Raviele A (1990) Tachicardia reciprocante idionodale insensibile alla profilassi farmacologica. Descrizione di un caso trattato con successo con la radiofrequenza. G Ital Cardiol 20:1168-1173
3. Haïssaguerre M, Gaita F, Fischer B et al (1992) Elimination of atrioventricular nodal re-entrant tachycardia using discrete slow potentials to guide application of radiofrequency energy. Circulation 85:2162-2175
4. Jackman WA, Beckman KJ, McClelland JH et al (1992) Treatment of supraventricular tachycardia due to atrioventricular nodal re-entry by radiofrequency catheter ablation of slow-pathway conduction. N Engl J Med 327:313-318
5. Hindricks G on behalf of the MERFS investigators of the Working Group on Arrhythmias of the European Society of Cardiology (1993) The Multicenter European Radiofrequency Survey (MERFS): complications of radiofrequency ablation of arrhythmias. Eur Heart J 14:1644-1653
6. Thakur RK, Klein GJ, Yee R, Stites HW (1993) Junctional tachycardia: a useful marker during radiofrequency ablation for atrioventricular node re-entrant tachycardia. J Am Coll Cardiol 22:1706-1710
7. Hintringer F, Hartikainen J, Davies W et al (1995) Prediction of atrioventricular block during radiofrequency ablation of the slow pathway of the atrioventricular node. Circulation 92:3490-3496

8. Anselme F, Hook B, Monahan K et al (1996) Heterogeneity of retrograde fast-pathway conduction pattern in patients with atrioventricular nodal re-entry tachycardia. Observations by use of simultaneous multisite catheter mapping of Koch's triangle. Circulation 93:960-968

9. Reithmann C, Hoffmann E, Grunewald A et al (1998) Fast pathway ablation in patients with common atrioventricular nodal reentrant tachycardia and prolonged PR interval during sinus rhythm. Eur Heart J 19:929-935

10. Ridgen LB, Klein LS, Mitrani RD et al (1995) Increased risk of heart block following slow pathway ablation for AV nodal re-entrant tachycardia in patients with marked PR interval prolongation during sinus rhythm. Pacing Clin Electrophysiol 18:II-918

11. Verdino RJ, Burke MC, Kall JG et al (1999) Retrograde fast pathway ablation for atrioventricular nodal re-entry associated with markedly prolonged PR intervals. Am J Cardiol 83:455-458

12. Delise P, Bonso A, Coro' L et al (1999) How to predict and avoid complete AV block complicating radiofrequency ablation of AV nodal slow pathway. In: Raviele A (ed), Cardiac arrhythmias. Springer, Milan, pp 176-184

13. Sra JS, Jazayeri MR, Blank Z et al (1994) Slow pathway ablation in patients with atrioventricular node re-entrant tachycardia and a prolonged PR interval. J Am Coll Cardiol 24:1064-1068

14. Natale A, Greenfield RA, Geiger MJ et al (1997) Safety of slow pathway ablation in patients with long PR intervals: further evidence of fast and slow pathway interaction. Pacing Clin Electrophysiol 20:1698-1703

15. Gianfranchi L, Brignole M, Delise P et al (1999) Modification of anterograde slow pathway is not crucial for successful catheter ablation of common atrioventricular nodal reentrant tachycardia. Pacing Clin Electrophysiol 22:263-267

16. Clague JR, Dagres N, Kottkamp H et al (2001) Targeting the slow pathway for atrioventricular nodal re-entrant tachycardia: initial results and long-term follow-up in 379 consecutive patients. Eur Heart J 22:82-88

17. Pelargonio G, Fogel RI, Knilans TK, Prystowsky EN (2001) Late occurrence of heart block after radiofrequency catheter ablation of the septal region: clinical follow-up outcome. J Cardiovasc Electrophysiol 12:56-60

18. Kottkamp H, Hindricks G, Borggrefe M et al (1997) Radiofrequency catheter ablation of the anterosuperior atrial approaches to the AV node for treatment of AV nodal re-entrant tachycardia: techniques for selective ablation of fast and slow AV node pathways. J Cardiovasc Electrophysiol 8:451-468

19. Delise P, Themistoclakis S, Coro' L et al (1997) Radiofrequency ablation of atrioventricular node re-entrant tachycardias: which results and predictors of success and recurrence? In: Raviele A (ed), Cardiac arrhythmias. Springer-Verlag Italia, Milan, pp 176-180

What Are the Accuracy and Limitations of Published Algorithms Using Surface ECG to Localize Overt AV Accessory Pathways?

J.A. SALERNO-URIARTE[1], F. CARAVATI[2], C.N. DAJELLI ERMOLLI[1], R. DE PONTI[2] AND M. TRITTO[2]

Introduction

Pre-excitation produces an anomalous ventricular activation through pathways other than His bundle, and so ventricular complexes observed in Wolff-Parkinson-White (WPW) syndrome during periods of sinoatrial rhythm are the results of fusion: the first phase of ventricular activation consists of excitation via the accessory pathway, while later forces result from the depolarization of residual portions of the ventricles via the His-Purkinje system [1-3].

Surgical resection in the 1980s and radiofrequency catheter ablation over the last few years are standardized treatments which can take advantage of an optimized pre-procedure assessment [4-7]. Electrophysiologic studies and radiofrequency ablations can be abbreviated, when presumptive localization of accessory pathways is available before the procedure: this allows advance planning of the most appropriate technique, shortening the time taken for information acquisition and reducing manipulations and, hence, mechanical damage to the heart chambers [8].

Normally, every electrocardiogram analysis is based on the presumption that the spatial orientation of the initial vector (delta wave, the first 0.03-0.04 s) and of the following QRS complex provide some insights into the pattern of ventricular pre-excitation in relation to the anatomic location of the accessory pathway [9]. Many electrocardiographic algorithms have been generated, but the proposed criteria for localization of accessory pathways generally provide only a crude indication of their position, and often they lack of sensibility and refined accuracy.

In this report, we will discuss the results obtained in the last 220 patients with a single pathway successfully treated in our laboratory in the last 4 years, and we will correlate the presumptive location of the anomalous pathway on the basis of various available algorithms with the true localization established at the time of ablation.

[1]Università degli Studi dell'Insubria, Dipartimento di Scienze Cardiovascolari, Ospedale di Circolo e Fondazione Macchi, Varese, Italy; [2]Dipartimento di Cardiologia, Istituto Clinico e Fondazione Mater Domini, Castellanza, Varese, Italy

Methods

We considered eight published algorithms that use only surface electrocardiogram recorded during sinus rhythm to localize accessory pathways in patients with a diagnosis of pre-excitation syndrome [10-17]. These algorithms were analyzed and their accuracy was tested in a population of patients with WPW syndrome.

The study population consisted of 220 subjects referred to our institution from 1997 up to today for management of arrhythmias associated with manifest WPW syndrome, who underwent successful radiofrequency catheter ablation. Patients with multiple accessory pathways, structural heart disease, or no electrocardiographic evidence of pre-excitation were excluded. All antiarrhythmic drug treatment was discontinued before the procedure.

The location of accessory pathways was classified into 14 regions (Fig. 1) and was defined as the site where endocardial mapping led to successful radiofrequency ablation with no recurrences of symptoms or ECG delta wave during a follow-up period of 45 days [18].

Left-sided accessory pathways were approached from the atrial aspect of the mitral annulus reached transseptally [19]. Right-sided accessory pathways were approached by positioning the catheter on the tricuspid valve annulus by way of the right femoral vein.

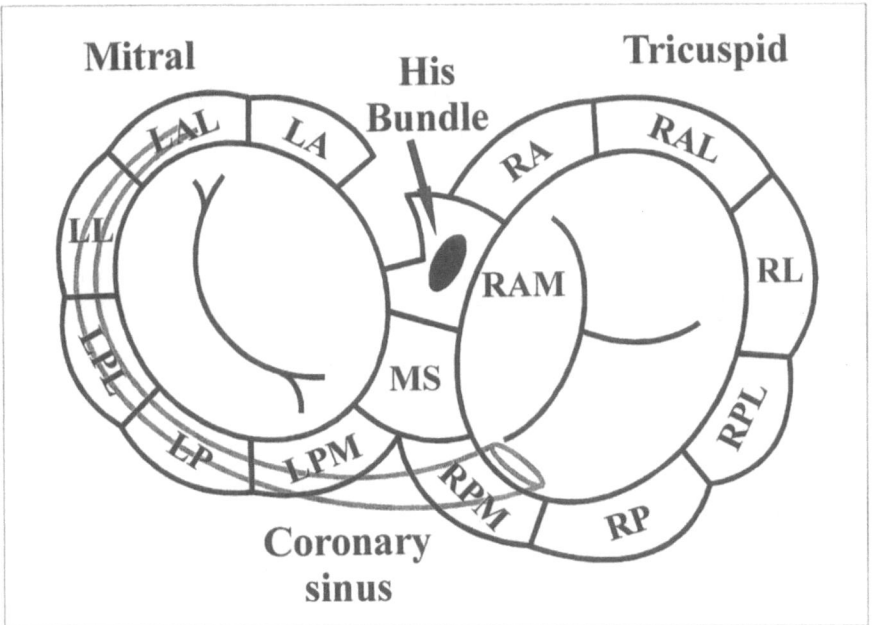

Fig. 1. Cross-sectional diagram for a classification of accessory pathway locations in a cranial view. The region is divided into 14 areas and the ostium and the course of the coronary sinus are shown. Abbreviations as in Table 2

During endocardial and, if necessary, epicardial mapping through the coronary sinus, particular care was taken to identify the atrial and ventricular insertion of the accessory pathway both on sinus rhythm and atrioventricular tachycardia prior to radiofrequency energy delivery. For the purpose of this study the location of the ventricular insertion of the accessory pathway was considered in case an oblique orientation was observed. When necessary, incremental atrial pacing and programmed atrial stimulation were used [20]. Electrocardiograms were recorded at a paper speed of 25 mm/s and evaluated by at least two independent observers, and errors of localization were reviewed and classified by consensus as failure of the algorithm when intraobserver and interobserver variability could be excluded.

Results

In the study population, accessory pathways were localized during endocardiac mapping in 75 patients in the left lateral wall (34.0%), 11 in the left posterior (5.0%), 13 in the left posterolateral (6.0%), 47 in the left posteroseptal (or, better, left posteromedial or left posteroparaseptal) (21.5%), 10 in the right posterior (4.5%), 6 in the right anterior (3.0%), 12 in the midseptal (5.5%), 1 in the right anterolateral (0.4%), 8 in the left anterolateral (3.5%), 7 in the right lateral (3.0%), 8 in the right posteroseptal (or, better, right posteromedial or right posteroparaseptal) (3.5%), 8 in the left anterior (3.5%), 2 in the right posterolateral (1.0%), and 12 in the right anteroseptal wall (or, better, right anteromedial or right anteroparaseptal wall) (5.5%). Pathway locations are shown in Fig. 1.

The success of the application of ECG-based algorithms is summarized in Table 1, while the detection power for the different locations of accessory pathways is reported in Table 2.

Table 1. Comparison of different algorithms based on surface 12-lead electrocardiogram in identifying accessory pathway location: published results and control techniques (applied to confirm site of anomalous pathway) were correlated with accuracy tested in 220 patients with WPW syndrome and successful ablation of accessory pathways

Author	Number of patients	Algorithm accuracy (%)	Control technique originally applied	Accuracy obtained with EPS (%)
Xie et al. [17] (St. George group)	106	86	EPS	80
Arruda et al. [15]	186	89	RFA	78
Milstein et al. [12]	141	90	EPS + SA	74
Chiang et al. [13]	182	93	RFA	80
Reddy and Schamroth [11]	-	-	No control	76
Gallagher et al. [10]	68	-	EPS + SA	80
Tavazzi et al. [16]	59	95	EPS	83
Lindsay et al. [14]	66	91	EPS + SA	83

EPS, electrophysiologic study; *RFA*, radiofrequency ablation; *SA*, surgical ablation

Table 2. Detection power of selected 12-lead electrocardiographic criteria in relation to different accessory pathway locations (expressed as percentages)

Site of accessory pathway	Number of patients	Xie et al. [17] (St. George group)	Arruda et al. [15]	Milstein et al. [12]	Chiang et al. [13]	Reddy and Schamroth [11]	Gallagher et al. [10]	Tavazzi et al. [16]	Lindsay et al. [14]
Left anterior (LA)	8	87	75	50	75	62	100	87	87
Left anterolateral (LAL)	8	75	62	75	75	37	75	62	75
Left lateral (LL)	75	84	73	87	96	93	91	93	91
Left posterolateral (LPL)	13	85	69	77	69	69	77	77	62
Left posterior (LP)	11	91	82	64	82	73	73	82	73
Left posteromedial (LPM)	47	79	85	64	68	66	77	83	87
Right posteromedial (RPM)	8	75	87	62	75	87	50	75	75
Right posterior (RP)	10	90	80	80	80	90	50	90	80
Right posterolateral (RPL)	2	50	50	50	50	100	50	50	100
Right lateral (RL)	7	86	57	86	43	71	57	86	71
Right anterolateral (RAL)	1	100	100	0	0	100	100	100	100
Right anterior (RA)	6	50	83	83	00	50	50	83	83
Right anteromedial (RAM)	12	58	100	75	92	67	83	83	75
Midseptal (MS)	12	75	83	58	67	58	92	83	75

Discussion

The algorithms proposed by Milstein et al. [12], Reddy and Schamroth [11], and Arruda et al. [15] achieved a poorer identification accuracy than the other methods, even though the number of areas they can discriminate was really limited. Thus, these criteria may be considered at the moment less adequate for pre-procedure assessment.

The classification of Gallagher et al. [10] was based on the initial direction of the delta wave and on ten possible accessory pathway locations around the tricuspid and mitral rings. It provided more discriminative power in comparison with previous algorithms, although its structure was quite complex.

The accuracy of the method proposed by Lindsay and his associates [14] proved to be usually superior to others in non-invasive assessment, but its practical value during evaluation of WPW patients appears to be compromised by the limited number of pre-selected anatomic regions considered (only five: left lateral, left posterior, posteroseptal with posteroparaseptal, right free wall, and right anteroparaseptal).

A similar accuracy was reached by the ECG criteria proposed by the authors of the St. George Hospital study [17], by Chiang et al. [13], and by our group [16], but the higher number of areas they discriminated (respectively 9, 13 and 14) permitted better direct accessory pathway identification. In particular, the last two algorithms, whose anatomic subdivisions were more fitted for electrophysiologic studies, probably represent the best available ECG-based approaches to non-invasive assessment before the ablation procedure.

Furthermore, ECG criteria based on results from surgical resection of anomalous pathways generally evidenced many differences from percutaneous assessment techniques in regard to the extension of dissection and then of the discrimination of the precise pathway site. However, any attempt at pathway localization using surface ECG is restricted by important limitations: first, ventricular pre-excitation must be present and, second, minor degrees of pre-excitation may sometimes mislead the ECG interpretation and the final determination of atrioventricular or bypass tract location. The presence of a second accessory pathway may not generally influence the surface ECG, since the bypass tract closer to the origin of the atrial rhythm should prevail. However, in this report we did not consider possible complex patterns related to the coexistence of multiple pathways (documented in up to 2% of patients with WPW syndrome), which can interfere with the correct diagnosis of the first anomalous bypass tract. Concomitant P wave modifications (e.g., changes in atrial repolarization) and QRS abnormalities (e.g., myocardial infarction, body configuration, orientation of the heart within the chest, and structural heart disease) may condition the final pre-excitation pattern.

At the moment, the ECG-based algorithms may be considered as a first non-invasive approach to WPW syndrome to guide the operator towards precise localization of an anomalous pathway by endocardial mapping, which is a prerequisite for success of catheter ablation. Thus, a simple method with good accuracy and an elevated discrimination power could represent the best help for electrophysiologic studies and catheter ablation.

References

1. Boineau JP, Moore EN, Spear JF, Sealy WC (1973) Basis of static and dynamic electro-cardiographic variations in Wolff-Parkinson-White syndrome. Anatomic and elec-trophysiologic observations in right and left ventricular preexcitation. Am J Cardiol 32:32-45
2. Gallagher JJ, Pritchett EL, Sealy WC et al (1978) The preexcitation syndromes. Prog Cardiovasc Dis 20:285-327
3. Tonkin AM, Wagner GS, Gallagher JJ et al (1975) Initial forces of ventricular depolari-zation in the Wolff-Parkinson-White syndrome. Analysis based upon localization of the accessory pathway by epicardial mapping. Circulation 52:1030-1036
4. Gallagher JJ (1997) Wolff-Parkinson-White syndrome: surgery to radiofrequency catheter ablation. Pacing Clin Electrophysiol 20:512-533
5. Willems JL, Robles de Medina EO, Bernard R et al (1985) Criteria for intraventricu-lar conduction disturbances and pre-excitation. World Health Organizatio-nal/International Society and Federation for Cardiology Task Force Ad Hoc. J Am Coll Cardiol 5:1261-1275
6. Scheinman MM, Wang YS, Van Hare GF, Lesh MD (1992) Electrocardiographic and electrophysiologic characteristics of anterior, midseptal and right anterior free wall accessory pathways. J Am Coll Cardiol 20:1220-1229
7. Bashir Y, Heald SC, Katritsis D et al (1993) Radiofrequency ablation of accessory atrioventricular pathways: predictive value of local electrogram characteristics for the identification of successful target sites. Br Heart J 69:315-321
8. Chiang CE, Chen SA, Wu TJ et al (1994) Incidence, significance, and pharmacological responses of catheter-induced mechanical trauma in patients receiving radiofre-quency ablation for supraventricular tachycardia. Circulation 90:1847-1854
9. Frank R, Fontaine G, Guiraudon G et al (1977) Correlation between the orientation of the delta wave and the topography of pre-excitation in the Wolff-Parkinson-White syndrome. Arch Mal Coeur 70:441-450
10. Gallagher JJ, Gilbert M, Svenson RH et al (1975) Wolff-Parkinson-White syndrome. The problem, evaluation, and surgical correction. Circulation 51:767-785
11. Reddy GV, Schamroth L (1987) The localization of bypass tracts in the Wolff-Parkinson-White syndrome from the surface electrocardiogram. Am Heart J 113:984-993
12. Milstein S, Sharma AD, Guiraudon GM, Klein GJ (1987) An algorithm for the electro-cardiographic localization of accessory pathways in the Wolff-Parkinson-White syn-drome. Pacing Clin Electrophysiol 10:555-563
13. Chiang CE, Chen SA, Teo WS et al (1995) An accurate stepwise electrocardiographic algorithm for localization of accessory pathways in patients with Wolff-Parkinson-White syndrome from a comprehensive analysis of delta waves and R/S ratio during sinus rhythm. Am J Cardiol 76:40-46
14. Lindsay BD, Crossen KJ, Cain ME (1987) Concordance of distinguishing electrocar-diographic features during sinus rhythm with the location of accessory pathways in the Wolff-Parkinson-White syndrome. Am J Cardiol 59:1093-1102
15. Arruda MS, McClelland JH, Wang X et al (1998) Development and validation of an ECG algorithm for identifying accessory pathway ablation site in Wolff-Parkinson-White syndrome. J Cardiovasc Electrophysiol 9:2-12
16. Tavazzi L, Salerno JA, Chimienti M et al (1978) Identificazione della sede della via anomala dall'elettrocardiogramma convenzionale nella pre-eccitazione ventricolare. In: Rovelli F et al (eds) Progressi in cardiologia. Pozzi, Rome, pp 71-78

17. Xie B, Heald SC, Bashir Y et al (1994) Localization of accessory pathways from the 12-lead electrocardiogram using a new algorithm. Am J Cardiol 74:161-165

18. Timmermans C, Rodriguez LM, Oreto G et al (1994) Recurrence rate after accessory pathway ablation. Br Heart J 72:571-574

19. De Ponti R, Zardini M, Storti C et al (1998) Transseptal catheterization for radiofrequency ablation of cardiac arrhythmias: results and safety of a simplified method. Eur Heart J 19:943-950

20. Salerno JA, Gavazzi L, Massacci E, Bobba P (1974) La stimolazione elettrica e la registrazione dei potenziali intracavitari applicate alla identificazione e localizzazione della via anomala nella sindrome di Wolff-Parkinson-White. Boll Soc Ital Cardiol 18:1154-1177

ATRIAL FIBRILLATION: ELECTROGENETIC, CLINICAL AND THERAPEUTICAL ASPECTS

Electrical and Mechanical Remodeling of the Atria: What Are the Underlying Mechanisms, the Time Course and the Clinical Relevance?

U. Schotten and M.A. Alessie

Introduction

The rapid and irregular atrial contractions during atrial fibrillation (AF) result in a depression of atrial transport function and contribute to the reduction of ventricular filling and cardiac output. The main clinical relevance of the loss of synchronized atrial contraction is the development of atrial thrombi, presumably due to increased stasis of blood near the atrial wall [1]. Accordingly, atrial fibrillation is a common cause of cerebral embolism, accounting for approximately 15% of all strokes [2]. Therefore, maintenance of sinus rhythm (SR) is of primary importance in the treatment of AF. Echocardiographic studies in patients have shown that after cardioversion, the contractile function of the atria is impaired. The degree of contractile dysfunction correlates with the previous duration of AF [3], and the recovery of atrial function can take months [4]. New thrombus formation after cardioversion to SR might therefore contribute to the thromboembolic risk associated with AF.

Mechanisms of Postcardioversion Atrial Contractile Dysfunction

The mechanisms responsible for the postfibrillatory dysfunction are still poorly understood. Initially, it was hypothesized that the application of electric energy during DC cardioversion might cause "atrial stunning" [5], but contractile dysfunction has also been demonstrated after pharmacological [3] and spontaneous cardioversion [6]. Studies in goats and humans with sustained AF have shown that AF is associated with alterations of the cellular ultrastructure and therefore suggest that a loss of myofibrils and fragmentation of the sarcoplasmic reticulum may also underlie the contractile abnormalities in remodeled atria (myolysis) [7]. In experimental and clinical studies verapamil was able to prevent part of the atrial dysfunction, indicating that the dysfunction was mediated by Ca^{2+} overload during AF [8, 9]. Several studies demonstrated that indeed altered Ca^{2+} metabolism contributes to the atrial dysfunction. In dogs with sustained atrial tachycardia atrial contractility has been shown to be reduced on the cellular level [10] and a pronounced reduction of the L-

Department of Physiology, University of Maastricht, The Netherlands

type Ca^{2+} current (I_{CaL}) was reported [11]. Recently, reduced I_{CaL} was confirmed in human atrial cardiomyocytes of patients with chronic AF [12, 13]. Since I_{CaL} triggers Ca^{2+} release from the sarcoplasmic reticulum and provides Ca^{2+} to maintain the Ca^{2+} load of the sarcoplasmic reticulum, it is a major determinant of myocardial force of contraction. Besides the importance of a reduced I_{CaL} for the AF-induced atrial contractile dysfunction, downregulation of I_{CaL} also causes electrical remodeling. In chronically instrumented goats AF was shown to produce a rapid shortening of the atrial effective refractory period (2-5 days) [14]. This was associated with a shortening of the AF cycle length and a progressive increase in the duration of AF (AF begets AF). A shortening of the atrial refractory period was also found in dogs undergoing prolonged rapid atrial pacing (42 days). In atrial cardiomyocytes of these animals I_{CaL} was found to be reduced by 70%, whereas repolarizing currents were less affected [11]. Inhibiting I_{CaL} of a control cell with nifedipine mimicked the action potential changes produced by atrial tachycardia, whereas increasing I_{CaL} with BayK8644 partly reversed action potential alterations in tachycardia-remodeled cardiomyocytes. These results strongly suggest that a reduction of I_{CaL} indeed underlies the tachycardia-induced shortening of the refractory period.

Electrical and Contractile Remodeling Go Hand in Hand

Since I_{CaL} is also one of the most important regulators of the atrial contractile function, electrical remodeling is expected to follow the same time course after the onset of AF as the AF-induced atrial contractile dysfunction. We recently tested this hypothesis using chronically instrumented goats. In six goats two pairs of electrodes were sutured on the epicardium of the right and the left atrium and sonomicrometer crystals were positioned in the groove between auricle and aortic root and on the free atrial wall of each side (Fig. 1). The crystals allowed the continuous recording of

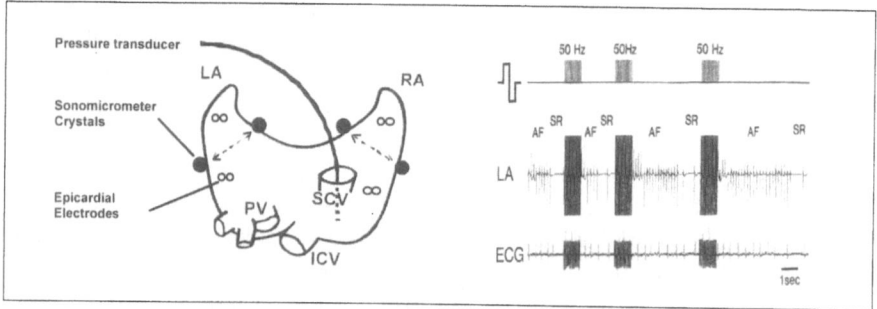

Fig. 1. Chronic instrumentation of the goat model of atrial fibrillation (AF). Two pairs of electrodes were sutured to the atrial epicardium of each side. Right and left atrial diameters were measured using implantable ultrasound probes (sonomicrometer crystals) positioned in the groove between auricle and aortic root and on the free atrial wall. Atrial pressure was monitored with a pressure transducer implanted in the right atrium via the jugular vein. AF was maintained by repetitive burst pacing of the atria

the right and the left atrial diameter. A pressure transducer was chronically implanted in the right atrium via one of the jugular veins. AF was induced with an external fibrillation pacemaker automatically delivering a burst of stimuli as soon as SR was detected. With this method AF was maintained 24 h a day. The mechanical function of the atria was studied 30 min after spontaneous cardioversion of AF during slow atrial pacing at a cycle length of 400 ms. The atrial pressure was plotted against the atrial diameter and the area enclosed by this pressure-diameter loop reflected the mechanical work performed during the atrial contraction (atrial work index). The atrial refractory period and the work index were measured once a day at a cycle length of 400 ms during the first 5 days of AF and during the first 5 days of SR. Figure 2 shows a representative example. As expected, AF shortened the refrac-

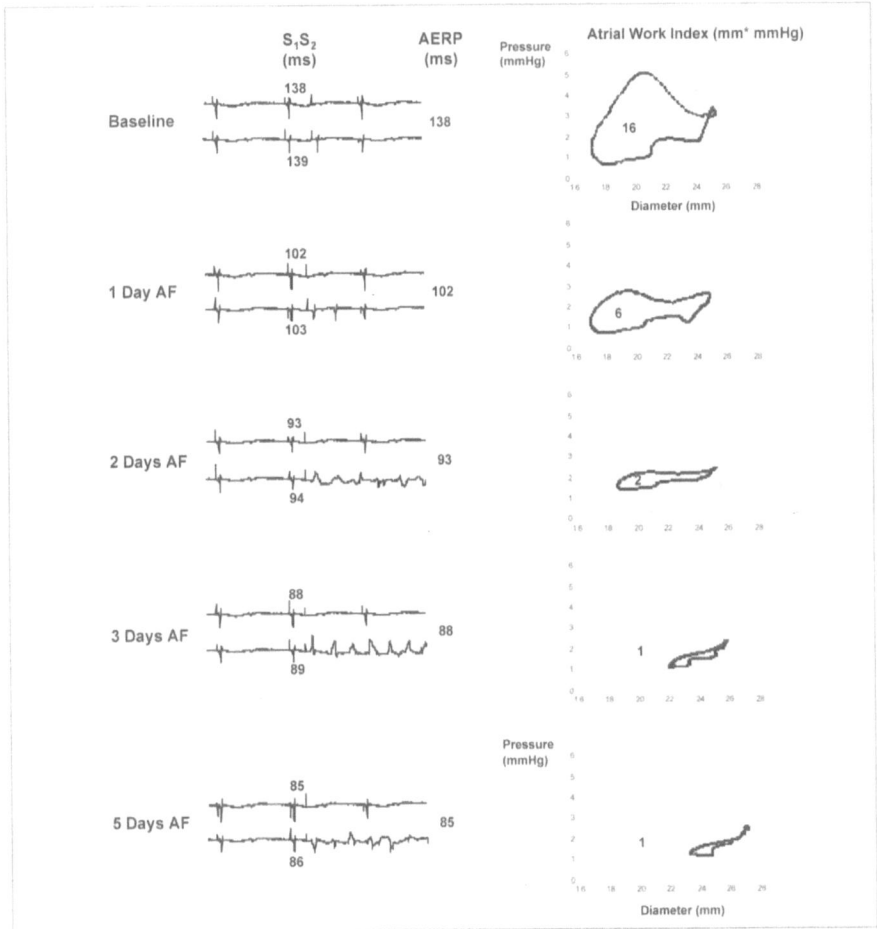

Fig. 2. Electrical and contractile remodeling of the atria during the first 5 days of AF. Pressure-diameter loops and atrial electrograms of a goat during slow atrial pacing at a cycle length of 400 ms. The refractory period (longest S₁S₂ interval failing to capture) shortened from 138 to 85 ms and the atrial work index (area enclosed by the pressure-diameter loop) declined from 16 to 1 mm mmHg

tory period from 138 ms to 85 ms during the first days of AF. Also, the strength of the atrial contractions declined. After only 2 days of AF the open pressure-diameter loop became closed, i.e., the atrial contractile function was nearly completely abolished. The atrial work index decreased from 16 mm mmHg to 2 mm mmHg and then remained constant until day 5. Also the reverse remodeling of the refractory period and the contractile function followed the same time course (Fig. 3). After 2 days of SR the open pressure-diameter loop had completely recovered and the refractory period increased from 85 ms to 133 ms. Obviously, the two phenomena are very closely linked and are probably due to the same underlying mechanism. Since the main cellular mechanism responsible for electrical remodeling is the reduction of I_{CaL}, it is reasonable to assume that the development of the atrial contractile dysfunction during the first 5 days of AF is also mainly caused by the reduction of the inward Ca^{2+} current.

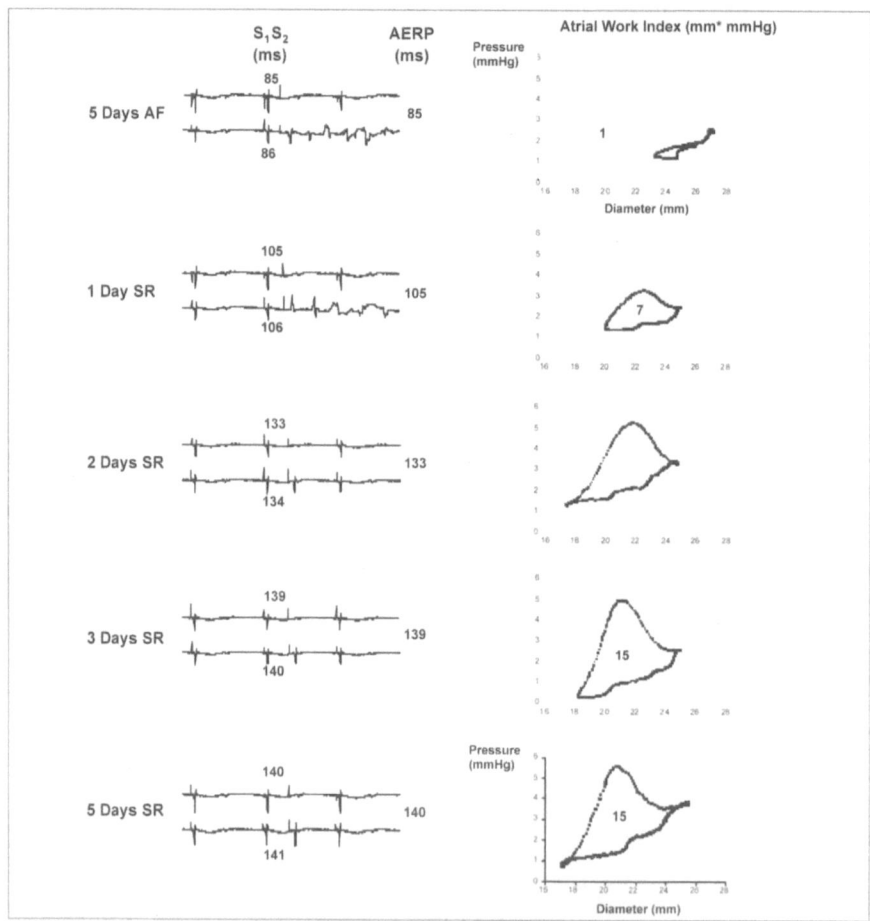

Fig. 3. Reverse electrical and contractile remodeling during the first 5 days after cardioversion. Pressure-diameter loops and atrial electrograms of a goat during slow atrial pacing at a cycle length of 400 ms. The refractory period and the contractile function recovered within 2-3 days of SR

Atrial Contractile Dysfunction in Patients with Chronic AF

Recent work has shown that in humans, too AF-induced electrical remodeling is reversible within a few days. This is true even after prolonged duration of AF (weeks to months) [15, 16]. By contrast, however, recovery of the contractile function after cardioversion in these patients takes weeks [3, 4]. This discrepancy strongly suggests that additional mechanisms beyond a reduction of I_{CaL} contribute to the contractile dysfunction of atrial myocardium in patients with chronic AF.

One possibility is that the observed atrial myolysis is the reason for the loss of contractility after chronic AF. Degradation and displacement of sarcomeres by glycogen has been described to occur during the first 1-4 months of AF [7]. The slow recovery of atrial contractility after cardioversion of chronic AF may reflect the resynthesis and reformation of sarcomeres. In a recent study we investigated the mechanism underlying the loss of force of contraction in isolated atrial trabeculae obtained from AF patients undergoing open chest surgery [17]. In these patients baseline contractile force was reduced by 75%

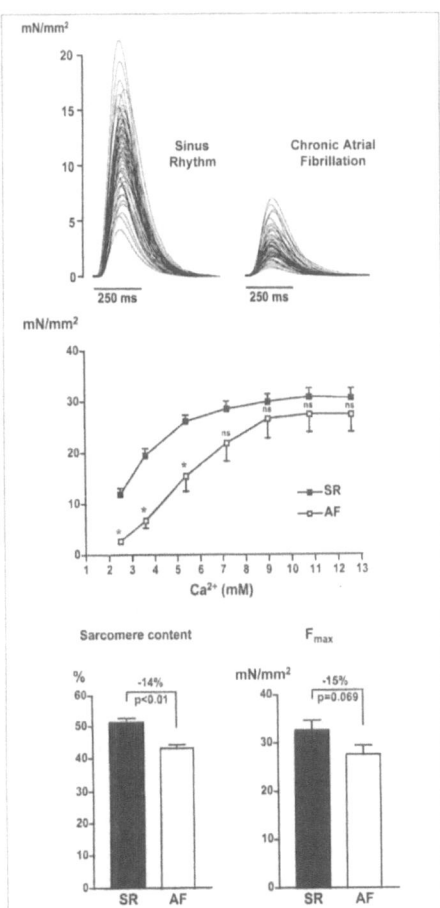

Fig. 4. Superimposed force recordings of isolated right atrial muscle preparations from 25 patients in SR (55 preparations) and from 22 AF patients (51 preparations) undergoing mitral valve surgery. In atrial myocardium of AF patients the force of contraction was reduced by ~75% (*top panel*). Increasing extracellular Ca^{2+} concentration elicited a strong positive inotropic effect in SR and AF preparations. In AF preparations the force of contraction at high Ca^{2+} concentrations was not lower than in SR preparations (*middle panel*). The sarcomere content and the contractile reserve (F_{max}, force of contraction at 10.8 mM Ca^{2+}) were equally reduced in AF preparations by 14%-15% (*bottom panel*).

(Fig. 4). An increase in extracellular Ca^{2+} concentration elicited a strong positive inotropic effect in both SR and AF patients and the contractile reserve (force of contraction at high $[Ca^{2+}]$) was reduced by only 15% in atrial myocardium of AF patients. Histological examination of the muscle bundles revealed that the degree of myolysis in the AF patients was limited. Only 14% of the sarcomeres had disappeared. Thus, structural changes (myolysis) can only partly explain the loss of atrial contractility. Dysfunction of the sarcoplasmic reticulum does not contribute to the AF-induced atrial contractile dysfunction either, since no alterations of the post-rest behavior of contractile force or the relaxation velocities of the muscle preparations were found. β-Adrenergic stimulation of contractile force was markedly impaired compared to the effect in SR patients. The reduced β-adrenergic response was due to an altered function and/or downregulation of the L-type Ca^{2+} channel which could be demonstrated by the loss of positive inotropic effect of the L-type Ca^{2+} channel agonist BayK8644. The loss of effect of BayK8644 emphasizes the key role of the L-type Ca^{2+} channel within the remodeling process, but on the other hand it might also mean that the direct spatial interaction between the L-type Ca^{2+} channel and the Ca^{2+} release channel of the SR is disturbed, as has been reported in an experimental model of heart failure [18]. A disturbed Ca^{2+} channel-ryanodine receptor interaction could provide a molecular basis for the delayed recovery of the contractile function following cardioversion. However, other potential contributors to the delayed recovery of the atrial function – such as dysfunction of the actin-myosin interaction – can certainly not been ruled out.

Clinical Relevance

Thromboembolism after cardioversion has been attributed to the dislodgement of a preformed atrial mural thrombus after the resumption of atrial contraction [19]. Although thromboembolic events often occur immediately after cardioversion, such events have been described several days to weeks after cardioversion in patients who have apparently maintained SR [20]. Indeed, transesophageal echocardiography studies have proven that new thrombus formation can also occur after cardioversion [5]. These findings emphasize the role of the atrial dysfunction in thrombus formation after cardioversion. Prevention of the atrial contractile dysfunction is therefore certainly desirable, but pharmacological tools to achieve this goal have so far only been shown to be effective during short episodes of AF. Some benefit in this respect was demonstrated with verapamil [8, 9] and the Na^+/H^+-exchange inhibitor HOE 642 [21]. So far, no therapeutic strategy exists for prevention of the atrial contractile dysfunction after prolonged AF, and anticoagulant therapy has to be continued after cardioversion for some time. In recent experiments we found that the force of contraction of isolated muscle preparations from patients with chronic AF could still be increased with the Ca^{2+} sensitizer EMD57033 at concentrations which could be administered clinically. This interesting finding might provide the basis of a new strategy to treat AF-induced atrial hypocontractility using positive inotropic agents. The intention of such a positive inotropic treatment would be to bridge the time span of depressed atrial function following cardioversion. This transient use of positive inotropic agents might provoke fewer side effects than the chronic use, e.g., in patients with heart failure. However, until such a treatment is established, early cardioversion within days and sufficient anticoagulant therapy are the only means of reducing the thromboembolic risk after cardioversion to SR.

References

1. Fatkin D, Kelly RP, Feneley MP (1994) Relations between left atrial appendage blood flow velocity, spontaneous echocardiographic contrast and thromboembolic risk in vivo. J Am Coll Cardiol 23:961-969
2. Wolf PA, Abbott RD, Kannel WB (1991) Atrial fibrillation as an independent risk factor for stroke: the Framingham Study. Stroke 22:983-988
3. Manning WJ, Silverman DI, Katz SE et al (1994) Impaired left atrial mechanical function after cardioversion: relation to the duration of atrial fibrillation. J Am Coll Cardiol 23:1535-1540
4. Manning WJ, Silverman DI, Katz SE et al (1995) Temporal dependence of the return of atrial mechanical function on the mode of cardioversion of atrial fibrillation to sinus rhythm. Am J Cardiol 75:624-626
5. Fatkin D, Kuchar DL, Thorburn CW, Feneley MP (1994) Transesophageal echocardiography before and during direct current cardioversion of atrial fibrillation: evidence for "atrial stunning" as a mechanism of thromboembolic complications. J Am Coll Cardiol 23:307-316
6. Grimm RA, Leung DY, Black IW et al (1995) Left atrial appendage "stunning" after spontaneous conversion of atrial fibrillation demonstrated by transesophageal Doppler echocardiography. Am Heart J 130:174-176
7. Ausma J, Wijffels M, Thone F et al (1997) Structural changes of atrial myocardium due to sustained atrial fibrillation in the goat. Circulation 96:3157-3163
8. Daoud EG, Marcovitz P, Knight BP et al (1999) Short-term effect of atrial fibrillation on atrial contractile function in humans. Circulation 99:3024-3027
9. Leistad E, Aksnes G, Verburg E, Christensen G (1996) Atrial contractile dysfunction after short-term atrial fibrillation is reduced by verapamil but increased by BAY K8644. Circulation 93:1747-1754
10. Sun H, Gaspo R, Leblanc N, Nattel S (1998) Cellular mechanisms of atrial contractile dysfunction caused by sustained atrial tachycardia. Circulation 98:719-727
11. Yue L, Feng J, Gaspo R et al (1997) Ionic remodeling underlying action potential changes in a canine model of atrial fibrillation. Circ Res 81:512-525
12. Van Wagoner DR, Pond AL, Lamorgese M et al (1999) Atrial L-type Ca^{2+} currents and human atrial fibrillation. Circ Res 85:428-436
13. Bosch RF, Zeng X, Grammer JB et al (1999) Ionic mechanisms of electrical remodeling in human atrial fibrillation. Cardiovasc Res 44:121-131
14. Wijffels MC, Kirchhof CJ, Dorland R, Allessie MA (1995) Atrial fibrillation begets atrial fibrillation. A study in awake chronically instrumented goats. Circulation 92:1954-1968

15. Hobbs WJ, Fynn S, Todd DM et al (2000) Reversal of atrial electrical remodeling after cardioversion of persistent atrial fibrillation in humans. Circulation 101:1145-1151
16. Yu WC, Lee SH, Tai CT et al (1999) Reversal of atrial electrical remodeling following cardioversion of long-standing atrial fibrillation in man. Cardiovasc Res 42:470-476
17. Schotten U, Ausma J, Stellbrink C et al (2001) Cellular mechanisms of depressed atrial contractility in patients with chronic atrial fibrillation. Circulation 103:691-698
18. Gomez AM, Valdivia HH, Cheng H et al (1997) Defective excitation-contraction coupling in experimental cardiac hypertrophy and heart failure. Science 276:800-806
19. Arnold AZ, Mick MJ, Mazurek RP et al (1992) Role of prophylactic anticoagulation for direct current cardioversion in patients with atrial fibrillation or atrial flutter. J Am Coll Cardiol 19:851-855
20. Resnekov L, McDonald L (1967) Complications in 220 patients with cardiac dysrhythmias treated by phased direct current shock, and indications for electroconversion. Br Heart J 29:926-936
21. Altemose GT, Zipes DP, Weksler J et al (2001) Inhibition of the Na^+/H^+ exchanger delays the development of rapid pacing-induced atrial contractile dysfunction. Circulation 103:762-768

"Lone" Atrial Fibrillation: How "Lone" Is It?

A.S. Montenero, D. Mangiameli, P. Franciosa, N. Bruno, A. Antonelli and F. Zumbo

Introduction

Among the varieties of supraventricular arrhythmias that confront electrophysiologists, atrial fibrillation (AF) is the most vexing. Not only is it extremely common, it is a progressive disorder that is often poorly controlled with antiarrhythmic medication and is associated with increased risk of cardiovascular morbidity and mortality. For this reason extensive efforts to cure AF are continuously ongoing even if the main goal of an effective treatment is still out of reach. At least in part, this may be due to both the heterogeneity of AF and our lack of complete understanding of the underlying electrophysiologic mechanisms.

Many different clinical situations lead to AF, so the electrophysiologic substrate may vary continuously as a consequence of this different pathophysiology. So far "lone AF" has been considered as a clinical situation in which there was no detectable heart disease, a pure form of electrical disease based on an unknown electrophysiologic mechanism. More recently, new concepts have been proposed that provide new insight into the initiation and perpetuation of AF that may help to explain this form of paroxysmal lone AF.

Anatomopathology of AF

AF has multiple disparate etiologies; conventionally associated with multiple organic heart disease, it may nevertheless occur in patients with no clinically evident abnormalities (lone AF). The higher incidence of AF in hypertensive, dilated, hypertrophic, ischemic or valvular patients can be explained by the presence of significant atrial enlargement and a high degree of atrial fibrosis, ranging from scattered foci to diffuse involvement [1]. For the idiopathic forms of AF, so far various pathological factors have been suggested, such as myocarditis [2], adipose replacement [3], and imbalance of autonomic tone [3].

Unità Operativa di Cardiologia, Policlinico MultiMedica, Sesto S.Giovanni, Milan, Italy

How Lone Is the AF?

The history of electrophysiologic intervention shows many examples where a cycle of clinical science and new interventional techniques is demonstrated. We start with a given hypothesis of arrhythmia mechanism or substrate; we intervene to alter what we believe to be the substrate (with surgery or catheter ablation); in the process of intervention we have an opportunity to garner further, more accurate insights into the mechanism and substrate and to develop subsets of what we thought was a single disorder, and this in turn allows us to develop better interventional tools and techniques. For example, all regular narrow complex tachycardias used to go by the moniker of "PAT". First with surgery and then with catheter ablation, we are now able to discern that "PAT" may actually be one of several specific arrhythmia substrates such as WPW, AV nodal reentry etc. Thus, our ability to intervene in patients with AF has begun to allow us to develop more detailed descriptions of mechanisms: AF as such may come to be recognized as the common surface manifestation of multiple potential mechanisms. At present, we can consider AF as having two mechanisms: one for perpetuation of multiple reentry loops [5], and one for initiation of the arrhythmia. The majority of investigative researches have focused on what is needed for maintenance of AF [6], but might it not be worth examining in addition what leads to its initiation? Studying transient events such as the spontaneous initiation of an arrhythmia is by its nature more difficult than studying the steady-state phenomenon, but in the case of AF, improving our knowledge of its initiation may help to identify a truly curative approach which targets the initiating event rather than the substrate of maintenance.

Is So-Called Focal AF the true "lone" AF?

For many years, electrophysiologic studies on AF have been limited to ongoing AF. However, as mentioned above, initiation is a very critical phase, both for our understanding and for the treatment of AF. Only recently has a new entity of AF been described: so-called "focal AF", which is electrophysiologically based on a sort of discharging foci triggering a rapid form of atrial tachycardia that leads to AF. From the pathologic point of view these foci are predominant in the pulmonary veins (in particular the left superior) and may be related to the presence of myocardial muscular sleeves that surround the orifices with variable extension. It has been demonstrated that atrial premature beats that initiate paroxysmal AF originate in the pulmonary veins in 94% of cases [7]. They trigger AF with bursts of rapid discharges and respond to local RF catheter ablation. The mechanism (abnormal automaticity versus microreentry versus triggered activity) is unknown and varying responses to different provocative maneuvers provide no further insights, so why pulmonary veins become arrhythmogenic is still unclear. The recorded spikes in the pulmonary veins reflect the physiologic activation of the muscular bands extending from the left atrium to the venous wall with complex pathways [8].

The pulmonary vein foci exhibited unique characteristics including deep venous origin, unpredictable firing, and complex delayed conduction to the left atrium with ectopic beats confined to the vein. This complex electrophysiologic behavior matches the complex anatomy of the surrounding venous muscular bands.

Based on these new electrophysiological insights, to define frequent paroxysmal AF in an apparently normal heart as "lone" may be sometimes misleading; in fact, although there is growing evidence that *something happens* around or within the pulmonary vein orifice, either in terms of anatomy or of pathophysiology, the electrophysiologic substrate is still not completely clear. Thus, even if the pulmonary vein triggers the majority of paroxysmal AF, other electrical disorders may also result in AF, such as atrial flutter or some sort of atrial tachycardia.

Therefore, based on certain clinical characteristics of this particular population of patients with a history of recurrent AF and a large number of atrial premature beats and atrial tachycardia documented by 24-h Holter recordings, we argue that so-called lone AF may be a sort of rapid atrial tachycardia that desynchronizes the atria, resulting in an electrocardiographic form of paroxysmal AF.

Conclusions

When dealing with frequent paroxysmal AF, we should investigate for any form of other atrial tachycardia before concluding the presence of "lone AF".

References

1. Ohtani K, Yutani C, Nagata S et al (1995) High prevalence of atrial fibrosis in patients with dilated cardiomyopathy. J Am Coll Cardiol 25:1162-1169
2. Frustaci A, Chimenti C, Bellocci F et al (1997) Histological substrate of atrial biopsies in patients with lone atrial fibrillation. Circulation 96:1180-1184
3. Guiraudon CM (1992) The pathology of intractable primary atrial fibrillation. Pacing Clin Electrophysiol 15:I-662 (abstr)
4. Coumel P (1994) Paroxysmal atrial fibrillation: role of the autonomic nervous system. Arch Mal Coeur Vaiss 87:55-62
5. Alessie MA, Lammers WJEP, Bonke FIM, Hollen J (1985) Experimental evaluation of Moe's multiple wavelet hypothesis of atrial fibrillation. In: Zipes DP, Jalife J (eds) Cardiac arrhythmias. Grune & Stratton, New York, pp 265-276
6. Ausma J, Wijffels M, Thone F et al (1997) Structural changes of atrial myocardium due to sustained atrial fibrillation in the goat. Circulation 96:3157-3163
7. Haïssaguerre M, Jaïs P, Shah DC et al (1998) Spontaneous initiation of atrial fibrillation by ectopic beats originating in the pulmonary veins. N Engl J Med 339:659-666
8. Zipes DP, Knope RF (1972) Electrical properties of the thoracic veins. Am J Cardiol 29:372-376

Focal Atrial Fibrillation: Which Clinical/Electrocardiographic Pattern?

D. C. Shah, M. Haïssaguerre, P. Jaïs, M. Hocini, T. Yamane, L. Macle, K.-J. Choi
and Jacques Clémenty

It has been shown that paroxysms of atrial fibrillation (AF) are consistently initiated by trains of spontaneous activity, originating in the majority of patients from the pulmonary veins (PVs). This spontaneous activity, much like programmed stimulation, is responsible for the transformation of sinus rhythm into AF.

However, spontaneous activity arising from the PVs (or other nonPV foci) can produce a range of different types of atrial arrhythmias [1]. Single discharges manifest as isolated extrasystoles, repetitive discharges with long cycle lengths manifest as an automatic rhythm (sometimes mimicking sinus rhythm, but with a different P wave), while shorter cycles result in organized monomorphic tachycardia or a pattern of focal "flutter". At short cycle lengths an ECG pattern of focal AF is produced, i.e. a rapid and irregular tachycardia without discrete P waves [2]. Sudden variations (up to 350 ms beat to beat) in the cycle length are the most characteristic pattern for a focal mechanism. Thus, a single arrhythmogenic focus may represent the sole abnormality in a few patients in whom the focus discharges for long periods (focal AF).

Our series now includes 16 patients with "focal AF" in whom a rapid atrial tachycardia mimicking AF has been cured by discrete RF ablation of the focus. These patients are young (40 ± 8 years) and without structural heart disease. Depending on the focus rate, the ECG tracings documented AF as well as monomorphic and irregular atrial tachycardia and extrasystoles of the same morphology. The ablation site was determined on the basis of earliest bipolar activity relative to a stable atrial electrogram reference during AF and, if the rate was slow enough to allow P wave identification on the surface ECG, the earliest bipolar activities relative to the P wave onset. Mapping during different types of atrial arrhythmia showed that they were due to the same focus firing irregularly. Long cycle lengths were responsible for the surface ECG morphology of organized monomorphic tachycardia or "focal" flutter, whereas at short cycle lengths (160-130 ms) an ECG pattern of AF was observed. Flecainide infusion (0.5-1 mg/kg) was found to facilitate mapping and ablation of the arrhyth-

Hôpital Cardiologique du Haut-Lévêque, Pessac, France

mia by slowing its rate. Focal AF suspected on the surface ECG was confirmed by endocardial mapping, showing a centrifugal and consistant activation of the atrium spreading from the focus. In most patients, the atrial activity during AF was organized (similar to type I AF). This is probably due to the fact that the atria of those patients are able to follow the very high rate imposed by the focus. In some patients, this daily paroxysmal AF could be traced back more than ten years without any evolution to a more disorganized AF (similar to type III) or to more persistent AF [3]. Four foci were found to be located in the right atrium: two near the sinus node, one at the ostium of the coronary sinus and one in the right appendage. All others were located in the left atrium: at the ostium of the right superior pulmonary vein [4] or right inferior pulmonary vein [5], and at the ostium of the left superior pulmonary vein [6] one patient had 2 foci. They were ablated with a mean of 5 ± 4 RF pulses; three had a clinically documented recurrence 7 days (two patients) and 20 days (one patient) after an initially successful procedure. Two of them underwent a definitively successful second ablation procedure. The third patient had, in fact, only one episode of arrhythmia, which never recurred subsequently with a follow-up of 1 year without antiarrhythmic drugs. A relatively normal atrial substrate was indicated by noninducibility (> 3 min) of sustained atrial arrhythmias after ablation in 12 patients, despite an agressive biatrial pacing protocol. When a young patient, usually without structural heart disease, presents with very frequent episodes of intermittent AF along with episodes of an irregular atrial tachycardia and monomorphic atrial extrasystoles, an electrophysiological study at the time of spontaneous episodes of arrhythmia is mandatory and frequently allows successful ablation.

More commonly, a short train of focal discharges trigger episodes of AF that subsequently continue independently of the initiating event (focally initiated AF) [1, 2, 7]. True intracardiac AF is initiated when the focus abruptly discharges in a very rapid train of impulses with a cycle length of 182 ± 57 ms (330 beats/min), leading to chaotic and practically unmappable atrial activity, which therefore cannot be linked to the PVs [1]. "Focal AF" includes only the small subset of AF patients in whom the focus discharges for long periods, while in actual fact, virtually 100% of paroxysmal AF - with or without ambient or isolated ectopy, with or without structural heart disease - have focal origins that can be targeted for ablation. These foci have a characteristically predominant anatomic location in the PVs, and unusual properties, including long conduction time to the left atrium (LA), unpredictable firing, and frequent occurrence of focal discharges confined within the vein. Less commonly, triggers originate from other veins (superior vena cava, ligament of Mashall, coronary sinus) or atrial tissue, notably the posterior LA [7, 3, 8-13]

In the clinical setting, paroxysms are frequently (although not always) preceded by isolated extrasystoles from the same source as the initiating trigger of AF. In instances where these extrasystoles are not evident, they may be blocked in the AV node and masked by the previous ST-T segment; or the extrasystolic activity may not capture the atrium, or each discharge(s) may directly trigger AF. Initiation of common atrial flutter, its degeneration into AF or its interruption are also frequently the result of PV discharges [14]. The first ectopic P wave – whether isolated or initiating AF – characteristically has a coupling interval that results in superimposition on the T wave of the previous QRS complex, producing a P-on-T pattern recognizable at first sight.

During an ablation procedure, any focus resulting in P-on-T ectopy is considered a target for ablation, even without documentation of its role in AF initiation, because when these foci are spared, the great majority of patients develop recurrences of AF originating from the unablated focus, requiring a new ablation session [15].

When one focus is identified, we cannot be sure that there is no other quiescent focus or foci that will be responsible for the recurrence of AF despite successful ablation of the targeted focus. One approach to identify all potential arrhythmogenic sources could be the use of 12 lead Holter recordings in order to analyze all the extrasystolic P wave morphologies inducing AF. The infrequent and variable manifestation of all foci mandates prolonged monitoring and analysis is compounded by difficulty in identifying the exact extrasystolic P wave morphology.

Another approach is to study the PV potentials recorded in sinus rhythm or during coronary sinus or left atrial appendage pacing. A careful analysis of the activity can be useful to discriminate normal vs arrhythmogenic pulmonary veins, notably in the absence of spontaneous or provocable arrhythmia. For this purpose, we studied the PV electrograms of 19 patients with drug-resistant paroxysmal AF and compared them to those of 19 age- and-sex matched control patients without AF and PV ectopy [17].

Different parameters were studied, including the duration from the atrial farfield to the local PV potential, the complexity of PV activity (number of high frequency deflections) and timing with respect to farfield atrial activity. Conduction times were also measured in sinus rhythm between the farfield atrial component and the local PV potential, as well as the conduction time during ectopy, spontaneous or mechanically provoked (for control patients).

Interestingly, PV potentials were recorded in 78% of PVs in controls and 87% in patients (p = NS), demonstrating a similar prevalence of muscular sleeves in PVs. However, the PVs activity was more complex (2.15 ± 0.8 vs 1.65 ± 0.78 PVP deflections, p = 0.01) and occurred later (terminal PVP = 69% vs 15%) in sinus rhythm in AF patients vs controls. The PV potential was superimposed with the atrial farfield potential in 19% in patients vs 84% in controls. The conduction times during ectopy were also significantly longer, suggesting anisotropic conduction in the arrhythmogenic veins in AF patients. The recording of a significantly late PV potential was found to be specific for arrhythmogenic veins.

Clinical Implications

Based on the above data, young patients without significant or severe structural heart disease and short incessant paroxysms of AF have a trigger-dominant arrhythmia, dependent on a usually single rapidly firing source for both initiation and maintenance. Typically the frequency of attacks permits ready documentation on 12 lead ECG, and these patients are excellent candidates for ablation of the triggering focus. Ablation characteristically terminates arrhythmia and renders it noninducible: nearly always a single focus, most frequently of intraPV or PV ostial origin, is documented. Particularly for intraPV foci, disconnection of the PV is easier and more effective than the latter strategy which may be more useful for ostial and nonPV foci. The medium-term follow-up is usually excellent.

The typical middle-aged male with paroxysms of longer-lasting AF (> 6-12 h), however, has multiple triggers – from more than one PV in most and additional nonPV foci in about one third. Paroxysms lasting days or even longer suggest marked substrate dominance – implying both widespread atrial remodeling as well as multiple triggers, including a significantly higher incidence of nonPV foci.

These patients should undergo disconnection of all four PVs and thereafter mapping and ablation of nonPV foci. Though the exact reasons are unclear, nonPV foci become manifest nearly always after PV ablation and their successful ablation is a major determinant of procedural success. In most situations, outcome after ablation can be readily appreciated by symptoms, prolonged telemetric monitoring, successive Holter recordings and stress tests. It is possible, however, that totally asymptomatic and short-lasting AF paroxysms may be missed, based on this form of assessment. Pacemaker memory switching may be a useful monitoring device in such a situation and a suitable implantable or portable device with a sufficiently large memory is required to definitely assess this question.

References

1. Haïssaguerre M, Jaïs P, Shah DC et al (1998) Spontaneous initiation of atrial fibrillation by ectopic beats originating in the pulmonary veins. N Engl J Med 339:659-666
2. Jaïs P, Haïssaguerre M, Shah DC et al (1997) A focal source of atrial fibrillation treated by discrete radiofrequency ablation. Circulation 95:572-576
3. Wharton JM, Vergara I, Shander G (1998) Identificaton and ablation of focal mechanisms of atrial fibrillation. Circulation 98(17):1-18 (abstr)
4. Cox JL, Boineau JP, Schuessler RB et al (1993) Five year experience with the Maze procedure for atrial fibrillation. Ann Thorac Surg 56:814-824
5. Wellens HJJ (1984) Atrial fibrillation, the last big hurdle in treating supraventricular tachycardia. N Engl J Med 331:944-945
6. Cox JL, Canavan TE, Schuessler RB et al (1991) The surgical treatment of atrial fibrillation II: intraoperative electrophysiologic mapping and description of the electrophysiologic basis of atrial flutter and fibrillation. J Thorac Cardiovasc Surg 101:406-426
7. Haïssaguerre M, Marcus FI, Fischer B, Clémenty J (1994) Radiofrequency catheter ablation in unusual mechanisms of atrial fibrillation: report of three cases. J Cardiovasc Electrophysiol 5:743-751

8. Chen SA, Tai CT, Yu WC (1999) Right atrial focal atrial fibrillation: electrophysiologic characteristics and radiofrequency catheter ablation. J Cardiovasc Electrophysiol 10:328-335

9. Chen SA, Hsieh MH, Tai CT (1999) Initiation of atrial fibrillation by ectopic beats originating from the pulmonary veins: electrophysiologic characteristics, pharmacologic responses, and effects of radiofrequency ablation. Circulation 100:1879-1886

10. Hwang C, Karagueuzian HS, Chen PS (1999) Idiopathic paroxysmal atrial fibrillation induced by a focal discharge mechanism in the left superior pulmonary vein: possible roles of the ligament of Marshall. J Cardiovasc Electrophysiol 10:636-648

11. Lau CP, Tse HF, Ayers GM (1999) Defibrillation-guided radiofrequency ablation of atrial fibrillation secondary to an atrial focus. J Am Coll Cardiol 33:1217-1226

12. Chen SA, Tai CT, Tsai CF et al (2000) Radiofrequency catheter ablation of atrial fibrillation initiated by pulmonary vein ectopic beats. J Cardiovasc Electrophysiol 11:218-227

13. Tsai CF, Tai CT, Hsieh MH et al (2000) Initiations of atrial fibrillation by ectopic beats originating from the superior vena cava: electrophysiological characteristics and results of radiofrequency ablation. Circulation 102:67-74

14. Shah DC, Haïssaguerre M, Jaïs P et al (1999) Atrial flutter: contemporary electrophysiology and catheter ablation. Pacing Clin Electrophysiol 22:344-359

15. Haïssaguerre M, Jaïs P, Shah DC et al (2000) Electrophysiological end point for catheter ablation of atrial fibrillation initiated from multiple pulmonary venous foci. Circulation 101:1409-1417

16. Shah DC, Jaïs P, Takahashi A et al (1999) Pulmonary vein electrogram from patients with focally initiated atrial fibrillation and controls. Pacing Clin Electrophysiol 22(II):709 (abstr)

17. Robbins IM, Colvin EV, Doyle TP et al (1998) Pulmonary vein stenosis after catheter ablation of atrial fibrillation. Circulation 98:1769-1775

Atrial Fibrillation Complicated by Heart Failure: First the Chicken or First the Egg?

G. Boriani[1], M. Biffi[1], C. Martignani[1], P. Bartolini[2], M. Gallina[1], C. Rapezzi[1] and A. Branzi[1]

Introduction

The hemodynamic consequences of atrial fibrillation (AF) are related to loss of atrial contribution to cardiac output, increase in heart rate, with shortening in the duration of diastole, and irregularity in diastolic intervals. The loss of atrial contribution to ventricular filling may be well tolerated in a healthy heart but may have adverse consequences in the presence of left ventricular dysfunction. Loss of atrial transport is particularly significant if there is impairment in left ventricular filling due to reduced diastolic compliance or mitral stenosis. Moreover, in patients of this kind, a high or irregular heart rate with frequent short diastolic intervals will be poorly tolerated. In the long term, sustained, uncontrolled tachycardia with a heart rate higher than 120 beats/min leads to impairment of left ventricular function with various degrees of ventricular dysfunction, which may result in significant worsening of the patient's clinical condition unless the heart rate can be controlled or sinus rhythm restored. This clinical condition has been called "tachycardiomyopathy" or "tachycardia-induced cardiomyopathy" [1-6].

AF and congestive heart failure are two common cardiac diseases, affecting 1%-2% of the population [7, 8] with a prevalence that rises steeply with age. AF and congestive heart failure have risk factors in common and frequently coexist [9]. The prevalence of left ventricular dysfunction and/or congestive heart failure among patients with AF may be up to 40% [10], and in the Framingham Study the presence of congestive heart failure implied a 6.6-fold increased risk of developing AF in a 2-year period. On the other side, the strong association between AF and congestive heart failure is reinforced by the high prevalence of AF found in major heart failure trials dealing with more advanced New York Heart Association (NYHA) functional class [9].

In clinical practice the relationship between AF and congestive heart failure or left ventricular dysfunction is intriguing. AF may in fact cause congestive

[1]Institute of Cardiology, University of Bologna, Italy; [2]Biomedical Engineering Laboratory, Istituto Superiore di Sanità, Rome, Italy

heart failure, particularly when there is a fast, uncontrolled ventricular response. This form of congestive heart failure may be reversible after rhythm or rate control [4]. At first observation of the patient it may be quite difficult to distinguish this condition from the more common phenomenon of AF facilitated by the mechanical, electrophysiological, and neurohormonal derangements caused by heart failure in a substrate characterized by primary ventricular dilation and ipokinesia.

Tachycardia-Induced Cardiomyopathy

The knowledge that incessant or chronic tachyarrhythmias may lead to reversible ventricular dysfunction is the result of a series of clinical observations and, in the last 10 years, of a focused interest that has produced clear experimental and clinical evidence.

In the 1930s some clinical observations documented complete resolution of congestive heart failure after cardioversion of AF to sinus rhythm [4, 5]. Later some authors reported that the pattern of dilated cardiomyopathy associated with AF with fast ventricular response was reversible when rate and rhythm control was obtained [1, 4]. Reversible cardiomyopathy was also described in cases treated medically or surgically for incessant atrial tachycardia, accessory pathway reciprocating tachycardia, or atrioventricular nodal re-entry tachycardia [2, 3]. The common findings in these observations were a chronic high heart rate (more than 120 beats/min) due to a persistent or permanent supraventricular arrhythmia, a clinical picture of dilated cardiomyopathy with congestive heart failure, and reversibility of this condition after the underlying arrhythmia had been treated or, at least, had been achieved adequate rate control [2-4].

Experimental Models of Tachycardia-Induced Cardiomyopathy

The first experimental model of tachycardia-induced cardiomyopathy was described by Whipple et al. in 1962 [11]. The models allow study of both the effects of chronic rapid pacing on ventricular function and the recovery phase associated with discontinuance of rapid pacing, mimicking the development and treatment of tachycardia-induced cardiomyopathy in humans. The most commonly used animals are pigs and dogs undergoing atrial or ventricular pacing at chronic rates of 210-240 beats/min for durations of 3-6 weeks [6]. Chronic pacing tachycardia results in progressive severe biventricular systolic and diastolic dysfunction over a 3- to 4-week period. Pacing at a slower rate or for a shorter duration results in a lesser degree of ventricular dysfunction.

The main hemodynamic changes observed in animal models are [5]: (1) markedly elevated ventricular filling pressures; (2) severe impairment of left ventricular (up to 55% reduction) and right ventricular systolic function; (3) severe reduction in cardiac output; (4) increase in left ventricular systolic wall stress; (5) reduction in intrinsic myocardial contractility; (6) impairment of intrinsic myocardial relaxation; (7) diminished cardiac sympathetic responsiveness; and (8) development of moderate mitral regurgitation.

Moreover, as in other forms of severe heart failure, the impairment in ventricular function is associated with intense neurohormonal activation [6]. In the early phases of ventricular dysfunction development, an increase in plasma catecholamines occurs, followed by a plateau associated with defects in the β-receptor transduction system. Elevation of atrial natriuretic peptide (ANP) is observed in the early phases but is followed by a depletion of the same in later stages. Activation of the systemic renin-angiotensin system does not occur until the later stages of left ventricular dysfunction progression. Endothelin increase, too, is detected only in the late stages of ventricular dysfunction.

In tachycardia-induced cardiomyopathy a series of cardiac structural changes occurs [5]. Left ventricular dilation is more marked for end-systolic than end-diastolic volumes and produces a spherical chamber geometry. This profound cardiac dilation is accompanied by right and left ventricular wall thinning or preservation of wall thickness without hypertrophy. A differential response between the ventricles has been demonstrated, with evidence of pacing-induced right ventricular hypertrophy without associated left ventricular hypertrophy. On the cellular level, both myocyte and extracellular matrix remodeling have been documented, with disruption of the extracellular matrix, altered myocyte alignment, myocyte loss, cellular elongation, fibril disalignment, and loss of sarcomeres [5]. In an experimental model [12], the extent of remodeling included a 39% loss of myocytes and a 61% increase in volume of remaining myocytes.

The development and recovery of hemodynamic impairment has a typical chronology of onset and recovery. After 24 h of rapid pacing, systemic arterial pressure and cardiac output are reduced. With longer pacing durations, cardiac filling and pulmonary artery pressures increase and systemic arterial pressures decrease, with a plateau at 1 week. Cardiac output, ejection fraction, and cardiac volumes may progressively deteriorate for up to 3-5 weeks, with development of end-stage heart failure [5].

The recovery from pacing-induced heart failure is the proof that the myopathic process associated with rapid heart rates is largely reversible. Within 48 h after termination of pacing, right atrial and mean arterial pressures, cardiac index, and systemic vascular resistance approach control levels [5, 13]. Left ventricular ejection fraction shows significant recovery by 24-48 h and normalizes after 1-2 weeks. Within 4 weeks, all hemodynamic variables return to control levels; yet end-systolic and end-diastolic volumes remain elevated at 12 weeks after termination of pacing, a finding indicating extensive ventricular remodeling. Diastolic dysfunction remains measurable 4 weeks after pacing [14]. Interestingly, left ventricular hypertrophy develops in the 4 weeks after discontinuance of pacing, and can be related to either the inability to respond to triggers for hypertrophy during pacing itself or to a compensatory remodeling [5].

The precise mechanisms responsible for the contractile dysfunction and structural changes of pacing-induced cardiomyopathy are not known. The following factors have been considered as causally related to the development of cardiac dysfunction [5, 6, 13]: (1) myocardial energy depletion and impaired energy utilization; (2) myocardial ischemia; (3) abnormalities of cardiac calcium regulation; and (4) myocyte and extracellular matrix remodeling. In fact, it is not known whether these factors have a causal role or are merely a secondary effect of pacing.

Tachycardia-Induced Cardiomyopathy in Humans

The effect of treating AF with fast ventricular response on cardiac function has been preliminarily investigated in studies dealing with the following treatments: (1) cardioversion to sinus rhythm; (2) pharmacologic ventricular rate control; and (3) atrioventricular junction ablation and permanent ventricular pacing.

The study of conversion of AF to sinus rhythm provides information on changes associated with the resumption of atrial contraction and atrioventricular synchrony. Van Gelder et al. [15] showed that electrical cardioversion of AF was associated with a discrepancy in the time course of recovery of atrial systole and ventricular function. Although the atrial contribution to ventricular filling normalized within 1 week after cardioversion, left ventricular ejection fraction continued to increase beyond that time, reaching peak values after 1 month. It was noteworthy that the increase in peak oxygen consumption was parallel to the increase in ejection fraction.

In recent years a relatively new technique, internal low energy cardioversion, has been employed for patients with chronic persistent AF [16-19]. This technique can restore sinus rhythm in patients refractory to conventional transthoracic cardioversion and may also be effective in patients with longstanding AF [18]. With internal cardioversion, the indications to restore sinus rhythm can be potentially widened to patients refractory to external cardioversion [19]. In a recent study [20], restoration of sinus rhythm by internal cardioversion in a group of patients with structural heart disease and persistent AF with normal ventricular response resulted in an improvement in cardiac performance that occurred later than recovery of left atrial mechanical function. This finding supports the suggestion that some forms of reversible occult myocardial dysfunction are associated with AF.

The effect of heart rate control alone on ventricular function, independently of atrioventricular synchrony, has been studied through the use of atrioventricular junction ablation and implantation of a VVIR pacemaker [21-23]. These studies have provided preliminary evidence that benefit can clearly occur without atrioventricular synchrony in patients with initial rapid ventricular responses, despite paced ventricular activation from the right ventricular apex. In patients with drug-refractory AF and mildly depressed ventricular function, rate control by radiofrequency atrioventricular junction ablation and implantation of a VVIR pacemaker induced a modest but significant increase in left ventricular ejection fraction without a significant change in treadmill exercise time [21]. In a series of 23 patients with AF and ventricular rates above 100 beats/min at rest, NYHA functional class and exercise time improved significantly with atrioventricular junction ablation and VVIR pacing [22]. Subgroup analysis demonstrated that in patients with decreased left ventricular systolic function, fractional shortening increased, whereas in subjects with normal baseline left ventricular systolic function, fractional shortening decreased significantly. Therefore, treatment of patients with AF can be considered as a balance between the benefits of rate control versus the possible deleterious hemodynamic effects of right ventricular pacing. In some cases, moderate to severe mitral regurgitation was observed in the follow-up of patients submitted to atrioventricular junction ablation and VVIR pacemaker implantation.

In patients who do not undergo junction ablation, the irregularity of AF despite "controlled" ventricular rates may contribute to ventricular dysfunction. This point is supported by the observation that atrioventricular junction ablation may improve symptoms, quality of life and left ventricular dysfunction even in patients with AF and "normal" ventricular response [24, 25].

In clinical practice a significant problem is the evaluation of patients with "chronic" AF with high ventricular rates and ventricular dysfunction: in several cases it remains unclear at first observation whether a left ventricular dysfunction results from chronic high rates or merely represents aggravation of a coexisting cardiomyopathy. This "chicken-egg dilemma" [3] has important practical implications because all the therapeutic possibilities currently available, including atrioventricular node radiofrequency ablation, are indicated to control ventricular rate in cases of tachycardia-induced cardiomyopathy. Proof that ventricular dysfunction is secondary to high ventricular rates may be obtained in the individual case only by treating the tachycardia [26]. However, complete reversal of a clinical picture of congestive heart failure has been reported [4] for patients with left ventricular dysfunction initially believed to have idiopathic dilated cardiomyopathy.

The diagnosis of tachycardiomyopathy remains a difficult issue in clinical practice. It may be suspected in the presence of coexisting chronic AF and left ventricular dysfunction when cardiac performance improves following rate control or rhythm control. In fact, even a lack of improvement does not prove that a tachycardiomyopathy component was not present, since it may reflect an advanced stage of irreversible tachycardia-related myocardial injury [26, 27]. The extent of regression of ventricular dysfunction with rate control depends on several factors and may be total, partial, or absent. An even more intriguing issue is the possibility that a tachycardiomyopathy component may exist in patients with heart failure dependent on a specific substrate but associated with AF with fast ventricular response. In these cases a vicious circle may develop with heart failure, facilitating AF with subsequent worsening of cardiac function by a rate-related mechanism. This condition facilitates arrhythmia persistence and atrial dilation.

Apart from clear cases of tachycardiomyopathy secondary to AF, there is also the possibility that AF may have a subtle long-term deleterious effect on left ventricular function [27]. In the V-HeFT II study [28] patients with AF had a significant decline in peak oxygen consumption compared with patients in sinus rhythm starting after 2 years of follow-up. A subtle form of cardiomyopathy secondary to chronic AF may be related to a series of factors including: (1) heart rate controlled at rest but disproportionately high (>120 beats/min) during minor exercise such as normal daily activity [27]; (2) lack of physiological rate response during daily activity; and (3) irregularity of ventricular cycle during AF. Patients with already impaired left ventricular function and with excessive sympathetic activation may be particularly prone to such a possible mechanism. The true prevalence of these forms of occult or latent tachycardiomyopathy among patients with chronic persistent AF is unknown, but a series of observation suggests that it is not negligible [23, 26-28].

The complex interplay between AF and congestive heart failure is also emphasized by the detrimental impact of AF on prognosis in patients with left ventricular dysfunction. In the SOLVD trial the presence of AF at baseline was a powerful independent predictor of pump failure death and rehospitalization for heart failure, and this adverse impact was independent of resting heart rate [29]. The latter finding suggests that the observed association between AF and progression of left ventricular dysfunction is not simply due to increased heart rate at rest (a "tachycardiomyopathy" component of left ventricular dysfunction) but is probably linked to other determinants of hemodynamic impairment such as RR variability. Recently [24, 25] an improvement in left ventricular function was demonstrated following atrioventricular model ablation even in patients with AF with normal "ventricular rate", suggesting that correction of RR interval irregularity may have positive implications for hemodynamics, symptoms, and quality of life.

Conclusions

Tachycardia-induced cardiomyopathy is now a well-recognized clinical entity, which emphasizes the complex interplay between AF and congestive heart failure. However, despite a large number of experimental studies, some important points still need to be clarified in clinical practice: (1) the minimum rate and duration of tachycardia required to induce ventricular dysfunction are unknown; (2) we do not know what factors modulate the predisposition to develop a tachycardia-induced cardiomyopathy and whether this disease is genetically influenced, as could be suspected on the basis of the different individual sensitivities to the adverse effects of a chronic high rate; (3) in the management of patients with stable AF and ventricular dysfunction, the optimum rates to be achieved at rest and during exercise have not been defined; (4) we do not know what role is played by RR irregularity, as a concurrent factor independent of heart rate, in developing the hemodynamic derangement of AF; and (5) the characterization of patients with pure reversible tachycardia-induced cardiomyopathy and their differentiation from other patients with dilated cardiomyopathy is really difficult a priori and constitutes the so-called "chicken-egg dilemma".

Until more precise clinical data from prospective controlled studies are available, rate control and rhythm control should be pursued in all patients with a clinical picture of unrecognized and unexplained ventricular dysfunction coupled with AF at relatively fast ventricular response. All the pharmacological and nonpharmacological treatments currently available can be considered for this purpose.

References

1. Peters KG, Kienzle MG (1988) Severe cardiomyopathy due to chronic rapidly conduced atrial fibrillation: complete recovery after restoration of sinus rhythm. Am J Med 85:242-244
2. Packer DL, Bardy GH, Worley SJ et al (1986) Tachycardia-induced cardiomyopathy: a reversible form of left ventricular dysfunction. Am J Cardiol 57:563-570
3. Gallagher JJ (1985) Tachycardia and cardiomyopathy: the chicken-egg dilemma revisited. J Am Coll Cardiol 6:1172-1173
4. Grogan M, Smith HC, Gersh BJ, Wood DL (1992) Left ventricular dysfunction due to atrial fibrillation in patients initially believed to have idiopathic dilated cardiomyopathy. Am J Cardiol 69:1570-1573
5. Shinbane JS, Wood MA, Jensen DN et al (1997) Tachycardia-induced cardiomyopathy: a review of animal models and clinical studies. J Am Coll Cardiol 29:709-715
6. Iannini JP, Spinale FG (1996) The identification of contributory mechanisms for the development and progression of congestive heart failure in animal models. J Heart Lung Transplant 15:1138-1150
7. Kannel WB, Abbott RD, Savage DD, McNamara PM (1982) Epidemiologic features of chronic atrial fibrillation. The Framingham Study. N Engl J Med 306:1018-1022
8. Krahn AD, Manfreda J, Tate RB et al (1995) The natural history of atrial fibrillation: incidence, risk factors, and prognosis in the Manitoba Follow-Up Study. Am J Med 98:476-484
9. Khand AU, Rankin AC, Kaye GC, Cleland JG (2000) Systematic review of the management of atrial fibrillation in patients with heart failure. Eur Heart J 21:614-632
10. Middlekauff HR, Stevenson WG, Stevenson LW (1991) Prognostic significance of atrial fibrillation in advanced heart failure. A study of 390 patients. Circulation 84:40-48
11. Whipple GH, Sheffield LT, Woodman EG (1962) Reversible congestive heart failure due to chronic rapid stimulation of the normal heart. Proc N Engl Cardiovasc Soc 20:39-40
12. Kajstura J, Zhang X, Liu Y et al (1995) The cellular basis of pacing-induced dilated cardiomyopathy. Myocyte cell loss and myocyte cellular reactive hypertrophy. Circulation 92:2306-2317
13. Schumacher B, Luderitz B (1998) Rate issue in atrial fibrillation. Consequences of tachycardia and therapy for rate control. Am J Cardiol 82 (8A):29N-36N
14. Tomita M, Spinale FG, Crawford FA, Zile MR (1991) Changes in left ventricular volume, mass, and function during the development and regression of supraventricular tachycardia-induced cardiomyopathy. Disparity between recovery of systolic versus diastolic function. Circulation 83:635-644
15. Van Gelder IC, Crijns HJGM, Blanksma PK et al (1993) Time course of hemodynamic changes and improvement of exercise tolerance after cardioversion of chronic atrial fibrillation unassociated with cardiac valve disease. Am J Cardiol 72:560-566
16. Levy S, Ricard P, Lau CP et al (1997) Multicenter low energy transvenous atrial defibrillation (XAD) trial results in different subsets of atrial fibrillation. J Am Coll Cardiol 29:750-755

17. Boriani G, Biffi M, Bronzetti G et al (1998) Efficacy and tolerability in fully conscious patients of transvenous low-energy internal atrial cardioversion for atrial fibrillation. Am J Cardiol 81:241-244
18. Boriani G, Biffi M, Pergolini F et al (1999) Low energy internal atrial cardioversion in atrial fibrillation lasting more than a year. Pacing Clin Electrophysiol 22:243-246
19. Boriani G, Biffi M, Camanini C et al (2001) Transvenous low energy internal cardioversion for atrial fibrillation: a review of clinical applications and future developments. Pacing Clin Electrophysiol 24:99-107
20. Boriani G, Biffi M, Rapezzi C et al (2000) Evaluation of atrial mechanical function recovery and ventricular performance improvement following internal atrial cardioversion. Eur Heart J 21 (abstr suppl):120
21. Twidale N, Sutton K, Bartlett L et al (1993) Effects on cardiac performance of atrioventricular node catheter ablation using radiofrequency current for drug-refractory atrial arrhythmias. Pacing Clin Electrophysiol 16:1275-1284
22. Brignole M, Gianfranchi L, Menozzi C et al (1994) Influence of atrioventricular junction radiofrequency ablation in patients with chronic atrial fibrillation and flutter on quality of life and cardiac performance. Am J Cardiol 74:242-246
23. Redfield MM, Kay GN, Jenkins LS et al (2000) Tachycardia-related cardiomyopathy: a common cause of ventricular dysfunction in patients with atrial fibrillation referred for atrioventricular ablation. Mayo Clin Proc 75:790-795
24. Natale A, Zimerman L, Tomassoni G et al (1996) Impact on ventricular function and quality of life of transcatheter ablation of the atrioventricular junction in chronic atrial fibrillation with a normal ventricular response. Am J Cardiol 78:1431-1433
25. Fenelon G, Wijns W, Andries E, Brugada P (1996) Tachycardiomyopathy: mechanisms and clinical implications. Pacing Clin Electrophysiol 19:95-106
26. Ueng KC, Tsai TP, Tsai CK et al (2001) Acute and long term effects of atrioventricular junction ablation and VVIR pacemaker in symptomatic patients with chronic lone atrial fibrillation and normal ventricular response. J Cardiovasc Electrophysiol 12:303-309
27. Van Den Berg MP, Tuinenburg AE, Crijns HJGM et al (1997) Heart failure and atrial fibrillation: current concepts and controversies. Heart 77:309-313
28. Carson PE, Johnson GR, Dunkman WB et al (1993) The influence of atrial fibrillation on prognosis in mild to moderate heart failure. The V-HeFT Studies. Circulation 87(suppl VI):102-110
29. Dries DL, Exner DV, Gersh BJ et al (1998) Atrial fibrillation is associated with an increased risk for mortality and heart failure progression in patients with asymptomatic left ventricular systolic dysfunction: a retrospective analysis of the SOLVD trials. J Am Coll Cardiol 32:695-703

Asymptomatic Atrial Fibrillation: How Frequent Is It ? What Are the Practical/Therapeutic Implications ?

P. Coumel

A survey conducted among cardiologists in France [1] showed a very large spectrum of symptoms in patients suffering from atrial fibrillation (AF) in its different forms: paroxysmal, permanent, or persistent or recent according to the now largely accepted definitions. The main data about symptoms in this study are presented in Tables 1 and 2, from which several observations can be drawn. In spite of the efforts made to relate symptoms to the clinical or ECG pattern of AF, it was difficult to correlate clinical manifestations with any other parameters such as the history, the paroxysmal or permanent character of the arrhythmia, the heart rate or even the treatment.

Of a total of 706 patients, AF was permanent in half and paroxysmal in one-fourth, the rest forming the intermediate class of persistent or recent AF. A cardiac disease was more frequently present in the chronic (three-quarters of cases) than in the paroxysmal form (one-half of cases), and dyspnea was more frequent in the former (47%) than in the latter (29%). It seems probable, however, that dyspnea was more frequent in the chronic form simply because of the more marked proportion of cardiac disease in this group compared to lone AF. Another points worth noting is that exercise limitation is obviously the major symptom taken into account to determine the NYHA functional class in AF, and one has to balance the former observation with the somewhat inconsistent finding that 38% of patients with paroxysmal AF were in class I, whereas only 22% of those with permanent AF were in the same class. If, on the other hand, one puts together the absence of symptoms and the presence of the mild symptoms forming class I, then the distribution is practically equal between the paroxysmal and the permanent forms, whereas there is clearly a greater proportion of class II-IV patients with permanent AF (almost two-thirds) than with paroxysmal AF (less than one-quarter), with an intermediate situation for patients with recent AF (one-half).

Further analysis of symptoms shows that silent AF is much less common in the paroxysmal (5%) and the persistent forms (only 7%) than in the permanent form (16%), and symptoms other than dyspnea also predominate in paroxys-

Hôpital Lariboisière, Paris, France

Table 1. Clinical characteristics of a cohort of 706 patients with AF

Form of AF (% of patients)	Patient with heart disease	Mean length of history (months)	Patients with embolic events	Patients with no symptoms	NYHA functional class			
					I	II	III	IV
Paroxysmal 24%	53%	39	8%	5%	38%	18%	4%	1%
Chronic 48%	76%	66	11%	16%	22%	40%	17%	4%
Recent 28%	72%	7	4%	7%	27%	35%	11%	3%

Table 2. Symptoms experienced in the various forms of AF

	AU patients ($n = 706$)		Patients with paroxysmal AF ($n = 167$; 24%)		Patients with permanent AF ($n = 339$; 48%)		Patients with recent AF ($n = 200$; 28%)	
	n	%	n	%	n	%	n	%
Palpitations	409	54	132	79	174	45	103	22
Chest pain	76	10	22	13	32	8	22	11
Dyspnea	336	44	38	29	182	47	116	58
Syncope	79	10	29	17	31	8	19	10
Fatigue	108	14	21	13	51	13	36	18
Other	7	1	0	0	7	2	0	0
None	86	11	9	5	63	16	14	7

mal AF. Palpitations are very frequent in paroxysmal AF (79%), whereas they form only 45% of the patients' complaints in the permanent form. This is certainly related to the very usual observation that palpitations tend to fade away as the AF continues after they were initially very marked at its onset, but the duration of this process is quite variable from patient to patient. Another very well-known fact is that the perception of palpitations by the patient closely depends on his or her activity at the time of arrhythmia (exercise or rest or even sleep), so that arrhythmia may or may not be perceived depending on these conditions as well as on treatment. The same type of remark applies to the presence of dizziness or syncope, observed in 17% of patients with paroxysmal AF versus 8% of those with permanent AF: the onset of AF is usually the occasion of these symptoms, the presence of which closely depends on the activity, and by definition patients with paroxysmal AF are more frequently exposed. They are also prone to have some cardiac pause or at least bradycardia at the termination of the attack. Finally, fatigue is equally distributed among the various forms (13%), as is chest pain. Although they are considered more often as complications than symptoms, the incidence of embolic events in the history was not different among the various forms (8% in paroxysmal AF, 11% in permanent AF), but these rather high numbers mainly cover transitory incidents rather than stroke. It should also be considered that in this survey the history averaged 39 months for paroxysmal AF and 66 months for permanent AF. Finally, concentrating on paroxysmal AF, the incidence of history of resistance to treatment, frequency of recurrences, and duration of attacks are quite variable and not related in any way to the symptoms.

The literature is not very abundant concerning the incidence of silent AF, and only 15 years ago or so did we begin to realize that it was much more frequent than previously believed [2]. This is probably related to the fact that for a long time clinical opinion and experience largely predominated over the systematic studies now available, for various reasons. The abnormal proportions of stroke in young adults is one of them, and there is most probably a direct relationship between the incidence of stroke and the paucity of the symptoms of AF, which deprives patients of preventive treatment for this serious complication, whether the profile of the AF is paroxysmal or permanent [3]. The necessary documenting of the effect of newly developed antiarrhythmic drugs was also a mechanism by which the significant proportion of silent attacks of AF was shown. Holter monitoring and transtelephonic monitoring studies have demonstrated that asymptomatic episodes of AF may exceed symptomatic paroxysms 12-fold or more [4].

Determining to what extent quality of life is impaired and why is a difficult matter that was dealt with in several studies recently. Impairment of the quality of life correlates poorly with more "objective" indices of AF disease severity in the experience of Dorian et al. [5], and this confirms our experience concerning the clinical pattern of AF, particularly its history. An interesting observation reported by Paquette et al. [6] in patients who participated in the Canadian Atrial Fibrillation Trial is that in a population with newly diagnosed, symptomatic, intermittent AF, quality of life is significantly more impaired in women than men despite comparable disease severity. This finding was not made, however, in a previous study by Hamer et al. [7], but cardiac symptoms and severity improved over time both for women and men – an observation by Hohnloser et al. [8] that only partly depends on the outcome: exercise tolerance is better with reversion to sinus rhythm than with control of ventricular rate, but hospital admission is more frequent.

Although the reasons why symptoms are present or absent in AF are unclear, at least our clinical experience with vagally or adrenergically mediated paroxysmal AF indicates that the tolerance to arrhythmia has to do with the autonomic nervous system. Clearly, vagally mediated paroxysmal AF are much better tolerated than adrenergic AF, although exceptions are not rare in either direction [9]. In this regard, very interesting observations were recently made by Crijns' group [10], which tried to determine the predictors of quality of life and the role of the autonomic function in this respect. Quality of life was assessed in 73 patients with paroxysmal AF and compared with age-matched controls, and the autonomic functions were assessed using heart rate variability and autonomic function tests. Curiously, structural heart disease did not predict quality of life, but scores were markedly lower in patients than in controls in four of the eight subscales: physical role function, emotional role function, vitality, and general health. Autonomic variables were predictive in all these subscales, depressed vagal function being predictive of low score. Symptoms, particularly severe perspiration, were also predictive of low score.

In conclusion, the main problem of silent AF is that it must be considered on the one hand as positive in terms of quality of life whatever the actual mechanism of the absence of symptoms, but on the other hand clearly the main complication, stroke, should be prevented in the same way as in symptomatic forms. Against the latter, rhythm control by antiarrhythmics should not justify discontinue action of anticoagulation treatment because one can never be certain of preventing recurrences.

References

1. Lévy S, Maarek M, Coumel P et al (1999) Characterization of different subsets of atrial fibrillation in general practice in France: the ALFA Study. Circulation 99:3028-3035
2. Savelieva I, Camm AJ (2000) Clinical relevance of silent atrial fibrillation: prevalence, prognosis, quality of life, and management. J Interv Card Electrophysiol 4:369-382
3. Hart RG, Pearce LA, Rothbart RM et al for the SPAF Investigators (2000) Stroke with intermittent atrial fibrillation: incidence and predictors during aspirin therapy. J Am Coll Cardiol 35:183-187
4. Bandhari AK, Anderson JL, Gilbert EM et al (1992) Correlation of symptoms with occurrence of paroxysmal supraventricular tachycardia or atrial fibrillation: a transtelephonic monitoring study. The flecainide supraventricular tachycardia study group. Am Heart J 124:381-386
5. Dorian P, Jung W, Newman D et al (2000) The impairment of health-related quality of life in patients with intermittent atrial fibrillation: implications for the assessment of investigational therapy. J Am Coll Cardiol 36:1303-1309
6. Paquette M, Roy D, Talajic M et al (2000) Role of gender and personality on quality of life impairment in intermittent atrial fibrillation. Am J Cardiol 86:764-768
7. Hamer ME, Blumenthal JA, McCarthy EA et al (1994) Quality of life assessment in patients with paroxysmal atrial fibrillation or paroxysmal supraventricular tachycardia. Am J Cardiol 74:826-829
8. Hohnloser SH, Kuck KH, Lilienthal J (2000) Rhythm or rate control in atrial fibrillation. Pharmacological Intervention in Atrial Fibrillation (PIAF): a randomized trial. Lancet 356:1789-1794
9. Coumel P (1996) Autonomic influences in atrial tachyarrhythmias. J Cardiovasc Electrophysiol 7:999-1007
10. Van den Berg MP, Hassink RJ, Tuinenburg AE et al (2001) Quality of life in patients with paroxysmal atrial fibrillation and its predictors: importance of the autonomic nervous system. Eur Heart J 22:247-253

Does Early Echocardiography-Guided Cardioversion of Atrial Fibrillation Prevent Electrical/Mechanical Remodeling of the Atria?

M. Disertori and M. Marini

Echocardiography-Guided Cardioversion of Atrial Fibrillation

Current guidelines for cardioversion of atrial fibrillation (AF) are mainly based on studies indicating that there is a substantial risk of embolic events in patients who have not received anticoagulant therapy which may be reduced by such therapy prior to cardioversion [1]. Some studies have shown that exclusion of left atrial appendage thrombus by transesophageal echocardiography indicates a low risk for embolic events after cardioversion of AF [2]. However, even if thrombi are absent on transesophageal echocardiography before cardioversion, they may yet form because of a reduction of atrial contractility that persists for up to 3 weeks after restoration of sinus rhythm, depending on the duration of AF [3].

To dissipate pre-existing left atrial thrombi and prevent new onset of thrombus formation after cardioversion, anticoagulation treatment should be maintained for a sufficient time. Current European guidelines [4] advocate anticoagulation with warfarin for at least 3 weeks before and 4 weeks after cardioversion for patients with AF lasting more than 48 h. Alternatively, a transesophageal echocardiography-guided approach may be used, with immediate heparinization, exclusion of a left atrial appendage thrombus before cardioversion, and subsequent anticoagulation with warfarin for at least 4 weeks. The just published results of ACUTE trial (1222 patients) show that there is no difference between the two strategies in the rate of embolic events [5]. In patients who need anticoagulation, transesophageal echocardiography guided cardioversion can reduce the AF duration of one month, with also a significant reduction of hemorragic events [5].

Electrical Remodeling of the Atria

Electrophysiological remodeling has been well described in experimental studies. The paper by Wijffels et al. [6] has demonstrated that, in goats, pacing-

Cardiology Department, S. Chiara Hospital, Trento, Italy

induced AF of up 2 weeks' duration induces a shortening of atrial refractoriness and a reverse adaptation of refractoriness to rate. The reduction of refractoriness reduces the wave length and then stabilizes the AF, and favors its recurrence after cardioversion. Reverse adaptation obviously cannot contribute to promoting maintenance of AF; on the contrary, it could have great importance in the induction and recurrence of AF, because the short refractory period during sinus rhythm increases the ability of premature beats to induce AF. Another experimental study by Gaspo et al. [7] showed that in dogs paced for 1-42 weeks, rapid atrial activation caused time-dependent decreases in the refractory period, in rate-dependent refractory period accommodation, and in conduction velocity and wave length, along with an increase in regional heterogeneity.

Several studies have addressed the presence and the characteristics of electrophysiological remodeling in humans. All the studies have shown a shortening of atrial refractory periods or monophasic action potential duration after cardioversion of persistent AF, while discordant results have been observed where refractoriness adapts to rate [8-11]. However, the extent of the electrical remodeling process seems to be more pronounced in animals than in humans [12]. AF-induced electrophysiological remodeling is reversible. In goats fibrillating for about 3 weeks, interposed periods of sinus rhythm prevent further AF-induced remodeling, so that subsequent AF episodes do not become chronic [13]. A day after cardioversion to sinus rhythm, the atrial effective refractory period remains short, but it returns to normal within a week.

In humans, prompt cardioversion by an implantable atrial defibrillator (IAD) progressively reduces the total time that patients are in AF and progressively increases the time between cardioverted episodes [14]. The latter result is attributable to prevention of long-lasting AF paroxysms and attendant remodeling, suggesting that prompt restoration of sinus rhythm will forestall progressive remodeling and the increase in duration and frequency of arrhythmic episodes. Because the time course of tachycardia-induced remodeling and subsequent reverse remodeling of the effective refractory period and action potential duration requires only 2 days, it is likely that not only electrophysiological but also other mechanisms, such as reverse mechanical and/or structural remodeling, are involved in the prevention of AF by prompt cardioversion [15].

Mechanical Remodeling of the Atria

Besides changes in electrophysiological atrial properties, AF induces structural modifications that could explain the impairment of contractile function after cardioversion of AF. The mechanisms responsible for this post-cardioversion atrial contractile dysfunction, frequently termed "atrial stunning", are not completely understood. It appears to be independent of the mode of conversion of sinus rhythm (spontaneous, pharmacological, or electrical) [16]. Potential mechanisms include relative Ca^{2+} depletion in the atrial myocardium caused by a "contractile remodeling" process imposed on the cells by the previous AF, or simple hemodynamic mechanisms such as a reduced left atrial appendage outflow velocity due to an increased afterload against which the left atrial appendage has to contract after restoration of sinus rhythm [17]. In the study published by Ausma et al. [18] AF was induced in goats and maintained for 9-23 weeks. After this time, myocytes showed marked changes in their cellular substructures, such as loss of myofibrils, accumulation of glycogen, changes in mitochondrial shape and size, fragmentation of sarcoplasmatic reticulum, and dispersion of nuclear chromatin. These changes were accompanied by an increase in the size of the myocytes.

It is interesting that these atrial structural changes due to prolonged AF are very similar to those seen in chronic hibernating ventricular myocardium as a result of low-flow ischemia. Thus hibernation of the atrial myocardium in response to prolonged AF might be an important long-term mechanism by which the cells protect themselves against a persistent high metabolic demand and Ca^{2+} influx resulting from an ultrarapid rate of activation. The loss of contractile material will markedly reduce the mechanical function and, thus, the oxygen consumption of the atria. This explains the poor atrial contractile function after cardioversion of AF and its slow recovery. The atrial transport function after AF will only normalize when the atrial contractile machinery has been rebuilt and the process of dedifferentiation reversed [19].

In humans, a recent study of 49 consecutive patients undergoing mitral valve surgery (23 with chronic AF and 26 in sinus rhythm) showed atrial contractility to be reduced by 75% after prolonged AF [20]. Failure of Bay K8644 to restore contractility suggested that the L-type Ca^{2+} channel was responsible for the contractile dysfunction. The restoration of contractile force by high extracellular Ca^{2+} showed that the contractile apparatus itself was nearly completely preserved after prolonged AF.

The definition of structural remodeling also includes extracellular changes that develop during long-term AF (months). The most important one is the development of interstitial fibrosis, which is probably promoted by increased expression of angiotensin-converting enzyme during AF [21].

To determine whether the timing of cardioversion of spontaneous AF with an IAD affects the time course of recovery of left atrial mechanical dysfunction seen after cardioversion, Tse et al. [22] studied 11 patients. The results demonstrated that significant left atrial mechanical dysfunction occurred after early and late cardioversion of AF using low-energy internal atrial defibrillation. Although there were no significant differences in the number of shocks delivered and the recurrence rate of AF between early versus late cardioversion of spontaneous AF with the IAD, cardioversion of AF episodes at more than 48 h was associated with an earlier onset and more delayed resolution of left atrial mechanical dysfunction. This finding suggests that prompt termination of AF episodes using the IAD may enhance the recovery from left atrial mechanical dysfunction seen after cardioversion and may also account for the low incidence of thromboembolic events after cardioversion of AF at less than 48 h. Moreover, in an other study, Tse et al. [23] have suggested that restoration and maintenance of sinus rhythm by repeated cardioversion of IAD may reverse the process of left atrial enlargement by reversing the mechanical remodeling process associated with AF (see Table 1).

Table 1. Four time domains in adaptation to heart rate [19]

Short-term (metabolic; second to minutes)	Ion concentrations Ion pump activities Phosphorylation of ionic channels
Moderate-term (electrical remodeling; hours to days)	Altered gene expression Synthesis/assembly
Long-term (contractile remodelling; weeks)	Hibernation
Very long-term (anatomical remodelling; months to years)	Irreversible structural damage (fibrosis, fatty degeneration, etc.)

Conclusions

In patients with AF who need anticoagulation before cardioversion, the use of transesophageal echocardiography-guided cardioversion can significantly reduce the duration of AF (of 1 month).

Although our knowledge of atrial electrophysiological and mechanical properties in patients with persitent or chronic AF is still incomplete, some preliminary studies suggest that prompt cardioversion of AF is associated with prompt resolution of electrical/mechanical remodeling of the atria. Thus, the incidence of AF relapses and the risk of embolic events could be reduced.

In recent-onset AF, echocardiography-guided cardioversion could prevent electrical/mechanical atrial remodeling; by contrast, in long-lasting AF (months) the gain in time related to the transesophageal echocardiography-guided approach could be of less importance.

References

1. Bjerkelund CJ, Orning OM (1969) The efficacy of anticoagulant therapy in preventing embolism related to DC electrical cardioversion of atrial fibrillation. Am J Cardiol 23:208-216
2. Manning WJ, Silverman DI, Gordon SPF et al (1993) Cardioversion from atrial fibrillation without prolonged anticoagulation with use of transesophageal echocardiography to exclude the presence of atrial thrombi. N Engl J Med 328:750-755
3. Manning WJ, Silverman DI, Katz SE et al (1994) Impaired left atrial mechanical function after cardioversion: relation to the duration of atrial fibrillation. J Am Coll Cardiol 23:1535-1540
4. Lévy S, Breithardt G, Campbell RWF et al on behalf of the Working Group of Arrhythmias of the European Society of Cardiology (1998) Atrial fibrillation: current knowledge and recommendations for management. Eur Heart J 19:1294-1320
5. Klein AL, Grimm RA, Murray D et al (2001) Use of transesophageal echocardiography to guide cardioversion in patients with atrial fibrillation. N Engl J Med 344:1411-1420

6. Wijffels M, Kirchhof C, Dorland R, Allessie MA (1995) Atrial fibrillation begets atrial fibrillation. A study in awake chronically instrumented goats. Circulation 92:1954-1968

7. Gaspo R, Bosch RF, Talajinc M, Nattel S (1997) Functional mechanisms underlying tachycardia-induced sustained atrial fibrillation in chronic dog model. Circulation 96:4027-4035

8. Pandozi C, Bianconi L, Villani M et al (1998) Electrophysiological characteristics of the human atria after cardioversion of persistent atrial fibrillation. Circulation 98:2860-2865

9. Franz MR, Karasik PL, Li C et al (1997) Electrical remodeling of the human atrium: similar effects in patients with chronic atrial fibrillation and atrial flutter. J Am Coll Cardiol 30:1785-1792

10. Tse H, Lau C, Ayers GM (1999) Heterogeneous changes in electrophysiologic properties in the paroxismal and chronically fibrillating human atrium. J Cardiovasc Electrophysiol 10:125-135

11. Lee SU, Yu WC, Chen SA (2000) Tachycardia induced changes of atrial electrophysiological properties. Pacing Clin Electrophysiol 23:2120-2127

12. Pandozi C, Santini M (2001) Update on atrial remodeling owing to rate. Does atrial fibrillation always beget atrial fibrillation? Eur Heart J 22:541-553

13. Garrat CJ, Duytschaever M, Killian M et al (1999) Repetitive electrical remodeling by paroxysms of atrial fibrillation in the goat: no cumulative effect on inducibility or stability of atrial fibrillation. J Cardiovasc Electrophysiol 10:1101-1108

14. Timmermans C, Rodriguez LM, Smeets JL (1998) Immediate reinitiation of atrial fibrillation following internal atrial defibrillation. J Cardiovasc Electrophysiol 9:122-128

15. Allessie MA, Boyden PA, Camm AJ et al (2001) Pathophysiology and prevention of atrial fibrillation. Circulation 103:769-777

16. Stellbrink C, Hanrath P (2000) The optimal management of cardioversion of atrial fibrillation or flutter: still a "stunning" problem. Eur Heart J 21:795-798

17. Zarse M, Waldmann M, Muehlenbruch G et al (1999) Left atrial appendage outflow is augmented during atrial fibrillation compared to sinus rhythm: insights from a pig model of pacing-induced atrial fibrillation. Eur Heart J 20 (Abstr Suppl):226

18. Ausma J, Wijffels M, Thonè F et al (1997) Structural changes of atrial myocardium due to sustained atrial fibrillation in the goat. Circulation 96:3157-3163

19. Allessie MA (1998) Atrial electrophysiologic remodeling: another vicious circle? J Cardiovasc Electrophysiol 9:1378-1393

20. Schotten U, Ausma J, Stellbrink C et al (2001) Cellular mechanisms of depressed atrial contractility in patients with chronic atrial fibrillation. Circulation 103:691-698

21. Goette A, Lendeckel U, Staak Y et al (1999) Increased expression of the angiotensin-converting enzyme in human atria during chronic atrial fibrillation. Circulation 100(Abstract) I-200

22. Tse HF, Wang Q, Yu CM, Ayers GM, Lau CP (2000) Time course of recovery of left atrial mechanical dysfunction after cardioversion of spontaneous atrial fibrillation with the implantable atrial defibrillator. Am J Cardiol 86:1023-1025

23. Tse HF, Lau CP, Yu CM et al (1999) Effect of the implantable atrial defibrillator on the natural history of atrial fibrillation. J Cardiovasc Electrophysiol 10:1200-1209

The "Pill in the Pocket" Approach for Paroxysmal Atrial Fibrillation: How Effective and Safe Is It?

M. Di Biase, R. Ieva, G. Mavilio, D. Casella and G. Maulucci

The occurrence of paroxysmal atrial fibrillation (AFib) is frequently associated with symptoms mainly due to the fast ventricular rate. In patients with nonvalvular AFib therapy is based on drugs which slow the ventricular rate and on anti-arrhythmic drugs which can restore the sinus rhythm and reduce the duration of the arrhythmic episodes. Most patients undergo this treatment in the emergency rooms, which is somewhat costly.

In this setting there are three needs:

1. To establish sinus rhythm as early as possible, in order to alleviate or reduce the patient's symptoms, lower the incidence of thromboembolisms, eliminate the need for long-term use of atrioventricular node blocking agents, reduce electrophysiological remodelling and increase the chances of successful cardioversion.
2. To avoid hospitalisation, in order to reduce costs and the time between the onset of the arrhythmia and the start of anti-arrhythmic treatment for sinus rhythm restoration.
3. To avoid prophylactic anti-arrhythmic treatment, which requires two or more administrations of the drug per day and is associated with a very high rate of recurrence of the arrhythmia: 66% at 1 year with class IA and IC anti-arrhythmic drugs.

To attain these three objectives a new therapeutic approach for paroxysmal AFib has been introduced: self-administration by the patient of the anti-arrhythmic drug a few minutes after the onset of the arrhythmia, without the support of hospital emergency rooms. Although this approach – known as the "pill in the pocket treatment" – has been utilised by many cardiologists in clinical practice, there is a lack of data on its efficacy and safety based on large and controlled clinical trials.

Department of Cardiology, University of Foggia, Italy

Avaible Data on the Efficacy, Safety and Side Effects of Paroxysmal AFib Treatment with Oral Anti-Arrythmic Drugs

Propafenone

Efficacy

The efficacy of a single oral loading dose of propafenone versus placebo for the treatment of recent onset AFib has been evaluated in various placebo-controlled trials [1-7]. The success rate was between 58% and 85%, depending on the duration of the AFib and the follow-up after the administration of the drug. The mean conversion time ranged between 110 ± 59 min and 287 ± 352 min. As regards dosage, 600 mg was the dose most frequently used, since 450-600 mg oral propafenone results in clinically effective plasma levels [8].

In one clinical study the propafenone dose was weight-titrated: 450 mg for 50-64 kg, 600 mg for 65-85 kg and 750 mg for > 85 kg body weight [3]. The efficacy of the drug versus placebo was confirmed, but the number of patients was not sufficient for an evaluation of the effects of weight-based adjustments on the efficacy.

As for the efficacy of propafenone compared to placebo, the incidence of conversion was statistically higher at 3 h and 8 h after drug administration, while at 24 h no statistically significant difference between propafenone and placebo was demonstrated [2].

Another study showed that a dose regimen of 600 mg was statistically more effective than one of 450 mg in restoring sinus rhythm at 2 h, while no statistically significant differences were found at 4 and 8 h after administration [3].

Safety

Adverse effects occurring after the single loading dose of propafenone were: transient supraventricular arrhythmias, widening of QRS complexes, transient hypotension and mild non-cardiac side effects. The supraventricular arrhythmias, appearing at the time of conversion, include atrial flutter (AFl), sinus bradycardia, sinus arrest and junctional rhythm [9]. No life-threatening ventricular arrhythmias were reported as a consequence of drug administration. The absence of pro-arrhythmic effects at ventricular level could be explained by the fact that the plasma concentration is significantly lower after a single oral dose than after chronic oral administration [10].

In most of the trials the incidence of supraventricular arrhythmias was similar to that for the placebo (7% versus 6%) [2]; the ventricular rate was mostly lower than 140 beats/min (frequently 2:1 atrioventricular conduction) and the duration of the arrhythmias did not exceed 30 s. Very few patients experienced sinus pauses or syncope. The Safety Antiarrhythmic Therapy Evaluation Trial, published in 1999 [7], showed that a 600 mg (> 60 kg body weight) or 450 mg (< 60 kg body weight) oral dose of propafenone, followed by 300 mg if AFib persisted, was not followed by serial clinical events, while the occurrence of

AFl, transient bundle branch block or asymptomatic transient sinus block was observed in a few patients. Mild transient hypotension, nausea, headache, paraesthesia and gastrointestinal disturbances were also observed in a very low percentage of cases.

No patient receiving an atrioventricular node blocking agent (β-blockers, calcium channel blockers) has been included in clinical trials with propafenone. From the theoretical point of view patients pre-treated with these drugs should be less prone to develop 1:1 conduction where there is AFl or atrial tachycardia before conversion. In clinical practice, most physicians administer low doses of β-blockers to patients being treated with loading doses of propafenone in order to avoid 1:1 conduction should AFl or tachycardia occur [11].

Since propafenone is principally metabolised by the liver, it was also possible to administer it in patients with renal failure.

In two studies propafenone was also administered in patients with structural heart disease (coronary heart disease, valvular heart disease, cardiomyopathy) and hypertension. No increase of side effects was observed in these patients, while its efficacy was almost the same as in patients without structural heart disease [3, 7, 12].

Flecainide

Efficacy

The efficacy of an oral loading dose of flecainide in converting recent-onset AFib has been evaluated in different clinical trials. The rate of conversion is between 59% and 91%, mainly depending on the duration of follow-up. After 3 h the conversion rate is 59%, and at 8 h it is higher (91%). A single oral loading dose of 300 mg was used. There was a statistically significant difference compared with the placebo [13, 14].

Safety

In the study of Capucci et al. [14], 1 out of 22 patients treated with a single oral loading dose of 300 mg experienced a sinus pause of 9 s, while the occurrence of AFl with a ventricular rate of less than 150 beats/min was observed in 2 patients. No significant adverse effects were reported [14].

Amiodarone

Efficacy

In the experience of Blanc et al. [15], amiodarone was administered to patients with recent-onset AFib at a dose of 30 mg/kg body weight for the first 24 h and, if necessary, a repeated dose of 15 mg/kg for the following 24 h. The median time to sinus restoration was 6.9 h and its incidence was 20% at 4 h, 30% at 13 h and 47%

at 24 h. In patients with persistent AFib after the first 24 h, a repeat dose of amiodarone for a further 24 h was followed by conversion to sinus rhythm in 63%.

Safety

Gastrointestinal side effects (digestive discomfort) were noted in 4% of cases, while one patient had supraventricular arrhythmia and another showed nonsustained ventricular tachycardia [15].

In conclusion, from the data in the literature it is possible to affirm that oral loading treatment of recent-onset AFib with anti-arrhythmic drugs is:
– Effective in a very high percentage of cases.
– More effective than placebo during the first 12 h.
– Safe in patients with structural heart disease, since there is no difference in the incidence of side effects (supraventricular tachycardias and sinus pauses) as compared to patients without evident heart disease.

Selection of Patients for "Pill in the Pocket" Treatment of AFib

According to the available clinical, electrophysiological and pharmacological data, patients with the following conditions should be excluded from "pill in the pocket" treatment: coronary heart disease; prophylactic anti-arrhythmic treatment on recurrence of AFib; heart failure (NYHA classes III and IV); valvular heart disease; dilated cardiomyopathy; hyperthyroidism; long QT syndrome; sick sinus syndrome; paroxysmal atrioventricular block; renal failure; myocarditis; pregnancy and hypokalaemia.

Need for a Large Multicentre Trial on the Efficacy and Safety of "Pill in the Pocket" Treatment of AFib

Because of the lack of data on "pill in the pocket" treatment coming from controlled clinical trials, there is a need for a large controlled multicentre clinical trial aimed at evaluating the efficacy and safety of this approach. For this reason Paolo Alboni [16], on behalf of the AIAC (Italian Society for Cardiac Pacing and Electrophysiology), has recently proposed a multicentre clinical trial utilising propafenone and flecainide for the treatment of recent-onset AFib to evaluate: (1) the safety of these two drugs administered as an oral loading dose outside the emergency department; (2) the need for admission to the emergency department during this type of treatment; and (3) the quality of life with this treatment. The trial will enrol 300 patients over 1 year and will probably be able to evaluate 100 episodes of AFib.

References

1. Capucci A, Boriani G, Rubino I et al (1994) A controlled study on oral propafenone versus digoxin plus quinidine in converting recent-onset atrial fibrillation to sinus rhythm. Int J Cardiol 43:305-313
2. Boriani G, Biffi M, Capucci A et al (1997) Oral propafenone to convert recent-onset atrial fibrillation in patients with and without underlying heart disease: a randomised, controlled trial. Ann Intern Med 126:621-625
3. Botto GL, Capucci A, Bonini W et al (1997) Conversion of recent onset atrial fibrillation to sinus rhythm using a single loading oral dose of propafenone: comparison of two regimens. Int J Cardiol 58:55-61
4. Botto GL, Bonini W, Broffoni T et al (1996) Conversion of recent onset atrial fibrillation with single loading oral dose of propafenone: is in hospital admission absolutely necessary? Pacing Clin Electrophysiol 19:1936-1943
5. Boriani G, Cappucci A, Lenzi T et al (1995) Propafenone for conversion of recent-onset atrial fibrillation: a controlled comparison between oral loading dose and intravenous administration. Chest 108:355-358
6. Botto GL, Bonini W, Broffoni T et al (1998) A randomized, crossover, controlled comparison of oral loading versus intravenous infusion of propafenone in recent-onset atrial fibrillation. Pacing Clin Electrophysiol 21:240-244
7. Capucci A, Villani GQ, Aschieri D, Piepoli M (1999) Safety of oral propafenone in the conversion of recent-onset atrial fibrillation to sinus rhythm: a prospective parallel placebo-controlled multicenter study. Int J Cardiol 68:187-196
8. Capucci A, Boriani G, Marchesini B et al (1990) Minimal effective concentration values of propafenone and 5-hydroxypropafenone in acute and chronic therapy. Cardiovasc Drug Ther 4:281-287
9. Khan IA (2001) Single oral loading dose of propafenone for pharmacological cardioversion of recent onset atrial fibrillation. Am J Cardiol 37:542-547
10. Hii JT, Duff HJ, Burgess ED (1991) Clinical pharmacokinetics of propafenone. Clin Pharmacokinet 21:1-10
11. Biffi M, Boriani G, Bronzetti G et al (1999) Electrophysiological effects of flecainide, propafenone on atrial fibrillation cycle and relation with arrhythmia termination. Heart 82:176-182
12. Ergene U, Ergene O, Cete Y et al (1998) Predictors of success in conversion of new-onset atrial fibrillation using oral propafenone. Eur J Emerg Med 5:425-428
13. Crijns HJ, Wijk MV, Glist HV et al (1998) Acute conversion of atrial fibrillation to sinus rhythm: clinical efficacy of flecainide acetate. Comparison of two regimens. Eur Heart J 9:634-638
14. Capucci A, Lenzi T, Boriani G et al (1992) Effectiveness of loading oral flecainide for converting recent-onset atrial fibrillation to sinus rhythm in patients without organic heart disease or with only systemic hypertension. Am J Cardiol 70:69-72
15. Blanc JJ, Voinov C, Maarket M, on behalf of the PARSIFAL study group (1999) Comparison of oral loading dose of propafenone and amiodarone for converting recent-onset atrial fibrillation. Am J Cardiol 84:1029-1032
16. Alboni P (2001) Trattamento episodico al di fuori dell'ospedale (pill in the pocket) in pazienti con fibrillazione atriale parossistica. Proceedings of the ANMCO, Congress, Florence

Class IC Drug Plus Ibutilide for Acute Cardioversion of Atrial Fibrillation: What Is the Rationale and What Are the Results?

S. Themistoclakis[1], A. Bonso[1], A. Rossillo[1], A. Corrado[1], G. Gasparini[1], A. Raviele[1] and M.M. Scheinman[2]

Atrial fibrillation is the most common cardiac arrhythmia, with a prevalence ranging from 2% to 4% in the general population over 60 years old and an incidence that increases with age.

This arrhythmia is also a significant social and financial burden. Indeed, in the US atrial fibrillation causes more hospital admissions than any other arrhythmia, accounting for nearly 1 million hospital days per year [1].

The clinical importance and the high cost of atrial fibrillation create the need for a rapidly effective drug treatment [2]. Various management strategies are currently employed [2], but there is general agreement that early cardioversion to sinus rhythm should be the mainstay of treatment. In patients without signs or symptoms of heart failure, antiarrhythmic drugs remain the first-line treatment. DC cardioversion, even though very effective (65%-90% conversion rate) [3], requires general anesthesia and is less used as the first choice of treatment in patients with well-tolerated atrial fibrillation.

Several randomized controlled trials have evaluated the efficacy of antiarrhythmic drugs for cardioversion of atrial fibrillation. Flecainide and propafenone appear to be two of the most effective drugs for this purpose. Currently, patients who remain in atrial fibrillation after acute class IC drug therapy are generally treated with electrical cardioversion. Thus, it could be important to have a drug to add to class IC antiarrhythmic therapy in order to improve its cardioversion rate.

Ibutilide is another antiarrhythmic drug used for the cardioversion of atrial fibrillation, even though it is less effective than flecainide and propafenone in the treatment of this arrhythmia. This drug has a so-called class III effect. Its primary mechanism is increased duration of the action potential, largely by blocking the rapid component of the cardiac delayed rectifier potassium current (I_{kr}) [4]. Flecainide, on the other hand, restricts the fast inward movement of sodium ions (class IC effect) and exerts a marked effect on intracardiac conduction and comparatively minor effect on the duration of repolarization [5].

[1]Cardiovascular Department, Division of Cardiology, Umberto I Hospital, Mestre-Venice, Italy; [2]Section of Cardiac Electrophysiology, University of California, San Francisco, California, USA

We hypothesize that combined therapy with flecainide and ibutilide, with their different mechanisms of action, could improve the pharmacological cardioversion rate in atrial fibrillation patients.

Study Design

This is a randomized study designed to evaluate the safety and efficacy of combined flecainide and ibutilide therapy compared with flecainide alone in patients with atrial fibrillation of recent onset. All patients are treated with flecainide given intravenously. Patients who still are in atrial fibrillation 2 h after flecainide administration are randomized to undergo ibutilide treatment (group 1) or clinical observation (group 2). The study enrolls consecutive patients who are hemodynamically stable with documented atrial fibrillation longer than 3 h and shorter than 48 h. Patients must not be receiving class I or III antiarrhythmic agents unless the medication has been discontinued more than five half-lives before enrollment.

The following exclusion criteria are applied: age below 18 years or over 80 years, pregnancy, congestive heart failure (NYHA class > II and/or LVEF $\leq$ 40%), history of ischemic heart disease, moderate to severe valvular heart disease, electrocardiographic evidence (present or past) of complete bundle branch block, second- or third-degree AV block, sick sinus syndrome or mean ventricular rate during atrial fibrillation < 70 bpm, history of torsade de pointes or ventricular tachycardia, corrected QT interval (QT_c) longer than 440 ms, weight < 50 kg or > 136 kg, hyperkalemia (K > 5 mEq/l) or hypokalemia (K < 3.5 mEq/l), and all clinical conditions in which acute cardioversion is contraindicated (recent stroke, hyperthyroidism, history of moderate or severe renal or hepatic failure, severe metabolic disturbances, etc.).

All patients, after providing informed consent, undergo baseline evaluation (history, physical examination, standard ECG), routine blood laboratory tests, and echocardiogram. All patients are treated with intravenous flecainide and are continuously monitored by telemetry.

Two hours after flecainide administration, patients who are still in atrial fibrillation are assigned randomly to either group 1, treated with ibutilide, or group 2, not treated but only clinically observed.

Flecainide is administered as follows: intravenously at a dosage of 2 mg/kg (maximum dose: 150 mg) in 100 ml 5% glucose over 10 min. Ibutilide is administered at a dosage of 1 mg over 10 min followed by 10 min observation and then, if sinus rhythm is not restored, one additional 1-mg dose given over 10 min.

Treatment with both drugs is discontinued if systolic blood pressure decreases to below 90 mmHg, a new left bundle branch block develops, QRS duration exceeds 50%, QT_c increases above 600 ms, and sustained or unsustained ventricular tachycardia appears. Both infusions are also discontinued if any change in rhythm or AV conduction occurs that in the investigator's opinion is a threat to patient safety. Ibutilide treatment is also terminated after sinus rhythm was achieved.

Cardiac rhythm is monitored by telemetry. Blood pressure is recorded every 2 min during infusion, every 10 min in the following 30 min, and every 30 min in the next 4 h.

A 12-lead ECG is recorded before flecainide administration, 10, 30 and 60 min after it, and every 60 min for the next 6 h. In group 1, ECGs are also recorded before ibutilide infusion, at the end of the first dose, before the second dose, at the end of the second dose, 10, 30, and 60 min afterward, and every 60 min for the next 4 h. ECGs are also recorded at termination of atrial fibrillation and at significant rhythm changes.

Venous blood is drawn to evaluate plasma flecainide concentration before ibutilide administration.

Successful cardioversion is defined as termination of atrial fibrillation for any length of time within 2 h after flecainide administration and within 1.5 h from ibutilide infusion.

Preliminary Results

From April to July 2001 fifty-nine consecutive patients, 31 male and 28 female (mean age 66 ± 14 years), with atrial fibrillation of recent onset were screened. Thirty patients (51%) were excluded from the study on the basis of the following criteria: age over 80 years (5/30; 17%), pretreatment with class I and III antiarrhythmic drugs (8/30; 27%), moderate to severe valvular heart disease (7/30; 23%), ischemic heart disease (5/30; 17%), congestive heart failure (3/30; 10%), and complete left bundle branch block (2/30; 7%). Twenty-nine patients were treated with intravenous flecainide and sinus rhythm was restored in 19 (65%) within 2 h. Ten patients, 7 male and 3 female (mean age 52 ± 19 years), remained in atrial fibrillation 2 h after flecainide infusion. Mean plasma flecainide concentration was in the therapeutic range (273 ng/ml) 2 h after drug administration. Nine patients had no structural heart disease, only one had chronic coronary artery disease. No patients had significant left atrial enlargement (mean left atrial size 38 ± 2 cm). Atrial fibrillation onset occurred a mean of 365 ± 527 min before enrolment. Five patients were randomized to group 1 (ibutilide infusion) and 5 to group 2 (clinical observation). All group 1 patients had restored sinus rhythm 25 ± 30 min after ibutilide infusion, two of them (40%) after single ibutilide dose. No group 2 patients were in sinus rhythm at the end of the observation period. Flecainide and ibutilide were well tolerated in all patients of both groups and treatment protocols were completed without side effects or complications. The QT intervals were 444 ± 50 ms and 439 ± 23 ms after flecainide and ibutilide administration, respectively. No patients of either group experienced atrial flutter or ventricular arrhythmia during or after treatment.

Discussion

Acute chemical conversion has recently enjoyed increasing popularity since need for direct/current cardioversion is obviated. To date, class IC agents (flecainide and propafenone) [6-12] and ibutilide [13-19] have been proven to be effective for acute cardioversion of patients with atrial fibrillation. The purpose of our study was to assess the safety and efficacy of combination IC therapy with ibutilide for patients with acute-onset atrial fibrillation. We found, in our preliminary data, that combination therapy resulted in 100% conversion to sinus rhythm without adverse side effects.

In patients with acute onset atrial fibrillation there is a high spontaneous conversion rate without drug therapy [3]. However, the sooner a positive effect is seen, the more likely it is to be related to true drug effects. We therefore decided to assess drug efficacy within 2 h of administration. In addition, it is well appreciated that the longer the duration of atrial fibrillation, the lower is positive response to drug therapy. For this reason we decided to assess drug effect for those with a recent onset of atrial fibrillation (3-48 h).

Prior studies have documented a wide variability of successful conversion in response to intravenous flecainide (51%-92%) [6-12]. The studies that enrolled a great number of patients with atrial fibrillation lasting less than 24 h showed the highest success rate. For instance, Crijns et al. [6] and Suttorp et al. [7] showed that the average efficacy of intravenous flecainide in restoring sinus rhythm was as high as 85% in patients with recent-onset atrial fibrillation (less than 24 h) compared to only 38% in patients with atrial fibrillation of longer duration. Similarly, ibutilide has been associated with increased conversion of atrial fibrillation depending on arrhythmia duration (35%-64%) [13-19]. Ellenbogen et al. [14] found a 42% efficacy rate for those with an arrhythmia duration of less than 30 days and 16% for those with a duration longer than 30 days. VanderLugt et al. [17] also observed a conversion success rate of 44% within 1.5 h in patients with recent-onset atrial fibrillation treated with ibutilide after cardiac surgery.

An increased risk of torsade de pointes has been observed in ibutilide-treated patients. In fact, ibutilide-induced torsade de pointes is reported in 4.3% of patients treated for conversion of atrial fibrillation [4]. For this reason, until now physicians have been advised against using ibutilide in association with other antiarrhythmic drugs. However, recently, Glatter et al. [19] reported a study on the concomitant use of ibutilide in patients receiving long-term amiodarone therapy for treatment of atrial fibrillation and atrial flutter. These authors observed that ibutilide converted 54% of patients with atrial flutter and 39% of patients with atrial fibrillation who were treated with amiodarone. Furthermore, one episode of nonsustained torsade de pointes (1.4%) was the only proarrhythmic event observed despite marked prolongation of the QT interval after combination therapy. These study data suggest that combined pharmacological therapy with amiodarone and ibutilide is safe and may be a useful adjunct to current cardioversion protocols for atrial flutter and atrial fibrillation. As the same authors observed, this study was biased toward the inclusion of patients with longer-duration arrhythmias (83% had had their arrhythmia for 1 week or more), which may have underestimated the true efficacy of combined therapy in patients with shorter-duration arrhythmias.

Reiffel et al. [20] observed the pharmacological effects of ibutilide and class IC drugs in six patients and concluded that pretreatment with class IC agents can reduce the prolongation of QT_c seen with ibutilide alone. In this study no patients experienced proarrhythmic events with the combination of flecainide and ibutilide.

Ours is the first study to evaluate in a prospective, randomized fashion the association of ibutilide with class IC antiarrhythmic drugs. The preliminary data seem to confirm that combined flecainide and ibutilide therapy is safe. Moreover, in patients with recent-onset atrial fibrillation the association of ibutilide and flecainide seems more effective than flecainide alone in the conversion to sinus rhythm. However, more data are needed to confirm these preliminary results.

References

1. Murgatroyd FD, Camm AJ (1993) Atrial arrhythmias. Lancet 341:1317-1322
2. Kowey PR, Marinchack RA, Rilas SJ et al (1998) Acute treatment of atrial fibrillation. Am J Cardiol 81:16C-22C
3. Lévy S, Breithard G, Campbell WF et al (1998) Atrial fibrillation: current knowledge and recommendations for management. Eur Heart J 19:1294-1320
4. Murray KT (1998) Ibutilide. Circulation 97:493-497
5. Estes M, Garan H, Ruskin JN (1984) Electrophysiologic properties of flecainide acetate. Am J Cardiol 53:26B-29B
6. Crijns HJGM, van Wijk LM, van Gilst WH et al (1988) Acute conversion of atrial fibrillation to sinus rhythm: clinical efficacy of two regimes. Eur Heart J 9:634-938
7. Suttorp MJ, Kingma HJ, Jessurun ER et al (1990) The value of class IC antiarrhythmic drugs for acute conversion of paroxysmal atrial fibrillation or flutter to sinus rhythm. J Am Coll Cardiol 16:1722-1727
8. Madrid AH, Moro C, Marin-Huerta E et al (1993) Comparison of flecainide and procainamide in cardioversion of atrial fibrillation. Eur Heart J 14:1127-1131
9. Kingma JH, Suttorp MJ (1992) Acute pharmacologic conversion of atrial fibrillation and flutter: the role of flecainide, propafenone and verapamil. Am J Cardiol 70:56A-60A
10. Donovan KD, Dobb GJ, Coombs LJ et al (1992) Efficacy of flecainide for the reversion of acute onset atrial fibrillation. Am J Cardiol 70:50A-54A
11. Boriani G, Biffi M, Capucci A (1998) Conversion of recent-onset atrial fibrillation to sinus rhythm: effects of different drug protocols. Pacing Clin Electrophysiol 21:2470-2474
12. Alp JN, Bell JA, Shahi M (2000) Randomized double blind trial of oral versus intravenous flecainide for cardioversion of acute atrial fibrillation. Heart 84:37-40
13. Roden DM (1996) Ibutilide and the treatment of atrial arrhythmias. Circulation 94:1499-1502
14. Ellenbogen KA, Stambler BS, Wood MA et al (1996) Efficacy of intravenous ibutilide for rapid termination of atrial fibrillation and atrial flutter: a dose-response study. J Am Coll Cardiol 28:130-136

15. Stambler BS, Wood MA, Ellenbogen KA et al (1996) Efficacy and safety of repeated intravenous doses of ibutilide for rapid conversion of atrial flutter or fibrillation. Circulation 94:1613-1621

16. Stambler BS, Wood MA, Ellenbogen KA (1997) Antiarrhythmic actions of intravenous ibutilide compared with procainamide during human atrial flutter and fibrillation. Circulation 96:4298-4306

17. VanderLugt JT, Mattioni T, Denker S et al (1999) Efficacy and safety of ibutilide fumarate for conversion of atrial arrhythmias after cardiac surgery. Circulation 100:369-375

18. Volgman AS, Carberry PA, Stambler B et al (1998) Conversion efficacy and safety of intravenous ibutilide compared with intravenous procainamide in patients with atrial flutter or fibrillation. J Am Coll Cardiol 31:1414-1419

19. Glatter K, Yang Y, Chatterjee K et al (2001) Chemical cardioversion of atrial fibrillation or flutter with ibutilide in patients receiving amiodarone therapy. Circulation 103:253-257

20. Reiffel JA, Blitzer M (2000) The actions of ibutilide and class IC drugs on the slow sodium channel: new insights regarding individual pharmacologic effects elucidated through combination therapies. J Cardiovasc Pharmacol Ther 5:177-181

What Is the Role of Internal Low-Energy Cardioversion Today, in the Era of External Biphasic Shock?

P. E. VARDAS AND E.M. KANOUPAKIS

Since atrial fibrillation (AF) may induce troublesome symptoms, embolic complications and deterioration in cardiac function, sinus rhythm restoration should be the main goal of treatment in most patients [1, 2].

For years, pharmacological cardioversion has formed the basic therapeutic approach to this aim [3-6]. However, it is only associated with a high success rate if AF is of recent onset. Apart from this, the problems that arise during the use of antiarrhythmic agents are normally the undesirable side effects, including the increased risk of proarrhythmia [7].

The next step in converting the arrhythmia is electrical cardioversion. In 1962 Lown et al. [8] first examined the method in which shocks are delivered transthoracically in an attempt to defibrillate the atria. Using an electrical charge ranging from 100-360 J, the external cardioversion has a success rate of 65-90%.

For those patients for whom external cardioversion of AF had failed and medications were unable to make arrhythmia bearable, new alternative techniques based on catheters that allow internal cardioversion of atrial fibrillation have been developed in recent years.

Advances on External Cardioversion

External direct-current cardioversion is the method most frequently used for restoration of sinus rhythm in patients with AF. It is available in all cardiological practices, in contrast to internal cardioversion.

An important determinant of external shock efficacy is the transthoracic impedance. To avoid high impedance, special attention needs to be paid to paddle pressure. Even shaving the hirsute chest in patients undergoing elective cardioversion may improve outcome [9]. Furthermore, self-adhesive pads, which are coated with a conducting gel, are preferred to metal paddles.

Cardiology Department, University Hospital of Heraklion, Crete, Greece

Another important factor is the polarity and the location of the pads used. In a study of 301 patients undergoing external cardioversion of AF, Botto et al. [10] found that an anteroposterior paddle position (right sternal body at the third intercostal space – angle of the left scapula) is superior to an anterolateral location of the pads and permits lower DC shock energy requirements.

Despite the widespread use of DC cardioversion, there is general disagreement on what should be the initial energy for elective cardioversion of persistent AF. In a recent study Joglar et al. [11] showed that an initial energy of 360 J was safe and significantly more effective than 100 or 200 J. Compared with the lower energies, fewer shocks and less total cumulative energy were required when 360 J was used initially [11].

Most defibrillators deliver a single monophasic shock. However, it has been shown that the defibrillation threshold is reduced in implantable defibrillators by delivering an internal biphasic shock instead of a monophasic shock. Currently this method is being applied to external defibrillators.

In a prospective randomized study, Mittal et al. [12] compared the efficacy of rectilinear biphasic waveform with a standard damped sine wave monophasic shock for the transthoracic cardioversion of AF. They showed that biphasic shocks have a significantly higher efficacy, which is achieved with significantly less delivered current than the monophasic shocks. In a recently published study, Ricard et al. [13] confirmed the superiority of biphasic shocks for AF external cardioversion.

The ability to cardiovert AF with fewer shocks and lower energy offers several advantages. Among them is the less negative inotropic effect of the shock, especially in heart failure patients, the lower risk of anesthesia-related complications, and the cost saving by reducing the time of the procedure.

Apart from this very useful new development, there are other techniques that may improve success rates to standard external shocks. Pretreatment with antiarrhythmic agents appears to be helpful. Ibutilide facilitates successful cardioversion of AF in patients who have failed conventional external cardioversion and may serve as an alternative to internal cardioversion [14, 15]. Finally, Saliba et al. [16] have shown that high-energy external shocks (720 J) increase the conversion rate for patients who fail initial attempts at direct current cardioversion.

Optimizing the external cardioversion technique, including the routine use of biphasic shocks and pretreatment with antiarrhythmic medications, may reduce the need for internal low-energy cardioversion. So, where does internal cardioversion stand?

Low-energy Internal Cardioversion Today

When internal cardioversion was proposed as a new technique to cardiovert AF in patients who had failed both pharmacological and external cardioversion, high-energy shocks were used. In 1992, in a randomized trial that compared classical external atrial defibrillation with 300-360 J to internal atrial defibrillation with 200-300 J, the success rates were 67% and 91%, respectively. The internal procedure was proved superior to conventional external cardioversion, with no more recurrences over long-term follow-up [17].

Since then a number of experimental and human studies [18-23] have enriched our knowledge and today low-energy endocardial defibrillation, an evolution of high-energy internal cardioversion, represents a new and extremely promising alternative for the treatment of atrial fibrillation. Extremely encouraging were the results of a large prospective study [24], which compared the low-energy intracardiac cardioversion and conventional external cardioversion in 187 consecutive patients with chronic atrial fibrillation. The restoration rate was 93% and 79%, respectively, with mean energy for successful cardioversion of 5.8 ± 3.2 J for the internal and 313 ± 71 J for the external cardioversion group. In this study, which involves a large number of patients, the authors demonstrate that internal low-energy defibrillation is not only feasible in humans, but is also of greater efficacy than the classical extracardiac transthoracic cardioversion. Another message from this study is that those patients who failed to restore sinus rhythm after an external DC shock, but were successfully treated by internal defibrillation, have no tendency for earlier relapse of their arrhythmia than others do [24].

Techniques using either two catheters or a single catheter have been developed. In a comparative evaluation of these systems, there was no difference in either the amount of energy used (8.4 ± 3 vs 7.2 ± 3 J) or the possible complications, while the primary success rate was as high (94% vs 93%) [25].

If we exempt the fact that temporary internal low-energy cardioversion of AF is an invasive method that requires catheterization in patients who are usually taking anticoagulants, the safety of the method remains very high. The advantages of low-energy transcatheter cardioversion include the avoidance of general anesthesia, which may be hazardous in some patients. It is also known that this procedure is safe and effective in patients with a history of heart failure and depressed left ventricular function. In a large multicenter trial, Andraghetti and Scalese [26] confirmed the safety and efficacy of internal cardioversion. It is important to know that over a half of their patients had failed to convert at external attempts.

Other selective indications are those patients with increased thoracic impedance, such as obese patients or those with pulmonary disease. Furthermore, it can be used in some acute settings, as in AF, that involve diagnostic electrophysiological studies and catheter ablations, and where the use of antiarrhythmic medication may make the procedure difficult. Moreover, the supportive pacing encompasses protections from possible bradycardiac phenomena in patients with longstanding atrial fibrillation whose sinus node function is undetermined.

Most importantly, internal cardioversion provides the opportunity to observe the clinical electrophysiology of AF, such as the electrical remodeling and the immediate recurrences of the arrhythmia [27, 28]. Finally, experience in the use of this technique may have important implications for the improvement of implantable atrial defibrillators for patients with paroxysmal AF.

References

1. Wolf PA, Dawber TR, Thomas HE Jr, Kannel WB (1978) Epidemiologic assessment of chronic atrial fibrillation and the risk of stroke: the Framingham study. Neurology 28:9973-9977
2. Shinbane J, Wood M, Jensen N et al (1997) Tachycardia - induced cardiomyopathy: a review of animal models and clinical studies. J Am Coll Cardiol 29:709-715
3. Stambler BS, Wood MA, Ellenbogen KA et al (1996) Efficacy and safety of repeated intravenous doses of ibutilide for rapid conversion of atrial flutter or fibrillation. Ibutilide Repeat Dose Study Investigators. Circulation 94:1613-1621
4. Capucci A, Boriani G, Botto GL et al (1994) Conversion of recent-onset atrial fibrillation by a single oral loading dose of propafenone or flecainide. Am J Cardiol 74:503-505
5. Tieleman RG, Gosselink AT, Grijns HJ et al (1997) Efficacy, safety and determinants of conversion of atrial fibrillation and flutter with oral amiodarone. Am J Cardiol 79:53-57
6. Kochiadakis GE, Igoumenidis NE, Parthenakis FI et al (1999) Amiodarone versus propafenone for cardioversion of chronic atrial fibrillation: results of a randomized controlled study. J Am Coll Cardiol 33:966-971
7. Falk RH (1992) Proarrythmia in patients treated for atrial fibrillation or flutter. Ann Intern Med 117:141-150
8. Lown B, Perlroth MG, Kaidbey S et al (1962) Cardioversion of atrial fibrillation. N Engl J Med 269:325-331
9. Bissing JW, Kerber RE (2000) Effect of shaving the chest of hirsute subjects on transthoracic impedance to self-adhesive defibrillation electrode pads. Am J Cardiol 86:587-589
10. Botto GL, Politi A, Bonini W et al (1999) External cardioversion of atrial fibrillation: role of paddle position on technical efficacy and energy requirements. Heart 82:726-730
11. Joglar JA, Hamdan MH, Ramaswamy K et al (2000) Initial energy for elective external cardioversion of persistent atrial fibrillation. Am J Cardiol 86:348-350
12. Mittal S, Ayati S, Stein KM et al (2000) Transthoracic cardioversion of atrial fibrillation: comparison of rectilinear biphasic versus damped sine wave monophasic shocks. Circulation 101:1282-1287
13. Ricard P, Levy S, Boccara G et al (2001) External cardioversion of atrial fibrillation: comparison of biphasic vs monophasic waveform shocks. Europace 3:96-99
14. Li H, Natale A, Tomassoni G et al (1999) Usefulness of ibutilide in facilitating successful external cardioversion of refractory atrial fibrillation. Am J Cardiol 84:1096-1098
15. Oral H, Souza JJ, Michaud GF et al (1999) Facilitating transthoracic cardioversion of atrial fibrillation with ibutilide pretreatment. N Engl J Med 340:1849-1854
16. Saliba W, Juratli N, Chung MK (1999) Higher energy synchronized external direct current cardioversion for refractory atrial fibrillation. J Am Coll Cardiol 34:2031-2034
17. Levy S, Lauribe P, Dolla E et al (1992) A randomized comparison of external and internal cardioversion of chronic atrial fibrillation. Circulation 86:1415-1420
18. Powell AC, Garan H, McGovern BA et al (1992) Low energy conversion of atrial fibrillation in the sheep. J Am Coll Cardiol 20:707-771
19. Cooper RA, Alferness CA, Smith WM, Ideker RE (1993) Internal cardioversion of atrial fibrillation in sheep. Circulation 87:1673-1686
20. Murgatroyd FD, Slade AKB, Sopher SM et al (1995) Efficacy and tolerability of transvenous low energy cardioversion of paroxysmal atrial defibrillation in humans. J Am Coll Cardiol 25:1347-1353
21. Alt E, Schmitt C, Ammer R et al (1994) Initial experience with intracardiac atrial defibrillation in patients with chronic atrial fibrillation. Pacing Clin Electrophysiol 17:1067-1078

22. Sopher SM, Murgatroyd FD, Slade AK et al (1996) Low-energy internal cardioversion of atrial fibrillation resistant to transthoracic shocks. Heart 75:635-638

23. Schmitt C, Alt E, Plewan A et al (1996) Low-energy intracardiac cardioversion after failed conventional external cardioversion of atrial fibrillation. J Am Coll Cardiol 28:994-999

24. Alt E, Ammer R, Schmitt C et al (1997) A comparison of treatment with low-energy intracardiac cardioversion and conventional external cardioversion. Eur Heart J 18:1796-1804

25. Alt E, Ammer R, Lehmann G et al (1998) Efficacy of a new balloon catheter for internal cardioversion of chronic atrial fibrillation without anaesthesia. Heart 79:128-132

26. Andraghetti A, Scalese M (2001) Safety and efficacy of low-energy cardioversion of 500 patients using two different techniques. Europace 3:4-9

27. Timmermans C, Rodriguez LM, Smeets JL, Wellens HJ (1998) Immediate reinitiation of atrial fibrillation following internal atrial defibrillation. J Cardiovasc Electrophysiol 9:122-128

28. Hobbs WJ, Fynn S, Todd DM et al (2000) Reversal of atrial electrical remodeling after cardioversion of persistent atrial fibrillation in humans. Circulation 101:1145-1151

Early Recurrences of Atrial Fibrillation: How to Predict and Avoid Them ?

G.L. BOTTO AND A. SAGONE

Introduction

Atrial fibrillation (AF) is the most common sustained tachyarrhythmia encountered in clinical practice [1, 2], causing the highest number of days of hospitalization for arrhythmia admission in the USA [3]. The overall prevalence in the adult population is 0.4% and its incidence increase with age and with the presence of heart disease [4, 5].

Management strategies for the treatment of AF include intravenous or oral rate control drugs, intravenous or oral pharmacologic conversion, direct current (DC) cardioversion, and drugs to maintain sinus rhythm after successful cardioversion [1, 2, 6]. With all of these options, embolic risk stratification and proper anticoagulation strategies are required for each patient [1, 2, 6, 7].

Electrical cardioversion is actually the more effective way to convert persistent atrial fibrillation to sinus rhythm. The procedure itself may restore sinus rhythm in approximately 75%-95% of patients with persistent AF [8, 9]. Unfortunately, because of the high recurrence rate, no more than 40%-50% of patients maintain sinus rhythm for 6 months or more, with antiarrhythmic drug prophylaxis different from amiodarone [10]. Indeed the most relevant clinical problem after successful cardioversion is represented by the risk of recurrence, which may occur in different time phases following the procedure.

Definition and Time Course Recurrences of Atrial Fibrillation

The etiology of early reinitiation of AF after external cardioversion is vague and its incidence is unknown. It can occur in a significant proportion of patients with AF following successful electrical cardioversion, using either internal [11, 12] or external [13] methods.

Department of Cardiology, Sant'Anna Hospital, Como, Italy

Indeed, it is a phenomenon which has only recently been described, partly because of the increasing use of internal electrical cardioversion [11], the catheters for which enable recording of atrial electrograms, and the employment of atrial defibrillator devices [12] that make the analysis of stored atriograms possible, providing the motive and the means for study of these phenomena which have acquired their own acronyms. The recurrence may occur: in a very early phase after electrical shock (minutes) (immediate recurrence of atrial fibrillation, IRAF); in an early phase (first 24-48 h to 5-7 days) (early recurrence of atrial fibrillation, ERAF); or in weeks to months following the successful procedure (late recurrence of atrial fibrillation, LRAF).

Recently, in a retrospective study of 85 patients with AF, the functional and pharmacological variables that could possibly influence the long-term outcome after the first electrical cardioversion were analysed [14]. Multivariate analysis confirmed that duration of the treated episode and age > 75 years were prognostic factors that predicted the persistence of sinus rhythm 100 days after successful cardioversion, while echocardiographic parameters and the presence of organic heart disease played no role. The phenomena of IRAF and ERAF are more difficult to characterize because they would require continuous monitoring of an AF patient's cardiac rhythm and, for this reason, only few studies are available concerning this subject.

Early Recurrences of Atrial Fibrillation

The phenomenon of early recurrence of AF following successful cardioversion is a clinical setting in which two important concepts are implicated and may strongly interact. The first concept is that an increasingly recognized and growing number of patients have AF initiated, and possibly maintained, by an ectopic focus of repetitive atrial activity [15]. The second concept is that AF itself causes changes in cellular electrophysiology that, at least in animal models, have the effect of further increasing the tendency to fibrillation [16, 17], and there is a reversal of this electrophysiological remodelling after a certain period of sinus rhythm [18]. The first of these two concepts relates to the triggers for initiation of the arrhythmia and the second to the myocardial substrate predisposing to and maintaining the arrhythmia.

However, the extent to which early recurrence of AF is due either to enhanced frequency of atrial ectopic activity as potential triggers or to enhanced vulnerability of the remodelled, recently defibrillated atrium to the effects of the atrial ectopy remains uncertain.

It has been demonstrated that prolonged atrial pacing in goats [16] and in dogs [17] at rates sufficiently rapid to produce AF causes reversible electrophysiological and structural changes in the atria. Whereas during the control condition no sustained AF could be induced, after several days to weeks of rapid pacing in these animals, AF had become sustained.

In the study of Wijffels et al. [16], the refractory period was measured at multiple sites by programmed electrical stimulation. AF was produced by burst pacing (1 s, 50 Hz). In the normal goat, electrically-induced AF lasted only for a short time and terminated promptly with a few seconds. After the baseline study was completed, the animals were connected to an external automatic atrial fibrillator. The device detected spontaneous cardioversion of AF and delivered a burst of stimuli to promptly reinduce the arrhythmia. Within the first 24 h of AF, both the duration and the rate of the arrhythmia increased significantly and the AF cycle length shortened progressively until, after about 4-6 days, a new steady state was reached. No changes in conduction velocity along Bachmann's bundle were found.

Simultaneously, Morillo et al. [17] performed a study on mongrel dogs equipped with a modified programmable pacemaker, allowing atrial pacing at a constant rate of 400 beats/min. Whereas at baseline sustained AF could not be induced in any dog, after 6 weeks of rapid atrial pacing, programmed atrial stimulation induced AF in 50% of the dogs. Marked bi-atrial enlargement was documented by echocardiography and the right atrial refractory period was significantly reduced from 150 ms to 127 ms.

The most important atrial parameter of AF-induced electrical remodelling is the refractory period. During control, early premature beats did not induce any arrhythmia. After a few hours of atrial fibrillation, the atrial refractory period was shortened and a premature stimulus was followed by a short run of rapid atrial responses. Twenty-four hours of AF further shortened the atrial refractory period, and now early premature beats triggered paroxysms of AF. Moreover, during control, the refractory period showed a short-term rate adaptation to pacing intervals. After hours of AF, the relationship between the refractory period and the rate become reversed, so that instead of lengthening at a slow rate, the refractory period actually shortens [16]. The loss of the physiological prolongation of the refractory period in response to a sudden decrease in rate has also been observed in other studies [19, 20].

In this condition, the physiological normalization of atrial refractoriness after sinus rhythm restoration was lost and it was recovered only after a few days of stable sinus rhythm. If atrial refractoriness requires a few days to revert completely, this could explain the high incidence of recurrences early after cardioversion.

With this hypothesis, some studies have tested the efficacy of drug treatment before cardioversion in preventing AF relapse, reducing atrial refractoriness maladaptation or preventing premature supraventricular beats.

Atrial Electrical Remodelling and Calcium-blocker Agents

The mechanisms sustaining electrophysiological remodelling are not completely known, but intracellular calcium overload seems to be involved [19].

Animal experiments have shown that verapamil infusion during rapid atrial pacing [19], or short episodes of artificially induced AF [20], significantly reduced the electrical changes of the atria. If, in humans also, electrical remodelling is related to intracellular calcium overload, the frequency of relapse might be lowered by drugs that lower the intracellular calcium concentration.

To date, two retrospective [21, 22] and only one prospective randomized study [23] have evaluated the role of intracellular calcium-lowering drugs in the clinical setting. Tieleman et al. [21], using transtelephonic monitoring in 61 patients cardioverted for chronic AF, documented that there was a peak incidence of relapse of AF during the first 5 days after cardioversion, suggesting a temporary vulnerable electrophysiologic state of the atria. Being on intracellular calcium-lowering medication, including verapamil, diltiazem, dihydropyridines and β-blocking agents, preceding the cardioversion was the only significant variable related to maintenance of the sinus rhythm. Botto et al. [22], in a retrospective study on 437 patients submitted to electrical cardioversion for persistent AF, observed a lower rate of unsuccessful procedures in patients treated with calcium blockers (verapamil, diltiazem, gallopamil and dihydropyridines) before the electrical shock. In contrast, they did not observe any difference in early recurrences of the arrhythmia in patients treated with calcium blockers compared to those who did not receive these drugs. In the Tieleman et al. study, antiarrhythmic medication was administered only in 30/61 patients (33%) while in the Botto et al. study, 291/437 patients (67%) received antiarrhythmic drugs during follow-up. Antiarrhythmic drugs are efficacious in reducing early recurrences after successful cardioversion [13], and this effect might conceal the action of calcium channel-blocking drugs in this setting.

De Simone et al. [23] first demonstrated, in a prospective randomized fashion, the beneficial effect of an oral pre-treatment with verapamil, associated with an antiarrhythmic drug, in reducing the incidence of early recurrences of AF after external or internal electrical cardioversion. They found a higher incidence of AF recurrences in patients who received propafenone alone, before electrical cardioversion, compared to patients in which propafenone was associated with verapamil, suggesting that intracellular calcium-lowering drugs reduce electrical remodelling, which may in turn lead to a more rapid recovery after cardioversion. The lack of benefits of long-term therapy with verapamil, shown in this study, strongly support the hypothesis that recovery from electrical remodeling occurs in a few days and that after this period intracellular calcium-lowering drugs might have only a marginal role in preventing AF recurrences.

Antiarrhythmic Drugs to Prevent Early Recurrences of Atrial Fibrillation

With respect to the triggers for the initiation of AF, there is evidence that any tendency to atrial ectopic activity is exaggerated in the early period following cardioversion.

In a recent study by Tse and co-workers [24], 91% of the episodes of early recurrence of AF were triggered by atrial premature complexes. Atrial ectopies that triggered AF were more premature than those that did not. In this study, sotalol infusion decreased the sinus rate and the frequency and prematurity of atrial premature beats, and prevented further early recurrence of AF in 83% of the patients.

Bianconi et al. [13] tested the efficacy of propafenone in a placebo-controlled study involving 100 patients, comparing two different strategies: pre-treatment with oral propafenone; or propafenone only after cardioversion. Pharmacological conversion before DC shock was obtained in 6% of the patients. Propafenone did not exert any significant effect on the total energy required for cardioversion or on the success rate of the procedure. Indeed, propafenone had differential effects requirements for successful cardioversion. It significantly decreased DC shock energy in those patients (22% of the propafenone pre-treatment group) in whom AF was transformed into a more stable arrhythmia, mimicking atrial flutter, whereas energy requirements were increased compared to control if the AF pattern did not change. Arrhythmia recurrence was significantly reduced within 10 min after cardioversion (0% vs 17% in the placebo group) and also within 24 h and 48 h. After cardioversion, the incidence of supraventricular ectopic beats was higher in the placebo patients.

Oral amiodarone is effective in the long-term maintenance of sinus compared to propafenone or sotalol [10]. However, its use around the electrical cardioversion of AF may be difficult, because amiodarone loading requires al least 4-6 weeks to reach therapeutic plasma levels, so that during the first weeks of treatment patients may be at risk of recurrences. Thus, it is mandatory to start amiodarone treatment at least 4-6 weeks before electrical cardioversion if we want patients completely protected from early recurrences of AF after successful electrical procedure.

Capucci et al. [25] randomized 92 patients with persistent AF and organic heart disease to pretreatment with oral amiodarone, 400 mg/day, 1 month before cardioversia, and 200 mg/day, 2 months after cardioversion, or oral diltiazem 180 mg/day 1 month before and 2 months after cardioversion. In the amiodarone group, 25% of patients reversed to sinus rhythm before DC cardioversion, and amiodarone pre-treatment increased DC-cardioversion efficacy. Twenty-four hours after cardioversion, the early recurrences of AF were similar in the different groups, with a slight trend in favour of amiodarone, while at 2 months the recurrence rate was lower in amiodarone-treated patients (32% vs 52%-56%). It is possible to suppose the beneficial effect of amiodarone, either on the prolongation of the atrial refractoriness and/or of the reduction in intracellular calcium concentration. Both these mechanisms may have affected the atrial remodelling phenomenon.

Therefore, there is evidence that both factors, triggers and substrate, contribute to the phenomenon of early recurrence of AF, and may interact in a dynamic manner [26]. The more premature the atrial ectopy, the shorter the time to relapse [21]. The finding that patients with the long-coupled atrial ectopic beats relapsed later would be consistent with the concept of progressive reversal of the remodelling of the atria after return to sinus rhythm.

Conclusions

The heterogeneous nature of AF dictates that a variety of treatment modalities should be used to manage this disease. The therapeutic efficacy of most of these treatment modalities is likely to be affected by early recurrences of AF noted soon after cardioversion. The mechanism underlying early recurrence of AF is unclear for the majority of patients, but is probably multifactorial. Contributing factors may include a complex electrophysiological remodelling, which strongly interacts with triggering factors such as atrial ectopic beats, both probably modulated by the autonomic nervous system.

The administration of Class IC and Class III antiarrhythmic drugs has a favourable effect in reducing early recurrences, mainly by reducing the incidence of premature atrial ectopic beats, which is counterbalanced by the possibility of postcardioversion bradyarrhythmias. An alternative approach could be a pretreatment with verapamil, alone or together with antiarrhythmic drugs, to reduce maladaptation of electrophysiological parameters induced by AF itself.

Ongoing, prospective, randomized studies with the aim of confirming these observations will be available in the near future [27, 28].

References

1. Pristowsky EN, Benson DW Jr, Fuster V et al (1996) Management of patients with atrial fibrillation: a statement for healthcare professionals for the subcommittee on the electrocardiography and electrophysiology, America Heart Association. Circulation 93:1262-1277
2. Lévy S, Breithard G, Campbell WF et al on behalf of the Working Group on Arrhythmias of the European Society of Cardiology (1998) Atrial fibrillation: current knowledge and recommendations for management. Eur Heart J 19:1294-1320
3. Bialy D, Lehmann MH, Schumacher DN et al (1992) Hospitalization for arrhythmias in the United States: importance of atrial fibrillation. J Am Coll Cardiol 19:41A (abstr)
4. Kannel WB, Wolf PA (1992) Epidemiology of atrial fibrillation. In: RH Falk, PJ Podrid (eds) Atrial fibrillation mechanisms and management. Raven, New York pp 81-92
5. Brand FN, Abbot RD, Kannel WB, Wolf PA (1985) Characteristics and prognosis of lone atrial fibrillation. J Am Med Assoc 254:3449-3516
6. Naccarelli GV, Dell' Orfano JT, Wolbrette DL et al (2000) Cost-effective management of acute atrial fibrillation: role of rate control, spontaneous conversion, medical and direct current cardioversion, transesophageal echocardiography, and anti-embolic therapy. Am J Cardiol 85:36D-45D
7. Laupacis A, Albers G, Dalen J et al (1998) Antithrombotic therapy in atrial fibrillation. Chest 114:579S-589S
8. Lown B (1967) Electrical reversion of cardiac arrhythmias. Br Heart J 29:469-489
9. Botto GL, Politi A, Bonini W et al (1999) External cardioversion of atrial fibrillation: role of paddle position on technical efficacy and energy requirements. Heart 82:726-730
10. Roy D, Talajic M, Dorian P et al, for the Canadian Trial of Atrial Fibrillation Investigators (2000) Amidarone to prevent recurrence of atrial fibrillation. N Engl J Med 342:913-920

11. Timmermans C, Rodriguez LM, Smeets JLRM, Wellens HJJ (1998) Immediate reinitiation of atrial fibrillation following internal defibrillation. J Cardiovasc Electrophysiol 9:122-128

12. Wellens HJJ, Lau CP, Luderiz B et al for the Metrix Investigators (1998) Atrioverter, an implantable device for the treatment of atrial fibrillation. Circulation 98:1651-1656

13. Bianconi L, Mennuni M, Lukic V et al (1996) Effects of oral propafenone administration before electrical cardioversion of chronic atrial fibrillation: a placebo-controlled study. J Am Coll Cardiol 28:700-706

14. Daytschaever M, Haerynck F, Tevernier R, Jordaens L (1998) Factors influencing long-term persistence of sinus rhythm after first electrical cardioversion of atrial fibrillation. Pacing Clin Electrophysiol 21:284-287

15. Jais P, Haissaguerre M, Shah DC et al (1997) A focal source of atrial fibrillation treated by discrete radiofrequency ablation. Circulation 95:572-576

16. Wijffels MCEF, Kirchhof CJHJ, Dorland R, Allessie MA (1995) Atrial fibrillation begets atrial fibrillation: a study in awake chronically instrumented goats. Circulation 92:1954-1968

17. Morillo CA, Klein GJ, Jones DL, Guirardon CM (1995) Chronic rapid atrial pacing: structural, functional, and electrophysiologic characteristics of a new model of sustained atrial fibrillation. Circulation 91:1588-1595

18. Yu WC, Lee SH, Tai CT et al (1999) Reversal of atrial electrical remodeling following cardioversion of long standing atrial fibrillation in man. Cardiovasc Res 42:470-476

19. Goette A, Honeycutt C, Langberg JJ (1996) Electrical remodeling in atrial fibrillation. Time course and mechanism. Circulation 94:2968-2974

20. Tieleman RG, De Langen CDJ, Van Gelder IC et al (1997) Verapamil reduces tachycardia-induced electrical remodeling of the atria. Circulation 95:1945-1953

21. Tieleman RG, Van Gelder IC, Crijins HJGM et al (1998) Early recurrence of atrial fibrillation after electrical cardioversion: a result of fibrillation-induced electrical remodeling of the atria? J Am Coll Cardiol 31:167-173

22. Botto GL, Bonatti R, De Nittis G et al (1999) Calcium-channel-blockers and efficacy of external cardioversion of persistent atrial fibrillation. Prevention of electrical remodeling? G Ital Cardiol 29[Suppl 5]:179-182

23. De Simone A, Stabile G, Vitale DF et al (1999) Pre-treatment with verapamil in patients with persistent or chronic atrial fibrillation who underwent electrical cardioversion. J Am Coll Cardiol 34:810-814

24. Tse HF, Lau CP, Ayers GM (1999) Atrial pacing for suppression of early reinitiation of atrial fibrillation after successful internal cardioversion. Heart 82:319-324

25. Capucci A, Villani GQ, Aschieri D et al (2000) Oral amiodarone increase the efficacy of DC-cardioversion in restoration of sinus rhythm in patients with chronic atrial fibrillation. Eur Heart J 21:66-73

26. Peters NS (2000) Post cardioversion atrial fibrillation: the synthesis of modern concepts? Eur Heart J 21:1119-1121

27. Van Noord T, Van Gelder IC, Tieleman RG et al (2000) The role of intracellular calcium lowering for maintenance of sinus rhythm after cardioversion of persistent atrial fibrillation, a randomized study. Pacing Clin Electrophysiol 4 (part II):577 (abstr)

28. Botto GL, Belotti G, Cirò A et al (2001) Verapamil pre-treatment before electrical cardioversion of persistent atrial fibrillation: the VERAF Study. Eur Heart J (in press) (abstr)

Reversal of Atrial Stunning After Cardioversion: What Are the Time Course and Clinical-Therapeutic Implications?

F. Rigo, V. Cutaia, P. Nicolin, A. Corrado, A. Bonso and A. Raviele

Introduction

Atrial fibrillation (AF) is one of the commonest types of arrhythmia, occurring in up to 4% of patients over 60 years of age [1-3]. Cardioversion is performed in patients with AF in an effort to improve cardiac function, relieve symptoms, and decrease the risk of thrombus formation. Successful cardioversion is associated with a 5%-7% incidence of embolism among patients who have not received adequate anticoagulation therapy [4-9]. The cardioversion of AF to sinus rhythm is associated with transient mechanical dysfunction of the left atrium (LA) and left atrial appendage (LAA) and the development of spontaneous echocardiographic contrast. This phenomenon has been termed "stunning" and is considered an important factor for thromboembolic stroke following cardioversion of AF to sinus rhythm [10-15].

Mechanism of Atrial Stunning

The exact mechanism by which conversion of AF results in LA and auricular mechanical dysfunction and predisposes to changes in the grade of spontaneous echocardiographic contrast is not clear [16]. Changes occurring in the atria during AF may have a deleterious effect on the atria once sinus rhythm is restored. The marked increase in the rate of atrial depolarization during AF might result in calcium loading, leading to desensitization or down-regulation of calcium receptors in the atria. Restoration of sinus rhythm and elimination of the calcium-loaded state might then result in a state of relative calcium deficiency and associated decrease in mechanical function, which would be expected to normalize as calcium receptors return to their baseline state [16]. Recently it has been demonstrated that the LAA shows a divergence in behavior compared with

Cardiovascular Department, Division of Cardiology, Umberto I Hospital, Mestre-Venice, Italy

the LA, as a whole and this may be related to intrinsic differences in LAA distensibility and shortening [17]. We are not aware of studies examining potential differences in calcium handling by atrial myocytes from the body of the LA and from the LAA during AF. The reduction in LAA contraction velocities has been identified as a risk factor for thrombus formation within the LAA [16, 17].

Time Course

The observation that thromboembolism after cardioversion may more often arise as a consequence of the effects of cardioversion on atrial function than from dislodgement of a preexistent thrombus [18] has highlighted the importance of the magnitude and duration of mechanical impairment of the LA. Recovery of atrial contractile function may vary greatly from patient to patient, depending on a number of factors [19, 20] and does not occur immediately after conversion of chronic AF, but proceeds gradually [20].

Mode of Cardioversion

Direct evidence of myocardial injury due to electrical cardioversion has been sustained by the initial evidence of organic damage demonstrated by transient ST changes [21], by CPKmb elevation, by evidence of myocyte necrosis [21], and by the presence of free radicals [22]. Fatkin et al. [18] and Grimm et al. [23] using transesophageal echocardiography during electrical cardioversion demonstrated new or increased spontaneous echo contrast in a considerable proportion of patients, an expression of subsequent LA mechanical dysfunction and a specific marker of thromboembolic risk. By contrast, Sparks et al. [24] recently demonstrated that endocardial and transthoracic DC shocks are not directly responsible for LA and LAA stunning and do not contribute to the stunning observed after the cardioversion of AF to sinus rhythm, and that moreover this is due to the function of the preceding arrhythmia itself rather than the mode of reversion. Abascal et al. [25] also found no significant difference in atrial mechanical recovery between electrically and pharmacologically cardioverted patients and concluded that the degree of LA dysfunction after cardioversion is independent of the mode of cardioversion.

Duration of AF

Harjal et al. [26] demonstrated that immediately after cardioversion and at 24 h and 1 week after cardioversion, atrial mechanical function is better in patients with AF of less than 2 weeks' duration than in those with AF of more than 6 weeks' duration. Although there was no difference in LA diameter between the groups with AF of "brief" (< 2 weeks), "moderate" (2-6 weeks), or "prolonged" (> 6 weeks) duration, other patient characteristics such as age, left ventricular ejection fraction, underlying cardiac diseases, concomitant antiarrhythmic therapy, and mode of cardioversion were not separately reported for the three groups. More recently Manning et al. [27] concluded that in patients with a clinical duration of AF of less than 5 weeks, recovery of atrial mechanical function appears related to the mode of cardioversion: a more prompt return of atrial mechanical function was seen in patients undergoing successful pharmacological cardioversion than in those undergoing successful electrical cardioversion after unsuccessful pharmacological cardioversion. Duration of AF of less than 24 h and normal LA size was also associated with early recovery of atrial function [28]. Sparks [29] more recently observed that LA stunning was not detected after brief duration of AF in patients with structural heart disease and therefore concluded that the thromboembolic risk is low after AF of brief duration that terminates either spontaneously or with an endocardial DC shock even in patients with significant structural heart disease. These findings have important implications for recipients of implantable devices that are capable of atrial defibrillation in response to AF.

Other Factors

Various clinical findings have been studied as risk factors responsible for postcardioversion atrial dysfunction. Blood hypertension, alcohol abuse, heart rate after conversion, cardiac loading conditions, drugs, the presence of valvular or myocardial diseases, LA size, left ventricular ejection fraction, and LAA contraction velocity have been studied [28, 30], but the associations remain unclear so far.

Clinical and Therapeutic Implications

Stroke is the third leading cause of death and long-term disability in the United States. Emboli arising from the heart are estimated to account for 15%-20% of all ischemic strokes, with a high reported prevalence of 34% [26]. It has been well documented that the thromboembolic risk in the pericardioversion period is very high [26-29]. For this reason the American College of Chest Physicians Consensus Committee on Antithrombotic Therapy Recommendations [31] stipulates that all patients with AF lasting less than 2 days should receive warfarin therapy for 3 weeks before and 4 weeks after cardioversion until sinus rhythm is maintained. There are several practical clinical problems with these recommendations, including bleeding complications related to warfarin, the requirement for a second hospital admission for cardioversion, and the delay in reversion of AF to sinus rhythm. A possible solution may be given by echocardiography, which shows good sensitivity in the screening before cardioversion to look for LA thrombus [18, 26]. Transesophageal echocardiography has clearly demonstrated superior sensitivity and specificity in detecting prethrombotic findings and LAA thrombus [32], and for this reason can be utilized to avoid long-term anticoagulation before cardioversion, especially in patients at high risk of bleeding. We believe that transesophageal echocardiography before cardioversion should be reserved for those patients with contraindication to anticoagulation, or who need to shorten their anticoagulation course, or have inadequate duration or extent of anticoagulation, or have poor documentation of anticoagulation status.

Thromboemboli have been known to occur after cardioversion in nonanticoagulated patients despite "negative" transesophageal echocardiograms immediately before cardioversion [33]. It is most likely that persistent or increased atrial stasis after cardioversion results in the formation of fresh, loosely adherent thrombi and subsequent embolism, and the lack of mechanical activity contributes to stasis in the LA and also in the LAA [21-24]. The occurrence of embolism in patients undergoing cardioversion is close to 7%; this finding in a large proportion of patients seems to be due to an increased thrombogenic milieu immediately after cardioversion, and the risk is present presumably until such time as "normal" atrial and appendage function resumes [24, 29]. It is unclear how long anticoagulation therapy should be continued after cardioversion, because there has been no safe demonstration of the recovery of atrial mechanical function and persistence of stunning, which may have a longer time course than overall atrial restoration [29]. Only the transesophageal approach allows clear demonstration of LAA function and subsequent potential thromboembolic risk. The cost-effectiveness of this approach needs to be better verified: we have no certain clinical findings about cost minimization and potential morbidity associated with anticoagulation. Future research should focus on identifying subsets of patients who do not require prolonged anticoagulation after cardioversion.

References

1. Ostrander LD, Brandt RL, Kjelsberg MO et al (1965) Electrocardiographic findings among the adult population of a total community, Tecumseh, Michigan. Circulation 31:888-898
2. Petersen P (1990) Thromboembolic complications in atrial fibrillation. Stroke 21:4-13
3. Kannel WB, Wolf PA (1992) Epidemiology of atrial fibrillation. In: Falk RH (ed) Atrial fibrillation: mechanism and management. Raven Press, New York, pp 81-92
4. Resnekov L, McDonald L (1967) Complications in 220 patients with cardiac dysrhythmias treated by phased direct current shock, and indications for electrocardioversion. Br Heart J 29:926-936
5. Bjerkelund CJ, Orning OM (1969) The efficacy of anticoagulation therapy in preventing embolism related to DC electrical conversion of atrial fibrillation. Am J Cardiol 23:208-216
6. Lown B, Perlroth MG (1963) Cardioversion of atrial fibrillation: a report on treatment of 65 episodes in 50 patients. N Engl J Med 269:325-331
7. Weinberg DM, Mancini GBJ, Goldberger AL (1989) Anticoagulation for cardioversion of atrial fibrillation. Am J Cardiol 63:745-746
8. Petersen P, Godtfredsen J, Andersen B (1986) Embolic complications in paroxysmal atrial fibrillation. Stroke 17:622-626

9. Rokseth R, Storstein O (1963) Quinidine therapy of chronic auricolar fibrillation: the occurrence and mechanism of syncope. Arch Intern Med 111:184-189
10. Grimm RA, Stewart WJ, Maloney JD et al (1997) Left atrial appendage "stunning" after electrical cardioversion of atrial flutter: an attenuated response compared with atrial fibrillation as the mechanism for lower susceptibility to thromboembolic events. J Am Coll Cardiol 29:582-589
11. Manning WJ, Silverman DI, Katz SE et al (1994) Impaired left atrial mechanical function after cardioversion: relation to duration of atrial fibrillation. J Am Coll Cardiol 23:1535-1540
12. Omram H, Jung W, Rabahich R et al (1997) Left atrial chamber and appendage function after internal atrial defibrillation: a prospective and serial transesophageal echocardiographic study. J Am Coll Cardiol 29:131-138
13. Irani WN, Grayburn PA, Limandri G et al (1997) Prevalence of thrombus, spontaneous echo contrast, and atrial stunning in patients undergoing cardioversion of atrial flutter. Circulation 95:962-966
14. Santiago D, Warshofsky M, Lei G et al (1994) Left atrial appendage function and thrombus formation in atrial fibrillation-flutter: a transesophageal echocardiographic study. J Am Coll Cardiol 24:159-164
15. O'Neill PG, Puleo PR, Botti R et al (1990) Return of atrial mechanical function following electrical conversion of atrial dysrhythmias. Am Heart J 120:353-359
16. Falcone RA, Morady F, Armstrong WF et al (1996) Transesophageal echocardiographic evaluation of left atrial appendage function and spontaneous contrast formation after chemical or electrical cardioversion of atrial fibrillation. Am J Cardiol 78:435-439
17. Hoit BD, Shao Y, Gabel M et al (1994) Influence of acutely altered loading conditions on left atrial appendage flow velocities. J Am Coll Cardiol 24:1117-1123
18. Fatkin D, Kuchar DL, Thorburn CW et al (1994) Transesophageal echocardiography before and during direct current cardioversion of atrial fibrillation: evidence for atrial stunning as a mechanism of thromboembolic complications. J Am Coll Cardiol 23:307-316
19. Murgatroyd FF, Camm AJ (1993) Atrial arrhythmias. Lancet 341:1317-1322
20. Jovic A, Troskot R, Arcan T et al (1997) Recovery of atrial systolic function after pharmacological conversion of chronic atrial fibrillation to sinus rhythm: a Doppler echocardiographic study. Heart 77:46-49
21. Daal CE, Ewy GA, Eshani A et al (1974) Myocardial necrosis from direct current countershock. Circulation 50:956-961
22. Caterine MR, Spencer KT, Lewis A et al (1994) Direct current countershocks generate free radicals. Circulation 90:1-5
23. Grimm RA, Stewart WJ, Maloney JD et al (1993) Impact of electrical cardioversion for atrial fibrillation on left atrial appendage function and spontaneous echo contrast: characterization by simultaneous TEE. J Am Coll Cardiol 22:1359-1366
24. Sparks PB, Kulkarni R, Alt G (1998) Effect of direct current shocks on left atrial mechanical function in patients with structural heart disease. J Am Coll Cardiol 31:1395-1399
25. Abascal VM, Dubrey S, Lewis F et al (1995) Electrical vs pharmacological cardioversion on atrial fibrillation: does the atrium really care? Circulation 92[Suppl-I]:I-591
26. Harjai KJ, Mobarek SK, Dimond F et al (1997) Clinical variables affecting recovery of left atrial mechanical function after cardioversion from atrial fibrillation. J Am Coll Cardiol 30:481-486

27. Manning WJ, Silverman DI, Katz SE et al (1995) Temporal dependence of the return of atrial mechanical function on the mode of cardioversion of atrial fibrillation to sinus rhythm. Am J Cardiol 75:624-626

28. Mattioli AV, Castellani ET, Vivoli D et al (1996) Restoration of atrial function after fibrillation of different etiological origins. Cardiology 87:205-211

29. Louie EK, Liu D, Dunn DE (1998) Stunning of the left atrium after spontaneous conversion of atrial fibrillation to sinus rhythm. J Am Coll Cardiol 32:2081-2086

30. Sparks PB, Jayaprakash S, Lee F et al (1999) Left atrial mechanical function after brief duration atrial fibrillation. J Am Coll Cardiol 33:342-349

31. Laupacis A, Albers G, Bird F (1992) Antithrombotic therapy in atrial fibrillation. Third ACCP Conference on Antithrombotic Therapy. Chest 102[Suppl]:426S-433S

32. Pearson AC (1995) Transesophageal echocardiographic screening for atrial fibrillation: when should we look before we leap? J Am Coll Cardiol 25:1362-1364

33. Black IW, Hopkins AP, Klein AL et al (1993) Evaluation of transesophageal echocardiography before cardioversion of atrial fibrillation and flutter in nonanticoagulated patients. Am Heart J 126:375-381

Signal-Averaged P-Wave: How Useful Is It in Identifying Patients at High Risk of Recurrences after Cardioversion?

K. Aytemir and A. Oto

Introduction

Atrial fibrillation (AF) is the most common sustained arrhythmia seen in clinical practice [1]. Its incidence increases with age and the presence of organic heart disease. Epidemiological studies have shown an incidence of 3%-5% in subjects over 65 years of age [2, 3] with an associated increase in mortality and risk of thromboembolism [4-6]. Although the relative benefits of the restoration of normal sinus rhythm compared to heart rate control and anticoagulation have yet to be defined, cardioversion remains an important tool in the treatment of patients with AF. Electrical cardioversion is effective for restoring normal sinus rhythm in 70%-90% of patients [7]. Unfortunately, AF will recur within 3 months in up to 50% of patients [8]. Irrespective of the institution of prophylactic antiarrhythmic drug treatment, during the first year only 20%-60% of patients maintain sinus rhythm after cardioversion of chronic AF [8-10].

Attempts to predict the patients who will have an early recurrence of AF after cardioversion have been dissappointing [7, 11-15]. Certain risk factors, such as duration of AF, left atrial size, and left ventricular ejection fraction, have been used to predict AF recurrences after direct current (DC) cardioversion. Recently, several groups have adapted the technology of signal-averaged ECG to the study of the P wave in an attempt to identify patients at risk for developing AF and AF recurrences after cardioversion [16-18].

Mechanism of Atrial Fibrillation and Signal Averaging

In 1959, Moe and Abildskov suggested the multiple wavelet hypothesis as a mechanistic explanation of AF [19]. According to this theory, several independent re-entrant circuits operate simultaneously in the atrial myocardium. Mapping studies generated in animals demonstrated that reduced conduction

Hacettepe University Faculty of Medicine, Department of Cardiology, Ankara, Turkey velocity, or "delay", facilitates the formation of multiple wavelets of AF [20]. Clinical studies have demonstrated intra-atrial conduction delay [21] and fragmentation of atrial electrograms [22] in patients with a history of AF, confirming the importance of slowed conduction. This relationship between conduction delay and the development of AF plays a central role in P wave signal averaging.

In ventricular tissue, signal averaging exposes microvolt-level signals called "late potentials", which arise from areas of delayed or fractionated conduction. It would seem that those same high-frequency, low-amplitude signals would be found by a simple application of signal averaging technique to the P wave. However, important modifications must be made to apply this high-resolution electrocardiography to atrial activity.

Signal averaging of P waves from the surface electrocardiogram (ECG) is performed in the same manner as standard signal averaging of the QRS. Silver-silver chloride electrodes are used to reduce noise. An orthogonal lead arrangement is used to record surface electrograms in three dimensions. Signals from each lead are amplified and digitized at sampling frequencies of 1000 to 2000 samples/s with A/D converters of at least 12-bit precision.

Most of the commercially available signal-averaging systems use the largest voltage deviation from baseline (QRS complex) as the trigger for alignment of the "window" used for template correlation and signal acquisition. For P wave signal averaging, the window width or duration is typically set between 100 ms and 150 ms. Within that window, the acquired digitized P wave is compared to an operator-selected sinus P wave template. P waves that do not match the template with a high degree of correlation are excluded from averaging: typical correlation coefficients range from 0.95 to 0.99. P waves are recorded until a noise endpoint of 0.3 μV is achieved in the TP interval (the interval between T wave and P wave): 200-500 beats are necessary to complete the signal averaging. P waves that fail to correlate with the template P wave are beats of ectopic origin, P waves with excessive noise, or misaligned P waves due to PR interval variations related to fluctuations in autonomic tone.

Signal Filtering

Before analysis can be performed, the ECG signal may be "processed" using a variety of filters (e.g. unidirectional/bidirectional, finite impulse response, least squares-fit, spectral). Filtering can serve in many ways: eliminate contamination by low frequency artefact, ensure isolated detection of depolarization (without contamination by repolarization) and enhance detection of onset and offset of the low-amplitude signals. The latter is particularly advantageous when analysing low-amplitude signals such as P waves. Various high-pass filtering frequencies, ranging from approximately 10 Hz to 100 Hz, have been used in signal averaging [23]. However, the optimal frequency has not yet been established. High-pass filtering removes signals of low frequency content that arise from two major sources: repolarization and respiratory motion artefact.

Analysis of the P Wave SAECG

P wave signal-averaged data is typically analysed in the form of a composite vector from the three bipolar leads by the formula $(X^2 + Y^2 + Z^2)^{1/2}$. The criteria for
an abnormal composite vector signal-averaged P wave have not yet been established and will clearly be technique-dependent. For example, Fukunami and
coworkers [16], comparing patients with paroxysmal AF to control subjects,
observed longer P wave signal-averaged ECG (SAECG) durations (137 ± 14 vs $119
\pm 11$ ms, $p < 0.0001$) in patients with AF than in normal subjects. They defined
vector P wave signal durations greater than 120 ms as abnormal. A significantly
longer P wave duration on the SAECG in patients with AF as compared to age-,
sex- and disease-matched control subjects (162 ± 15 vs 140 ± 12 ms, $p < 0.01$) was
also demonstrated by Guidera and Steinberg [24]. These authors defined a filtered vector P wave signal duration of more than 155 ms as abnormal.

Another method used to specifically quantify the degree of atrial conduction delay is measurement of the amplitude (RMS voltage) of the terminal segment of the signal-averaged P wave; low voltage in this segment suggests a low-
amplitude late potential [16].

Predicting the Development of Atrial Fibrillation

The most commonly identified risk factors for the recurrence of AF after cardioversion are rheumatic mitral valve disease [25], atrial size [12, 15], age [12]
and the duration of AF prior to cardioversion [14]. None of these variables has
proved very useful in clinical practice. Atrial size is the variable most often
cited as predictive of the risk of recurrence. Unfortunately, studies that have
excluded patients with valvular AF have not found atrial size to be very helpful
in predicting the risk of AF after cardioversion [11, 13, 26]. Dittrich et al. [11]
examined the predictors of the recurrence of AF in the first month after cardioversion in 65 patients who had undergone their first cardioversion for AF.
Patients who had been in AF > 12 months prior to cardioversion were at
increased risk for recurrence. No other clinical variables were useful in predicting recurrence. Standard echocardiographic measurement of left atrial size did
not correlate with the risk of recurrence.

AF is a re-entrant rhythm and one factor that can facilitate AF is depressed
intra-atrial conduction, which could manifest as lengthening of the P wave
duration recorded on the ECG [27, 28]. The P wave SAECG can enhance detection of conduction delay within the atria, especially if it occurs late in relatively
small portions of the atria [24]. Studies on the duration of P wave SAECG have
shown it to be useful not only for the detection of patients at risk of paroxysmal AF [16, 24] but also for the development of chronic AF in patients with
paroxysmal AF [29]. Abe et al. [29] observed in a prospective study of patients
with paroxysmal AF with a P wave duration > 145 ms and amplitude of the last

30 ms (RMS) of P wave < 3.0 µV as useful criteria for prediction of transmission from paroxysmal to chronic AF. When these two criteria were combined, sensitivity, specificity and predictive accuracy for transition to chronic atrial fibrillation were 71%, 91% and 89%, respectively.

Studies on P-wave SAECG also suggested its predictive importance in the recurrence of AF after cardioversion. Opolsky et al. [30] measured signal-averaged P wave duration in 35 patients after cardioversion and found that P wave duration was longer in the 11 patients who had a recurrence of AF over a 6 month follow-up than in patients who maintained sinus rhythm (145 ± 12 vs 130 ± 11 ms, $p < 0.001$). Root mean square voltage of the last 20 ms was significantly lower in the group with recurrence (1.6 ± 0.6 vs 2.2 ± 0.9 µV, $p < 0.03$). A filtered P wave duration of > 137 ms associated with a RMS 20 ms < 1.9 µV had a sensitivity of 73% and specificity of 71% for the detection of patients with recurrence of AF after successful DC electrical cardioversion of AF. In a similar prospective study, Raitt et al. [31] showed a significantly longer signal-averaged P wave duration in patients who had a recurrence of AF within 3 months after electrical cardioversion, compared to patients who did not (148 ± 17 vs 135 ± 20 ms, $p = 0.005$). In the study of Aytemir et al. [32], filtered P wave duration 128 ms associated with root mean square voltage for the last 20 ms of the P wave < 1.9 µV had a sensitivity of 73% and specificity of 71% for the AF recurrence after cardioversion. In contrast, Stafford et al. [18] performed P wave signal averaging after 75 cardioversions in 31 patients not taking antiarrhythmic medications and found no difference in P wave duration between patients who had a recurrence after > 4 weeks compared to those who did not (156 ± 2 vs 151 ± 4 ms, $p = ns$). The negative result in this study may have been related to differences in the patients studied and signal-averaged ECG P wave technique and left atrial dilatation. They included patients at very high risk for recurrence (only three of 75 cardioversions resulted in normal sinus rhythm that persisted > 3 months). Stafford et al. [18] used a finite impulse response filtering technique which in previous studies did not give any discrimination between AF and those without it [33, 34].

Turitto et al. [35] examined the value of P wave signal averaging performed up to a month after spontaneous, medical, or electrical cardioversion of AF for predicting recurrent arrhythmias over a 1 year follow-up in 60 patients. There was no difference in P wave duration between patients with and without recurrence. There are a few possible reasons for the negative result in this study: inclusion of patients with atrial flutter; the use of antiarrhythmic medications, long follow-up period. The effect of antiarrhythmics on the predictive value P wave SAECG was studied by Raitt et al. [31]. In this study, among patients not taking antiarrhythmic medications, signal-averaged P wave duration was significantly longer, with a recurrence of AF after cardioversion. In contrast, in patients taking antiarrhythmic medication at the time or after cardioversion, signal-averaged P-wave duration did not correlate with the risk of recurrence of AF. A very long follow-up might adversely affect the predictive value, because late recurrences could be due to changes in atrial electrophysiology over time that are not reflected in the initial P wave study.

In conclusion, the duration of P wave SAECG and the amplitude of RMS voltage of the terminal segment of the vector magnitude of the P wave may be helpful for the identification of patients with recurrence of AF after successful DC cardioversion and patients at risk for transition from paroxysmal AF to chronic AF. However, the effect of antiarrhythmic medications and the signal-averaged ECG method used should be taken into account, and the results derived from one signal-averaged ECG technique could not be applied directly to results from other signal-averaged ECG P wave techniques for determination of AF recurrences after cardioversion.

References

1. Prystowsky EN, Benson DW, Fuster V et al (1996) Management of patients with atrial fibrillation. Circulation 93:1262-1277
2. Kannel WB, Abbot RD, Savage DD et al (1982) Epidemiologic features of chronic atrial fibrillation: the Framingham Study. N Engl J Med 306:1018-1022
3. Cairns JA, Connolly SJ (1991) Nonrheumatic atrial fibrillation: risk of stroke and role of antithrombotic therapy. Circulation 84:469-479
4. Wiener I (1987) Clinical and echocardiographic correlates of systemic embolisation in non rheumatic atrial fibrillation. Am J Cardiol 59:177-181
5. Gajewski J, Singer RB (1981) Mortality in the insured population with atrial fibrillation. J Am Med Assoc 245:1540-1544
6. Peterson P, Godtfredsen J (1984) Atrial fibrillation, a review of course and prognosis. Acta Med Scand 216:5-9
7. Van Gelder IC, Crijns HJ, Van Gilst WH et al (1991) Prediction of uneventful cardioversion and maintenance of normal sinus rhythm from direct-current electrical cardioversion of chronic atrial fibrillation and flutter. Am J Cardiol 68:41-46
8. Coplen SE, Antman EM, Berlin JA et al (1990) Efficacy and safety of quinidine therapy for maintenance of sinus rhythm after cardioversion. Circulation 82:1106-1116
9. Van Gelder IC, Crijns HJ, Van Gilst WH et al (1989) Efficacy and safety of flecainide acetate in the maintenance of sinus rhythm after electrical cardioversion of chronic atrial fibrillation or atrial flutter. Am J Cardiol 64:1317-1321
10. Lundstrom T, Ryden L (1988) Chronic atrial fibrillation-long-term results of direct current conversion. Acta Med Scand 223:53-59
11. Dittrich HC, Erickson JS, Schneiderman T et al (1989) Echocardiographic and clinical predictors for outcome of elective cardioversion of atrial fibrillation. Am Heart J 63:193-197
12. Alt E, Ammer R, Lehmann G et al (1997) Patient characteristics and underlying heart disease as predictors of recurrent atrial fibrillation after internal and external cardioversion in patients treated with oral sotalol. Am Heart J 134:419-425
13. Perez Y, Duval AM, Carville C et al (1997) Is left atrial appendage flow a predictor for outcome of cardioversion of nonvalvular atrial fibrillation? A transthoracic and transesophageal echocardiographic study. Am Heart J 134:745-751
14. Verhorst PMJ, Chassat C, Roy D et al (1997) Transesophageal echocardiographic predictors for maintenance of sinus rhythm after electrical cardioversion of atrial fibrillation. Am J Cardiol 79:1355-1359
15. Dethy M, Chassat C, Roy D et al (1998) Doppler echocardiographic predictors of recurrence of atrial fibrillation after cardioversion. Am J Cardiol 62:723-726

16. Fukunami M, Yamada T, Ohmori M et al (1991) Detection of patients at risk for paroxysmal atrial fibrillation during sinus rhythm by P wave-triggered signal-averaged electrocardiogram. Circulation 83:162-169

17. Opolsky G, Stanislawska J, Stomka K et al (1991) Value of the signal averaged electrocardiogram, in identifying patients with paroxysmal atrial fibrillation. Int J Cardiol 30:315-319

18. Stafford PJ, Kamalvand K, Tan K et al (1998) prediction of maintenance of sinus rhythm after cardioversion of atrial fibrillation by analysis of seria signal-averaged p waves. Pacing Clin Electrophysiol 21:1387-1395

19. Moe GJ, Abildskov JA (1959) Atrial fibrillation and self sustaining arrhythmia independent of focal discharge. Am Heart J 58:59

20. Allessie MA, Lammers WJ, Bonke FI, Hollin J (1985) Experimental evaluation of Moe's multiple wavelet hypothesis of atrial fibrillation. In: Zipes D, Jalife J (eds) Cardiac electrophysiology arrhythmias. Grune Stratton, New York, pp 265-276

21. Simpson RJ, Foster JR, Gettes ls (1982) Atrial excitability and conduction in patients with intra-atrial conduction defects. Am J Cardiol 50:1331-1337

22. Ohe T, Matsuhisa M, Kamakura S et al (1983) Relation between the widening of the fragmented atrial activity zone and atrial fibrillation. Am J Cardiol 53:1219-1222

23. Gomes JA, Winters SL, Stewart D et al (1987) Optimal bandpass filters for time-domain analysis of the signal averaged electrocardiogram. Am J Cardiol 60:1290-1298

24. Guidera SA, Steinberg JS (1993) The signal-averaged P wave duration. A rapid and non-invasive marker of atrial fibrillation. J Am Coll Cardiol 21:1645-1651

25. Van Gelder IC, Crijns HJ, Van Gilst WH et al (1991) Prediction of uneventful cardioversion and maintenance of normal sinus rhythm from direct-current electrical cardioversion of chronic atrial fibrillation and flutter. Am J Cardiol 68:41-46

26. Duytschaever M, Haerynck F, Tavernier R et al (1998) Factor influencing long-term persistence of sinus rhythm after a first electrical cardioversion for atrial fibrillation. Pacing Clin Electrophysiol 21:284-287

27. Buxton AE, Waxman HL, Marchlinski FE et al (1984) Atrial conduction: effects of extra stimuli with and without atrial dysrhythmias. Am J Cardiol 54:755-761

28. Leier CV, Meacham JA, Schall SF (1978) Prolonged atrial conduction: a major predisposing factor for atrial flutter. Circulation 57:213-216

29. Abe Y, Fukunami M, Ohmori M et al (1993) Prognostic significance of P wave-triggered signal-averaged electrocardiogram in predicting paroxysmal atrial fibrillation: a prospective study. Circulation 88:1-312

30. Opolski G, Scislo P, Stanislawska J et al (1997) Detection of patients at risk for recurrence of atrial fibrillation after successful electrical cardioversion by signal-averaged P wave ECG. Int J Cardiol 60:181-185

31. Raitt M, Ingram K, Thurman M (2000) Signal-averaged P wave duration predicts early recurrence of atrial fibrillation after cardioversion. Pacing Clin Electrophysiol 23:259-265

32. Aytemir K, Aksoyek S, Yildirir A et al (1999) Prediction of atrial fibrillation recurrence after cardioversion, by P wave electrocardiography. Int J Cardiol 70:15-21

33. Chan E, Steinberg JS, Santoni-Rugiu F, Gomes A (1998) P wave signal-averaged electrocardiography techniques. Ann Noninvasive Electrocardiol 3:147-152

34. Ehlert FA, Korenstein D, Steinberg JS (1997) Evaluation of P wave signal-averaged electrocardiographic filtering and analysis methods. Am Heart J 134:985-993

35. Turitto G, Bandarizadeh B, Salciccioli L et al (1998) Risk stratification for recurrent tachyarrhythmias in patients with paroxysmal atrial fibrillation and flutter: role of signal-averaged electrocardiogram and echocardiography. Pacing Clin Electrophysiol 21:197-201

Prevention of Atrial Fibrillation: Is Amiodarone a First Choice?

P. Dorian

Atrial fibrillation is the most common sustained cardiac arrhythmia. Patients with atrial fibrillation have a substantially impaired quality of life [1], suffer from impaired exercise tolerance and cardiac symptoms which may be disabling, may be at increased risk for the development of heart failure and ventricular arrhythmias, and are at a markedly higher risk of stroke than age-matched controls without atrial fibrillation [2]. For these reasons, many physicians believe that, in general, attempts should be made to restore and maintain sinus rhythm in patients with atrial fibrillation. In situations where sinus rhythm cannot be maintained, physicians may choose to control the rapid and irregular ventricular response to minimize symptoms. It must be noted that there is no proof from randomized clinical trials that the strategy of sinus rhythm maintenance is necessarily superior to the strategy of ventricular rate control, in particular with respect to mortality or the development of heart failure and other major clinical endpoints [3]. This question is currently being addressed by several large-scale, randomized, clinical trials, in particular the AFFIRM trial, which will be completed in October 2001, and will test the hypothesis that sinus rhythm maintenance reduces mortality compared to ventricular rate control [4].

Paroxysmal or Persistent Atrial Fibrillation

In most large studies of patients with symptomatic atrial fibrillation eligible for sinus rhythm maintenance, approximately half suffer from *paroxysmal* atrial fibrillation, defined as atrial fibrillation episodes that stop spontaneously without medical intervention. Generally, these episodes last hours to days at most. The other half suffer from *persistent* atrial fibrillation, defined as episodes that do not spontaneously terminate, but will require drug therapy or

Division of Cardiology, St. Michael's Hospital, Toronto, Ontario, Canada cardioversion to restore sinus rhythm. In general, the efficacy of antiarrhythmic drugs in paroxysmal or persistent atrial fibrillation is similar, although drug therapy is less effective in restoring sinus rhythm (in cases of persistent atrial fibrillation) than it is in preventing recurrences, either in paroxysmal atrial fibrillation or following electrical cardioversion for persistent atrial fibrillation.

Many trials have compared the efficacy of a variety of antiarrhythmic drugs to maintain sinus rhythm, i.e. prevent its recurrence, and the drugs below can all be shown to be superior to placebo with respect to the usual primary endpoint used in investigational studies, the time to first recurrence of symptomatic atrial fibrillation after study onset. Effective drugs include quinidine, disopyramide and procainamide (Class Ia drugs); propafenone and flecainide (Class Ic drugs), sotalol, dofetilide and amiodarone (Class III agents or with primarily Class III mechanism of action) [2]. Until recently, the relative efficacy of these drugs has been difficult to assess. Most direct comparative trials have shown approximately equal efficacy when any of the drugs in the above list were paired, except for retrospective or nonrandomized analyses, which suggested that amiodarone was associated with a lower risk of recurrence [5]. The majority of trials showed an approximately 50% recurrence rate after 6-12 months following the drugs on the above list, with the exception of amiodarone, associated with an approximately 35% recurrence rate at 6-12 months.

It should be noted that there is relatively little controlled trial information on the effect of drugs on "total recurrences over time", since most studies arbitrarily stop after the first recurrence of symptomatic atrial fibrillation. There is some evidence that the time to first recurrence is not well correlated with the average interevent interval (or the total number of episodes over a given time period, say 1 year) if the drug is continued for the long term. Nevertheless, the "time to first recurrence" information gives a reasonable estimate of overall drug efficacy that can be used to guide clinical decision making.

The Canadian Trial of Atrial Fibrillation (CTAF) [6] was the first large-scale, randomized, multicentre, controlled clinical trial of amiodarone compared to alternative, commonly used drugs. Patients with paroxysmal or persistent atrial fibrillation were randomized in a 1:1 ratio to receive either amiodarone (n = 202) or one of sotalol (n = 101) or propafenone (n = 101), with the choice of the latter drugs being randomized, and followed within 21 days by cardioversion if atrial fibrillation was persistent. If sotalol or propafenone were ineffective or could not be tolerated, the alternative drug between these two could be started. After 21 days of "run-in therapy", the evaluation period began and all subsequent symptomatic recurrences were documented by 12 lead or event monitor electrocardiograms, the primary endpoint being time to first recurrence of symptomatic atrial fibrillation.

There was a statistically significant reduction in the probability of atrial fibrillation recurrence in the amiodarone vs sotalol/propafenone group, with a 35% recurrence rate following amiodarone vs a 63% recurrence rate with propafenone or sotalol, after 468 ± 150 days of follow-up (hazard ratio = 0.43,

$p < 0.001$). There were no differences in recurrence rates between sotalol- and propafenone-treated patients. All drugs were relatively well tolerated and discontinuation rates were very similar for all of the drugs studied. Serious adverse events were rare. Therapy could be continued in this study despite a recurrence, and overall discontinuation rates of therapy allow some estimate of "clinical efficacy", as judged by the treating physician. By the end of follow-up, 34% of amiodarone patients had therapy discontinued because of inefficacy or adverse effects, whereas 46% had therapy discontinued in the sotalol/propafenone arm ($p = 0.01$). The secondary analysis suggests that amiodarone is clinically more efficacious, as well as more effective, in preventing first recurrences of atrial fibrillation than the alternative therapies in this study [6].

Quality of life was also assessed in this study. There was overall improvement in both generic measures of quality of life and symptoms of atrial fibrillation over the first 3 months of study, similar in the amiodarone and propafenone/sotalol groups. Patients without recurrence of atrial fibrillation had significantly more improvement in quality of life than those with recurrences [7]. Atrial fibrillation "burden", measured as the atrial fibrillation symptom score (AFSS), a composite measure of frequency, duration and severity of atrial fibrillation, was significantly lower in the amiodarone-treated group vs the propafenone/sotalol treated group at 3 months ($p = 0.001$) [7].

In the management of patients with persistent atrial fibrillation, the clinician is faced with the choice of initiating therapy with an antiarrhythmic agent, followed by cardioversion if atrial fibrillation does not revert, as compared to beginning with cardioversion and following with antiarrhythmic drug therapy to maintain sinus rhythm. For patients with persistent atrial fibrillation of more than approximately 30 days duration, it is generally not expected to be successfully converted by oral antiarrhythmic drug therapy. However, pretreatment, for example with oral propafenone, has been shown to reduce the risk of early recurrences of atrial fibrillation following cardioversion [8]. Another potential benefit of pretreatment with antiarrhythmic drugs is an increase in the probability of successful cardioversion, as has been shown with intravenous ibutilide [2, 9].

In a recent study comparing pretreatment with amiodarone vs oral diltiazemplus intravenous potassium/insulin/glucose 24 h pre-cardioversion, vs oral diltiazem alone, in 92 patients with approximately 16 weeks of atrial fibrillation prior to treatment, amiodarone was associated with a higher rate of *chemical* cardioversion (25%, vs 6% or 3% in the latter two groups, respectively, $p < 0.005$) [10]. Furthermore, electrical cardioversion was more successful following 1 month of amiodarone pretreatment (88%) than following 1 month of diltiazem with or without potassium/insulin/glucose pretreatment (56% and 65% respectively; $p < 0.05$). The strategy of pretreatment with an antiarrhythmic drug such as amiodarone prior to cardioversion thus seems reasonable, especially in patients expected to have a high risk of recurrence following sinus rhythm restoration.

Proarrhythmia and other adverse effects of antiarrhythmic therapy are more common in heart failure patients than in those with normal ventricular function [2, 11, 12]. Partly for this reason, the Atrial Fibrillation and Congestive Heart Failure (AF-CHF) study, which began in April 2001, will compare the strategy of sinus rhythm restoration and maintenance to the strategy of ventricular rate control in patients with heart failure, poor ejection fraction (EF < 35%) and symptomatic atrial fibrillation. The primary endpoint is all-cause mortality; the antiarrhythmic therapy of choice in the rhythm control group will be amiodarone, compared to rate control with β-blockers and digoxin in the rate control group, with innovative and ancillary therapies (e.g. pacing, AV node ablation, other ablative procedures, other antiarrhythmic drugs) used as necessary. This important large trial (n = 1450) will provide important information on the best strategy on managing atrial fibrillation in heart failure patients. In the meantime, it is reasonable to assume that sinus rhythm restoration and maintenance are desirable in most patients with heart failure and symptomatic atrial fibrillation, provided that it can be done safely and effectively.

As with any therapy, the potential benefit from antiarrhythmic therapy, particularly amiodarone, needs to be balanced against its potential risk. Most of the randomized trials of amiodarone involved a loading dose of 400-800 mg/day for approximately 2 weeks, followed by eventual dose reduction to maintenance doses of 200 mg/day. At this dose, adverse effects requiring drug discontinuation occur in approximately 18% of patients (over a follow-up of 468 ± 150 days) [6], and serious adverse effects such as pulmonary toxicity and serious neurological toxicity occur in less than 3% of patients. Amiodarone has a very low risk of causing proarrhythmia [13], but may cause both sinus bradycardia or very slow ventricular response during atrial fibrillation should the latter recur, occasionally leading to the need for pacemaker therapy. All patients on amiodarone require ongoing and careful clinical and laboratory follow-up to monitor for amiodarone toxicity. Physicians following such patients need to be thoroughly familiar with the range of adverse effects from amiodarone and their management.

Conclusions

The varied manifestations of atrial fibrillation, a lack of consistently effective therapies and the paucity of large-scale, controlled clinical trials makes the evidence-based management of atrial fibrillation a particular challenge. Current evidence suggests that amiodarone is an effective and relatively safe drug for many patients with atrial fibrillation of various patterns, and with varying associated heart diseases. The ideal management of patients with atrial fibrillation will be importantly influenced by large-scale clinical trials which are currently under way or soon to be published.

References

1. Dorian P, Jung W, Paquette M et al (2000) The impairment of health-related quality of life in patients with intermittent atrial fibrillation: implications for the assessment of investigational therapy. J Am Coll Cardiol 36:1303-1309
2. Falk RH (2001) Atrial fibrillation. N Engl J Med 344:1067-1078
3. Hohnloser SH, Kuck KH, Lilienthal J, for the PIAF Investigators (2000) Rhythm or rate control in atrial fibrillation - pharmacological intervention in atrial fibrillation (PIAF): a randomised trial. Lancet 356:1789-1794
4. The Planning and Steering Committees of the AFFIRM Study for the NHLBI AFFIRM Investigators (1997) Atrial fibrillation follow-up investigation of rhythm management - the AFFIRM study design. Am J Cardiol 79:1198-1202
5. Gosselink ATM, Crijns HJGM, Van Gelder IC et al (1992) Low-dose amiodarone for maintenance of sinus rhythm after cardioversion from atrial fibrillation or flutter. J Am Med Assoc 267:3289-3293
6. Roy D, Talajic M, Dorian P et al for the Canadian Trial of Atrial Fibrillation Investigators (2000) Amiodarone to prevent recurrence of atrial fibrillation. N Engl J Med 342:913-920
7. Dorian P, Paquette M, Newman D et al (1999) Quality of life improves following treatment in the Canadian Trial of Atrial Fibrillation. Circulation 100:1-502(abstr)
8. Bianconi L, Mennuni M, Lukie V et al (1996) Effects of oral propafenone administration before electrical cardioversion of chronic atrial fibrillation: a placebo-controlled study. J Am Coll Cardiol 28:700-706
9. Oral H, Souza JJ, Michaud GF et al (1999) Facilitating transthoracic cardioversion of atrial fibrillation with ibutilide pretreatment. N Engl J Med 340:1849-1854
10. Capucci A, Villani GQ, Aschieri D et al (2000) Oral amiodarone increases the efficacy of direct-current cardioversion in restoration of sinus rhythm in patients with chronic atrial fibrillation. Eur Heart J 21:66-73
11. Roden DM (1998) Mechanisms and management of proarrhythmia. Am J Cardiol 82:49I-57I
12. Flaker GG, Blackshear JL, McBride R et al (1992) Antiarrhythmic drug therapy and cardiac mortality in atrial fibrillation. The Stroke Prevention in Atrial Fibrillation Investigators. J Am Coll Cardiol 20:527-532
13. Hohnloser S, Klingenheben T, Singh BN (1994) Amiodarone-associated proarrhythmic effects: a review with special reference to torsades de pointes tachycardia. Ann Intern Med 121:529-538

Antiarrhythmic Drug Prophylaxis to Avoid Permanent Atrial Fibrillation: Is it Worthwhile?

M. Brignole[1] and C. Menozzi[2]

Atrial Fibrillation and Mortality

Epidemiological and observational studies have shown that the development of permanent atrial fibrillation (AF) is associated with an adverse outcome [1, 2]. However, owing to the design of those studies, a direct cause-effect relationship between AF and outcome has not yet been proven, and it is a matter of debate whether AF independently affects survival. It has recently been suggested that patients with and without AF have comparable survival rates [3, 4]. However, the ultimate question is not whether AF increases mortality, but rather whether the strategy of maintaining sinus rhythm can reduce the risk. A recent long-term follow-up study [5] has shown that, in the absence of underlying heart disease, survival among patients with AF after ablation of the atrioventricular junction was similar to expected survival in the general population; survival was similar for patients with AF whether they received ablation or drug therapy. Until large trials such as the Atrial Fibrillation Follow-up Investigation of Rhythm Management study (AFFIRM) [6] report their results on mortality, no definite answer can be given and it seems appropriate to choose the best therapeutic strategy for the improvement of the patients' quality of life.

Rhythm Control vs Rate Control in AF

Restoration and maintenance of sinus rhythm is believed by many physicians to be superior to rate control only. This assumption is derived from observational and uncontrolled studies and remains largely unproven. To date, there are only two prospective randomized trials that compare the two therapeutic strategies, the Pharmacological Intervention in Atrial Fibrillation (PIAF) [7] and the paroxysmal atrial fibrillation (PAF) studies [8].

[1]Department of Cardiology and Arrhythmologic Center, Ospedali Riuniti, Lavagna; [2]Department of Interventional Cardiology and Arrhythmologic Center, Ospedale S. Maria Nuova, Reggio Emilia, Italy

Pharmacological Intervention

The PIAF study [7] is the only randomized multicenter trial to compare two different therapeutic strategies, rate versus rhythm control, in patients with symptomatic AF. The results indicate that neither of the two therapeutic strategies is superior in terms of improvement in AF-related symptoms. These results may have important implications for the care of individual patients, most of whom are treated mainly for symptomatic reasons.

In brief, the trial was a randomized study of 252 patients with AF of 7-360 days' duration, which compared rate control (group A, 125 patients) with rhythm control (group B, 127 patients). In group A, diltiazem was used as first-line therapy and amiodarone was used in group B. Amiodarone pharmacologically restored sinus rhythm in 23% of patients, the remaining majority undergoing at least one direct current cardioversion; 56% of patients who were successfully cardioverted were successfully maintained in sinus rhythm on continued low-dose amiodarone treatment over the observation period. The primary study endpoint was improvement in symptoms related to AF. Over the entire observation period of 1 year, a similar proportion of patients reported improvement in symptoms in both groups (76 responders at 12 months in group A vs 70 responders in group B, $p = 0.317$). Walking distance in a 6-min walk test was better in group B than in group A, but assessment of quality of life showed no differences between the groups. The incidence of hospital admission was higher in group B [87 (69%) out of 127 vs 30 (24%) out of 125 in group A, $p = 0.001$]. Adverse drug effects more frequently led to a change in therapy in group B [31 (25%) patients compared with 17 (14%) in group A, $p = 0.036$].

The interpretation of the study results is that patients randomized to treatment for rhythm control had a better exercise tolerance than patients who underwent rate control. This finding may be due to improvement in hemodynamics after restoration of sinus rhythm. However, the improved exercise tolerance did not translate to an overall improved quality of life compared to the other group. Rate control has the advantage that antiarrhythmic drug therapy, and hence its potential side effects, can be avoided. Symptomatic improvement was similar in patients randomized to rate control. This finding re-emphasizes the point that careful control of the ventricular rate in AF can result in a substantial benefit to the patient. The strategy of rate control was associated with significantly fewer hospital admissions in our patients, which shows that rate control in AF may be associated with significant cost savings – a fact that is particularly relevant given the number of people who have this rhythm disturbance.

Rhythm Control vs Rate Control After "Ablate and Pace"

In patients with paroxysmal AF that is not controlled by pharmacological therapy, ablation and pacing therapy has proved highly effective in controlling symptoms, although chronic AF develops in many patients shortly after ablation. For example, in one study [9] chronic AF was present 1 and 2 years after ablation in 22% and 40% of patients, respectively. In one randomized prospective study [10], antiarrhythmic drugs were able to prevent the development of chronic AF in the first 6 months after ablation. However, the long-term efficacy of antiarrhythmic drug therapy is unknown, and the potential advantage of maintaining sinus rhythm with antiarrhythmic drugs must be weighed against the potential negative impact of these drugs on quality of life and cardiac performance.

The aim of the Paroxysmal Atrial Fibrillation 2 study (PAF2) [8] was to evaluate the effect of antiarrhythmic drug therapy on long-term maintenance of normal sinus rhythm after ablation and pacing therapy and to evaluate its clinical efficacy. As it was expected that some patients would not be able to maintain sinus rhythm in the long term, this study was actually an evaluation of a strategy that initially allowed patients to remain in AF versus a strategy that initially attempted to restore and maintain normal sinus rhythm.

Briefly, in this multicenter randomized trial, 141 patients affected by severely symptomatic paroxysmal AF were assigned, after successful atrioventricular junction ablation and DDDR mode-switching pacemaker treatment, to antiarrhythmic drug therapy with amiodarone, propafenone, flecainide or sotalol (71 patients) or to no antiarrhythmic drug therapy (70 patients). The patients were followed up for 12-24 months (mean 16 ± 4). The drug arm patients had a 57% reduction in the risk of developing chronic AF (21% vs 37%, $p = 0.02$). Evaluation after 12 months revealed similar quality of life scores and echocardiographic parameters in the two groups, but the drug arm patients had more episodes of heart failure and hospitalizations, which showed 2.5-fold and 2.7-fold relative increases, respectively ($p = 0.047$ and 0.055, respectively). The outcome was similar for the 40 patients who developed chronic AF and the 97 who did not.

The interpretation of the study results is that a conventional antiarrhythmic drug therapy is able to reduce the risk of development of chronic AF after ablation and pacing therapy for at least 2 years, even in a selected population with frequent recurrences of paroxysmal AF that had been considered to be resistant to multiple pharmacological treatment. Despite the higher percentage of patients who remained in sinus rhythm, however, the study was unable to show any clinical benefit in patients treated with antiarrhythmic therapy in addition to that already obtained with ablation and pacing alone; on the contrary, in some patients we observed serious adverse clinical events, as evidenced by the higher number of episodes of heart failure and hospitalization. Thus, the excellent control of ventricular rhythm provided by ablation and pacing seems to be the most important objective to obtain and probably reduces the importance of preserving atrial contraction. In short, conventional antiarrhythmic therapy reduces the risk of development of chronic AF after ablation and pacing therapy, but the present data do not support the concept that the development of chronic AF is related to an adverse outcome when perfect control of heart rate is achieved by ablation and pacing.

Conclusions

The findings of the two randomized controlled studies are consistent with the suggestion that careful control of the ventricular rate in AF can result in substantial benefit for the patient at least as well as rhythm control and with fewer complications and hospitalizations.

References

1. Kannel WB, Abbott RD, Savage DD et al (1982) Epidemiologic features of chronic atrial fibrillation: the Framingham study. N Engl J Med 306:1018-1022
2. Middlekauff H, Stevenson WG, Stevenson LW (1991) Prognostic significance of atrial fibrillation in advanced heart failure. A study of 390 patients. Circulation 84:40-48
3. Carson PE, Jonhson G, Dunkman W et al (1993) The influence of atrial fibrillation on prognosis in mild to moderate heart failure. The V-HeFT studies. The V-HeFT VA Cooperative Studies Group. Circulation 87 (suppl 6):102-110
4. Stevenson WG, Stevenson LW, Middlekauff H et al (1996) Improving survival for patients with atrial fibrillation and advanced heart failure. J Am Coll Cardiol 28:1458-1463
5. Ozcan C, Jahangir A, Friedman P et al (2001) Long-term survival after ablation of the atrioventricular node and implantation of a permanent pacemaker in patients with atrial fibrillation. N Engl J Med 344:1043-1051
6. The Planning and Steering Committees of the AFFIRM study for the NHLBI AFFIRM Investigators (1997) Atrial fibrillation follow-up investigation of rhythm management – the AFFIRM study design. Am J Cardiol 79:1198-1202
7. Hohnloser S, Kuck KH, Lilienthal J (2000) Rhythm or rate control in atrial fibrillation. Pharmacological Intervention in Atrial Fibrillation (PIAF): a randomized trial. Lancet 356:1789-1794
8. Brignole M, Menozzi C, Gasparini M et al (2001) An evaluation of the strategy of maintenance of sinus rhythm by antiarrhythmic drug therapy after ablation and pacing therapy in patients with paroxysmal atrial fibrillation. Eur Heart J (in press)
9. Gianfranchi L, Brignole M, Menozzi C et al (1998) Progression of permanent atrial fibrillation after atrioventricular junction ablation and dual-chamber pacemaker implantation in patients with paroxysmal atrial tachyarrhythmias. Am J Cardiol 81:351-354
10. Brignole M, Gianfranchi L, Menozzi C et al (1997) An assessment of atrioventricular junction ablation and DDDR mode-switching pacemaker versus pharmacological treatment in patients with severely symptomatic paroxysmal atrial fibrillation. A randomized controlled study. Circulation 96:2617-2624

Antiplatelet Agents for Prevention of Thromboembolism in Atrial Fibrillation: When, Why, and Which One?

G. Di Pasquale, E. Cerè, S. Biancoli, B. Sassone, A. Lombardi, F. Serafini, G.F. Tortorici, R. Vandelli and L.G. Pancaldi

Atrial fibrillation (AF) carries a high risk of systemic embolism, in particular stroke. This is true not only when AF is associated with valvular heart disease, but also in patients with nonvalvular AF, which represents 70% of all cases of AF [1]. However, the risk of stroke is not uniform, widely ranging between 0.4% and 12% per year, with an average of 4.5% per year observed in the pooled analysis of five randomized controlled trials [2].

The principal mechanism for stroke in AF is emboli resulting from stasis-related left atrial thrombi (associated with enlarged atria, and thrombi in the left atrial appendage or atrial septal aneurysm), or stasis-related left ventricular thrombi (associated with left ventricular enlargement). Because of stasis of blood flow, activation of the coagulation system with fibrin formation predominates over platelet activation as the principal mechanism in the development of intracavitary thrombi. On the basis of the pathogenetic mechanism, oral anticoagulant treatment (OAT) seems the most appropriate prophylactic treatment [3]. Alternative mechanisms for stroke in patients with nonvalvular AF include structural abnormalities of the mitral valve (including myxomatous or thickened valvular leaflets or mitral annular calcification), coexisting atherosclerotic carotid artery disease (noted in approximately 20% of AF-associated strokes), or atherosclerotic plaques in the ascending aorta and proximal arch. In these conditions sources of embolism are represented by platelet-fibrin thrombi and therefore platelet inhibition may be effective [4].

Adjusted-Dose Warfarin

The effectiveness of OAT for the prevention of thromboembolism and stroke has been definitely assessed by a number of randomized clinical trials [5-11]. Overall adjusted-dose warfarin (six trials, 2900 participants) reduced stroke by 62% (95% CI, range 48%-72%); absolute risk reductions were 2.7% per year for primary prevention [number needed to treat (NNT) for 1 year to prevent one stroke = 37] and 8.4% per year (NNT = 12) for secondary prevention (Table 1).

Unità Operativa di Cardiologia, Ospedale di Bentivoglio, Bologna, Italy

Table 1. Adjusted-dose warfarin compared with placebo. (Modified from [5])

Study	Type of prevention	No. of patients	Target INR	Relative risk reduction (%)[a]	Absolute risk reduction (% per year)
AFASAK [6]	Primary	671	2.8-4.2	54	2.6
SPAF [7]	Primary	421	2.0-4.5	60	4.7
BAATAF [8]	Primary	420	1.5-2.7	78	2.4
CAFA [9]	Primary	378	2.0-3.0	33	1.2
SPINAF [10]	Primary	571	1.4-2.8	70	3.3
EAFT [11]	Secondary	439	2.5-4.0	68	8.4
All trials		2900	-	62 (48 to 72)	3.1

[a] Ninety-five percent confidence interval

The risk of bleeding in patients receiving warfarin in these studies was quite low. The annual frequency of major bleeding events was 1.3% in warfarin-treated patients (vs 1.0% in patients receiving placebo or controls, and 1.0% in aspirin-treated patients). However, the bleeding risk is likely to be higher in patients treated in general clinical practice. Patients included in the clinical trials were carefully selected (representing only 7%-39% of the screened patients) and followed up carefully according to strict protocols. This could explain the low bleeding risk during warfarin treatment. Moreover, the safety and tolerability of long-term anticoagulation to conventional levels has not been completely defined among patients older than 75 years. In the AFASAK study [6] involving AF patients older than those enrolled in every other trial (mean age of 75 years) the withdrawal rate from warfarin was 38% after 1 year. In the SPAF II study [12] (International Normalized Ratio, INR 2.0-4.5, mean 2.7) the risk of major hemorrhage, mainly cerebral, was substantially higher among AF patients older than 75 years.

Despite the strong evidence for efficacy of OAT, the use of warfarin for stroke prevention in patients with AF is still low in general clinical practice [13-15]. Major reasons for the underuse of OAT are the difficulty of high-quality monitoring of OAT, especially in older patients, and the fear of bleedings. Therefore, new thromboprophylactic strategies for patients with AF are warranted.

Low-Dose Warfarin

The possibility of low-intensity antithrombotic strategies seemed attractive and plausible, but three studies, SPAF III [16], MIWAF [17], and AFASAK II [18], have unanimously demonstrated poor efficacy of this therapeutic strategy.

The first of these studies was SPAF III [16], a study of fixed-dose mini-intensity warfarin (INR 1.2-1.5) in combination with aspirin (325 mg per day). The study was withdrawn after 1 year of follow-up because the annual incidence of stroke and systemic embolism was much lower (1.9% per year) with adjusted-dose warfarin in comparison with combination therapy (7.9% per year).

The Italian study MIWAF [17] confirmed the failure of fixed minidose warfarin to prevent thromboembolism in patients with nonrheumatic AF. In this study 303 patients aged over 60 years with nonvalvular AF were randomized to adjusted-dose warfarin (INR 2.0-3.0) or fixed minidose warfarin (1.25 mg per day). In a mean follow-up of 14 months the annual incidence of primary events was 6.2% in the adjusted-dose group and 3.6% in the fixed-dose group. In particular the annual incidence of ischemic stroke was significantly higher in the fixed minidose warfarin group (3.7% vs 0%).

The AFASAK-II trial [18] compared fixed-minidose warfarin 1.25 mg, warfarin 1.25 mg plus aspirin 300 mg, aspirin 300 mg, and adjusted-dose warfarin (INR 2.0 - 3.0) in chronic nonvalvular AF. Among 677 patients the cumulative primary event rate after 1 year was 5.8% in patients receiving minidose warfarin, 7.2% warfarin + aspirin, 3.6% aspirin and 2.8% adjusted-dose warfarin, which suggests a trend towards superiority of adjusted-dose warfarin over the other treatment strategies.

Finally, in the PATAF study [19], 729 patients were assigned to receive aspirin 150 mg, warfarin (INR 2.5-3.5), or warfarin (INR 1.1-1.6). After a mean follow-up of 2.7 years, the event rate was similar (2% per year) in the three groups; however, among patients with contraindications for OAT, the event rate was 10% per year in the aspirin and low-dose warfarin groups. This study excluded high-risk patients (older than 78 years, heart failure, hypertension, valve disease, previous cerebrovascular event) and thus merely suggests that aspirin may suffice in low-risk patients and that low-intensity or adjusted-dose warfarin did not bring further advantages.

Antiplatelet Therapy

The fears regarding full-dose OAT and the risk of bleeding, mainly in older patients, and the failure of minidose warfarin explain the hopes pinned on antiplatelet agents among physicians.

Aspirin Compared with Placebo

Six trials (AFASAK [6], SPAF I [7], EAFT [11], ESPS II [20], LASAF [21], and UK TIA [22]) compared antiplatelet therapy with placebo. In these trials, 3119 participants experienced a total of 349 strokes while randomly assigned to receive antiplatelet therapy or placebo. In five trials assignment was double-blind. Aspirin dosage ranged from 25 mg twice daily to 1300 mg/day. Mean duration of follow-up in these trials ranged from 1.2 to 4 years (overall average = 1.5 years per participant). Meta-analysis of all six trials showed that aspirin reduced the incidence of stroke by 22% (95% CI, 2%-38%). On the basis of these six trials, the absolute risk reduction was 1.5% per year (NNT = 67) for primary prevention and 2.5% per year (NNT = 40) for secondary prevention (Table 2).

Table 2. Antiplatelet agents compared with placebo. (Modified from [5])

Study	Type of prevention	No. of patients	Relative risk reduction (%)[a]	Absolute risk reduction (% per year)
Aspirin vs placebo[b]				
AFASAK [6]	Primary	672	17	0.9
SPAF I [7]	Primary	1 120	44	2.5
EAFT [11]	Secondary	782	11	1.9
ESPS II [20]	Secondary	211	29	6.9
LASAF [21]	Primary[c]	195	-17	-0.5
		181	67	1.6
UK TIA [22]	Secondary[d]	28	17	0.9
		36	14	0.7
All aspirin trials	-	3 225	22 (2 to 38)	1.7
Dipyridamole vs placebo				
ESP II [20]	Secondary	221	22 (-60 to 62)	5.7
Dipyridamole + aspirin vs placebo				
ESPS II [20]	Secondary	211	43 (-24 to 74)	9.7
All antiplatelet trials	-	3 657	24 (7 to 39)	1.9

[a] Ninety-five percent confidence interval
[b] Aspirin dosage 75-1200 mg/day; dipyridamole dosage 200 mg b.i.d.
[c] One hundred ninety-five patients randomized to aspirin 125 mg/day and 181 patients randomized to aspirin 125 mg every other day
[d] Twenty-eight patients randomized to aspirin 300 mg/day and 36 patients randomized to aspirin 1200 mg/day

A subgroup of patients with AF that has a particularly large reduction in stroke incidence from aspirin therapy was not convincingly identified.

Although all six trials showed trends toward reduced stroke with aspirin, this result was statistically significant only in the SPAF I study [7]. This trial had the highest proportion of nondisabling stroke (52%); the effect of aspirin was qualitatively different for nondisabling stroke (relative risk reduction 62%; $p = 0.008$) than for disabling stroke (relative risk reduction 17%; $p > 0.2$). When disabling stroke from the three largest trials [6, 7, 11] that reported stroke severity was considered, aspirin use was associated with a relative risk reduction of only 13% (95% CI, -19% to 36%).

The effect of antithrombotic therapy varies according to the ischemic stroke mechanism in AF patients. Aspirin reduces noncardioembolic strokes more than cardioembolic strokes in AF patients, whereas adjusted-dose warfarin is much more efficacious than aspirin for the prevention of cardioembolic strokes. Using clinical and neuroradiological criteria Miller et al. [23] categorized strokes in the SPAF I study as definitely cardioembolic, probably cardioembolic, atherothrombotic, lacunar, of other specific cause, and of uncertain etiology. The preventive effect of aspirin therapy was different for cardioembolic and noncardioembolic ischemic strokes. Aspirin was associated with a risk reduction in noncardioembolic strokes of 100% (95% CI, 60%-100%; $p = 0.001$), but with a risk reduction of only 31% for cardioembolic strokes (95% CI, -35% to 65%; $p = 0.31$). The differential effect of antithrombotic therapies according to stroke mechanism in AF explains the discrepant results from clinical trials and is important for the choice of antithrombotic prophylaxis in the individual patient.

Aspirin Compared with Warfarin

A direct comparison between adjusted-dose warfarin and aspirin has been done in five nonblinded randomized trials [6, 11, 12, 18, 19] involving 2837 patients who had a total of 205 strokes during a mean follow-up of 2.2 years per participant. When only ischemic strokes were considered, adjusted-dose warfarin was associated with a 46% (CI, 27%-60%) relative risk reduction compared with aspirin (Table 3).

Table 3. Adjusted-dose warfarin compared with other antithrombotic regimens. (Modified from [5])

Study	Type of prevention	No. of patients	Relative risk reduction (%)[a]	Absolute risk reduction (% per year)
Adjusted-dose warfarin vs aspirin				
AFASAK [6]	Primary	671	45	1.7
SPAF II [12]	Primary	1100	10	0.2
EAFT [11]	Secondary	455	67	7.0
AFASAK II [18]	Primary	339	-23	-0.6
PATAF [19]	Primary	272	20	0.3
All trials	-	2837	36 (14 to 52)	0.8
Adjusted-dose warfarin vs low or fixed-dose warfarin + aspirin				
SPAF III [16]	Primary + Secondary	1044	73	6.2
AFASAK II [18]	Primary	341	-1	-0.2
Adjusted-dose warfarin vs indobufen				
SIFA [24]	Secondary	916	21 (-54 to 60)	1.0
Adjusted-dose warfarin vs low or fixed-dose wafarin				
AFASAK II [18]	Primary	337	24	0.8
MIWAF [17]	Primary	303	81	2.2
PATAF [19]	Primary	253	31	0.4
All trials	-	893	38 (-20 to 68)	1.0

[a] Ninety-five percent confidence interval

Other Antiplatelet Agents

One small randomized trial compared dipyridamole and dipyridamole plus aspirin with placebo; however the data were insufficient to allow assessment of the individual efficacy of dipyridamole [20].

In the Italian study SIFA [24] the efficacy and safety of the antiplatelet drug indobufen, a reversible cyclooxygenase inhibitor (100-200 mg b.i.d.) has been compared with warfarin (INR 2.0-3.5) in patients with nonvalvular AF and a recent (≤ 14 days) transient ischemic attack (TIA) or stroke. In this multicenter open trial 916 AF patients were randomized to receive anticoagulation or indobufen. At the end of treatment after 1 year follow-up the frequency of primary outcome events (nonfatal stroke, systemic embolism, nonfatal myocardial infarction, or vascular death) was 10.6% and 9.0% and that of vascular death 6.7% and 6.2% in the indobufen and warfarin groups respectively, with no statistical difference between the treatments. Major bleeding events (0.9%) were observed only on warfarin. In comparison with the EAFT study [11], the efficacy of antiplatelet treatment was substantially higher.

In another recent meta-analysis [25] of randomized controlled trials of direct comparison between warfarin and antiplatelet treatment (aspirin/indobufen) in patients with nonvalvular AF the superiority of OAT was attenuated, with a borderline significant difference of -32% relative reduction in nonfatal stroke in favour of OAT. In this systematic review, which included the SIFA comparative study of warfarin and indobufen, the EAFT study was not considered. This may explain the different results found in the previous meta-analysis [5].

Choice of Antithrombotic Therapy

Considering that warfarin is more effective than aspirin but associated with a higher risk of hemorrhage, the choice of antithrombotic treatment should be based on: (1) thromboembolic risk stratification; (2) the ability to provide high-quality monitoring if OAT is chosen; (3) the patient's inherent risk of bleeding with OAT; and (4) the patient's preference.

Thromboembolic Risk Stratification

In patients with nonvalvular AF embolic risk stratification can be done on the basis of clinical and echocardiographic risk factors [26, 27]. Clinical features independently associated with a high stroke rate in AF patients have been defined and integrated into several risk stratification schemes. The two major schemes are those developed by the Atrial Fibrillation Investigators (AFI) group [2] and by the SPAF Investigators [28].

The AFI [2] analyzed the data from the pooled control group of the five primary prevention trials (1236 patients) and found the following independent risk factors for stroke in AF: prior stroke or TIA (relative risk, RR = 2.5), age (RR =

1.6/decade), history of hypertension (RR = 1.6), and diagnosis of diabetes mellitus (RR = 1.7). A subsequent AFI analysis [26] of echocardiograms done in three of the original trials found that moderate-to-severe left ventricular dysfunction was an additional strong risk factor (RR = 2.5). Patients younger than 65 years who have none of these predictive factors (15% of all patients in the randomized clinical trials) have a low annual rate of stroke, approximately 1%, in the absence of any antithrombotic prophylaxis. These results confirm a previous observation that patients with "lone" AF (defined also by the absence of hypertension and diabetes) younger than 60 years have a risk for stroke of less than 0.5% per year [29]. Moreover, the SPAF II study [12] demonstrated that patients with AF aged ≤ 75 years without clinical risk factors and treated with aspirin had a low incidence of stroke. In this subgroup of patients anticoagulant treatment instead of aspirin would give only marginal incremental benefit.

The SPAF Investigators recently published an analysis of risk factors for stroke among the 2012 patients allocated to the aspirin arms of the SPAF I, SPAF II, and SPAF III randomized trials (in SPAF III aspirin was combined with very low-intensity anticoagulation) and the SPAF III aspirin cohort study [28]. Six features were found to be significant independent risk factors: prior stroke or TIA (RR = 2.9), age (RR = 1.8/decade), history of hypertension (RR = 2.0), systolic BP > 160 mmHg (RR = 2.3), female gender (RR = 1.6), and alcohol consumption of ≥ 14 drinks/week (RR = 0.4, i.e. protective).

Despite marginal differences the AFI and SPAF risk stratification schemes are largely consistent with each other. Putting together these two schemes and prior information from the literature, the recent Sixth American College of Chest Physicians' 2001 Consensus Conference on antithrombotic therapy [30] has defined high risk factors (consistent independent predictors) and moderate risk factors (possible independent predictors which are not as strong or consistent as the high risk factors). High risk factors include age > 75 years, prior stroke/TIA or systemic embolism, history of hypertension, congestive heart failure or poor left ventricular systolic function, rheumatic mitral valve disease, and prosthetic heart valves. Moderate risk factors include age 65-75 years, diabetes mellitus, and coronary artery disease with preserved left ventricular systolic function.

The efficacy of aspirin in patients without risk factors has been confirmed in the open arm of the SPAF III study [31]. In this part of the study 892 patients with nonvalvular AF, defined as low-risk because of the absence of specific risk factors (recent congestive heart failure or left ventricular dysfunction, prior TIA/stroke or systemic embolism, systolic blood pressure greater than 160 mmHg, or female sex at age older than 75 years), were followed-up under treatment with aspirin 325 mg per day. The annual incidence of stroke was 2.0%, with a significant difference between patients with (3.6%) and without a history of hypertension (1.1%).

Transesophageal echocardiography provides further markers of embolic risk, i.e. left atrial and left atrial appendage thrombi, spontaneous echocontrast, and left atrial appendage dysfunction [32]. The predictive value of these markers has been investigated in two large prospective studies, SPAF III [33] and FASTER [34]. In the SPAF III study the echocardiographic variables independently associated with a higher thromboembolic risk were: left atrial appendage thrombi, spontaneous echocontrast, low emptying left atrial appendage flow velocity (≤ 20 cm/s), and complex aortic plaques [33]. In the FASTER study, transesophageal echocardiography allowed the detection of patients with AF at very low risk of stroke and death during treatment with antiplatelet agents (aspirin or indobufen). In particular the absence of left atrial appendage thrombi and enlargement of atrial septal aneurysm combined with left atrial appendage flow velocity > 25 cm/s identified patients at very low risk of events [34].

Feasibility of Monitoring

A high-quality monitoring of OAT is the key to minimizing the risk of bleeding. A systematic approach to anticoagulation management, as offered by anticoagulation clinics, can improve the safety and effectiveness of warfarin therapy by reducing related and unrelated complications. In most cases coordinated care can be defined as a specialized program of patient management focused predominantly, if not exclusively, on managing OAT. A program is often directed by a single physician and the actual management is usually conducted by nurses, pharmacists, or physician assistants. This care can be contrasted with that provided by a patient's own physician, without systematic coordination (routine medical care).

Available data indicate that coordinated care will reduce the incidence of adverse outcomes and also the burden on financial resources. In a meta-analysis of six studies comparing coordinated versus routine anticoagulation, the reduction of bleeding events was roughly five episodes averted per 100 patient-years by coordinated care [35]. Chiquette et al. [36] also demonstrated that anticoagulation clinics, in comparison with usual medical care, improved anticoagulation control, reduced bleeding and thromboembolic events rates, and saved $162 058 per 100 patients annually in reducing hospitalization and emergency department visits.

Patient's Risk of Bleeding

Bleeding is the most important complication of OAT. In particular, conventional intensities of anticoagulation increase the risk of intracranial hemorrhage seven- to ten-fold. Therefore cerebral bleed is often a major concern in relation to anticoagulation treatment for stroke prevention in elderly patients. The key issue in using warfarin to prevent stroke and systemic embolism in AF patients is whether the benefit of therapy outweighs the risk of bleeding in the individual patient. Risk factors for bleeding during OAT include intensity of anticoagulation, advanced age, recent initiation of warfarin therapy, and comorbid conditions [37-40].

The quality of laboratory control of anticoagulation treatment is also affected by the mental ability of the patient. Palareti et al. [41] found an unsuspected reduction of mental ability or attention levels in a number of elderly patients receiving OAT; these patients went through longer periods of either under- or over-anticoagulation and were therefore exposed to a higher risk of thrombotic or bleeding complications.

In a recent prospective Italian collaborative study (ISCOAT) the frequency of bleeding complications has been studied in outpatients treated routinely in anticoagulation clinics [42]. The rate of fatal, major, and minor bleeding events was quite low, 0.25, 1.1 and 6.2 per patient-years of follow-up respectively. The rate was higher in older patients and during the first 90 days of treatment compared with later. The risk of bleeding was related to the intensity of anticoagulation, even if a fifth of the bleeding events occurred at INR < 2.0.

A subsequent analysis [43] performed in patients aged 75 years or more included in the ISCOAT showed a nonsignificant trend toward a higher rate of both bleeding and thrombotic complications in elderly versus matched younger patients. However, intracranial bleedings and fatal thrombotic events were more frequent in the elderly. The results of this analysis also indicated that lower than 2.0 INR neither precludes bleeding in the elderly nor offers adequate protection from thrombotic events.

In the subset of patients with AF, major bleeding occurred more frequently in patients over 75 years of age (5.1% per year) than in younger patients (1.0% per year). Univariate analysis revealed a higher frequency of major bleeding in females, in diabetics, and in those who had suffered a previous thromboembolic event [44].

Safe anticoagulation requires monitoring with the INR that corrects for varying thromboplastin sensitivities. Studies of the optimal intensity of OAT provide information about the target for each of the indications for this therapy. In AF patients the risk of stroke increases at INR below 2.0 [45], while the risk of hemorrhage increases at INR above 4.5 [46].

Patient's Preference

In patients at moderate risk of thromboembolism the choice betwee OAT and aspirin should be made on the basis of the risk/benefit ratio of the two treatments. However, the decision process should also take into account the patient's preference. The guidelines for management of AF should be modified to incorporate patients' preferences in the treatment decisions, particularly with regard to the consequences of OAT.

In a recent British observational study on elderly patients with AF, the patients' treatment preferences regarding OAT were compared with other treatment guidelines and current prescriptions [47]. The treatment alternatives and their possible consequences (protection from thromboembolism, side effects) were clearly explained to the patients who then expressed their preference. Given clear information, the participants were able to weigh up the benefits and drawbacks of the intervention and make a personal choice. Of the 38 participants whose decision analysis indicated that they preferred not to be treated with warfarin, 17 (45%) were in fact being prescribed warfarin. Of the remaining 59 participants, 28 (47%) were not being prescribed warfarin, i.e., contrary to their decision. This study shows that when patients are actively involved in clinical decision making, their preference could strongly influence treatment decisions. Successfully involving patients in clinical decisions requires good information. Videos and information booklets about AF can improve patient's understanding of the benefits and risks of treatment choices [48]. It is likely that a shared decision-making tool would have an important impact on patient's knowledge, satisfaction, and compliance with OAT.

Future Perspectives

The hope for the future is the discovery of new efficient, inexpensive, convenient, and safe antithrombotic strategies, beyond aspirin therapy.

New antiplatelet agents might be an interesting option. The promising results with indobufen in the SIFA study, where indobufen was compared with warfarin in secondary prevention, prompted the design of a SIFA II study in which indobufen is being compared with aspirin in patients with AF not eligible for OAT. This ongoing double-blind study will include 2000 patients with nonvalvular AF (900 patients in secondary prevention and 1300 patients in primary prevention) randomized to receive aspirin 300 mg and indobufen 100 or 200 mg; the follow-up is 42 months.

The combination of antiplatelet therapy could be another solution, since regimens such as aspirin-ticlopidine have been shown to be superior to anticoagulation in the prevention of coronary artery stent thrombosis. Recently the association of clopidogrel plus aspirin in the CURE study [49] showed a striking 20% reduction of primary events, in comparison with aspirin alone, in patients with acute coronary syndromes.

Oral thrombin inhibitors represent another option which is under evaluation in a large prospective randomized trial (SPORTIF III) in which melagatran is being compared with warfarin in patients with nonvalvular AF.

Hopefully, from these studies effective alternatives to OAT could be derived with a more convenient profile in respect of the risk of bleeding and ease of management. If these alternative regimens to OAT are demonstrated to be effective and safe, it is likely that antithrombotic prophylaxis could be extended to a larger number of older patiens with AF for whom OAT is often problematic and aspirin is not sufficient.

Conclusions

The ultimate choice of antithrombotic prophylaxis depends on the factors already mentioned (Table 4). Recommendations for treatment based on thromboembolic risk stratification have been reconfirmed in the Sixth 2001 Consensus Conference on Antithrombotic Therapy of the American College of Chest Physicians [30].

OAT is mandatory in high-risk AF patients (those with any high risk factor or with more than one moderate risk factor), provided that a high-quality monitoring of OAT is possible and no risk factors for bleeding are present. These

Table 4. Guidelines for antithrombotic prophylaxis in patients with atrial fibrillation. (Modified from [30])

Category	Treatment
High-risk patients (any age): 　Any high-risk factor[a] 　One moderate risk factor[b]	OAT (INR 2.0-3.0)
Moderate-risk patients (65-75 years): 　No high risk factors 　One moderate risk factor	OAT (INR 2.0-3.0) or aspirin 325 mg
Low-risk patients: 　No high risk factors 　No moderate risk factors	Aspirin 325 mg

[a] *High-risk factors*: age > 75 years, prior stroke or systemic embolism, history of hypertension, congestive heart failure or left ventricular dysfuncton, rheumatic mitral valve disease, prosthetic heart valves
[b] *Moderate risk factors*: age 65-75 years, diabetes mellitus, coronary artery disease with preserved left ventricular function
OAT, oral anticoagulant treatment

two last requirements are particularly important when deciding about OAT in patients older than 75 years.

Aspirin is a possible and acceptable alternative to OAT in moderate-risk patients (those without high risk factors and with only one moderate risk factor). In this group of patients the choice between aspirin and OAT is based on the assessment of the risk/benefit ratio of OAT and also on the patient's preference.

Finally, aspirin is the treatment of choice in low-risk patients (those without high or moderate risk factors). This group is represented by patients with no clinical or echocardiographic evidence of cardiovascular disease.

It is evident from these guidelines that older age (> 75 years) per se is a high risk factor for thromboembolism and all patients older than 75 years should receive OAT for effective prophylaxis. This represents a therapeutic dilemma because of the higher risk of life-threatening hemorrhages, in particular cerebral hemorrhage, in these patients during OAT. A safer and effective antithrombotic regimen is warranted particularly for older patients, who represent a substantial proportion of the AF population.

References

1. Hart RG, Halperin JL (2001) Atrial fibrillation and stroke. Concepts and controversies. Stroke 32:803-808
2. Atrial Fibrillation Investigators (1994) Risk factors for stroke and efficacy of antithrombotic therapy in atrial fibrillation: analysis of pooled data from five randomized controlled trials. Arch Intern Med 154:1449-1457

3. Stein B, Fuster V, Halperin JL, Chesebro JH (1989) Antithrombotic therapy in cardiac disease. An emerging approach based on pathogenesis and risk. Circulation 80:1501-1513

4. Chesebro JH, Fuster V, Halperin JL (1991) Atrial fibrillation: risk marker for stroke. N Engl J Med 323:1556-1558

5. Hart RG, Benavente O, McBride R, Pearce LA (1999) Antithrombotic therapy to prevent stroke in patients with atrial fibrillation: a meta-analysis. Ann Intern Med 131:492-501

6. Petersen P, Boysen G, Godtfredsen J et al (1989) Placebo-controlled, randomised trial of warfarin and aspirin for prevention of thromboembolic complications in chronic atrial fibrillation. The Copenhagen AFASAK Study. Lancet 1:175-179

7. The Stroke Prevention in Atrial Fibrillation Investigators (1991) The Stroke Prevention in Atrial Fibrillation trial: final results. Circulation 84:527-539

8. The Boston Area Anticoagulation Trial for Atrial Fibrillation Investigators (1990) The effect of low-dose warfarin on the risk of stroke in patients with nonrheumatic atrial fibrillation. N Engl J Med 325:1505-1511

9. Connolly SJ, Laupacis A, Gent M et al for the CAFA study coinvestigators (1991) Canadian Atrial Fibrillation Anticoagulation (CAFA) study. J Am Coll Cardiol 18:349-355

10. Ezekowitz MD, Bridgers SL, James KE et al for the Veterans Affairs Stroke Prevention in Nonrheumatic Atrial Fibrillation Investigators (1992) Warfarin in the prevention of stroke associated with nonrheumatic atrial fibrillation. N Engl J Med 327:1406-1412

11. European Atrial Fibrillation Trial (EAFT) Study Group (1993) Secondary prevention in nonrheumatic atrial fibrillation after transient ischaemic attack or minor stroke. Lancet 342:1255-1262

12. Stroke Prevention in Atrial Fibrillation Investigators (1994) Warfarin versus aspirin for prevention of thromboembolism in atrial fibrilllation: Stroke Prevention in Atrial Fibrillation II Study. Lancet 346:687-691

13. Stafford RS, Singer DE (1996) National patterns of warfarin use in atrial fibrillation. Arch Intern Med 156:2537-2541

14. Bungard TJ, Ghali WA, Teo KK et al (2000) Why do patients with atrial fibrillation not receive warfarin? Arch Intern Med 160:41-46

15. Cohen N, Sarafian DA, Alon I et al (2000) Warfarin for stroke prevention still underused in atrial fibrillation. Stroke 31:1217-1222

16. Stroke Prevention in Atrial Fibrillation Investigators (1996) Adjusted-dose warfarin versus low-intensity, fixed-dose warfarin plus aspirin for high risk patients with atrial fibrillation: Stroke Prevention in Atrial Fibrillation III randomised clinical trial. Lancet 348:633-638

17. Pengo V, Zasso A, Barbero F et al (1998) Effectiveness of fixed minidose warfarin in the prevention of thromboembolism and vascular death in nonrheumatic atrial fibrillation. Am J Cardiol 82:433-437

18. Gullov AL, Koefoed BG, Petersen P et al (1998) Fixed minidose warfarin and aspirin alone and in combination vs adjusted-dose warfarin for stroke prevention in atrial fibrillation. Arch Intern Med 158:1513-1521

19. Hellemons BS, Langenberg M, Lodder J et al (1999) Primary prevention of arterial thromboembolism in nonrheumatic atrial fibrillation in primary care: randomised control trial comparing two intensities of coumarin with aspirin. Br Med J 319:958-964

20. Diener HC, Lowenthal A (1997) Antiplatelet therapy to prevent stroke: risk of brain hemorrhage and efficacy in atrial fibrillation. J Neurol Sci 153:112

21. Posada IS, Barriales V for the LASAF pilot Study Group (1999) Alternate-day dosing of aspirin in atrial fibrillation. Am Heart J 138:137-143

22. Benavente O, Hart RG, Koudstal P et al (1999) Antiplatelet therapy for preventing stroke in patients with nonvalvular atrial fibrillation and no previous history of stroke or transient ischemic attacks. In: Warlow C, Van Gijn J, Sandercock P (eds) Stroke module of the Cochrane database of systematic reviews. BMJ Publishing Group, London

23. Miller VT, Rothrock JF, Feinberg WM et al, on behalf of the Stroke Prevention in Atrial Fibrillation Investigators (1993) Ischemic stroke in patients with atrial fibrillation: effect of aspirin according to stroke mechanism. Neurology 43:32-36

24. Morocutti C, Amabile G, Fattapposta F et al (1997) Indobufen versus warfarin in the secondary prevention of major vascular events in nonrheumatic atrial fibrillation. Stroke 28:1015-1022

25. Taylor FC, Cohen H, Ebrahim S (2001) Systematic review of long term anticoagulation or antiplatelet treatment in patients with nonrheumatic atrial fibrillation. Br Med J 322:321-326

26. The Stroke Prevention in Atrial Fibrillation Investigators (1992) Predictors of thromboembolism in atrial fibrillation: I. Clinical features of patients at risk. Ann Intern Med 116:1-5

27. Atrial Fibrillation Investigators (1998) Echocardiographic predictors of stroke in patients with atrial fibrillation. A prospective study of 1066 patients from 3 clinical trials. Arch Intern Med 158:1316-1320

28. Hart RG, Pearce LA, Mc Bride R et al, on behalf of the Stroke Prevention in Atrial Fibrillation (SPAF) Investigators (1999) Factors associated with ischemic stroke during aspirin therapy in atrial fibrillation. Analysis of 2012 participants in the SPAF I-III clinical trials. Stroke 30:1223-1229

29. Kopecky SL, Gersh BJ, McGoon MD et al (1987) The natural history of lone atrial fibrillation: a population-based study over three decades. N Engl J Med 317:669-674

30. Albers GW, Dalen JE, Laupacis A et al (2001) Antithrombotic therapy in atrial fibrillation. Sixth ACCP Consensus Conference on Antithrombotic Therapy. Chest 119[Suppl]:194S-206S

31. The SPAF III Writing Committee for the Stroke Prevention in Atrial Fibrillation Investigators (1998) Patients with nonvalvular atrial fibrillation at low risk of stroke during treatment with aspirin. JAMA 279:1273-1277

32. Di Pasquale G, Urbinati S, Pinelli G (1995) New echocardiographic markers of embolic risk in atrial fibrillation. Cerebrovasc Dis 5:315-322

33. Zabalgoitia M, Halperin JL, Pearce LA et al (1998) Transesophageal echocardiographic correlates of clinical risk of thromboembolism in nonvalvular atrial fibrillation. J Am Coll Cardiol 31:1622-1626

34. The Investigators of FASTER Study (1996) Fibrillazione Atriale Studio Transesofageo Emiliano-Romagnolo, Italy: Transesophageal echocardiographic correlates of prior thromboembolism in non-valvular atrial fibrillation: a multicentre study. Eur Heart J 17[Suppl]:442 (abstr)

35. Ansell JE, Hughes R (1996) Evolving models of warfarin management: anticoagulation clinics, patient self-monitoring, and patient self-management. Am Heart J 132:1095-1100

36. Chiquette E, Amato MG, Bussey HI (1998) Comparison of an anticoagulation clinic with usual medical care: anticoagulation control, patient outcomes, and health care costs. Arch Intern Med 158:1641-1647

37. Levine MN, Raskob G, Landefeld S, Kearon C (2001) Hemorrhagic complications of anticoagulant treatment. Sixth ACCP Consensus Conference on Antithrombotic Therapy. Chest 119[Suppl]:108S-121S

38. Landefeld CS, Goldman L (1989) Major bleeding in outpatients treated with warfarin. Incidence and prediction by factors known at the start of outpatient therapy. Am J Med 87:144-152
39. Fihn SD, Mc Donell M, Martin D et al (1993) Risk factors for complications of chronic anticoagulation: a multicenter study. Ann Intern Med 118:511-520
40. Hylek EM, Singer DE (1994) Risk factors for intracranial hemorrhage in outpatients taking warfarin. Ann Intern Med 120:897-902
41. Palareti G, Poggi M, Guazzaloca G et al (1997) Assessment of mental ability in elderly anticoagulated patients: its reduction is associated with a less satisfactory quality of treatment. Blood Coagul Fibrinolysis 8:411-417
42. Palareti G, Leali N, Coccheri S et al, on behalf of the Italian Study on Complications of Oral Anticoagulant Therapy (1996) Bleeding complications of oral anticoagulant treatment: an inception-cohort, prospective collaborative study (ISCOAT). Lancet 348:423-428
43. Palareti G, Hirsh J, Legnani C et al (2000) Oral anticoagulation treatment in the elderly: a nested prospective, case-control study. Arch Intern Med 160:470-478
44. Pengo V, Legnani C, Noventa F, Palareti G, on behalf of the ISCOAT Study Group (2001) Oral anticoagulant therapy in patients with nonrheumatic atrial fibrillation and risk of bleeding. Thromb Haemost 85:418-422
45. Hylek EM, Skates SJ, Sheehan MA, Singer DE (1996) An analysis of the lowest effective intensity of prophylactic anticoagulation for patients with nonrheumatic atrial fibrillation. N Engl J Med 335:540-546
46. The European Atrial Fibrillation Study Group (1995) Optimal oral anticoagulant therapy in patients with nonrheumatic atrial fibrillation and recent cerebral ischemia. N Engl J Med 333:5-10
47. Protheroe J, Fahey T, Montgomery AA, Peters TJ (2000) The impact of patient's preferences on the treatment of atrial fibrillation: observational study of patient based decision analysis. Br Med J 320:1380-1384
48. Man-Son-Hing M, Laupacis A, O'Connor AM et al, for the Stroke Prevention in Atrial Fibrillation Investigators (1999) A patient decision aid regarding antithrombotic therapy for stroke prevention in atrial fibrillation. JAMA 282:737-743
49. Anonimous (2001) Presentation of the 50th Annual Scientific Session of the American College of Cardiology, Orlando, Florida

Self-management of Oral Anticoagulants by Patients with Atrial Fibrillation: How Effective and Safe Is It?

R. Cazzin[1], P. Serra[1] and C. Lestuzzi[2]

Atrial Fibrillation and Thromboembolism

Atrial fibrillation (AF) is the most frequent arrhythmia. Its frequency is constantly increasing together with the life span of the general population, since the incidence of AF rises with age. This arrhythmia should not be underestimated, because it leads to a significant increase of mortality [1] and of clinical events with a high medical cost: heart failure and systemic thromboembolism. Hence the rising involvement of health structures in order to manage the arrhythmia and its complications, with the contribution of different medical operators.

AF is the main cause of 20% of ischemic strokes [2]; moreover, an increasing number of cases of silent brain ischemia has been observed (about 15% of patients with AF without clinically evident cardiovascular events). Silent cerebral accidents may cause progressive brain damage, with worsening of life quality [3].

Oral Anticoagulant Therapy in Atrial Fibrillation

The benefits of oral anticoagulant therapy with warfarin for patients with mitral valve disease or atrial thrombi are evident, widely accepted and need no further confirmation. In patients with AF without valve disease, an indication of anticoagulant therapy is linked to the evaluation of thromboembolic risk. According to data from large population studies, the main risk factors are previous thromboembolism, recent acute heart failure, left ventricular dysfunction, systemic hypertension, diabetes and age over 65 [4-8]. If one or more of these factors are present, oral anticoagulant therapy is recommended. The efficacy of such therapy in primary prevention of stroke has been evaluated in five large controlled studies [4-8], whose combined results suggest a 69% reduction of cerebrovascular events in patients with chronic AF.

[1]Unità Operativa di Cardiologia, Ospedale di Portogruaro, Venezia; [2]Servizio di Cardiologia, Centro di Riferimento Oncologico, IRCCS, Aviano, Pordenone, Italy

In secondary prevention of the thromboembolic risk, warfarin use has gained unanimous consensus [9]. In patients with previous ischemic stroke the recurrence rate has been lowered by 70%. This result is widely superior to that obtained with aspirin, which probably prevents mainly extracranial embolism. Despite these results, in clinical practice there are some concerns about oral anticoagulant therapy, which is often considered dangerous and difficult to manage [10]. The most threatening complication is major hemorrhage, whose incidence is about 0.9%-2.5%/year [11, 12]. Use of warfarin can be difficult to manage because of the presence of renal or hepatic failure, advanced age, low compliance of the patient and interaction with other drugs. In order to overcome this problem, warfarin therapy is often substituted by aspirin, whose benefit is markedly reduced in patients at high risk as compared to those at low risk (subjects less than 65 years old, without cardiac disease and previous embolism).

Management of Anticoagulant Therapy

The incidence of hemorrhagic or embolic events depends mainly on the quality control of anticoagulant therapy, which requires efficient organization to manage such therapy. This organization should try to obtain the most favorable results and the best cost:benefit ratio. To do so, cooperation between the patient, the physician and the laboratory is most important.

The physician who prescribes anticoagulant therapy independently or following the specialist's advice should know the problems regarding anticoagulant therapy, anticoagulant drugs and the patient's disease; he should be able to follow-up the therapy using a reliable and easily accessible laboratory, and he must inform and encourage a responsible attitude in the patient and his relatives through a continuous treatment education program [3].

In order to help the general physician in the difficult management of anticoagulant therapy, many countries have created operative units to give patients direct access and complete follow-up of anticoagulant therapy [13-15]. Patients monitored by these units have an hemorrhage rate 50%-75% lower than those followed routinely by other physicians (13, 16, 17).

Self-management of Anticoagulant Therapy

Despite the presence of a wide net for the management of anticoagulant therapy, with reliable laboratories organized with computerized prescription of warfarin dosage, some patients still remain for long periods out of the therapeutic range. And it should be stressed that complications are related to the extent of time the patients are out of the INR range suggested [17, 18]. Several causes may be involved, but most often the main reason is low patient compliance, due to several factors: problems related to the laboratory organization, to blood-sample ambulatory accessibility, to the time required to obtain the INR result and then to the final assessment of warfarin dosage. These difficulties may affect the patient's lifestyle and even lead to a significant worsening of his quality of life.

Recently, portable equipment able to measure the INR from capillary blood has been produced [19-21]. With the aid of this equipment, the patient may be able, after specific training, to self-manage warfarin dosage. The self-management of anticoagulant therapy, through the direct control of the patient without the need of a laboratory, markedly improves both patient compliance and the final quality of anticoaugulation treatment. Most studies about the self-management of anticoagulation suggest that about 50%-70% of patients are able to apply this procedure [22-28].

The first study on 50 patients randomized between self-management, and traditional management, with an 8 week follow-up of the INR range, was published in 1998 [24]. Nearly all patients in the self-management group maintained the therapeutic range, in contrast with less than two-thirds in the group followed by an external laboratory. Since the follow-up was short, significant differences in hemorrhagic or embolic complications could not be detected.

Sawiki and co-workers [29], for a 6-month period, compared 82 patients whose anticoagulant therapy was followed by their general physician and 83 patients enrolled in a self-management program after a training period. The self-managed group showed a better accuracy in INR control and a higher score in a questionnaire on quality of life. Similar results were reported in a recent Dutch study on 50 patients [30], who clearly preferred the self-management of anticoagulant therapy.

Ansell and co-workers [16] evaluated the expense of various kinds of anticoagulation checking, laboratory-centered, self-managed or traditional: the costs of laboratory-centered and self-managed checking were 50% lower of those of the traditional checking. Self-management still has this better costs:benefits ratio, even tough the INR dosage is used more often than in the other systems.

These studies have opened the way to a new approach to anticoagulant therapy with wide possibilities, although larger studies and longer follow-up are needed. House self-management helps the frequent use of the test with immediate results and then an easier adaptation of warfarin dosage. The possibility of remaining for a longer period within the therapeutic range allows a reduction of both hemorrhagic and embolic complications. Whenever patients are not able to manage the method by themselves, the use of the equipment may be left to the relatives, to the home-care nurse or to the general physician.

Conclusions

Self-management of anticoagulant therapy in atrial fibrillation is feasible, effective and with a good cost:benefit ratio, comparable to that of central laboratories. It represents a system better accepted by, and more satisfying for, patients who must receive anticoagulant therapy for a long time. The good results and the simpler checking of anticoagulant therapy through self-management may lead more general physicians to prescribe this therapy to patients affected by AF, with a good outcome in the prevention of thromboembolism.

References

1. Benjamin EJ, Wolf PA, D'Agostino RB et al (1998) Impact of atrial fibrillation on the risk of death. The Framingham heart study. Circulation 98:946-952

2. Atrial Fibrillation Investigators (1994) Risk factors for stroke and efficacy of antithrombotic therapy in atrial fibrillation. Analysis of pooled data from five randomized controlled trials. Arch Intern Med 154:1449-1457

3. Ezekowitz MD, James KE, Nazarian SM et al (1995) Silent cerebral infarction in patients with nonrheumatic atrial fibrillation. The Veterans Affairs Stroke Prevention in Nonrheumatic Atrial Fibrillation Investigators. Circulation 92:2178-2182

4. Petersen P, Boisen G, Godtfredsen J et al (1989) Placebo-controlled, randomized trial of warfarin and aspirin for prevention of thromboembolic complications in chronic atrial fibrillation. The Copenhagen AFASAK Study. Lancet 1:175

5. The Boston Area Anticoagulation Trial for Atrial Fibrillation Investigators (1990) The effect of low-dose warfarin on the risk of stroke in patients with nonrheumatic atrial fibrillation. N Engl J Med 323:1505

6. Stoke Prevention in Atrial Fibrillation Investigators (1991) Stroke Prevention in Atrial Fibrillation Study: Final results. Circulation 84:527

7. Connolly SJ, Laupacis A, Gent M et al (1991) Canadian Atrial Fibrillation Anti-Coagulation (CAFA) Study. J Am Coll Cardiol 18:349

8. Ezekowitz MD, Bridgers SL, James KE et al (1992) Warfarin in the prevention of stroke associated with nonrheumatic atrial fibrillation (SPINAF). N Engl J Med 327:1406-1412

9. EAFT (European Atrial Fibrillation Trial) Study Group (1993) Secondary prevention in nonrheumatic atrial fibrillation after transient ischemic attack or minor stroke. Lancet 342:1255

10. Scardi S, Mazzone C (1997) La profilassi anticoagulante: dai grandi trial alla pratica clinica. G Ital Cardiol 28:171-183

11. Levine MN, Roaskob G, Landefeld S et al (1998) Haemorrhagic complications of anticoagulant treatment. Chest 114:511-523

12. Landefeld Cs, Beyth RJ (1993) Anticoagulant-related bleeding: clinical epidemiology, prediction and prevention. Am J Med 95:315-328

13. Palareti G, Leali N,Coccheri S et al (1997) Complicanze emorragiche della terapia anticoagulante orale: risultati dello studio prospettico multicentrico ISCOAT. G Ital Cardiol 27:231-243

14. Cortellazzo S, Finazzi G, Viero P et al (1993) Thrombotic and hemorrhagic complications in patients with mechanical heart valve prosthesis attending an anticoagulation clinic. Thromb Haemostasis 69:316-320

15. Bussey HL, Chiquette E, Amato M (1995) Anticoagulation clinic care versus routine medical care: a review and interim report. J Thomb Thrombolysis 2:315-319

16. Ansell JE (1998) Anticoagulation management as a risk factor for adverse events: grounds for improvement. J Thromb Thrombolysis 5[Suppl]:S13-S18

17. Rosendaal FR (1996) The Scylla and Charybdis of oral anticoagulant treatment. N Engl J Med 335:587-589

18. Saour JN, Sieck JO, Mamo LAR et al (1990) Trial of different intensities of anticoagulation in patients with prosthetic heart valves. N Engl J Med 322:428-432

19. Leaning KE, Ansell JE (1996) Advances in the monitoring of oral anticoagulation: point-of-care testing, patient self-monitoring, and patient self-management. J Thromb Thrombolysis 3:377-383

20. Kitchen S, Preston FE (1997) Monitoring oral anticoagulant treatment with the TAS near-patient test system: comparison with conventional thromboplastins. J Clin Pathol 50:951-956

21. Ansell JE (1999) Empowering patients to monitor and manage oral anticoagulation therapy. J Am Med Assoc 281:182-183

22. Andrew M, Marzinotto V, Leakar M et al (1997) Home monitoring of pediatric patients. Scientific Symposium: self-management of oral anticoagulation, State of the art, Florence, pp 20-25

23. Hasenlam M, Knudsen L, Kimose HH et al (1997) Practicability of patient self testing of oral anticoagulation therapy by the international normalized ratio using a portable whole blood monitor. Thrombosis Res 85:77-82

24. White RH, McCurday SA, Von Marensdorff H et al (1998) Home prothrombin time monitoring after the initiation of warfarin therapy. A randomized, prospective study. Ann Intern Med 111:730-737

25. Ansell JE, Patel N, Ostrovsky D et al (1995) Long-term patient self-management of oral anti coagulation. Arch Intern Med 155:2185-2189

26. Kaatz SS, White RH, Hill J et al (1995) Accuracy of laboratory and portable monitor international normalized ratio determinations. Comparison with a criterion standard. Arch Intern Med 155:1861-1867

27. Hasenkam JM, Kimose L, Gronnesby H et al (1997) Self -management of oral anticoagulant therapy after heart valve replacement. Eur J Cardio Thorac Surg 11:935-942

28. Bernardo A (1992) Home prothrombin estimation. In: Butchart EG, Bodnar E (eds) Thrombosis, embolism and bleeding. ICR, London pp 325-330

29. Sawicki PT (1999) A structured teaching and self-management program for patients receiving oral anticoagulation. A randomized controlled trial. J Am Med Assoc 281 (2)

30. Cromheecke ME, Levi M, Colly LP et al (2000) Oral anticoagulation self-management and management by a specialist anticoagulation clinic: a randomised cross-over comparison. Lancet 356:97-102

ATRIAL FIBRILLATION:
NON-PHARMACOLOGICAL THERAPY

Focal Atrial Fibrillation: The Bordeaux Experience

D. C. SHAH, M. HAÏSSAGUERRE, P. JAÏS, M. HOCINI, T. YAMANE, L. MACLE, K. J. CHOI
AND J. CLÉMENTY

Initial attempts at linear ablation for atrial fibrillation (AF) indicated that creating continuous linear lesions to duplicate surgical atriotomies was difficult, that right atrial lesions alone were safe but ineffective, and that left atrial lesions improved success rates, although at a significant morbidity (including proarrhythmic left atrial reentry) and even mortality cost – but, most importantly perhaps, these studies showed the feasibility of cure by catheter-based techniques in patients with paroxysmal and persistent AF [1-3].

Linear ablation also afforded the possibility of observing shortened paroxysms of AF at close quarters with mapping catheters in the left atrium. Stereotyped initiations were traced in nearly all patients to sleeves of atrial myocardium encasing the ostia of one or more pulmonary veins (PVs) [4, 5].

The typical patient with paroxysmal atrial fibrillation has frequent involvement of two or three PVs and may have additional nonPV-initiating sources. It is frequently difficult to identify each of the multiple focal sources. Therefore, a practical and expeditious solution is to systematically ablate and disconnect the myocardial sleeve of all the PVs during sinus rhythm.

Anatomical considerations dictate that the more proximal the level of ablation for the PVs, the greater the extent of disconnected myocardium, but this requires more extensive ablation because of increasing diameter and myocardial coverage proximally. Electrophysiologically definable sites of preferential inputs to the veins, however, enable disconnection to be achieved at the ostia without circumferential ablation in the majority [6, 7].

Activation of the vein can best be appreciated with some form of circumferential mapping - as opposed to longitudinal mapping, typified by a multi-electrode catheter placed along the length of the vein. Because of the cul-de-sac nature of electrical activation in the PV, the disappearance of all distal (circumferentially recordable) potentials is a clear and unarguable indicator of conduction block.

Distinguishing target PV potentials from far field atrial potentials is, however, important in order to avoid unnecessary ablation which could result in vein stenosis or avoidable collateral damage (e.g. to the lung or the phrenic nerve).

Hôpital Cardiologique du Haut-Lévêque, Pessac, France

Typically, circumferential mapping allows electrophysiologically-guided disconnection of the four PVs to be accomplished successfully in nearly 100% of patients, and quite rapidly - at times within 1 h. In this context, the potential role of circumferential ablation devices is debatable, since the gain in efficacy (if any) would be limited. Ablative energy could be unnecessarily delivered at bystander sites, with resulting collateral damage, or may not be sufficiently concentrated or focused to ablate a discrete fascicle.

This strategy of expeditious PV disconnection without documented proof of arrhythmogenicity can only be justified by a sufficiently low risk of side effects, notably PV stenosis. The use of limited RF power, minimizing the circumferential extent of ablation and targeting the most proximal segment (usually the largest diameter) are all important in limiting the frequency of this difficult-to-treat complication to 1%-2% of ablated PVs. Nonocclusive stenosis limited to a single PV (typically draining about half of one lung) usually has no significant clinical consequences.

After PV Disconnection

Following disconnection, provocative maneuvers in the form of isoprenaline infusion and rapid atrial pacing are performed. Spontaneous arrhythmia at this juncture is necessarily of nonpulmonary venous origin. Unlike the PVs, with their relatively constant location and arborizing structure – which is what allows anatomic disconnection – these focal sources present specific problems. Initiation of sustained AF, coupled with the limited electrode coverage possible through the transseptal route of left atrial access, makes their localization difficult. Most frequently located in the left atrium, they are preferentially found in the posterior left atrium and surrounding the ostia of the PVs.

Supplemental ostial ablation aimed at late or fractionated potentials may eliminate some of these recurrences; for some others, opportune mapping during periods of nonsustained (and thus mappable) arrhythmia can allow successful ablation. When these nonPV sources are multiple or trigger sustained atrial fibrillation, they are difficult to map during the brief and few opportunities offered by early or immediate reinitiation following cardioversion, and different options may have to be tried. Better mapping techniques based on the noninvasive analysis of surface ECG P waves, multi-electrode basket-type catheters designed for the left atrium, or projection of intracardiac or body surface potentials to modeled endocardial boundaries (based on Laplace's equation) may allow localization and elimination by wide or even anatomical ablation of these nonPV sources. Adjuvant linear ablation – probably a necessary component for ablation of chronic AF – can also terminate or reduce the duration of paroxysms and facilitate mapping, although at the cost of possible left atrial proarrhythmia (in case of incomplete lines) and perhaps a variable effect on left atrial contractile function. Previously ineffective antiarrhythmic drug therapy, though, can eliminate residual AF in about 30%-40% of these patients.

Results

One hundred consecutive patients underwent catheter ablation for drug-resistant paroxysmal AF. Guided by a 10 pole Lasso catheter, 1, 2, 3 and 4 PVs were ablated in 6, 14, 40 and 38 patients, respectively. Two patients required only nonPV foci ablation. Successful distal PV disconnection was achieved in 302/306 PVs (99%) and complicated by three acute PV stenoses (50% narrowing, all without gradient) and two pericardial effusions. Provoked (with Isuprel and burst pacing) or spontaneous ectopics or AF initiations after PV ablation were mapped with two or three multi-electrode catheters.

After PV disconnection, remaining foci were often difficult to map precisely because of sporadic discharges and repeated induction of sustained AF. These 'nonPV' foci originated: (a) from the PV ostia, within 1 cm proximal to the level of previous ablation in 25 cases (nine left superior, nine right superior and seven inferior PVs), usually from the adjacent posterior wall; (b) from the atrial tissue in 23, posterior left atrium in 13, other parts of the left atrium in six, right atrium or septum in four; (c) from the coronary sinus or left superior vena cava in one each. Nine foci could not be localized.

After ablation of these foci, AF was eliminated without drug in 68 patients. Only 27% of cured patients had 'nonPV' foci vs 86% of the unsuccessfully ablated group ($p < 0.01$).

Conclusions

Electrical disconnection of PVs is easily demonstrable and routinely possible, with a low risk of PV stenosis, which compares favourably with the risk of persistent AF, antiarrhythmic and anticoagulant drug therapy and eliminates AF in 70% of patients with paroxysmal AF (which is particularly easy in patients with frequent paroxysms), freeing the patient not only from antiarrhythmic treatment but also from oral anticoagulation. This procedure, though, does not eliminate paroxysmal atrial fibrillation in about 30% of patients, who typically have longer duration of AF and nonpulmonary focal sources. Thus, at present, resistance to antiarrhythmic drugs should determine when this therapeutic option should be offered to a specific patient with paroxysmal AF. With future reduction in the risk profile of the procedure and more complete elimination of nonpulmonary venous foci and/or more efficient and safe deployment of linear lesions, the majority of patients with paroxysmal AF could become amenable to catheter-based curative treatment.

References

1. Haïssaguerre M, Jaïs P, Shah DC et al (1996) Right and left atrial radiofrequency catheter therapy of paroxysmal atrial fibrillation. J Cardiovasc Electrophysiol 7:1132-1144

2. Swartz JF, Pellersels G, Silvers J et al (1994) A catheter-based curative approach to atrial fibrillation in humans. Circulation 90(II):I-335 (abstr)
3. Ernst S, Shluter M, Ouyang F et al (1999) Modification of the substrate for maintenance of idiopathic human atrial fibrillation: efficacy of radiofrequency ablation using nonfluoroscopic catheter guidance. Circulation 100:2085-2092
4. Haïssaguerre M, Jaïs P, Shah DC et al (1998) Spontaneous initiation of atrial fibrillation by ectopic beats originating in the pulmonary veins. N Engl J Med 339:659-666
5. Jaïs P, Haïssaguerre M, Shah DC et al (1997) A focal source of atrial fibrillation treated by discrete radiofrequency ablation. Circulation 95:572-576
6. Haïssaguerre M, Jaïs P, Shah DC, et al (2000) Electrophysiological end point for catheter ablation of atrial fibrillation initiated from multiple pulmonary venous foci. Circulation 101:1409-1417
7. Haïssaguerre M, Shah DC, Jaïs P et al (2000) Electrophysiological breakthroughs from the left atrium to the pulmonary veins. Circulation 102:2463-2465

Milan Experience of Catheter Ablation for Atrial Fibrillation

C. Pappone[1], S. Rosanio[1], G. Oreto[2], M. Tocchi[1], F. Gugliotta[1], A. Salvati[1], C. Dicandia[1], P. Mazzone[1], V. Santinelli[1], S. Gulletta[1] and G. Vicedomini[1]

Introduction

Until very recently, physicians considered atrial fibrillation (AF) as a benign arrhythmia which either did not require any treatment or could be managed adequately with some digoxin. During the last decade, however, epidemiological studies have shown that AF carries considerable morbidity and mortality. The concept that "AF begets AF" has further strengthened the need for a more aggressive approach towards prevention and treatment of AF. At the same time, the evolution of cardiac mapping technologies has allowed the development of new, nonsurgical strategies to cure this common arryhythmia.

Linear Ablation for AF

The past 5 years have witnessed a steady and continuous evolution in the catheter-based treatment of AF. Very recently, the possibility of treating AF by linear radiofrequency (RF) lesions has been reported. Linear ablation therapies for AF originate from the multiple reentrant hypothesis originally proposed by Moe to explain the genesis of the arrhythmia, and the assumption that an adequate spatial extent of contiguous electrically active tissue is necessary for fibrillatory wavelets to perpetuate AF. These electrophysiologic concepts initially led to the development of surgical techniques to restore sinus rhythm in patients with AF undergoing mitral valve operations. The so-called MAZE operation and its variants consisted of placing incisions in specific areas of both atria, an approach that was effective in restoring adequate atrial systole and preventing AF recurrences in over 80% of the patients [1].

These favorable results stimulated attempts to reproduce the surgical technique using a less invasive, transcatheter approach. The first clinical study by

[1]Division of Cardiac Electrophysiology, Department of Cardiology, San Raffaele University Hospital, Milan; [2]Division of Cardiology, University of Messina, Italy

Haïssaguerre et al. described the application of RF lesions in both atria to treat patients with paroxysmal, drug-refractory AF [2]. In the right atrium (RA), three lines were deployed (one septal intercaval line and two lines in the RA free wall, one longitudinal and one transverse). In the left atrium (LA), the investigators attempted to create a long line encircling the four pulmonary veins (PVs) and connected to the mitral annulus on both sides. The results of the study suggested that ablation restricted to the RA is a safe technique, but the success rate was only 13% without antiarrhythmic drugs, increasing to 40% after the procedure was extended to the LA. Furthermore, the procedure was particularly challenging because fluoroscopy was used to guide navigation of the ablation catheter, and it was not possible to obtain objective evidence that conduction block across the lines was achieved. Incomplete electrical separation between contiguous areas could allow impulse conduction as well as propagation of the fibrillatory wavefront, and even provide the substrate for atrial reentry, thus compounding the problem of AF with that of atrial flutter. On the other hand, efforts to achieve and verify local block result in long fluoroscopy times, potentially increasing the risk of embolism.

In our earliest experience, we demonstrated that creation of the long continuous RF linear lesions necessary to compartmentalize the atria is facilitated by the use of a 3D nonfluoroscopic electroanatomic mapping system (CARTO, Biosense/Webster) [3]. Complex linear lesions can be generated using the ability of the CARTO system to navigate the catheter precisely to predefined sites, to monitor electrogram changes during RF delivery, and to tag ablated sites. In addition, postablation remapping allows evaluation of lesion completeness on the basis of specific quantitative criteria such as conduction delay and double potentials across the line, which have been shown to correlate closely with pathological evidence of continuous and transmural lesions. However, the electroanatomical definition of "complete" block for linear lesions does not imply total absence of conduction, but rather indicates that the route of propagation of the impulse front is different compared with the baseline condition. Theoretically, therefore, a circulating wavefront could still cross the line of block despite a significant postablation change in the activation map, which might account for some recurrences of the arrhythmia after the creation of continuous lines.

Results of studies of linear ablation for AF using standard fluoroscopic or electroanatomical guidance are reported in Table 1. These results underline how extension of the procedure to the LA uniformly increased the success rates, with the exception of the study by Ernst et al., in which 100% recurrence rates with both LA and biatrial ablation were accompanied by very long fluoroscopy times and difficulties in achieving continuous block despite the use of electroanatomical guidance. This emphasizes the operator dependency of the technique and the presence of a learning curve effect. In our own experience at a single institution where CARTO-guided atrial ablation procedures have been performed since early 1996, we have witnessed a progressive increase in physician and staff confidence with different linear ablation strategies, resulting in a significant decrease in procedure duration and fluoroscopy use over time.

Table 1. Ablation studies in atrial fibrillation

Author	Year	AF type	Guidance	Atrial chamber	Freedom from AF[a] (%)	Follow-up (months)
Haïssaguerre et al. [2]	1996	Paroxysmal	Fluoro	RA	33	11 ± 4
				RA+LA	60	
Jaïs et al. [4]	1998	Paroxysmal	Fluoro	RA	37	26 ± 5
Maloney et al. [5]	1998	Chronic	Fluoro	RA+LA	81	23 ± 10
Garg et al. [6]	1999	Paroxysmal	Fluoro	RA	67	12 ± 13
Pappone et al. [3]	1999	Paroxysmal	CARTO	RA	50	11 ± 3
				LA	60	
				RA+LA	85	
Ernst et al. [7]	1999	Paroxysmal	CARTO	LA	0	1 ± 1
				LA+RA	0	
Pappone et al. [8]	2000	Paroxysmal and chronic	CARTO	LA (PV isolation)	85%	9 ± 3

RA, right atrium; *LA*, left atrium; *PV*, pulmonary vein
[a]Percentage of patients free from atrial fibrillation (AF) are maximum success reported, with or without drug therapy

New Lesion Paradigms

The field of ablation for AF is still evolving. Landmark studies have recently demonstrated the dominance of the LA in the PV region for the initiation as well as the maintenance of AF [9-11]. This has led to a paradigm shift in catheter-based approaches for AF. Focal ablation of PV triggers has been shown to be able to suppress AF in selected patients. However, the feasibility of this technique is limited by the difficulty in mapping the focus if the patient is in AF or has no consistent firing, the frequent existence of multiple foci (69%) causing high recurrence rates, and an incidence of PV stenoses as high as 42% [10, 11]. To circumvent these limitations, we recently developed an anatomic approach, in which circumferential lines of conduction block are created using CARTO guidance around the ostia of each PV, with the aim of isolating these veins from the LA while reducing the risk of PV stenosis [8].

As far as evaluation of conduction block is concerned, the criteria used for objective validation of circular lines are different from those used for linear lesions. In fact, theoretically no activation should be present beyond a complete circular line. To verify this phenomenon we use the electroanatomical voltage map, which displays the peak-to-peak bipolar signal amplitude superimposed on the 3D anatomical map. Our criterion for defining absence of impulse penetration through the line is the detection of signal amplitudes below 0.1 mV at all points inside the circular line. Although such low amplitude signals are not likely to represent propagated potentials, they are sensed by the mapping system and displayed as "activation", resulting in blue-purple color shades in isochronal maps. The activation delay was considered satisfactory when it was greater than 30 ms. However, detection of delayed conduction across the line required pacing from a site close to the lesion. Therefore, our initial approach required two postablation maps acquired during coronary sinus (CS) and RA appendage pacing to validate the lesions around the septal and lateral PVs, respectively.

Later on, we modified our strategy for line validation in that we abandoned the activation delay criterion [12, 13]. We now consider a lesion as "complete" if peak-to-peak bipolar electrogram amplitude is less than 0.1 mV inside the line and no double potentials are present. To verify this, only one postablation map is necessary, because local amplitude signals from points inside the ablated areas are similar during pacing from different sites. This evolution of our technique has resulted in a significant reduction in procedure duration because of the shorter mapping times.

PV Isolation: Long-Term Outcome

We evaluated the clinical outcome of the PV isolation procedure described above in a large consecutive series of patients with paroxysmal ($n = 179$) or permanent ($n = 72$) AF [12]. Circular RF lesions were deployed transseptally during sinus rhythm or AF at 5 mm or more from PV ostia. Procedural and mapping times were 112 ± 32 min and 75 ± 27 min, respectively, with 29 ± 11 min of fluoroscopy. Thus, procedure duration is quite acceptable, as most cases require 2 h or less, with fluoroscopy times below 30 min in all cases. Complete lesions were achieved in 85% of the veins treated. The extent of the ablated area was 4.9 ± 0.5 cm^2, accounting for $28 \pm 9\%$ of the total LA map surface. Sinus rhythm was restored during RF delivery in 52% of cases and by DC shock in the rest. As for as adverse events, major complications (cardiac tamponade) occurred in 3%, which demonstrates that this ablation technique can be considered quite safe. However, the availability of a specifically designed catheter capable of deploying ring lesions with a single energy application, as is currently under development, would increase the feasibility of RF PV isolation.

Regarding long-term outcome, our most important result is that freedom from AF without antiarrhythmic drugs was obtained for 85% of patients with paroxysmal and 68% of patients with permanent AF after 11 ± 5 months. The success rate in paroxysmal AF is higher than that obtained in our previous experience with linear LA ablation alone (60%) and comparable to that obtained with biatrial linear ablation (85%) [3]. No PV stenoses were detected. By univariate analysis, an increased risk of recurrence was predicted by LA dilation (diameter > 50 mm), AF duration, and a small ablated area (< 15% of total LA surface). After adjustment, only the latter variable continued to be significant (odds ratio 3.5, 95% confidence interval, 1.6-5.8), suggesting that patients with an enlarged LA may require wider lesions to achieve AF suppression.

Compared with focal ablation, our anatomic PV isolation approach has the advantage of not requiring mapping of arrhythmogenic triggers, a complex task using combinations of physiologic maneuvers, intravenous drugs, atrial pacing, and electrical cardioversion to elicit premature atrial contractions, with the risk of inducing AF requiring cardioversion [10, 11]. On the other hand, although 89%-94% of AF triggers have been shown in the PVs, the arrhythmia can be initiated by ectopic beats from other sites, such as the crista terminalis, CS ostium, and atrial free wall [10, 11]. Therefore, a limitation to a purely anatomic map is that a complex PV isolation procedure can be performed and yet the source of AF may not be the PVs. However, ablation may still be effective through other mechanisms, such as (1) the interruption of pathways crucial in the maintenance of AF located at the PV-LA junction, a region comprised of highly anisotropic, electrically active fibers; (2) modification of the arrhythmogenic substrate, as suggested by the profound changes in intra-atrial impulse conduction; and (3) atrial debulking and/or denervation.

Conclusions

RF ablation for AF represents the frontier of arrhythmia research. Given the relative dissatisfaction with pharmacologic therapy, and the encouraging results seen with ablation in selected patients, it is understandable that so much energy is being focused on identifying a feasible methodology that can be widely applied with a good degree of safety.

Enough evidence has now accumulated that proves the safety of LA catheter ablation after appropriate screening and prophylactic antithrombotic treatment. As far as clinical efficacy is concerned, it must be emphasized that most of the available studies were in patients with paroxysmal AF, who were predominantly young and without any underlying heart disease. At present, few data are available for patients with persistent or permanent AF, those with cardiac disease, and the elderly.

So far, AF ablation has been considered an investigational technique, but our large experience suggests that it is ready to become a routine clinical tool. The feasibility of the procedure has been enhanced by the use of electroanatomical mapping, which allows the 3D atrial anatomy to be defined, the lesions to be accurately generated, and their effect on intra-atrial conduction to be assessed in real time. With the development of newer lesion paradigms for PV isolation and simplification of techniques for line validation, AF ablation is now practicable not only by the electrophysiologist but even by a cardiologist experienced in transseptal puncture and atrial navigation. Given the high success rates and good safety profile, it could be expected that the application of catheter ablation for AF with electroanatomical guidance will soon be broadly applied in patients with AF.

References

1. Cox JL, Boineau JP, Schuessler RB et al (1993) Five-year experience with the maze procedure for atrial fibrillation. Ann Thorac Surg 56:814-823
2. Haïssaguerre M, Jaïs P, Shah D et al (1996) Right and left atrial radiofrequency catheter therapy of paroxysmal AF. J Cardiovasc Electrophysiol 7:1132-1144
3. Pappone C, Oreto G, Lamberti F et al (1999) Catheter ablation of paroxysmal atrial fibrillation using a 3D mapping system. Circulation 100:1203-1208
4. Jaïs P, Shah DC, Takahashi A et al (1998) Long-term follow-up after right atrial radiofrequency catheter treatment of paroxysmal atrial fibrillation. Pacing Clin Electrophysiol 21:2533-2538
5. Maloy JD, Milner L, Barold S et al (1998) Two-staged biatrial linear and focal ablation to restore sinus rhythm in patients with refractory chronic atrial fibrillation: procedure experience and follow-up beyond 1 year. Pacing Clin Electrophysiol 21:2527-2532
6. Garg A, Finneran W, Mollerus M et al (1999) Right atrial compartmentalization using radiofrequency catheter ablation for management of patients with refractory atrial fibrillation. J Cardiovasc Electrophysiol 10:763-771
7. Ernst S, Schluter M, Ouyang F et al (1999) Modification of the substrate for maintenance of idiopathic human atrial fibrillation: efficacy of radiofrequency ablation using nonfluoroscopic catheter guidance. Circulation 100:2085-2092
8. Pappone C, Rosanio S, Oreto G et al (2000) Circumferential radiofrequency ablation of pulmonary vein ostia. A new anatomic approach for curing atrial fibrillation. Circulation 102:2619-2628
9. Sueda T, Nagata H, Horihashi K et al (1997) Efficacy of a simple left atrial procedure for chronic atrial fibrillation in mitral valve operations. Ann Thorac Surg 63:1070-1075
10. Haïssaguerre M, Jaïs P, Shah DC et al (2000) Electrophysiological end-point for catheter ablation of atrial fibrillation initiated form multiple pulmonary venous foci. Circulation 101:1409-1417
11. Chen SA, Hsieh MH, Tai TC et al (1999) Initiation of atrial fibrillation by ectopic beats originating from the pulmonary veins. Circulation 100:1859-1866
12. Pappone C, Rosanio J, Tocchi M et al (2001) Circumferential radiofrequency ablation of pulmonary vein ostia for curing atrial fibrillation: long-term results from a large, single center experience. J Am Coll Cardiol 37:107A
13. Pappone C, Rosanio J, Tocchi M et al (2001) Effects of circumferential radiofrequency ablation of pulmonary vein ostia on sympathovagal balance in patients with atrial fibrillation. J Am Coll Cardiol 37:132A

Catheter Ablation of Focal Atrial Fibrillation: Taiwan Experience

S.A. Chen, C.T. Tai, M.H. Hsieh, Y.K. Lin, H.M. Tsao, W.C. Yu and C.F. Tsai

Atrial fibrillation (AF) is the most common sustained arrhythmia seen in clinical practice. Recently, several reports have demonstrated that most paroxysmal AF is initiated by ectopic beats from the thoracic veins or atria, and radiofrequency catheter ablation can effectively cure it [1-11]. These ectopic foci include the pulmonary veins (PVs), superior vena cava (SVC), ligament of Marshall, crista terminalis, coronary sinus, and atrial wall [1-11]. Several critical points learned from more than 300 experiences from the last 5 years in this laboratory will be discussed here.

Inclusion Criteria

Because this focal ablation technique is still under investigation, the criteria used to select patients for focal ablation of the ectopic beats initiating AF vary in different laboratories. In most laboratories (including ours), only the patients with atrial premature beats related to bursts of rapid repetitive atrial depolarization or initiation of AF were considered to undergo radiofrequency ablation.

Performance of a Simple and Delicate Mapping

1. The different anatomic variations of thoracic veins should be considered.
2. Simultaneous mapping of multiple PVs using regular size, micro size, basket, Lasso or spiral multielectrode catheters around the ostium and the distal PVs, also the SVC, coronary sinus, crista terminalis, and vein of Marshall help accurate observation of the activation pattern of focal AF.
3. Intracardiac ultrasound imaging during the procedure, and spiral CT and MR angiography before the procedure, would be useful for a more precise

National Yang-Ming University and Taipei Veterans General Hospital, Taipei, Taiwan

delineation of the venoatrial junction area than that provided by angiography. Recently, a noncontact mapping system has demonstrated semplicity and high efficiency in localizing the ectopic focus for the initiation of focal AF, including ectopy from a non-PV area [12-16].

Although some investigators prefer an anatomic approach to isolating PV from atrial tissues, practice in this laboratory is to try to find the arrhythmogenic foci before the isolation procedure.

Target Sites and Procedural End-Point

Circumferential, segmental, or discrete radiofrequency lesions around the PV (or SVC) ostium, with disconnection between the PV (or SVC) and atrial tissues, can create a conduction barrier, so that rapid PV (or SVC) depolarization cannot be conducted to the left (right) atrium via the PV (or SVC) ostium. For patients with focal AF from the ligament of Marshall, it is necessary to disconnect the ligament from the atrial tissues or CS. However, it is a difficult procedure in patients with multiple connections between this ligament and the left atrium.

Recurrence, Safety, and Complications

The success rate of focal ablation may depend on the number of ectopic foci initiating AF and on the ablation techniques. In general, the acute success rate in AF patients with a single ectopic focus is around 90%-95%; however, it may decrease to 50%-70% in patients with multiple AF initiators [1-11]. Recently, we found the success rate may be higher in patients with ectopic foci from the right atrial area, including the SVC and crista terminalis; perhaps most of these foci initiate the typical type of focal AF (burst depolarization from the ectopic focus with normal substrate). Furthermore, a significantly lower recurrence rate was demonstrated in patients who underwent the PV isolation technique. Major complications may include cerebral emboli, cardiac perforation, and PV stenosis. Yu et al. used transesophageal echocardiography to assess the effects of radiofrequency ablation on PV, and found that 30%-40% of the ablated PV had an increase in PV flow velocity [17]. Applying the radiofrequency energy at lower power and a lower preset temperature around the PV ostium may reduce the risk of PV stenosis [18, 19]. Isolation of PV from the left atrium with the ablation lesion around the PV ostium-atrial junction would reduce the risk of PV narrowing or stenosis [19]. However, the correlation between patients' symptoms of pulmonary hypertension (during rest and exercise) and the degree of narrowing or stenosis (assessed by transesophageal echocardiography, CT or MR angiography) needs further assessment.

Note: part of the content of this article appears also in the following publications:
  - Chen SA (2001) Cathether ablation of focal AF using different technology. In: Capucci A (ed) Proceedings of Atrial Fibrillation International Conference, Bologna. Monduzzi, Bologna
  - Chen SA (2001) Current progress of ablation of focal AF. In: Liam LB, Downar E (eds) Progress in Catheter Ablation. Kluwer, Norwall, USA

References

1. Jaïs P, Haïssaguerre M, Shah DC et al (1997) A focal source of atrial fibrillation treated by discrete radiofrequency ablation. Circulation 95:572-576
2. Haïssaguerre M, Jaïs P, Shah DC et al (1998) Spontaneous initiation of atrial fibrillation by ectopic beats originating in the pulmonary veins. N. Engl J Med 339:659-666
3. Wharton JM, Vergara I, Shander G et al (1998) Identification and ablation of focal mechanisms of atrial fibrillation. Circulation 98:I-18 (abstr)
4. Lau CP, Tse HF, Ayers GM (1999) Defibrillation guided mapping and radiofrequency ablation of focal atrial fibrillation. J Am Coll Cardiol 33:1217-1226
5. Hsieh MH, Chen SA, Tai CT et al (1999) Double multielectrode mapping catheters facilitate radiofrequency catheter ablation of focal atrial fibrillation originating from pulmonary veins. J Cardiovasc Electrophysiol 10:136-144
6. Chen SA, Tai CT, Yu WC et al (1999) Right atrial focal atrial fibrillation – electrophysiologic characteristics and radiofrequency catheter ablation. J Cardiovasc Electrophysiol 10:328-335
7. Chen SA, Hsieh MH, Tai CT et al (1999) Initiation of atrial fibrillation by ectopic beats originating from the pulmonary veins – electrophysiologic characteristics, pharmacologic responses, and effects of radiofrequency ablation. Circulation 100:1879-1886
8. Tsai CF, Tai CT, Hsieh MH et al (2000) Paroxysmal atrial fibrillation initiated by ectopic beats originating in the superior vena cava: electrophysiologic findings and radiofrequency ablation results. Circulation 102:67-74
9. Natale A, Pisano E, Beheiry S et al (2000) Ablation of right and left atrial premature beats following cardioversion in patients with chronic atrial fibrillation refractory to antiarrhythmic drugs. Am J Cardiol 85:1372-1377
10. Hwang C, Wu TJ, Doshi RN et al (2000) Vein of Marshall cannulation for the analysis of electrical activity in patients with focal atrial fibrillation. Circulation 101:1503-1508
11. Tai CT, Hsieh MS, Tsai CF et al (2000) Differentiating the ligament of Marshall from the pulmonary vein musculature potentials in patients with paroxysmal atrial fibrillation: electrophysiological characteristics and results of radiofrequency ablation. Pacing Clin Electrophysiol 23:1493-1501
12. Schneider MAE, Ndrepepa G, Zrenner B et al (2000) Noncontact mapping-guided catheter ablation of atrial fibrillation associated with left atrial ectopy. J Cardiovasc Electrophysiol 11:475-479
13. Friedman PA, Grice S, Munger TM et al (2000) Spot welding the trigger in focal atrial fibrillation ablation. J Cardiovasc Electrophysiol 11:1091
14. Wahl MR, Roman-Gonzalez J, Asirvatham S et al (2000) Spatial fusion of ultrasound with computed tomographic imaging of the heart to facilitate 3D mapping. Pacing Clin Electrophysiol 23:626 (abstr)

15. Tsao HM, Tai CT, Lin YK et al (2000) An unperceived pulmonary vein: role of right middle pulmonary vein for catheter ablation of paroxysmal atrial fibrillation. Circulation 102: 2157 (abstr)

16. Mangrum JM, Mounsey JP, DiMarco JP, Haines DE (2000) Intracardiac echocardiography-guided, anatomically-based ablation of focal atrial fibrillation originating from pulmonary veins. Pacing Clin Electrophysiol 23:625 (abstr)

17. Yu WC, Hsu TL, Cheng HC et al (2001) Focal stenosis of pulmonary vein after application of radiofrequency energy in patients with paroxysmal atrial fibrillation. J Cardiovasc Electrophysiol (August issue), in press

18. Jaïs P, Shah D, Haïssaguerre M et al (1999) Pulmonary vein patency after radiofrequency ablation. Pacing Clin Electrophysiol 22: 38 (abstr)

19. Tsao HM, Yu WC, Wu MH et al (2001) Application of magnetic resonance angiography to detect pulmonary vein stenosis after focal ablation of atrial fibrillation. Pacing Clin Electrophysiol 24:289 (abstr)

Ablation of Atrial Fibrillation: The Cleveland Clinic Experience

N.F. Marrouche and A. Natale

Introduction

Atrial fibrillation (AF) is the most common arrhythmia in clinical practice, with an overall prevalence in the general population of 0.4% [1]. Initial therapy of AF is directed toward the return to and maintenance of sinus rhythm, usually with the addition of antiarrhythmic drug therapy. However, even the best antiarrhythmic therapy is associated with only a 50%-60% success rate of maintaining sinus rhythm after 1 year, and is associated with significant side effects including proarrhythmia, drug toxicity, and possibly an increase in mortality [2]. Catheter ablation of the atrioventricular node with subsequent pacemaker implantation can be useful to facilitate ventricular rate control, but atrial systole is not restored and the thromboembolic risk is unchanged.

As our understanding of the mechanisms of arrhythmias progresses, so does our ability to treat arrhythmias with catheter-based interventions [2]. As we have seen in the past few years, each change in the mechanistic understanding of AF has corresponded to an advance in the treatment options.

The proposal of a multiple wavelet theory of AF [3, 4] led to the development of the surgical maze procedure [5, 6]. By making multiple linear scars in the atrium, the atrial chambers are compartmentalized into smaller regions unable to sustain AF. This technique, although successful, requires general anesthesia and open heart surgery. These important limitations have encouraged the development of catheter-based maze procedures.

For the catheter-based maze a variety of tools have been used to make linear lesions in the atrium and interrupt the propagation of the wavelets [7-10]. Several different approaches have been considered, including epicardial linear lesions [11], the creation of right-sided-only linear lesions [9, 12], both right- and left-sided linear lesions [7], and the use of different proprietary catheters. The use of three-dimensional electroanatomical mapping has been suggested to facilitate line placement and to insure continuity of the lesions as well [12, 13]. Due to the risk of

Division of Pacing and Electrophysiology, Department of Cardiology, The Cleveland Clinic Foundation, Cleveland, Ohio, USA

stroke with left-sided ablation, there was initial interest in right-sided-only ablation [9, 10, 14]. The initial enthusiasm, however, was mitigated by the overall poor results and long procedure time. Ultimately, despite the use of a variety of specially designed catheters, the linear lesion approach has been nearly abandoned.

That AF could be triggered from a rapidly firing single focus was first suggested by Scherf [15]. However, it was not until recently that this concept was more fully explored. We now have evidence that, in addition to the substrate needed for multiple wavelets, there is a rapidly firing focus that initiates AF in the majority of cases, if not all. This is based on the pioneering work of Haïssaguerre et al. [16], who have demonstrated that in some patients atrial ectopic beats within the pulmonary veins (PVs) are responsible for the initiation of spontaneous paroxysms of AF. This finding paved the way for different catheter-based treatment approaches. Initially, focal ablation of the ectopic focus was considered.

Haïssaguerre and coworkers described their experience with their first 45 patients in a landmark study published in 1998 [16]. Of the 45 patients, a single point of origin of atrial ectopic beats was found in 29 patients, 2 points in 9 patients, and 3 or 4 points in 7 patients, giving a total of 69 foci. One of the foci was in the posterior left atrium, 3 were in the right atrium, but the majority (94%) originated from the PVs. Of those originating from the PVs, about half were from the left superior vein, a third from the right superior vein, and the rest from the inferior veins, with a predominant number coming from the left inferior vein. Sixty-two percent of the patients had no recurrence of their AF in the 8 ± 6 months of follow-up after ablation.

Natale et al. reported their results with 48 patients who underwent focal AF ablation [17]. All of the patients had had persistent or chronic drug-refractory AF for a median of 3 years (range 1-6 years). In nearly two-thirds of the patients, the site of earliest activation of the atrial ectopic beats was from the PVs, with the left superior PV the most common. However, in 37% of the patients the earliest activation was in the right atrium, predominantly in the high and mid crista terminalis. During follow-up, sinus rhythm was successfully maintained in 40 patients (83%), but only 4 patients (8%) maintained sinus rhythm without any drug therapy. One patient experienced a transient ischemic attack 5 days after the ablation. Two different mainly strategies had been developed to map and eliminate PV triggers: focal ablation targeting single or multiple foci in the arrhythmogenic PV trunk, or electrical isolation of the PV by circumferential PV lesions.

PV Isolation: Clinical Series

Recently, isolation of the PV by applying segmental lesions at the site of the earliest conduction identified by circumferential mapping has been suggested to be effective [16]. In our institution we have attempted isolation with three different approaches: (1) lesions guided by a three-dimensional nonfluoroscopic mapping system (CARTO) [18]; (2) circumferential isolation delivering through-the-balloon ultrasound energy [19] (Fig. 1); and (3), more recently, circumferential mapping of the PV [20]. The acute and chronic results with each approach are shown in Table 1. Overall isolation with the CARTO system and the through-the-balloon ultrasound catheter achieved similar results. However, stenosis of the PV was higher in the CARTO group. The most encouraging results were observed with circular mapping. With this approach 115 patients (80 men, mean age 53 ± 10 years) with symptomatic paroxysmal (65 patients), persistent (25 patients), or chronic (25 patients) AF (duration 5 ± 3 years) underwent catheter ablation. All antiarrhythmic drugs (3 ± 0.8 drugs) were discontinued five half-lives prior to the ablation. Immediately prior to the procedure transesophageal echocardiography was performed in all study patients. Spiral CT was performed 2 months after the procedure.

Sixty-three patients presented to the electrophysiology laboratory in sinus rhythm (SR), 44 were in AF, and 8 in atrial flutter/fibrillation. In 20 out of 63 patients in SR, spontaneous ectopies and AF were documented. DC cardioversion was followed by spontaneous reinitiation of AF in 31 of the 48 patients with sustained AF or flutter. Isoproterenol was required in 65% of patients (74/115) to initiate ectopies triggering AF. These included 44 patients presenting in SR and 17 patients initially in atrial flutter/fibrillation. Table 2 gives a profile of patients' characteristics.

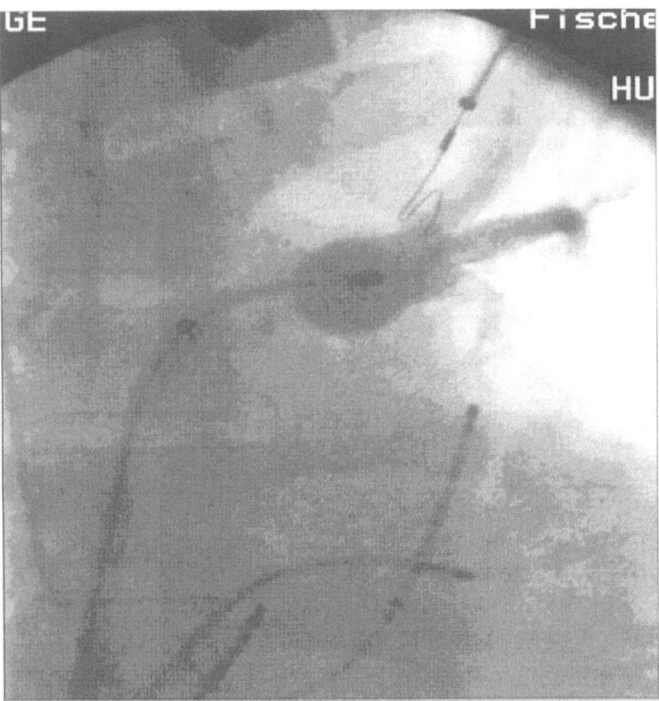

Fig. 1. Isolation of the left upper pulmonary vein using the through-the-balloon ultrasound energy delivery system (CUVA)

Table 1. Cleveland Clinic results with different ablation strategies

	CARTO guided	CUVA	Circular mapping
No. of patients	48	30	115
Mean follow-up	16 ± 6 months	12 ± 6 months	6 ± 4 months
Acute success	97% (47/48)	77% (23/30)	97% (113/115)
Chronic success	59% (28/48)	53 % (16/30)	85% (98/115)
Chronic control with AAD	29% (14/48)	30% (9/30)	12% (14/115)
No benefit	12.5% (6/48)	17% (5/30)	2.5% (3/115)
Chronic stenosis	35% (17/48)	0%	4% (4/115)

AAD, antiarrhythmic drugs; *CUVA*, through-the-balloon ultrasound energy delivery

Table 2. Patient characteristics

Patient Characteristics	
No. of patients	115
Age, years	53 ± 11 (24-65)
Sex, male/female	80/35
AF: paroxysmal/persistent/chronic	65/25/25
Duration of AF (years)	4 ± 2.2 (0.5-12)
Structural heart disease	10% (12/115)
Hypertensive heart disease	18% (21/115)
Sick sinus syndrome	5% (6/115)
Left atrial diameter, mm	4.1 ± 0.6
Left ventricular ejection fraction, %	54 ± 7

Pulmonary Vein Ectopy

Arrhythmogenic ectopic foci originated from a single vein in 64 patients. Firing from 2 veins occurred in 30 patients, from 3 veins in 17 patients, and from 4 veins in 4 patients, giving a total of 191 arrhythmogenic PV foci in 115 patients. This included 70 right upper PVs (RUPVs), 90 left upper PVs (LUPVs), 9 right lower PVs (RLPVs), and 20 left lower PVs (LLPVs).

After defining the arrhythmogenic PV, a custom-made circular mapping catheter was deployed into that specific vein (Fig. 2). Simultaneous circular and longitudinal mapping of the same PV appeared to support spiral conduction of activation during sinus rhythm and APCs distal to the ostium and a more uniform longitudinal activation at the ostium.

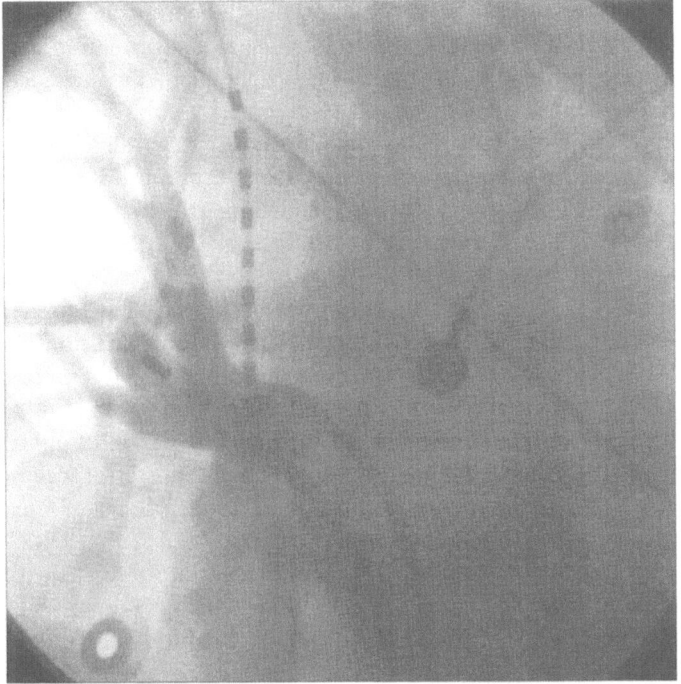

Fig. 2. Circular mapping of the distal right upper pulmonary vein

Distal and Ostial Isolation

Distal isolation ($\geq$ 5 mm from LA-PV junction) was performed in the first 21 patients. This approach was considered because the circular catheter was more stable when distally deployed. Lesions were delivered targeting the site with the earliest PV local activation on the circular mapping catheter in 34 arrhythmogenic PVs. Radiofrequency energy was delivered 6 ± 2 mm into the RUPV, 5 ± 2 mm into the LUPV, 7 mm into the RLPV, and 6 ± 1 mm into the LLPV. A mean of 5 ± 2 radiofrequency lesions (3 ± 1 min) were needed for distal isolation.

Ostial isolation was performed in 348 of the 360 treated PVs. In the initial 21 patients (34 PVs) ostial isolation was only performed in veins still capable of initiating ectopies and AF after distal isolation (24 out of 34 PVs). In 1 LUPV ostial isolation was not attempted due to evidence of nearly complete occlusion after distal ablation. In another patient the procedure was terminated due to evidence of a neurologic embolic event before proximal isolation of the RUPV was achieved. In 10 PVs distal isolation eliminated ectopies initiating AF. Ostial isolation required a mean of 14 ± 4 radiofrequency lesions (8.6 ± 2 min) with a 4-mm-tip ablation catheter, a mean of 5 ± 2 radiofrequency lesions (2 ± 1 min) with an 8-mm-tip ablation catheter, and a mean of 7 ± 4 radiofrequency lesions with the Chilli ablation catheter.

After distal isolation, PV ectopies initiating AF from the treated vein were still present in 15 (71%) out of 21 patients. After ostial isolation no APCs triggering AF were initiated from any but one PV, despite an average isoproterenol infusion rate of 14.3 ± 4.7 μg/min. In one patient isolation of a large RUPV ostium appeared difficult and was abandoned due to evidence of a neurologic embolic event. Mean procedure and fluoroscopy time were 4 ± 1 h and 90 ± 30 min, respectively. The procedure time included the transesophageal echocardiogram performed in the laboratory before the ablation. Distal and ostial isolation data are represented in Table 2.

Seventy-five percent of patients (56 out of 75 patients) requiring isoproterenol for initiation of ectopies triggering AF needed an infusion rate above 10 μg/min. After isolation of the primary arrhythmogenic PV in 26 out of 115 patients (23%), APCs and AF from other foci were seen only during a mean isoproterenol infusion rate of 15.2 ± 4.2 μg/min (range 10-20 μg/min). These arrhythmogenic APCs originated from the left atrial posterior wall in the proximity of the RUPV in 4 patients, from the superior vena cava in 4 patients, and from a different PV in 18 patients.

The ostial circumference of the PVs was divided into 16 sectors based on the maximum number of electrodes present on the 2-cm loop catheter. The number of sectors showing PVPs on the circular catheter, at which radiofrequency energy was delivered to complete ostial isolation, were documented. PVPs were seen and required ablation in all infero-anterior sectors of the RUPV ostia. In the LUPV the superior and inferior segments appeared critical for PV activation in all patients. No sector consistently showed preferential conduction around the circumferences of the distal and ostial LLPVs and RLPVs. No correlation between the distally and ostially ablated sectors was observed. In order to perform ostial isolation ablation of all 16 sectors was needed in 65% of RUPVs, 76% of LUPVs, 45% of LLPVs, and 2% of the RLPVs.

Complications and Follow-Up

PV venograms performed immediately after distal ablation lesions showed more than 50% narrowing of the RUPV in one patient, the LUPV in two patients, and both LUPV and LLPV in one patient. Narrowing of less than 25% was seen in two LUPV and three RUPV. No further narrowing was seen following ostial isolation. The spiral CT scan performed in all patients 2 months after PV isolation showed thickening of the posterior wall extending to the LUPV and causing moderate to severe stenosis (60%-50% narrowing) in two asymptomatic patients. Severe stenosis (≥ 70% narrowing) of both LUPV and LLPV was seen in another patient. Two of these three patients underwent dilatation by balloon angioplasty. One patient undergoing ostial isolation showed 50%-60% ostial narrowing at the 2-month follow-up. Anticoagulation therapy was continued in the two patients with greater than 50% PV narrowing. Another patient developed aphasia documented at the end of the ablation, which nearly resolved after 48 h.

During a mean follow-up time of 5.3 ± 1.4 month AF recurrence was documented in 26 patients (22%). Twenty-four patients experienced recurrence of AF within 2 weeks after ablation and two patients had recurrence after 3 weeks. Five patients presented with firing from the previously isolated PV. The reasons for recurrence were found to be recovery of the PV ostium (2 patients) and a large PV ostium (2 LLPVs and 1 RUPV). These PVs were successfully isolated in a second procedure. Nine of these patients underwent a repeat procedure during which recurrence appeared associated with firing from veins not targeted during the first procedure in five patients and with firing from a focus in the posterior wall of the left atrium in the vicinity of the RUPV ostium in two patients. Twelve patients responded to previously ineffective drug therapy. In one of them, following isolation of three PVs, firing from the posterior wall of the left atrium close to the left PVs was documented during the first procedure and could not be abolished. One patient with recurrence had a large single ostium right PV, which could not be proximally isolated during the initial procedure. After ablation only 3 of the 115 patients continued to have AF despite drug therapy and are scheduled for reablation.

In conclusion, the reported recurrence rates of AF after focal ablation have been quite high, with the majority of patients requiring two or more procedures to achieve cure [16, 21, 22]. In our experience, circular mapping guided lesions appeared to provide the highest probability of cure with the first procedure. We documented a 23% early recurrence rate, associated with (1) an arrhythmogenic PV not seen at the time of the initial ablation, (2) foci originating from the posterior wall of the left atrium in the vicinity of the RUPV, and (3) conduction recovery of ablated PVs. The main advantage of isolation with the ultrasound system was the lack of PV stenosis. Design flaws were responsible for nearly 50% of the recurrences seen after ultrasound ablation, and if properly resolved could improve the cure rate achieved with this system. Isolation with the CARTO mapping system appeared to result in an unacceptable rate of PV stenosis. Circular mapping guided ablation appeared to simplify and facilitate isolation of the PVs. Although distal isolation can be achieved by limited ablation lesions, it appears to have a higher risk of stenosis and may be effective in only one-third of the patients. It appears imperative that an effort is made to deliver lesions only at the ostium to avoid or limit PV stenosis, which remains a problem if one applies radiofrequency at the sites where the circular catheter is more stable.

References

1. Wolf PA, Dawber TR, Thomas HE Jr, Kannel WB (1978) Epidemiologic assessment of chronic atrial fibrillation and risk of stroke: the Framingham study. Neurology 28:973-977
2. Coplen SE, Antman EM, Berlin JA et al (1990) Efficacy and safety of quinidine therapy for maintenance of sinus rhythm after cardioversion. A meta-analysis of randomized control trials. Circulation 82:1106-1116

3. Moe GK (1975) Evidence for reentry as a mechanism of cardiac arrhythmias. Rev Physiol Biochem Pharmacol 72:55-81
4. Moe GK (1968) A conceptual model of atrial fibrillation. J Electrocardiol 1:145-146
5. Cox JL, Schuessler RB, Boineau JP (2000) The development of the Maze procedure for the treatment of atrial fibrillation. Semin Thorac Cardiovasc Surg 12:2-14
6. Cox JL, Sundt TM 3rd (1997) The surgical management of atrial fibrillation. Annu Rev Med 48:511-523
7. Jaïs P, Shah DC, Haïssaguerre M et al (1999) Efficacy and safety of septal and left-atrial linear ablation for atrial fibrillation. Am J Cardiol 84:139R-146R
8. Haïssaguerre M, Jaïs P, Shah DC et al (1996) Right and left atrial radiofrequency catheter therapy of paroxysmal atrial fibrillation. J Cardiovasc Electrophysiol 7:1132-1144
9. Haïssaguerre M, Marcus FI, Fischer B, Clementy J (1994) Radiofrequency catheter ablation in unusual mechanisms of atrial fibrillation: report of three cases. J Cardiovasc Electrophysiol 5:743-751
10. Natale A, Leonelli F, Beheiry S et al (2000) Catheter ablation approach on the right side only for paroxysmal atrial fibrillation therapy: long-term results. Pacing Clin Electrophysiol 23:224-233
11. Elvan A, Pride HP, Eble JN, Zipes DP (1995) Radiofrequency catheter ablation of the atria reduces inducibility and duration of atrial fibrillation in dogs. Circulation 91:2235-2244
12. Pappone C, Oreto G, Lamberti F et al (1999) Catheter ablation of paroxysmal atrial fibrillation using a 3D mapping system. Circulation 100:1203-1208
13. Schwartzman D, Kuck KH (1998) Anatomy-guided linear atrial lesions for radio-frequency catheter ablation of atrial fibrillation. Pacing Clin Electrophysiol 21:1959-1978
14. Garg A, Finneran W, Mollerus M et al (1999) Right atrial compartmentalization using radiofrequency catheter ablation for management of patients with refractory atrial fibrillation. J Cardiovasc Electrophysiol 10:763-771
15. Scherf D (1966) The mechanism of flutter and fibrillation. Am Heart J 71:273-280
16. Haïssaguerre M, Jaïs P, Shah DC et al (1998) Spontaneous initiation of atrial fibrilla-tion by ectopic beats originating in the pulmonary veins. N Engl J Med 339:659-666
17. Natale A, Pisano E, Beheiry S et al (2000) Ablation of right and left atrial premature beats following cardioversion in patients with chronic atrial fibrillation refractory to antiarrhythmic drugs. Am J Cardiol 85:1372-1375
18. Kanagaratnam L, Tomassoni G, Schweikert R, Pavia P et al (2000) Empirical pulmonary vein isolation in patients with chronic atrial fibrillation using a three dimensional non-fluoroscopic mapping system: long-term follow-up. Pacing Clin Electrophysiol
19. Natale A, Pisano E, Shewchik J et al (2000) First human experience with pulmonary vein isolation using a through-the-balloon circumferential ultrasound ablation system for recurrent atrial fibrillation. Circulation 102:1879-1882
20. Haïssaguerre M, Shah DC, Jaïs P et al (2000) Electrophysiological breakthroughs from the left atrium to the pulmonary veins. Circulation 102:2463-2465
21. Chen SA, Hsieh MH, Tai CT et al (1999) Initiation of atrial fibrillation by ectopic beats originating from the pulmonary veins: electrophysiological characteristics, pharmacological responses, and effects of radiofrequency ablation. Circulation 100:1879-1886
22. Lin WS, Prakash VS, Tai CT et al (2000) Pulmonary vein morphology in patients with paroxysmal atrial fibrillation initiated by ectopic beats originating from the pulmo-nary veins: implications for catheter ablation. Circulation 101:1274-1281

Worldwide Experience in Surgical Treatment of Atrial Fibrillation

J.Q. Melo[1] and T. Santiago[2]

Surgical treatment for atrial fibrillation started in 1980. In those early days the techniques aimed at controlling patients' heart rate. Left atrial isolation and the corridor procedure are good examples of these approaches.

In 1991, Cox described the maze 1 operation and later the maze 2 and maze 3 operations [1, 2]. The latter became the gold standard for the surgical treatment of atrial fibrillation. Because it is a complex operation [3] requiring a long ischemic time and with major potential for bleeding, however, it never became a widespread technique. Other limitations of this operation relate to its effects on the hemodynamic function of the left atrium (which are still debated), the requirement of a significant number of pacemaker implants, and the difficulties encountered in reproducing published results [4].

Since 1996 various approaches [5, 6] have emerged in the attempt to address the issues of this complex disease and to avoid the drawbacks of the maze operation.

These approaches involve an alternative to using a scalpel to create scars in the atrial wall, and a surgical technique that avoids extensive scars in the atrium, so that the hemodynamic condition of the atrium will be as little compromised as possible. The search for the least possible imposition of lesions to successfully eliminate atrial fibrillation is an issue for ongoing research. Still, many surgical groups have started to treat atrial fibrillation in patients with concomitant atrial fibrillation, using either radiofrequency currents or microwave emission for intraoperative ablation of atrial fibrillation [7-12].

The results obtained by these pioneer groups are very encouraging and their techniques are currently used all over the world. Although the success rate is variable, the number of complications is extremely low provided the safety protocols for the different forms of energy are properly observed.

The patients who can benefit from these techniques are those with lone atrial fibrillation and those who have atrial fibrillation and are subjected to a concomitant cardiac operation. The latter cases are becoming routine in surgical practice.

Table 1 summarizes published papers reporting atrial fibrillation treatment using a surgical scalpel to perform the maze operation. Table 2 describes the

[1]Division of Cardiac Surgery, Leiden University Medical Center, The Netherlands;
[2]Instituto do Coracáo, Lisboa, Portugal

same procedures performed with alternative forms of energy: radiofrequency currents (dry and irrigated) and microwave emission. It is noteworthy that, during a period of 10 years, only around 700 maze operations were reported in Europe and America, whereas a fast-growing number of procedures involving the intraoperative use of alternative energies has been reported in the last 3 years. There are very few papers reporting surgical ablation in the treatment of lone atrial fibrillation patients. Nevertheless, several groups are currently performing it, with early results that are superior to these achieved in mitral patients (Table 3).

At present several crucial issues remain to be answered. The first is how to create transmural lesions that will ensure that the scar actually creates an electrical block in the atrium.

Table 1. Results of the maze 3 procedure in mitral patients

Author	Year	Patients (n)	Mortality (%)	Ischemic time (min)	AF- (%)	RA+ (%)	LA+ (%)	PM (%)
Cox [13]	2000	79	6		99	98	93	24
Handa et al. [14]	1999	39	3	122	74			3
Nitta et al. [15]	1999	13		165	92	100	100	15
Izumoto et al. [16]	2000	100	4		53			6
Jatene et al. [17]	2000	20	10	125	76			
Szalay et al. [18]	1999	7		127	73			
Melo et al. [3]	1997	17	0		62	80	50	6
Schaff et al. [19]	2000	83	2		72/82			3
Kosakay et al. [20]	1994	90	0	142	84	84	71	

AF-, patients out of atrial fibrillation; *RA+*, patients with right atrial contraction; *LA+*, patients with left atrial contraction; *PM*, patients requiring a pacemaker

Table 2. Atrial fibrillation surgery in mitral patients

Technique	Author	Year	Patients (n)	Mortality (%)	Ischemic time (min)	AF- (%)	RA+ (%)	LA+ (%)	PM (%)
LA isolation	Vigano et al. [21]	1996	252	4		75		16	0
Partial LA exclusion	Melo et al. [10]	1999	48	0		56	86	54	0
Minimaze	Szalay et al. [18]	1999	45		87	71		79	
DresMW	Spitzer et al. [22]	1999	46	2	18*	72			0
Radial	Nitta et al. [15]	1999	13	8	174	90	100	100	10
BIPV, RF	Melo et al. [10]	1998	43	0	7*	64	85	76	0
BIPV, RF	Melo et al. [23]	1999	35	0	12*	60	81	81	0
BIPV+, RF	Benussi et al. [24]	2000	40	3	77	77	100	93	0
BIPV, RF	Melo et al. [7]	2000	46	0	22*	75	100	91	0

DresMW, microwave; *BIPV*, bilateral isolation pulmonary veins; *BIPV+*, bilateral isolation pulmonary veins with additional line. Other abbreviations as in Table 1.
* Duration of the atrial fibrillation procedure

Table 3. Lone atrial fibrillation surgery

Technique	Author	Year	Patients (n)	Mortality (%)	CPB	AF- (%)	RA+ (%)	LA+ (%)	PM (%)
Maze 3	Cox et al. [25]	1999	222	2		100	99	99	24
Maze 3	McCarthy [26]	1997	31				81	71	
Maze	Feinberg et al. [27]	1995	46			87	83	61	
BIPV, RF	Melo et al. [7]	2000	10	0	0	90	100	100	0

CPB, time of cardiopulmonary bypass. Other abbreviations as in Tables 1 and 2

It also remains to be shown whether these scars need to be created in the right atrium. It is clear that the pulmonary veins are a major component in the origin or perpetuation of atrial fibrillation. But is there need for additional lines and, if so, where should they be created? What is the role of the left atrial appendage in atrial fibrillation? Does it have any arrhythmic potential? What is the role of the autonomic nervous system in the origin and/or perpetuation of atrial fibrillation?

These are some of the issues that require a solid answer. The next years will be very rich in research into surgery for the treatment of atrial fibrillation. The ultimate goal is to develop a procedure that will be performed on the beating heart using small incisions or ports. If and when that technology is available, the challenge will be to decide with our electrophysiologist colleagues on the easiest and safest way to create the lines. In the meantime, it is crucial that surgeons and electrophysiologists work in close cooperation to provide answers to the questions described here.

References

1. Cox JL (1991) The surgical treatment of atrial fibrillation. IV. Surgical technique. J Thorac Cardiovasc Surg 101:584-592
2. Cox JL, Jaquiss RD, Schuessler RB, Boineau JP (1995) Modification of the maze procedure for atrial flutter and atrial fibrillation. II. Surgical technique of the maze III procedure. J Thorac Cardiovasc Surg 110:485-495
3. Melo J, Neves J, Abecasis M et al (1997) Operative risks of the maze procedure associated with mitral valve surgery. Cardiovasc Surg 5:112-116
4. Cox JL, Schuessler RB, Lappas DG, Boineau JP (1996) An 8 1/2-year clinical experience with surgery for atrial fibrillation. Ann Surg 224:267-275
5. Melo JQ, Adragão P, Neves J et al (1998) Surgery for atrial fibrillation using intra-operative radiofrequency ablation. Rev Port Cardiol 17:377-379
6. Alfieri O, Benussi S, Nascimbene S, Pappone C (1998) The ablation of chronic atrial fibrillation during mitral valve surgery: a realistic prospect. G Ital Cardiol 28:1317-1321
7. Melo J, Adragão P, Neves J et al (2000) Endocardial and epicardial radiofrequency ablation in the treatment of atrial fibrillation with a new intra-operative device. Eur J Cardiothorac Surg 18:182-186

8. Knaut M, Spitzer SG, Karolyi L et al (1999) Intraoperative microwave ablation for curative treatment of atrial fibrillation in open heart surgery – The MICRO-STAF and MICRO-PASS pilot trial. Thorac Cardiovasc Surg 47:379-384

9. Spitzer SG, Richter P, Knaut M, Schüler S (1999) Treatment of atrial fibrillation in open heart surgery – the potential role of microwave energy. Thorac Cardiovasc Surg 47:374-378

10. Melo J, Adragão P, Neves J et al (1999) Surgery for atrial fibrillation using radiofrequency catheter ablation: assessment of results at 1 year. Eur J Cardiothorac Surg 15:851-855

11. Adragão P, Melo J, Teles R et al (1999) Postoperative electrophysiologic evaluation of radiofrequency pulmonary vein isolation. Pacing Clin Electrophysiol 22:892

12. Sie HT, Beukema WP, Ramdat Misier AR et al (2001) The radiofrequency modified maze procedure. A less invasive surgical approach to atrial fibrillation during open-heart surgery. Eur J Cardiothorac Surg 19:443-447

13. Cox J (2000) Current status of the maze procedure for the treatment of atrial fibrillation. Semin Thorac Cardiovasc Surg 12:15-19

14. Handa N, Schaff HV, Morris JJ et al (1999) Outcome of valve repair and the Cox maze procedure for mitral regurgitation and associated atrial fibrillation. J Thorac Cardiovasc Surg 118:628-635

15. Nitta T, Ishii Y, Ogasawara H et al (1999) Initial experience with the radial incision approach for atrial fibrillation. Ann Thorac Surg 68:805-810

16. Izumoto H, Kawazoe K, Eishi K, Kamata J (2000) Medium-term results after the modified Cox/maze procedure combined with other cardiac surgery. Eur J Cardiothorac Surg 17:25-29

17. Jatene MB, Marcial MB, Tarasoutchi F et al (2000) Influence of the maze procedure on the treatment of rheumatic atrial fibrillation – evaluation of rhythm control and clinical outcome in a comparative study. Eur J Cardiothorac Surg 17:117-124

18. Szalay ZA, Skwara W, Pitschner H-F et al (1999) Midterm results after the mini-maze procedure. Eur J Cardiothorac Surg 16:306-311

19. Schaff HV, Dearani JA, Daly RC et al (2000) Cox-maze procedure for atrial fibrillation: Mayo Clinic experience. Semin Thorac Cardiovasc Surg 12:30-37

20. Kosakay Y (2000) Treatment of atrial fibrillation using the maze procedure: the Japanese experience. J Thorac Cardiovasc Surg 12:44-52

21. Vigano M, Graffigna A, Ressia L et al (1996) Surgery for atrial fibrillation. Eur J Cardiothorac Surg 10:490-497

22. Spitzer SG, Richter P, Knaut M, Schuler S (1999) Treatment of atrial fibrillation in open heart surgery – the potential role of microwave energy. Thorac Cardiovasc Surg 47[Suppl 3]:374-378

23. Melo J, Adragão P, Neves J et al (1999) Electrosurgical treatment of atrial fibrillation with a new intraoperative radiofrequency ablation catheter. Thorac Cardiovasc Surg 47[Suppl]:370-372

24. Benussi S, Pappone C, Nascimbene S et al (2000) A simple way to treat atrial fibrillation during mitral valve surgery: the epicardial radiofrequency approach. Eur J Cardiothorac Surg 17:524-529

25. Cox JL, Ad N, Palazzo T (1999) Impact of the maze procedure on the stroke rate in patients with atrial fibrillation. J Thorac Cardiovasc Surg 118:833

26. McCarthy P, Gillinov AM, Castle L et al (2000) The Cox-maze procedure: the Cleveland Clinic experience. J Thorac Cardiovasc Surg 12:25-29

27. Feinberg MS, Waggoner AD, Kater KM et al (1994) Restoration of atrial function after the maze procedure for patients with atrial fibrillation. Assessment by Doppler echocardiography. Circulation 90:II285-II292

Surgical Treatment of Atrial Fibrillation: The Japanese Experience

T. SUEDA[1] AND Y. KOSAKAI[2]

Introduction

Cox and colleagues devised the Maze procedure in 1991, in which both atria and all pulmonary veins were incised and sutured, in addition to excision of both atrial appendages [1, 2]. The idea behind the Maze procedure was to separate all possible areas for macroreentry and restore atrial contractility [3]. Although the Maze procedure was devised as a procedure for idiopathic atrial fibrillation (AF), it has been used for surgical ablation of chronic AF associated with mitral valve disease and proved effective in curing chronic AF as well as idiopathic AF [4]. In Japan, more than 2500 Maze procedures have performed to cure chronic or paroxysmal AF. The original Maze II and Maze III procedures have been modified and simplified in recent years. I have performed several procedures to eliminate AF in over 100 patients and simplified the procedure from the original Cox Maze III procedure to sole isolation of the pulmonary vein orifice. In this study, I investigated the results of different procedures in Japan and give new insights into surgical procedures for AF.

Survey of the Treatment of AF in Japan

In 2000, Dr. Kosakai performed a survey of AF surgery in Japan [5]. He sent a questionnaire to 517 Japanese hospitals that perform cardiac surgery. Answers were returned from 288 hospitals, stating that 2547 procedures had been performed to eliminate chronic or paroxysmal AF with or without concomitant cardiac surgery.

In the analysis of the results of this questionnaire, the patients were divided into four groups: lone AF, chronic AF with mitral valve disease (mitral AF group), AF with congenital heart disease (congenital AF group), and "other AF",

[1]First Department of Surgery, Hiroshima University, School of Medicine, Hiroshima;
[2]Department of Cardiovascular Surgery, Tarazuka, City Hospital, Japan

a group which contains patients with aortic valve disease or coronary heart disease. The procedure was defined as successful when persistent AF disappeared at discharge or during the follow-up period, even if paroxysmal AF occurred postoperatively or sick sinus syndrome appeared. Operative procedures used were the Cox Maze II procedure, the Cox Maze III procedure, the cryo-Maze procedure (Kosakai procedure), the left atrial procedure (Sueda procedure), the right atrial Maze procedure, the compartment procedure, and the radial aproach.

Results

In the lone AF group, 52 underwent AF surgery. The success rates were 69% (11/16) for the Cox Maze II and Cox Maze III procedures, 85% (29/34) for the cryo-Maze (Kosakai) procedure, and 66% (2/3) for the left atrial procedure. There were no significant differences among these procedures.

In the mitral AF group, 2094 patients underwent AF surgery. The success rates were 89% (17/19) for the Cox Maze II procedure, 76% (558/735) for the Cox Maze III procedure, 74% (707/956) for the cryo-Maze procedure, 73% (221/304) for the left atrial procedure, and 77% (58/75) for other modified Maze procedures. There were no significant differences among these results.

In the congenital AF group, 208 patients underwent AF surgery. The success rates were 67% (2/3) for the Cox Maze II procedure, 91% (51/56) for the Cox Maze III procedure, 87% (65/67) for the cryo-Maze procedure, 49% (20/41) for the right atrial Maze procedure, 55% (11/20) for compartment operation, and 58% (7/12) for other modified Maze procedures. The success rates of the right atrial Maze procedure, compartment operation, and other modified Maze procedure were significantly lower than those of the Cox Maze III procedure and the cryo-Maze procedure ($p < 0.05$).

In the other AF group, 206 patients underwent AF surgery. The success rates were 74% (23/31) for the Cox Maze III procedure, 80% (43/54) for the cryo-Maze procedure, 80% (4/5) for the left atrial procedure, and 79% (11/14) for other modified Maze procedures. There were no significant differences in results among these procedures.

Personal Experience and Insight into the Essence of AF Surgery

Between February 1993 and April 2001, 100 patients were treated with several AF procedures at Hiroshima University Hospital. Among these, there was 1 hospital death (mortality 1%). The cause of death was cerebral embolism, where severe cerebral embolism by a left atrial thrombus occurred during the preoperative stay in the intensive care unit. The average age of the patients was 60.6 ± 7.3 years. There were 98 patients with sustained AF, and 2 with paroxysmal AF.

Several procedures were performed. The Cox Maze III procedure or cryo-Maze procedure were applied in 6 patients with lone AF and 10 with mitral valvular AF. The left atrial procedure was applied in 2 patients with lone AF and 77 with mitral valvular AF. The original left atrial procedure consisted of isolation of all pulmonary veins, excision of the left atrial appendage, and concomitant cryoablation to the posterior mitral valvular annulus (Fig. 1). This procedure was applied in 54 patients with mitral valve disease. However, recently the left atrial procedure was simplified and became a procedure of sole isolation of all pulmonary vein orifices (Fig. 2). Sole isolation of pulmonary vein orifices was performed in 22 patients with mitral AF and 3 with lone AF. Right atrial separation was performed in 5 patients with congenital AF due to atrial septal defect.

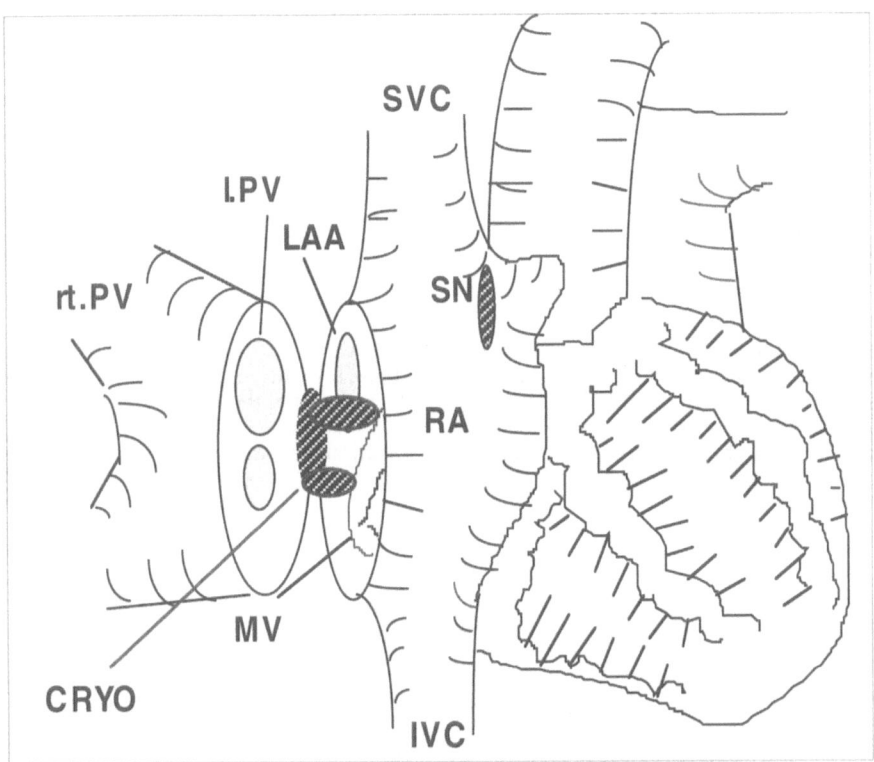

Fig. 1. Left atrial procedure. A right-sided vertical atriotomy of the left atrium was extended toward the left margin of the left pulmonary veins. After the excision of the left atrial appendage, cryoablation was delivered at –60°C for 2 min to the posterior wall of the left atrium. The cryoablation was directed toward the incision edges between the upper and lower left pulmonary veins, and to two areas of the posterior left atrial wall, from the left upper atrial incision edge into the posterior mitral valvular annulus, and from the left lower atrial incision edge into the center of the posterior mitral valvular annulus. *SN*, sinus node; *RA*, right atrium; *MV*, mitral valve; *LAA*, left atrial appendage; *LPV*, left pulmonary vein; *rt. PV*, right lower pulmonary vein; *SVC*, superior vena cava; *IVC*, inferior vena cava; *CRYO*, cryoablation

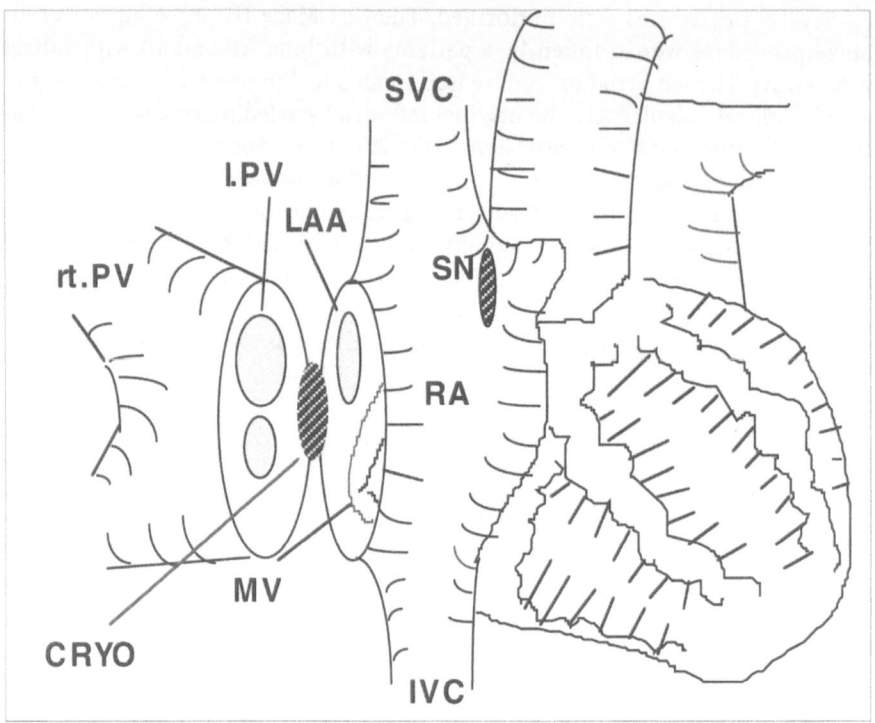

Fig. 2. Pulmonary vein orifice isolation. A right-sided vertical atriotomy of the left atrium was extended to the left margin of the left pulmonary vein orifices. Complementary cryoablation (-60°C for 2 min) was delivered to the remnant of the left atrial wall between the left upper pulmonary vein orifice and the left lower pulmonary vein orifice. *SN*, sinus node; *RA*, right atrium; *MV*, mitral valve; *LAA*, left atrial appendage; *LPV*, left pulmonary vein; *rt. PV*, right lower pulmonary vein; *SVC*, superior vena cava; *IVC*, inferior vena cava; *CRYO*, cryoablation

The success rate of the right atrial separation procedure was 60% (3/5) in the congenital AF group. In the lone AF group, success rates were 83% (5/6) for the Cox Maze III or the cryo-Maze procedure and 67% (2/3) for pulmonary vein isolation. In the mitral AF group, success rates were 80% (8/10) for the Cox Maze III procedure and the cryo-Maze procedure, 74% (40/54) for the left atrial procedure, and 77% (17/22) for pulmonary vein orifice isolation. There were no significant differences among these procedures in the mitral AF group.

Discussion

The Maze procedure has been used for surgical ablation of chronic AF associated with mitral valve disease, and has proved to be effective for conversion to sinus rhythm in this condition as well as in idiopathic AF. In Japan, more than

2500 procedures for AF have been performed, because the Japanese health insurance system completely covers patients' expenses. The Japanese experiences of the Maze procedure may be the largest in the world.

The majority of the patients underwent the Cox Maze III procedure or the cryo-Maze procedure. However, other procedures have been devised and applied in Japan. We attempted to simplify the original Maze procedure and devised the left atrial procedure [6]. Our most recent procedure is pulmonary vein orifice isolation. This newest procedure is simpler than the left atrial procedure [7]. The success rates for curing chronic AF by this simple procedure are no different from the success rates of the Maze procedure.

Why are the success rates the same among these different procedures?

Recently, Haïssaguerre and coworkers reported spontaneous initiation of AF due to ectopic beats originating from the pulmonary veins [8], and reported the successful application of radiofrequency ablation at these focal sources. We also observed repetitive activation originating from the left atrium during chronic AF with mitral valve disease [9]. In this study, we hypothesized that these regular activations might originate from the pulmonary veins, similar to the activation in cases of paroxysmal AF, and might similarly trigger AF. For this reason, we simplified our previous left atrial procedure and performed a simple pulmonary vein orifice isolation for treatment of chronic AF associated with mitral valve disease. Chronic AF was effectively eliminated in most cases.

Although our atrial mapping did not show the exact mechanisms underlying the chronic AF, because of limitations due to lack of extensive atrial mapping and interelectrode conduction-time data, our clinical experience suggests that the pulmonary veins act as a driver to maintain chronic AF, and that simple isolation of the pulmonary vein orifices might be adequate for elimination of the AF, even in patients with chronic AF associated with mitral valve disease.

References

1. Cox JL, Canavan TE, Schuessler RB et al (1991) The surgical treatment of atrial fibrillation. II. Intraoperative electrophysiologic mapping and description of the electrophysiological basis of atrial flutter and atrial fibrillation. J Thorac Cardiovasc Surg 101:406-426
2. Cox JL (1991) The surgical treatment of atrial fibrillation: IV. Surgical technique. J Thorac Cardiovasc Surg 101:584-592
3. Cox JL, Schuessler RB, Boineau JP (1991) The surgical treatment of atrial fibrillation: I. Summary of the current concepts of the mechanisms of atrial flutter and atrial fibrillation. J Thorac Cardiovasc Surg 101:402-405
4. Kosakai Y, Kawaguchi A, Isobe F et al (1994) Cox Maze procedure for chronic atrial fibrillation associated with mitral valve disease. J Thorac Cardiovasc Surg 108:1049-1055
5. Kosakai Y (2000) Treatment of atrial fibrillation using the Maze procedure: The Japanese experience. Semin Thor Cardiovasc Surgery 12:44-52
6. Sueda T, Nagata H, Orihashi K et al (1997) Efficacy of a simple left atrial procedure for chronic atrial fibrillation in mitral valve operations. Ann Thorac Surg 63:1070-1075

7. Sueda T, Imai K, Ishii O et al (2001) Efficacy of pulmonary vein isolation for the elimination of chronic atrial fibrillation in cardiac valvular surgery. Ann Thorac Surg 71:1189-1193
8. Haïssaguerre M, Jaïs P, Shah DC et al (1998) Spontaneous initiation of atrial fibrillation by ectopic beats originating in the pulmonary veins. N Engl J Med 339:659-666
9. Sueda T, Nagata T, Shikata H et al (1996) Simple left atrial procedure for chronic atrial fibrillation associated with mitral valve disease. Ann Thorac Surg 62:1796-1800

Intraoperative Radiomaze for Atrial Fibrillation Patients Undergoing Heart Surgery: Which Acute and Long Term Results?

A. Venturini[1], A. Asta[1], D. Mangino[1], R. Moretti[1], E. Polesel[1], F. Rigo[2], A. Corrado[2] and C. Zussa[1]

Introduction

Studies have revealed that chronic atrial fibrillation (AF) not only impairs cardiac function but also (together with paroxysmal AF) increases the risk of thromboembolic complications [1, 2]. A recent retrospective study by Obadia et al. [3] underlined the importance of the restoration of sinus rhythm in the mid-term follow-up of patients who had undergone mitral valve repair: 4 years postoperatively 94% of the patients in sinus rhythm were alive, while the survival rate of the patients in chronic AF was only 77%.

Therefore, several surgical techniques have been designed to ablate the arrhythmia, e.g. the corridor operation, the left atrial isolation, the Cox-Maze procedure [4-9]. However, most surgeons are reluctant to expose their patients to the risk of the Maze procedure because of the significantly increased aortic cross-clamping time and postoperative bleeding.

To simplify the Maze procedure, intraoperative radiofrequency energy has been used according to two different techniques to eliminate chronic or paroxismal AF in patients undergoing heart surgery.

Materials and Methods

Patient Characteristics

Between November 1999 and March 2001 32 patients with AF were operated upon for valve or coronary artery disease. Two groups were formed, according to the different Radiomaze technique used. Group I consisted of two men (12.5%) and 14 women (87.5%) aged 57-77 years (mean 62 years); while Group II consisted of seven men (43.7%) and nine women (56.3%) aged 49-80

Cardiovascular Department, [1]Division of Cardiac Surgery and [2]Division of Cardiology, Umberto I Hospital, Mestre-Venice, Italy

years (mean 63 years). Most of the patients (73%) in both groups were in NYHA Class II. Concomitant cardiac pathologies were: mitral regurgitation (seven patients, 43.7%, in both groups), mitral stenosis (six patients, 37.5%, in Group I, and four patients, 25%, in Group II), combined aortic and mitral valve disease (three patients, 18.7%, in both groups), aortic stenosis (one patient, 6.2%, in Group II), and coronary artery disease (one patient, 6.2%, in Group II). Five patients (31.2%) in Group I and nine (56.2%) in Group II had concomitant tricuspid valve regurgitation. Groups I and II did not differ in regard to the type of AF (chronic, 66%; paroxismal, 34%) and duration of AF (Group I, median 12 months, range 6-200; Group II, median 14 months, range 3-240). Most of the patients in both groups were in digoxin therapy before the operation.

Surgical Procedure

The ablation was performed using a temperature-controlled multipolar radio frequency catheter (Thermaline, Boston Scientific, USA). Radiomaze Type I procedure (Group I, $n = 16$ patients) was performed by creating epicardial bilateral, encircling isolation of the ostia of the pulmonary veins, an endocardial linear lesion connecting the previous lines and another lesion connecting the left pulmonary veins to the mitral valve annulus.

Radiomaze type II procedure (Group II, $n = 16$ patients) was performed by creating epicardial (or, if not feasible, partial endocardial) bilateral, circumferential isolation of the pulmonary veins only. The right epicardial lesion was performed without cardiopulmonary bypass (CPB); the left lesion with CPB and beating heart; the endocardial lesion of Radiomaze type I with aortic cross-clamping and cardioplegic cardiac arrest. Concomitant cardiac procedures were mitral valve repair, using Gore-Tex neochordae implantation and pericardial anuloplasty (seven patients, 43.7%, in both groups), mitral valve replacement (six patients, 37.5%, in Group I, and four patients, 25%, in Group II), aortic valve replacement (one patient, 6.2%, in Group II), mitral and aortic valve replacement (three patients, 18.7%, in both groups) and CABG (1 patient, 6.2%, in Group II). Tricuspid valve repair according to de Vega was performed in five patients (31.2%) of Group I and nine (56.2%) of Group II.

Follow-up

Early postoperative care was similar to that for routine heart surgery. Amiodarone infusion (900 mg in 24 h) was started in the intensive care unit in most of the patients. Postoperative early atrial arrhythmias were treated with i.v. amiodarone (300 mg in 30 min + 900 mg in 24 h), sometimes associated with low-dose (25 mg) oral atenolol. At discharge the majority of patients ($n = 30$; 93.7%) were in oral amiodarone therapy. DC cardioversion, if necessary, was planned 1 month after operation and was performed in seven patients (43.7%) of both groups. Patients were seen in the outpatient clinic 3 and 12 months after operation. Doppler echocardiography was performed 2 and 12 months after surgery to assess atrial systolic function.

Results (Table 1)

Table 1. Results

	Group I ($n = 16$ patients)	Group II ($n = 16$ patients)
In-hospital DC-Cardioversions	0	0
Presence of Sinus Rhythm at discharge	56.2% ($n = 9$ patients)	56.2% ($n = 9$ patients)
n° DC-Cardioversions 1 month postop.	7	7
Presence of Sinus Rhythm at follow-up	81.2% ($n = 13$ patients)	81.2% ($n = 13$ patients)
Early (In-hospital) mortality	0	0
Late mortality	6.2% ($n = 1$ patient)	0
Systolic left atrial function at final follow-up	19% ± 5%	18.3% ± 4.6%

In-hospital Mortality and Morbidity

There were no in-hospital deaths. No patients required re-exploration for bleeding. In-hospital morbidity included low-output syndrome (one patient, 3.1%), respiratory failure (one patient, 3.1%) and complete A-V block (one patient, 3.1%). One patient in Group II with triple valve disease required the insertion of an intra-aortic balloon pump for a few days after surgery. One patient in Group I with rheumatic mitral valve disease required a prolonged period of mechanical ventilation. One patient in Group II who underwent mitro-aortic valve replacement required pacemaker insertion because of a complete A-V block.

Survival

Mean follow-up was 9.8 months (range 5-16 months) in Group I and 2.8 months (range 2-4 months) in Group II. One patient in Group I with a dilated cardiomyopathy died suddenly 8 months after operation.

Cardiac Rhythm and Atrial Function

At discharge seven patients (43.7%) in both groups were in AF: all of them were in oral amiodarone and DC cardioversions were performed 1 month after operation. At final follow-up, the presence of stable sinus rhythm was identical in both groups (13 patients; 81.2%). Doppler echocardiography was performed in all patients at follow-up and showed no major or minor left atrial thrombosis and only a mild impairment of the systolic left atrial function (percentages of the diastolic ventricular filling given by the atrial contraction: Group I, 19% ± 5%; Group II, 18.3% ± 4.6%; normal values, 25% ± 5%). In the group of 26 patients who were free of AF at follow-up, antiarrhythmic therapy was maintained in the majority: 16 patients (61.5%) were in amiodarone therapy, while the remaining were in sotalol (n = three patients; 11.5%) or digoxin (n = seven patients; 27%).

Conclusions

Intraoperative radiofrequency ablation is a fast, simple, safe and highly effective treatment to restore sinus rhythm in patients with AF undergoing cardiac surgery. Moreover, the restoration of an only mildly impaired left atrial function is advantageous, and no further anticoagulation is required in patients receiving a mitral valve repair or a bioprosthetic valve replacement.

References

1. Selzer A (1960) Effects of atrial fibrillation upon the circulation in patients with mitral stenosis. Am Heart J 59:518-526
2. Wolf PA, Dawber TR, Thomas Jr HE, Kannel WB (1978) Epidemiologic assessment of chronic atrial fibrillation and risk of stroke: the Framingham study. Neurology 28:973-977
3. Obadia JF, El Farra M, Bastien OH et al (1997) Outcome of atrial fibrillation after mitral valve repair. J Thorac Cardiovasc Surg 114:179-185
4. Cox JL, Schuessler RB, D'Agostino HJ Jr et al (1991) The surgical treatment of atrial fibrillation. (III) Development of a definitive surgical procedure. J Thorac Cardiovasc Surg 101:569-583
5. Cox JL, Boineau JP, Schuessler RB et al (1993) Five year experience with the Maze procedure for atrial fibrillation. Ann Thorac Surg 56:814-824
6. Cox JL, Jaquiss RDB, Schuessler RB, Boineau JP (1995) Modification of the Maze procedure for atrial flutter and atrial fibrillation. II. Surgical technique of the Maze III procedure. J Thorac Cardiovasc Surg 110:485-495
7. Williams JM, Ungerleider RM, Lofland GK, Cox JL (1980) Left atrial isolation: new technique for supraventricular arrhythmias. J Thorac Cardiovasc Surg 80:373-380
8. Scheinmann MM, Morady F, Hess DS, Gonzalez R (1982) Catheter-induced ablation of the atrioventricular junction to control refractory supraventricular arrhythmias. J Am Med Assoc 248:851-855
9. Defauw JJAMT, Guirardon JM, van Hemel NM et al (1992) Surgical therapy of paroxismal atrial fibrillation with the "corridor" operation. Ann Thorac Surg 53:564-571

Implantable Atrial Defibrillator: Where Are We and Where Are We Going?

B. Lüderitz

Introduction

Atrial fibrillation (AF) is a frequent and costly health care problem, the most common arrhythmia resulting in hospital admission. The overall prevalence of AF in the United States ranges from < 1% in young, otherwise healthy individuals up to nearly 9% in elderly patients. AF can cause disabling symptoms and serious adverse effects such as impairment of cardiac function or thromboembolic events (Fig. 1). Due to the limited efficacy of antiarrhythmic drugs for AF, several nonpharmacologic options have evolved, including pacemaker therapy, transvenous catheter ablation techniques, surgical procedures, and treatment with an implantable atrial defibrillator (IAD) (Table 1). The high prevalence of AF and its clinical complications, the poor efficacy of medical therapy for preventing recurrences in many cases, and dissatisfaction with alternative modes of therapy stimulated interest in an IAD [3].

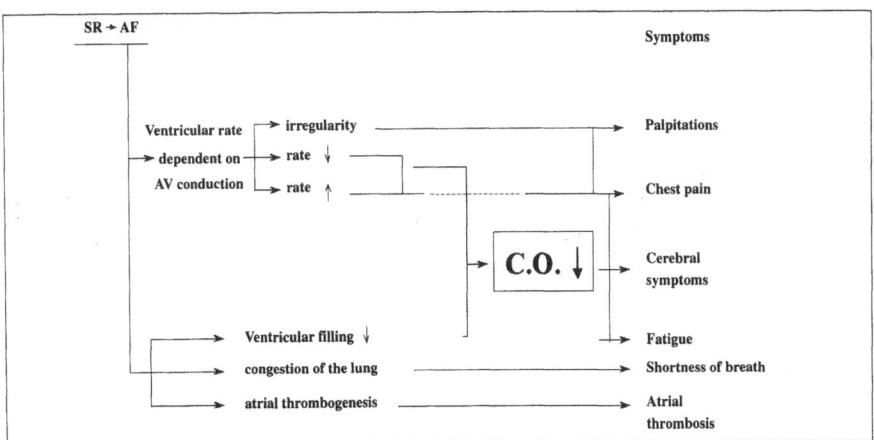

Fig. 1. Genesis of symptoms in AF: relationship of symptoms to hemodynamic change during AF. *CO*, cardiac output; *SR*, sinus rhythm

Department of Medicine-Cardiology, University of Bonn, Germany

Table 1. Nonpharmacologic treatment of atrial fibrillation (AF)

DC cardioversion/defibrillation
Atrioventricular node ablation (or modification)
        Electrical catheter
        Laser
        Cryogenics
        Surgery
        Alcohol or phenol ablation
        RFC isolation of pulmonary veins
        Linear right atrial ablation
Pacemaker
        (Pause-dependent AF, biatrial pacing, multisite pacing, DDD-R mode switch,
        DDDRP preventive pacing algorithms)
Antiarrhythmic surgery
        Corridor procedure [1]
        Maze procedure [2]
Atrial (internal) defibrillation
Implantable atrial defibrillator
Atrioventricular cardioverter/defibrillator

RFC, radio frequency current

Implantable Atrial Defibrillator

The development of an implantable cardioverter-defibrillator for the management of ventricular tachyarrhythmias had stimulated investigation of a similar approach to AF. A device for the management of recurring AF should have several characteristics [4]: low thresholds using only transvenous electrodes, small size with several years of implant life, freedom from ventricular proarrhythmia, a minimum of patient discomfort, limited thromboembolic risk, and high sensitivity and specificity for AF detection. Furthermore, cost-effectiveness and improvement in quality of life will have to be demonstrated when such a device is introduced for clinical management of patients with AF [5-7].

Patients with symptomatic recurrences of AF despite antiarrhythmic drug therapy represent potential candidates for an IAD. The number and duration of AF episodes should be taken into account in determining the indication. Patients with frequent episodes must be excluded as candidates for implantation of an atrial defibrillator on the grounds of too frequent discharges, patient discomfort, and rapid battery depletion. Similarly, patients with episodes of short duration and spontaneous termination may not be good candidates. Thus, selected patients with infrequent, symptomatic attacks of long-lasting episodes of AF despite antiarrhythmic drug therapy may benefit from an IAD.

The first atrial defibrillator was implanted on 30 October 1995 in London, UK. Initial clinical experience with human implants has been recently reported [8, 9]. As of the end of 1998, 220 atrial defibrillators have been implanted in patients around the world.

In a government relations editorial, the rationale for an IAD, potential problems, and the risk-to-benefit ratio of such a new electrotherapeutic treatment have been critically discussed [10]. Several considerations have to be taken into account before an automatic IAD could be widely accepted for the clinical management of patients with AF. These issues include accurate detection of AF, safe and effective termination of AF, patient tolerability, risk of thromboembolism, quality of life, and costs (Table 2) [11].

Table 2. Specific considerations of internal AF

Detection: sensitivity and specificity
Efficacy: energy requirements
Safety: ventricular proarrhythmia
Patient tolerability: pain
Thromboembolic risk: left atrial appendage function
Quality of life: repeated shocks
Cost-effectiveness: health reform

Quality of Life

The efficacy of a therapy has been based primarily on objective criteria such as mortality and morbidity. Besides these objective criteria, there has been increased interest in recent years in measuring quality of life in relation to health care. Multidimensional endpoints such as quality of life present particular problems of design, analysis, and interpretation [12]. Besides efficacy and safety, any new therapy should improve the patient's quality of life, particularly if it is a palliative or symptomatic treatment such as therapy with the IAD. AF often remains a poorly tolerated disorder resulting in palpitations, dyspnea, fatigue, chest pain, and limited exercise capacity. Alleviation or suppression of AF-related symptoms is an essential objective of any new therapeutic option. Thus, for a new treatment such as the IAD, it is imperative to demonstrate improvement in quality of life despite the potential negative impact on patient tolerability caused by recurrent atrial defibrillation shocks [13].

Patient Tolerability

In a prospective study, we evaluated the tolerability of internal atrial defibrillation in 35 consecutive patients with chronic AF. Biphasic shocks were delivered between transvenous catheters located in the right atrial appendage and the coronary sinus using a step-up voltage protocol starting at 60 V. Voltage was usually increased in 40-V steps until an energy of 180 V was reached. All patients were conscious at the beginning of the study and were asked to report pain perception after each shock delivery. Since the majority of patients reported severe pain at shock energies below 1 J, pain perception may have a major impact on quality of life in patients with an IAD [14, 15].

Future Perspectives

Without any doubt, the IAD was a milestone in the evolution of atrial defibrillation towards advanced electrotherapeutic devices (Fig. 2). Concern has been raised as to whether a stand-alone IAD is safe enough or whether ventricular back-up defibrillation should be provided for the rare case of shock-induced ventricular proarrhythmia. Some years ago, a new dual chamber defibrillator [Arrhythmia Management Device (AMD), model 7250, Medtronic Inc., Minneapolis, MN, USA] has entered clinical investigation. On 10 January 1997, a 61-year-old woman suffering from recurrent, drug-refractory supraventricular and ventricular tachycardia was the first patient in the world to receive a multi-programmable dual chamber implantable defibrillator [16]. As of May 2001, more than 75 devices of this type (7250 Jewel AF) have been implanted in our institution. The availability of a dual chamber defibrillator has reactivated the discussion about the safety of a stand-alone IAD. A dual chamber defibrillator

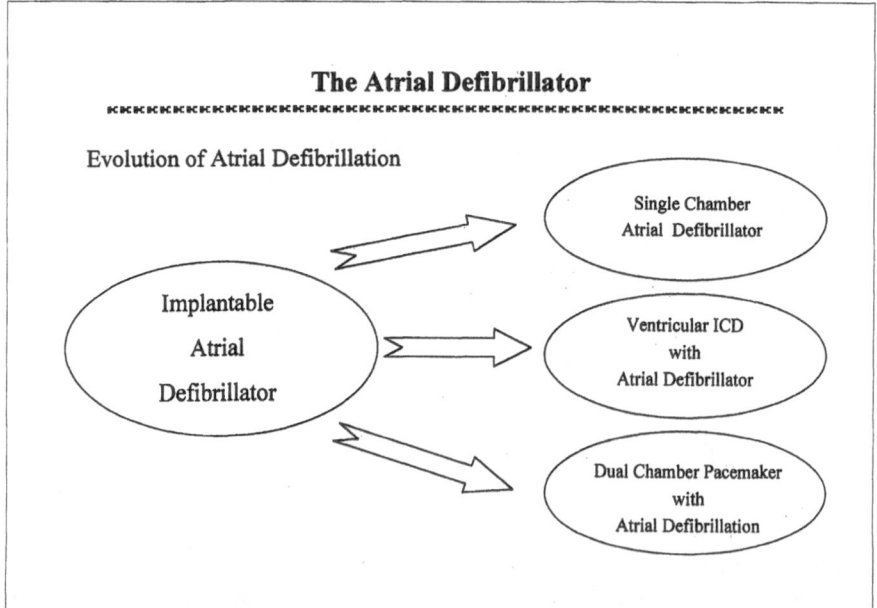

Fig. 2. Schematic interpretation of the implantable atrial defibrillator as a milestone in the evolution of atrial defibrillation towards new, more advanced electrotherapeutic devices

providing ventricular back-up defibrillation might meet the "pure" safety criteria in terms of ventricular proarrhythmia somewhat more easily than a stand-alone atrial defibrillator. However, the former device is larger, more complex, probably less specifically optimized to AF, and more costly than a single chamber device using a similar design and technology. On the other hand, there certainly will be a role for a dual chamber defibrillator for the subset of patients suffering from both atrial and ventricular arrhythmias. Future large studies and the upcoming clinical trials with both devices will teach us more about the safety issues of these new electrotherapeutic strategies in the management of patients with AF. Furthermore, a future IAD ideally should provide dual chamber pacing capabilities, especially for the subgroup of patients with sick sinus syndrome and AF. Moreover, some specialized forms of pacing might be beneficial for selected patients for the prevention of AF [17, 18].

References

1. Guiraudon GM, Klein GJ, Guiraudon CM, Yee R (1994) Treatment of atrial fibrillation: preservation of sinoventricular impulse conduction (the corridor operation). In: Olsson SB, Allessie MA, Campbell RWF (eds) Atrial Fibrillation. Mechanisms and Therapeutic Strategies. Futura Publishing, Armonk, NY, pp 349-371
2. Cox JL, Chuessler RB, D'Agostino jr J et al (1991) The surgical treatment of atrial fibrillation. J Thorac Cardiovasc Surg 101:569-583
3. Hillsley RE, Wharton JM (1995) Implantable atrial defibrillators. J Cardiovasc Electrophysiol 6:634-638
4. Griffin JC, Ayers GM, Adams J et al (1996) Is the automatic atrial defibrillator a promising approach? J Cardiovasc Electrophysiol 7:1217-1224
5. Dorian P, Jung W, Newman D et al (2000) The impairment of health-related quality of life in patients with intermittent atrial fibrillation: implications for the assessment of investigational therapy. J Am Coll Cardiol 36:1303-1309
6. Savelieva I, Paquette M, Dorian P et al (2001) Quality of life in patients with silent atrial fibrillation. Heart 85:216-217
7. Lüderitz B, Jung W (2000) Quality of life in patients with atrial fibrillation. Arch Intern Med 160:1749-1757
8. Lau CP, Tse HF, Lok NS et al (1997) Initial clinical experience with an implantable human atrial defibrillator. Pacing Clin Electrophysiol 20:220-225
9. Wellens HJJ, Lau CP, Lüderitz B et al for the METRIX investigators (1997) Atrioverter: an implantable device for the treatment of atrial fibrillation. Circulation 98:1651-1656
10. Jung W, Lüderitz B (1997) Implantable atrial defibrillator: quo vadis? (editorial) Pacing Clin Electrophysiol 20:2141-2145
11. Griffin JC (1997) The automatic atrial defibrillator: state of the art and future directions. In: Santini M (ed) Progress in clinical pacing. Futura Media Services, Armonk, NY, pp 279-288
12. Jung W, Lüderitz B (1998) Quality of life in patients with atrial fibrillation. J Cardiovasc Electrophysiol 9:S177-S186
13. Lüderitz B, Jung W (2000) Quality of life in atrial fibrillation. J Interv Card Electrophysiol 4:201-209

14. Jung W, Pfeiffer D, Schumacher B et al (1996) A prospective evaluation of pain per-
     ception in patients undergoing internal atrial defibrillation (abstract). Eur Heart J
     17:493
15. Lüderitz B, Jung W (1999) Intra-atrial defibrillation in humans. Thorac Cardiovasc
     Surg 47:342-346
16. Jung W, Lüderitz B (1997) Implantation of a new arrhythmia management system in
     patients with supraventricular and ventricular tachyarrhythmias. Lancet 349:853-854
17. Daubert C, Mabo P, Berder V (1990) Arrhythmia prevention by permanent atrial
     resynchronization in advanced interatrial block. Eur Heart J 11:237-242
18. Prakash A, Saksena S, Hill M et al (1997) Acute effects of dual-site right atrial pacing
     in patients with spontaneous and inducible atrial flutter and fibrillation. J Am Coll
     Cardiol 29:1007-1014

Atrial Pacing to Prevent Atrial Fibrillation: Is There Any Evidence of Its Real Efficacy?

S. Saksena[1,2,3] and A. Filipecki[1,3]

Introduction

Atrial pacing has been widely but intermittently reported to reduce the recurrence of atrial fibrillation (AF) and progression to permanent AF in a wide variety of observational reports, with the vast majority of these involving retrospective analyses [1-3]. In addition, a variable patient population with respect to AF and underlying cardiac disease has often characterized these reports. The subject has received substantial attention since the follow-up report of the Danish Trial of Physiologic Pacing in sick sinus syndrome reported reduction in the incidence of persistent or permanent AF with atrial-based pacing in patients with sick sinus syndrome [4]. Clinical investigation of atrial pacing techniques for management of AF in symptomatic or high-risk populations has been examined in a series of prospective clinical trials [5-9]. Serious investigative interest has now focused on the electrophysiologic effects of different atrial pacing methods in experimental and clinical laboratory AF models. Analysis of the benefit of atrial pacing is complicated by the interactions of this apparently simple intervention with a heterogeneous AF population and our limited knowledge of the natural history of the arrhythmia in its different substrates. Finally, the appropriate endpoints for demonstration of device clinical efficacy and safety have been unclear, leading to increasing difficulty in defining and quantifying clinical benefit [10, 11].

Issues in Clinical Trial Analysis

For the analysis of recently completed clinical trials, several important issues should be clearly recognized in data analysis. First and foremost of these is appropriate definition of the patient population. Progress has been recently

[1]Cardiovascular Institute, Arrhythmia and Pacemaker Service, Atlantic Health System, Passaic, New Jersey; [2]Robert Wood Johnson School of Medicine, New Brunswick, New Jersey; [3]Electrophysiology Research Foundation, Millburn, New Jersey, USA

made on this front. In essence, patients will be categorized as having initial or new-onset AF, or paroxysmal, persistent and permanent forms of the arrhythmia. Permanence of AF is no longer defined solely on the basis of resistance to or recurrence after direct current cardioversion, but may also be diagnosed based on physician judgment. The clinical relevance of this classification is that studies have delineated the higher prevalence of symptomatic palpitations in paroxysmal AF than in more persistent AF [12]. Thus, studies relying solely on symptom endpoints before or without ECG verification in persistent AF are more likely to underestimate AF events, or the burden and measurement of asymptomatic AF may be particularly important in this patient group.

Progression to permanent AF may also vary in patient populations based on types of asymptomatic or symptomatic AF. In the CTOPP study of sick sinus syndrome patients, the incidence of AF was 5.3% annually in the physiologic-pacing group, while it averaged only 1.2% in the Danish trial [4, 5]. Gianfranchi et al. reported persistent AF at 1 year in 22% of patients with paroxysmal AF with high right atrial (RA) pacing in the DDD mode after atrioventricular (AV) junctional ablation [13]. In the PA3 trial, 43% of patients developed persistent AF [14]. In studies that permit both population groups, this progression could only be assessed either if the population was kept homogeneous and matched to a historical control or if a control group with minimal or no pacing was available. Finally, another important factor now recognized from device-based studies in AF populations is the enormous variability in frequency of AF. In the Medtronic Jewel AF-only and Dual Site Atrial Pacing for Permanent Atrial Fibrillation (DAPPAF) studies, identical entry criteria were used for AF event frequency, namely two symptomatic episodes in the 3 months prior to study entry [7, 15]. In the former study, AF frequency among patients varied from single digits to thousands of events. In the latter study, one-third of patients actually had one or more AF events per day. Thus, event frequency may remain an important and potentially unmatched variable in such randomized trials without a crossover design. Even crossover designs may not fully address this issue and may require a priori measurement of this variable in patient inclusion criteria in the future.

Endpoints for Efficacy Assessment

A firmer basis for selecting endpoints in AF trials is emerging. For symptomatic paroxysmal AF, time to initial AF has been a gold standard. Recently, it has been suggested that patterns of AF recurrences may fit other models such as a Weibull distribution in small samples [16]. Such mathematical modeling may be overly simplistic and quite inapplicable to these multiple AF populations or the widely varying clinical substrates. In our view, favorable effects on the initial recurrence may imply salutary effects on the AF trigger and/or substrate, and may be a harbinger of future rhythm control. The converse – no change in time to initial AF recurrence – may not predict eventual outcome. Intercurrent clinical events, particularly heart failure and chest infections, which may activate AF triggers, can produce a temporary resurgence of AF. Cluster arrhythmic events have been well delineated in malignant ventricular arrhythmias. It is likely, and clinical experience seems to validate, that similar behavior exists in AF. Similarly, introduction of any antiarrhythmic therapy, such as drugs, may modify outcome and represent an important variable to be controlled in such studies.

Is Atrial Pacing Efficacious in AF Populations?

In the light of the above considerations, a series of clinical trials have now become available for analysis. Initial prospective studies of high RA pacing in patients with sick sinus syndrome without antecedent AF have noted that relatively long follow-up periods show lower incidence of AF as compared to ventricular pacing [4]. However, proarrhythmia with ventricular pacing could not be excluded. These data have been reconfirmed in the analyses of the CTOPP and MOST trials [5, 6]. Both trials show a substantial reduction in the incidence of persistent and permanent AF with dual-chamber pacing. This benefit could be seen within 2 years of follow-up in the MOST study, with a hazard ratio of 0.79. In addition, a very high incidence of failure to remain in the randomized arm was noted in the ventricular demand pacing group, with a crossover rate of 30% within 1 year. Thus, in the sick sinus syndrome population, atrial-based pacing can improve tolerance and compliance with the mode, and perhaps reduce progression to persistent or permanent AF.

More recent studies have become available in patients with bradycardias requiring pacing and symptomatic AF. In the ADOPT-A study, a new pacing algorithm – dynamic atrial overdrive – was used and AF frequency assessed by symptomatic AF events validated by ECG transmissions [9]. This study permitted paroxysmal and persistent AF, and required two events in 6 months with one ECG-documented event in the prior 3 months. The study actually enrolled patients with an average of eight events in the preceding 6 months. Drug refractoriness was not required, and whether new or previously ineffective drugs were used is unclear. The control group had DDDR pacing alone with 68% atrial pacing and the active algorithm arm had 93% pacing. Use of class I and III antiarrhythmic drugs was 45%-50% in the two arms. Approximately 52% of patients in the dynamic overdrive arm and 56% in the DDDR-only arm experienced recurrent AF. There was a trend to reduced AF frequency in both groups, with an incidence of 4.44% in the first month in the control group and 1.73% at 6 months. The overall event rate was halved in the DDDR arm as compared to the pre-pacing period and reduced by 25% further by the algorithm. While a control arm with no pacing was not present, it would be reasonable to assume that the reduced event rate would be related to the institution of atrial pacing rather than chance. Furthermore, this study reported reduced AF frequency with the addition of the new algorithm by approximately 28% in the first month and 21% in the 6-month period. There was no reduction in the percentage of patients experiencing recurrences in the dynamic overdrive arm, indicating that this type of high RA pacing does not eliminate recurrent AF. The event rate in the patient cohort without AF recurrences (approximately one-half) could not be compared with the event rate in those without any atrial pacing due to the variables of antiarrhythmic drug therapy and frequency variability as indicated earlier. However, the conclusion that a higher level of atrial pacing reduced event rates in patients who would have recurrent AF is supported by this data.

The DAPPAF study compared high RA, dual site RA, and support pacing in patients with recurrent, symptomatic AF and bradycardias in the presence or absence of antiarrhythmic drugs in a crossover study design [7]. One hundred twenty patients with symptomatic AF and bradycardias were randomly assigned to 6-month periods in the each of the three pacing modes for a projected total follow-up period of 18 months. Patient tolerance and adherence to the pacing mode was superior with dual RA pacing as compared to support (p < 0.001) and high RA pacing (p = 0.006). Freedom from any symptomatic AF recurrence trended to be greater with dual RA (hazard ratio 0.715, p = 0.07) but not with high RA pacing (p = 0.19) compared to support pacing. When dual RA pacing was compared to high RA pacing there was a reduced relative risk of recurrent AF (hazard ratio 0.835), but this did not achieve significance, probably owing to reduced event rates due to crossover and other factors (p = 0.17). Combined symptomatic and asymptomatic AF frequency in patients measured by device datalogs was significantly reduced during dual RA pacing as compared to high RA pacing (p < 0.01). However, in antiarrhythmic drug-treated patients, dual RA pacing increased symptomatic AF free survival compared to support pacing (p = 0.011) and high RA pacing (hazard ratio 0.669, p = 0.06). In drug-treated patients with ≤ 1 AF event per week, dual RA pacing significantly improved AF suppression compared to support pacing (hazard ratio 0.464, p = 0.004) and high RA pacing (hazard ratio 0.623, p = 0.006). Finally, echocardiographic data from the three treatment arms showed superior left atrial filling and prevention of the reduction in left ventricular ejection fraction seen with high RA pacing in the DDDR mode with dual site RA pacing [17]. Lead dislodgement was uncommon (1.7%), with coronary sinus and high RA lead stability being comparable.

Analysis of this study shows that dual RA pacing had comparable safety and was better tolerated than high RA and support pacing for long-term application. Furthermore, dual RA pacing increased freedom from recurrent AF when combined with class I or III antiarrhythmic drugs in patients with symptomatic AF with a frequency of one event per week or less. Finally, dual site RA pacing reduced the incidence of symptomatic and asymptomatic AF events compared to standard pacing modes in the entire population. Thus, the novel pacing mode combined with overdrive pacing could improve adherence to the pacing mode for long-term use, reduce the proportion of patients with recurrent AF when previously ineffective drug therapy was continued in patients with one or fewer symptomatic events per week, and, finally, prolong the time to recurrence in patients with recurrences or reduce the number of recurrences in these patients. These benefits are strongly supported by physiologic data relative to left heart hemodynamics [17].

Another proposed modality is the use of septal pacing. Bailin et al. showed that progression to persistent AF is reduced to 25% in the first year after high septal pacing [8]. This is still a fairly high progression rate, and longer-term results will be of importance to assess further progression. The number of recurrent AF events, as assessed by the device recorded mode switch frequency, were similar between RA appendage and high septal pacing. Thus, neither method appeared particularly efficacious in suppression of recurrent AF. It is therefore likely that monotherapy with single site pacing techniques alone is unlikely to achieve clinical outcomes in symptomatic AF populations, which could lead to a paradigm shift in AF management.

The efficacy of pacing therapy in patients without primary bradycardias has often been a subject of controversy. Our own center data, reported previously, and data reported more recently from the DAPPAF database show that the presence of more persistent AF and the use of sotalol were associated with better outcomes with dual RA pacing than with high RA pacing or support pacing [18, 19]. This was largely due to poorer outcomes of high RA and support pacing, with dual RA pacing maintaining efficacy. In our long-term study database in patients with drug-refractory AF with follow-up up to 7 years, 23% of patients did not present with primary bradycardia but with symptomatic AF. Over 90% of these patients are free of persistent or permanent AF at 4 years [18]. Thus, it is reasonable to infer that a hybrid approach using drug and dual RA pacing is effective in this population with paroxysmal AF to prevent progression to persistent or permanent AF. More recently, our own data with dual site atrial pacing in combination with drug and/or ablation therapies in patients with permanent or persistent AF have shown greater than 90% freedom from persistent or permanent AF at 5 years. Thus, it may be necessary to institute hybrid therapies to achieve the outcomes necessary to change clinical practice.

Conclusions

We can conclude that atrial pacing is associated with a reduced progression to permanent or persistent AF in high-risk populations with bradycardias and is better tolerated than ventricular pacing. Whether there is an absolute reduction in AF recurrence or progression remains uncertain in this population. However, in patients with symptomatic AF with bradycardias there is limited benefit with high RA or septal pacing; novel algorithms such as dynamic atrial or other overdrive modes and dual site RA pacing are required to achieve efficacy that can result in long-term arrhythmia burden reduction or AF suppression.

References

1. Saksena S, Prakash A, Krol RB et al (1997) Prevention of atrial fibrillation with single and multisite atrial pacing. In: Murgatroyd FD, Camm AJ (eds) Nonpharmacological management of atrial fibrillation. Futura, Armonk, NY, pp 339-353

2. Saksena S, Giorgberidze I, Delfaut P et al (1997) Pacing in atrial fibrillation. In: Rosenqvist M (ed) Cardiac pacing: new advances. WB Saunders, London, pp 39-59

3. Saksena S, Mehra R (1998) Pacing for prevention of atrial fibrillation. In: Ellenbogen K, Kay GN, Wilkoff B (eds) Clinical cardiac pacing and implantable cardioverter defibrillator. WB Saunders, Philadelphia, pp 461-496

4. Andersen HR, Nielsen JC, Thomsen et al (1997) Long-term follow-up of patients from a randomized trial of atrial versus ventricular pacing for sick sinus syndrome. Lancet 350:1210-1216

5. Connolly SJ, Kerr CR, Gent M et al (2000) Effects of physiologic pacing versus ventricular pacing on the risk of stroke and death due to cardiovascular causes. Canadian Trial of Physiologic Pacing Investigators. N Engl J Med 342:1385-1391

6. Lamas GA, Lee K, Sweeney M et al (2000) The Mode Selection Trial (MOST) in sinus node dysfunction: design, rationale, and baseline characteristics of the first 1000 patients. Am Heart J 140:541-551

7. Saksena S, Prakash A, Ziegler P et al (2001) The Dual Site Atrial Pacing for Permanent Atrial Fibrillation Trial: improved suppression of drug refractory atrial fibrillation with dual site atrial pacing and antiarrhythmic drugs. Presented at Late Breaking Clinical Trials Session, American College of Cardiology, Orlando, Florida, 20 March 2001

8. Bailin SJ, Adler S, Guidici M (2001) Prevention of chronic atrial fibrillation by pacing in the region of Bachmann bundle: results from a multicenter randomized trial. J Cardiovasc Electrophysiol (in press)

9. Carlson MA for the ADOPT-A investigators (2001) The Atrial Dynamic Overdrive Pacing Trial (ADOPT-A). Presented at Late Breaking Clinical Trials Session, North American Society of Pacing and Electrophysiology, Boston, Massachussets, 5 May 2001

10. Saksena S (1997) Definitions and endpoints for device clinical trials in atrial fibrillation – a pressing need. J Interv Card Electrophysiol 1:173-174

11. Camm AJ, Levy S, Saksena S, Wyse DG (2000) Don't you agree, or what part of the problem don't you understand? J Interv Card Electrophysiol 4:559-560

12. Levy S, Maarek M, Coumel P et al (1999) Characterization of different subsets of atrial fibrillation in general practice in France: the ALFA study. The College of French Cardiologists. Circulation 99:3028-3035

13. Gianfranchi L, Brignole M, Menozzi C et al (1998) Progression of permanent atrial fibrillation after atrioventricular junction ablation and dual-chamber pacemaker implantation in patients with paroxysmal atrial fibrillation. Am J Cardiol 81:351-354

14. Gillis AM, Connolly SJ, Lacombe P et al (2000) Randomized crossover comparison of DDDR versus VDD pacing after atrioventricular junction ablation for prevention of atrial fibrillation. The atrial pacing peri-ablation for paroxysmal atrial fibrillation (PA3) study investigators. Circulation 102:736-742

15. Saksena S, Sulke N, Manda V et al on behalf of the Worldwide Jewel AF Investigators (2000) Reduction in frequency of atrial tachyarrhythmia episodes using novel prevention algorithms of an atrial pacemaker defibrillator. Pacing Clin Electrophysiol 23:581 (abstr)

16. Kaemmerer WF, Rose S, Mehra R (2001) Distribution of patients' paroxysmal atrial tachyarrhythmia episodes: implications for detection of treatment efficacy. J Cardiovasc Electrophysiol 12:121-130

17. Prakash A, Saksena S, Ziegler P et al (2001) Dual site atrial pacing for prevention of atrial fibrillation [DAPPAF] trial: echocardiographic evaluation of atrial and ventricular function during a randomized trial of support, high right atrial and dual site right atrial pacing. Pacing Clin Electrophysiol 24:553 (abstr)

18. Prakash A, Lin WH, Saksena S et al (2001) Survival, stroke and cardioversion after dual site atrial pacing for atrial fibrillation: long-term results of pilot and main clinical studies. Pacing Clin Electrophysiol 24:641 (abstr)

19. Saksena S, Prakash A, Krol RB, Sroczynski H (2001) Randomized trial of dual site, high right atrial and support pacing modes in patients with recurrent atrial fibrillation with bradyarrhythmias: a single center experience. Circulation 2001 (submitted)

Is Overdrive Pacing Useful for the Prevention of Paroxysmal Atrial Fibrillation?

P. Attuel*, D. El Allaf, K.H. Konz, I. Szendey, J. Brachmann, V. Schibgilla, D. Danilovic, on behalf of the "Suppression of Atrial Fibrillation by Overdrive Pacing with Inos^2 CLS" Study Investigators

Introduction

Earlier observations that a high percentage of atrial pacing was associated with a reduced incidence of atrial tachyarrhythmia in selected patients paved the way to the development of pacemaker algorithms for the prevention of atrial fibrillation (AF) by pacing the atrium slightly above the intrinsic atrial rate [1-4]. Dynamic atrial overdrive pacing could decrease atrial ectopic activity involved in the onset of AF, prevent prolonged postextrasystolic pauses following premature atrial beats, and be efficient in the prevention of AF associated with absolute or relative bradycardia.

The therapeutic efficacy of different atrial overdrive algorithms is currently under investigation [2-7]. This article reports on the interim results of the "Suppression of Atrial Fibrillation by Overdrive Pacing with Inos^2 CLS" study. This prospective and randomized crossover study is being carried out at 19 centers in Germany, Belgium, France, and Brazil, with the aim of evaluating the clinical utility of the "DDD+ mode" overdrive algorithm implemented in Inos^2 closed loop stimulation (CLS) pacemakers (Biotronik, Germany).

Methods

In the DDD+ mode, sensing of an atrial event outside the postventricular atrial refractory period triggers pacing rate increase by the overdrive step size (nominal =10 beats/min; programmable range = 1-32). In the absence of sensed atrial events, the pacing rate is decreased by 1 beat/min each time the overdrive plateau length expires (nominal = 20 cycles; programmable range = 1-32 cycles). The atrial pacing rate cannot exceed the programmed maximum overdrive rate. The algorithm has been described in detail elsewhere [3].

*Centre Médico – Chirurgical Parly 2, le Chesnay, France

Patient eligible for enrollment in the DDD+ study were those who had received a bipolar atrial lead and an Inos^2 CLS or Inos^2 DR pacemaker for conventional pacing indications. The patients had to have exhibited a history of paroxysmal AF. The major exclusion criteria were chronic AF (> 18 h/day), unresolved atrial sensing problems, and unstable antiarrhythmic drug therapy. The patients were actively enrolled in the study at 1-9 months after pacemaker implantation, when the pacemaker mode was randomized to DDD or DDD+. Pacemaker mode crossover was scheduled for 6 months after mode randomization. To monitor the medical condition of the patients and the success of the overdrive therapy, the follow-up controls were performed every 3 months. AF data stored in the pacemaker memory were retrieved at each hospital visit.

The results for DDD+ vs DDD mode were compared in view of the mean number of sustained AF episodes per day, mean duration of sustained AF in hours per day, and the mean delay until the first recurrence of AF (in weeks), as recorded in the pacemaker diagnostic memory based on the mode-switch function. Mode-switch in Inos^2 CLS is activated when five out of eight consecutive atrial beats (P-P intervals) are faster than the mode-switch intervention rate, which is programmable to 100-180 beats/min. Following the mode switch, the pacemaker operates in the VDI mode until eight out of eight consecutive atrial beats are paced or sensed below the programmed intervention rate [8, 9].

Differences between the mean values were evaluated on the intrapatient basis using the paired two-tailed t-test. p values < 0.05 were considered significant. Data in the text are presented as mean value ± standard deviation and in Fig. 1 as mean value ± standard error of the mean.

Results

A total of 111 patients, aged 70.2 ± 10.4 years, were referred to their hospitals for enrollment in the study. Atrial leads were mostly positioned in the right atrial appendage (51%), onto the right atrial lateral wall (33%), in the high right atrium (4%), and at the right atrial anterior wall (3%). The basic rate was programmed to 62 ± 4 beats/min (DDD+ mode) or 62 ± 6 beats/min (DDD mode). Overdrive step size was programmed to 9 ± 2 beats/min (range 5-15) and the overdrive plateau length to 20 ± 3 cycles (range 10-32). The maximum overdrive rate was 129 ± 14 beats/min. These settings resulted in atrial pacing of 98% ± 5% (range 80%-100%) in the DDD+ mode and 62% ± 32% (range 1%-100%) in the DDD mode ($p < 0.05$).

From 111 eligible patients, ten were excluded at the time of mode randomization due to permanent AF, absence of AF after pacemaker implantation, or poor medical condition. From the 101 enrolled patients, five were excluded during the study due to the development of permanent AF (three in DDD mode and two in DDD+ mode), four due to death or significant change in medical condition or medication regime, and two patients due to violation of study protocol resulting in loss of crossover data.

   Patients referred to their hospitals 111 times for pacemaker control while
being in DDD+ mode. In 108 cases, programmed overdrive parameters were
well tolerated, and in the remaining three cases reprogramming of the overdrive step size or plateau length amended a certain discomfort initially caused
by atrial overdrive.
   Study results for 41 patients in whom crossover data have been available are
summarized in Fig. 1 and reviewed for each individual in Table 1.

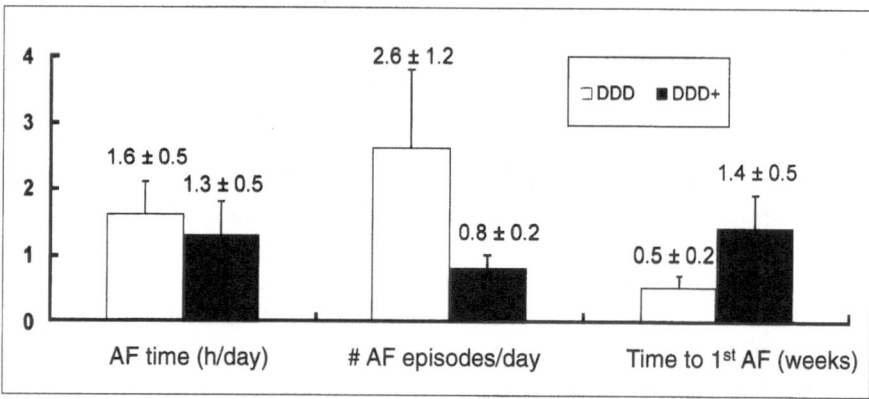

Fig. 1. Crossover data on atrial fibrillation (AF) recurrence following mode randomization
(mean value ± standard error of the mean). None of the differences reached statistical
significance (from left to right: $p = 0.43, p = 0.16, p = 0.09$)

Table 1. Burden of sustained atrial fibrillation in individual patients*

Patient	AF (h/day)		Difference (h/day)	AF (episodes/day)		Difference (episodes/day)
No.	DDD	DDD+	DDD – DDD+	DDD	DDD+	DDD – DDD+
1	10.97	1.38	9.59	0.138	0.137	0.001
2	4.28	0.47	3.81	49.43	2.29	47.14
3	14.89	11.19	3.70	0.06	1.03	-0.97
4	3.20	0.54	2.66	3.62	0.99	2.63
5	2.33	0.00	2.32	9.97	0.01	9.96
6	4.24	1.94	2.30	0.37	0.08	0.29
7	2.35	0.56	1.78	6.45	1.54	4.91
8	1.65	0.00	1.65	2.04	0.03	2.02
9	1.07	0.12	0.95	0.10	0.34	-0.24
10	0.46	0.08	0.38	7.82	0.72	7.10
11	1.22	0.91	0.31	10.89	5.90	5.00
12	0.23	0.00	0.23	0.023	0.016	0.007
13	0.43	0.22	0.21	4.42	1.51	2.91
14	0.05	0.00	0.05	0.80	0	0.80
15	0.005	0.002	0.003	0.14	0.05	0.09
16	0.001	0	0.001	0.01	0	0.01

Cont. Table 1.

Patient	AF (h/day)		Difference (h/day)	AF (episodes/day)		Difference (episodes/day)
No.	DDD	DDD+	DDD – DDD+	DDD	DDD+	DDD – DDD+
17	0	0.0002	-0.0002	0	0.01	-0.01
18	0.00	0.03	-0.03	0.032	0.016	0.016
19	0.01	0.05	-0.04	0.06	0.21	-0.15
20	0.06	0.22	-0.16	1.90	0.13	1.77
21	0.11	0.32	-0.21	2.15	3.86	-1.71
22	0.02	0.31	-0.29	0.32	4.11	-3.79
23	0.09	0.43	-0.34	0.09	0.40	-0.31
24	0.00	0.47	-0.47	0.02	0.71	-0.68
25	0.00	1.43	-1.43	0	0.03	-0.03
26	9.58	11.31	-1.73	3.03	6.42	-3.39
27	0.13	2.18	-2.05	0.02	0.57	-0.54
28	5.99	9.27	-3.28	0.22	0.20	0.01
29	1.05	8.95	0-7.90	0.38	2.44	-2.06

*Twelve patients without atrial fibrillation (AF) after mode randomization are not shown

Discussion

The interim data analysis based on the available crossover data in 41 patients indicated that DDD+ pacing was more effective than conventional dual-chamber pacing in 16 patients (39%) in terms of reduced AF time by 25%-100%. The results were neutral in 12 patients (29%) in whom there were no AF episodes in either mode, while 13 patients (32%) had more AF in DDD+ than in DDD mode. In 1994, Murgatroyd et al. [10] had already demonstrated that overdrive pacing reduced the number of premature atrial contractions in 18 patients, but also increased it in eight patients, atrial salvos were less frequent in 12 but more frequent in four patients, and AF incidence was reduced in 11 but increased in eight patients treated by overdrive pacing. This mixed response - an improvement observed in some patients and aggravation in others - may explain the controversial results of clinical studies that included patients with documented paroxysmal AF without any other considerations.

Recently, Wiberg et al. [11] reported on the efficacy of right atrial overdrive pacing in the prevention of symptomatic AF attacks in 35 patients. The number of sustained, symptomatic, ECG-documented episodes of paroxysmal AF was significantly lowered during medium- and high-rate pacing (1.4 and 1.3 episodes/week) compared with no pacing (2.5 episodes/week, $p < 0.006$). Funck et al. [7] published preliminary results of the PROVE study in 78 patients, which combined atrial overdrive pacing with an algorithm maintaining an elevated basic rate during active periods of the day and a lower basic rate during the night. This algorithm combination provided, on average, 84% of atrial pacing and led to a 34% reduction in the number of mode-switch episodes and to a 48% shortening of the total AF duration. However, there was no reduction in the mean number of atrial runs consisting of more than five beats. In the PIPAF study [12], the sinus rate overdrive and the suppression of the post-extrasystolic compensatory pause did not translate into a reduction in the total mode-switch time. However, the number of mode-switch episodes was reduced from 20 to ten in nine patients during a follow-up period of 13 months.

Earlier observations that atrial ectopic activity is often involved in the onset of AF led to the development of a range of atrial overdrive pacing algorithms aimed at suppression of atrial ectopic activity [3]. Not quite in agreement with this, Hnatkova et al. [13] found that irregular intervals during the last three cycle lengths before the onset of AF were present in 22% of the total number of studied onset sequences, while classical short-long-short patterns were seen in only 6% of the sequences. This implies that the suppression of premature atrial activity is probably only one of the possible mechanisms underlying the prevention of paroxysmal AF by overdrive pacing; a diminution of refractory period dispersion (often associated with vagally mediated AF) and facilitation of the pre-excitation of certain anisotropic areas may play an equally important role [14]. As Garrigue et al. [1] demonstrated, the increased percentage of pacing achieved by atrial overdrive contributes to the homogeneity of the atrial activation front. It is also known that local anatomical factors may play a role in the initiation of AF [15]. Prolonged and fractionated atrial electrogram characteristics can be closely related to the vulnerability of the atrial muscle, particularly in patients with both paroxysmal AF and sick sinus syndrome [16]. Thus, it is essential to evaluate the nature of the predominant factors responsible for the initiation and the perpetuation of AF if we want to target the responder patients to overdrive atrial pacing.

Clinical Investigators: D. El Allaf (Huy, Belgium); K.H. Konz and I. Szendey (Mönchengladbach, Germany); J. Brachmann and V. Shibgilla (Coburg, Germany); P. Attuel (St. Cloude Ceex, France); C. Gomes (Taguatinga, Brazil); S. Löscher (Leipzig, Germany); C. John (Dresden, Germany); U. le Blanc, S. Rupp and M. Klutmann (Düren, Germany); T. Scheibner (Löbau, Germany); K. Malinowski (Aue, Germany); L. Griesbach (Kirchberg, Germany); H. Müller-Dieckert (Rochtliz, Germany); K. Göhl and C. Huber (Nuremberg, Germany); G. Lascault (St. Denis Cedex, France); R.U. York (Hartmannsdorf, Germany); T. Walter (Greiz, Germany); B. Hailer and H. Schäfer (Essen, Germany); D. Stockmann (Antwerpen, Belgium); S. Schüssler (Kaufbeuren, Germany).

References

1. Garrigue S, Barold SS, Cazeau S et al (1998) Prevention of atrial arrhythmias during DDD pacing by atrial overdrive. Pacing Clin Electrophysiol 21:1751-1759
2. Israel CW (2000) Prevention of atrial tachyarrhythmias: promise of new pacing algorithms. Herzschrittmacher 20:8-11

3. Attuel P (2000) Therapy and prevention of atrial fibrillation by overdrive stimulation? Herzschrittmacher 20:104-111
4. Begemann MJS, Boute W (2000) Novel preventive pacing algorithms aiming to stop atrial fibrillation from starting. Herzschrittmacher 20:47-58
5. Poezevara Y, Hümmer A, Lazarus A (2000) Dedicated therapeutic tools in the prevention of atrial arrhythmias by means of pacing. Herzschrittmacher 20:26-33
6. Israel CW, Lawo T, Lemke B et al (2000) Atrial pacing in the prevention of paroxysmal atrial fibrillation: first results of a new combined algorithm. Pacing Clin Electrophysiol 23:1888-1890
7. Funck RC, Adamec R, Lurje L et al (2000) Atrial overdriving is beneficial in patients with atrial arrhythmias: first results of the PROVE study. Pacing Clin Electrophysiol 23:1891-1893
8. Israel CW, Lawo T (1999) Introduction to a new "X out of Y" mode-switching algorithm in Inos[2] CLS and Logos dual-chamber pacemakers. Prog Biomed Res 4:117-125
9. Israel CW (2001) Mode-switching algorithms: programming and usefulness. Herz. 26:2-17
10. Murgatroyd F, Nitzsche R, Slade AK et al (1994) A new pacing algorithm for overdrive suppression of atrial fibrillation. Pacing Clin Electrophysiol 17:1966-1973
11. Wiberg S, Lonnerholm S, Jensen S et al (2001) Effect of right atrial overdrive pacing on symptomatic attacks of atrial fibrillation: a multicenter study. Pacing Clin Electrophysiol 24:554 (abstr)
12. Anselme F, Saoudi N, Cribier A (2000) Pacing in prevention of atrial fibrillation: the PIPAF studies. J Int Card Electrophysiol 4:177-184
13. Hnatkova K, Waktare J, Murgatroyd F et al (1998) Analysis of the cardiac rhythm preceding episodes of paroxysmal atrial fibrillation. Am Heart J 135:1010-1019
14. Attuel P, Pelerin D, Mujica J et al (1988) DDD pacing: an effective treatment modality for recurrent atrial arrhythmias. Pacing Clin Electrophysiol 11:237-242
15. Roithinger F, Karch MR, Steiner PR et al (1999) The spatial dispersion of atrial refractoriness and atrial fibrillation vulnerability. J Int Card Electrophysiol 3:311-319
16. De Sisti A, Attuel P, Manot S et al (2000) Electrophysiological characteristics of the atrium in sinus node dysfunction with and without post pacing atrial fibrillation. Pacing Clin Electrophysiol 23:303-308

Which Patients with Atrial Fibrillation Benefit Most from Overdrive Pacing?

K.H. Konz*, I. Szendey, D. El Allaf, C. Gomes, P. Attuel and D. Danilovic on Behalf of the "Suppression of Atrial Fibrillation by Overdrive Pacing with Inos² CLS" Study Investigators

Introduction

A range of basically similar atrial overdrive pacing algorithms have been recently designed to prevent the onset of atrial tachyarrhythmia (AT) in patients with conventional indications for pacing [1-10]. These algorithms aim at achieving a high percentage of atrial pacing by a dynamic, slight overdrive of the sinus rhythm, without significantly increasing the mean atrial rate. The available literature indicates a high success of the overdrive algorithms in terms of reduced total AT burden in a portion of a patient cohort, while a considerable number of patients still see no benefit from such algorithms [2, 3, 11-13]. Current research is therefore focusing on identifying clinical predictors of success or failure of atrial overdrive pacing therapy.

In this article we utilize the available crossover data from the Suppression of Atrial Fibrillation by Overdrive Pacing With Inos² CLS trial to evaluate the predictive value of a range of clinical variables, in view of the success of the DDD+ mode (overdrive algorithm in Inos pacemakers) in the prevention of AT.

Methods and Results

A total of 101 patients with the history of paroxysmal AT and conventional indications for pacing were enrolled in the study. The patients received a bipolar atrial lead and an Inos² CLS or Inos² DR pacemaker (Biotronik, Germany). One to nine months after pacemaker implantation, the patients were randomized to DDD or DDD+ mode. In the DDD+ mode, sensing of an atrial event triggers pacing rate increase by the programmed overdrive step size (nominal value = 10 beats/min, range 1-32). If there are no sensed atrial events, the pacing rate is decreased by 1 beat/min after each overdrive plateau length (nominal value = 20 cycles, range 1-32 cycles). The mode crossover is scheduled for 6 months after mode randomization. Details of the

---

*Kliniken Maria Hilf, Med. Klinik II-Kardiologie, Mönchengladbach, Germany

DDD+ algorithm and study protocol have been published elsewhere [8,13].

To date, crossover data have been available in 41 patients followed for 164 ± 60 days in the DDD+ and 168 ± 61 days in the DDD mode [13]. DDD+ mode was associated with a reduced AT burden in 16 patients, in whom mean duration of the sustained AT was reduced from 3.0 ± 4.2 h/day (DDD) to 1.1 ± 2.7 h/day (DDD+). An increased AT burden with DDD+ pacing was seen in 13 patients: 1.3 ± 3.0 h/day (DDD) vs 2.7 ± 4.2 h/day (DDD+). Twelve patients had no AT after mode randomization. To distinguish responders from non-responders to DDD+ therapy, we applied the χ^2 goodness of fit test to a number of clinical variables (Table 1).

The expected values for the χ^2 test for the "DDD+ success" group and "DDD+ failure" group were calculated as the probabilities of 0.552 [= 16/(16 + 13)] and 0.448 [= 13/(16 + 13)] multiplied by the total occurrence of the

Table 1. Predictors for success or failure of DDD+ therapy*

Potential clinical predictor	DDD+ success (n = 16)		DDD+ failure (n = 13)		χ^2 test
	Parameter present in # of patients	Expected value for χ^2 test	Parameter present in # of patients	Expected value for χ^2 test	p
NYHA Class					
I	9	7.7	5	6.3	0.49
II	5	6.6	7	5.4	0.35
III	2	1.7	1	1.3	0.69
IV	0	0	0	0	-
Gender					
Male	9	8.8	7	7.2	0.93
Female	7	7.2	6	5.8	0.92
Age					
> 70 years	8	6.6	4	5.4	0.42
≤ 70 years	8	9.4	9	7.6	0.50
Drugs					
Class I antiarrhythmics	2	1.7	1	1.3	0.69
Class II antiarrhythmics[**]	3	7.2	10	5.8	0.02[**]
Class III antiarrhythmics	9	7.7	5	6.3	0.49
Class IV antiarrhythmics[**]	5	3.3	1	2.7	0.17[**]
ACE inhibitors[**]	2	3.9	5	3.1	0.16[**]
Nitrates	4	3.9	3	3.1	0.92
Other cardiac drugs	5	5.0	4	4.0	0.98
Electrode position[+]					
Right atrial appendage	9	8.8	7	7.2	0.93
High right atrium	1	0.6	0	0.4	0.37
Right lateral wall	4	4.4	4	3.6	0.77
Right anterior wall	0	0	0	0	-

Cont.

Cont. Table 1.

Potential clinical predictor	DDD+ success (n = 16)		DDD+ failure (n = 13)		χ^2 test
	Parameter present in # of patients	Expected value for χ^2 test	Parameter present in # of patients	Expected value for χ^2 test	$p =$
Conduction and heart disease					
Bradycardia	7	5.5	3	4.5	0.35
Sick-sinus syndrome	11	11.0	9	9.0	0.99
Brady-tachycardia	5	3.9	2	3.1	0.39
Atrioventricular block	5	4.4	3	3.6	0.68
Cardiomyopathy	1	2.2	3	1.8	0.22
Cardiac ischemia	4	3.9	3	3.1	0.92
Fibrosis of conduction system	2	1.7	1	1.3	0.69
Order of mode programming					
DDD first	10	10.5	9	8.5	0.82
DDD+ first	6	5.5	4	4.5	0.76
Progressive increase in AF time[**] [#]	1	2.8	4	2.2	0.11[**]

*The analysis involved data of 29 patients in whom there was a difference between results in DDD and DDD+ mode. **Currently most significant findings. +There is no information on electrode position in two patients in each group. #Patients with a progressive increase in the prevalence of atrial fibrillation (AF) between successive follow-up visits (i.e., AF progressively increased with time)

observed parameter in the "DDD+ success" and "DDD+ failure" groups, respectively. The χ^2 test was carried out separately for each parameter and was considered significant for p values < 0.05.

In this interim data analysis, only the use of Class II antiarrhythmics reached a significant predictive value for failure of atrial overdrive pacing to suppress AT. There was also a tendency for Class IV drugs to be associated with a successful DDD+ treatment, and for ACE inhibitors and a progressive increase in AT time to be associated with a less successful DDD+ treatment.

Discussion

Half-way through our prospective, randomized study, atrial overdrive pacing effectively decreased the AT burden in 39% of the patients, who had less AT in the DDD+ than in the DDD mode. An additional 29% of patients had no recurrence of atrial fibrillation (AF) in either pacing mode following mode randomization. The recently published data on the single-site AAI pacing from the right atrial appendage imply that a fixed overdrive stimulation at a rate 10-19 beats/min faster than the mean intrinsic atrial rate extracted from 24 h Holter ECGs may be equally, if not more, effective in the suppression of symptomatic AF episodes than overdrive pacing [14]. The authors, however, did not report on patient tolerance of the used basic pacing rates of 70-90 beats/min, which may be poorly tolerated during the night.

As in previous studies [11], we found no correlation between the success of overdrive pacing and clinical variables such as patient age, gender, NYHA functional class, atrial lead position, conduction disorders, concomitant heart disease, and the sequence of mode programming. Table 1 suggests, however, that the concomitant drug therapy may have better predictive value than other variables. In particular, Class II antiarrhythmic drugs were taken significantly more frequently by the patients in whom atrial overdrive pacing led to little clinical success ($p < 0.02$).

In 13 patients specified to use β-blockers in Table 1, the mean heart rate in the DDD mode was 67.8 beats/min, and 74.0 beats/min in the DDD+ mode ($p < 0.05$). These values did not significantly differ from the mean heart rates in 16 patients using no β-blockers: 65.8 beats/min in the DDD mode (p = ns compared with the DDD mode in the β-blocker group) and 70.7 beats/min in the DDD+ mode (p = ns compared with the DDD+ mode in the β-blocker group, $p < 0.05$ compared with the DDD mode in the no β-blocker group).

In almost all studies to date has the evaluation of AF prevalence been based on the diagnostic data collected in the pacemaker memory in relation to the mode-switching function. For correct pacemaker functioning and data interpretation, proper pacemaker sensing is of crucial importance. Far-field R wave sensing is a major factor influencing the risk of oversensing. In our study, the atrial sensitivity was typically programmed to 0.5 mV and the blanking period was 125 ms. By comparison, a 3% incidence of atrial oversensing was reported for the atrial sensitivity of 0.5 mV in patients in whom far-field R wave sensing from the right atrial appendage occurred at 117 ± 16 ms after the ventricular pacing stimulus [15]. Another study revealed a 9% incidence of far-field R wave sensing in conditions when atrial sensitivity and blanking time were programmed to 0.6 ± 0.2 mV and 127 ± 9 ms, respectively, and the (ventricular stimulus to far-field R wave sensing) coupling interval was 141 ± 10 ms [16].

A suboptimal pacing site might be another factor limiting the success of atrial overdrive pacing, although the AAI-mode overdrive pacing from the right atrial appendage did significantly reduce the incidence of symptomatic AF episodes [14]. It has been suggested that the degree of atrial tachyarrhythmia organization, rather than the cycle length, predicts the success of automatic atrial antitachycardia pacing [17]. Different pacing sites within the atrium, as well as dual-site atrial pacing, may significantly alter the total atrial activation time and the P wave duration. For instance, pacing from the Bachmann's bundle or coronary sinus ostium shortens the total atrial activation time compared with pacing from the high right atrium, whereas a major effect is attainable with dual-site pacing [18]. It is, however, not clear which pacing site is more beneficial in conjunction with hemodynamic alterations [18, 19].

A small but recognized group of patients in our study exhibited increasing AF prevalence over time. This may be explained by the results of the recent study that evaluated the influence of type (spontaneous or paced) and duration of atrioventricular delay on the incidence of AF, congestive heart failure and mortality, in patients with sick sinus syndrome [20]. The study showed that patients paced in the ventricle developed a significantly higher incidence of AF than those treated with AAI pacing.

Study Limitations

AF is a complex disease with no consensus with respect to classification and terminology used to characterize AF (syndromes). Most studies may therefore be a mixture of different entities.

The occurrence of AF episodes was assumed to coincide with the sustained (> 60 s) mode-switching episodes recorded in the pacemaker memory. This assumption relies on the adequate pacemaker sensing of AF. Cited studies [15, 16] indicated that atrial oversensing due to far-field R waves (the most frequent atrial sensing disturbance) is likely to occur in 3-9% of patients with parameters similar to those used in our study. Nevertheless, the presentation of crossover data should minimize any influence of atrial over- and undersensing on the comparative results for the two pacing modes.

This chapter has utilized data in 41 of 101 enrolled patients. The expected inflow of clinical results until the end of the study may override some of the present observations. In the final data analysis, currently insignificant improvements associated with DDD+ overdrive pacing in the total patient population may become significant, and additional clinical variables may be identified as having a significant predictive value of the success or failure of the therapy. Finally, a carry-over effect due to the sequence of mode programming may play an important role and will be evaluated.

Clinical Investigators: D. El Allaf (Huy, Belgium); K.H. Konz and I. Szendey (Mönchengladbach, Germany); J. Brachmann and V. Shibgilla (Coburg, Germany); P. Attuel (St. Cloude Cedex, France); C. Gomes (Taguatinga, Brazil); S. Löscher (Leipzig, Germany); C. John (Dresden, Germany); U. le Blanc, S. Rupp and M. Klutmann (Düren, Germany); T. Scheibner (Löbau, Germany); K. Malinowski (Aue, Germany); L. Griesbach (Kirchberg, Germany); H. Müller-Dieckert (Rochtliz, Germany); K. Göhl and C. Huber (Nuremberg, Germany); G. Lascault (St. Denis Cedex, France); R.U. York (Hartmannsdorf, Germany); T. Walter (Greiz, Germany); B. Hailer and H. Schäfer (Essen, Germany); D. Stockmann (Antwerpen, Belgium); S. Schüssler (Kaufbeuren, Germany).

References

1. Murgatroyd FD, Nitzsche R, Slade AK et al (1994) A new pacing algorithm for overdrive suppression of atrial fibrillation. Chorus Multicentre Study Group. Pacing Clin Electrophysiol 17:1966-1973
2. Garrigue S, Barold SS, Cazeau S et al (1998) Prevention of atrial arrhythmias during DDD pacing by atrial overdrive. Pacing Clin Electrophysiol 21:1751-1759

3. Israel CW (2000) Prevention of atrial tachyarrhythmias: promise of new pacing algorithms. Herzschrittmacher 20:8-11
4. Poezevara Y, Hümmer A, Lazarus A (2000) Dedicated therapeutic tools in the prevention of atrial arrhythmias by means of pacing. Herzschrittmacher 20:26-33
5. Begemann MJS, Boute W (2000) Novel preventive pacing algorithms aiming to stop atrial fibrillation from starting. Herzschrittmacher 20:47-58
6. Hess MF (2000) New device therapy for atrial tachyarrhythmias: the Medtronic AT500. Herzschrittmacher 20:68-75
7. Levine PA, Sperzel J, Florio J et al (2000) Device management of paroxysmal atrial fibrillation using the dynamic atrial overdrive algorithm. Herzschrittmacher 20:86-95
8. Attuel P (2000) Therapy and prevention of atrial fibrillation by overdrive stimulation? Herzschrittmacher 20:104-111
9. Klesius A, Simon A (2000) "Atrial Pacing Preference (APPTM)": a new pacing algorithm to reduce the incidence of atrial fibrillation. Herzschrittmacher 20:118-125
10. Funck RC, Pomsel K, Grimm W et al (2001) Prevention of atrial arrhythmias by pacing. Herz 26:18-29
11. Israel CW, Lawo T, Lemke B et al (2000) Atrial pacing in the prevention of paroxysmal atrial fibrillation: first results of a new combined algorithm. Pacing Clin Electrophysiol 23:1888-1890
12. Funck RC, Adamec R, Lurje L et al (2000) Atrial overdriving is beneficial in patients with atrial arrhythmias: first results of the PROVE study. Pacing Clin Electrophysiol pp 23:1891-1893
13. Attuel P, El Allaf D, Konz KH et al (2001) Is overdrive pacing useful for the prevention of paroxysmal atrial fibrillation? In: Raviele A (ed) Cardiac Arrhythmias 2001, Springer-Verlag Italia, Milan, pp 492-497
14. Wiberg S, Lonnerholm S, Jensen S et al (2001) Effect of right atrial overdrive pacing on symptomatic attacks of atrial fibrillation: a multicenter randomized study. Pacing Clin Electrophysiol 24(abstr):554
15. van Erven L, de Melker R, Schalij MJ (2001) Atrial antitachycardia algorithms: factors influencing the risk of oversensing. Pacing Clin Electrophysiol 24(abstr):566
16. Geraux L, Cazeau S, Mabo P (2001) True incidence of far-field R wave sensing during chronic DDD Pacing. Pacing Clin Electrophysiol 24(abstr):566
17. Israel CW, Ehrlich JR, Plock KC et al (2001). Degree of atrial tachyarrhythmia organization rather than cycle length predicts success of automatic atrial antitachycardia pacing. Pacing Clin Electrophysiol 24(abstr):555
18. Choe W, Rankovic V, Passman R et al (2001) Atrial pacing side alters atrial activation times: a comparison of 5 pacing locations. Pacing Clin Electrophysiol 24(abstr):645
19. von Dryander S, Lemke B, Deneke T et al (2001) Differences in hemodynamics in AAIR and DDDR pacing in sick sinus syndrome. Pacing Clin Electrophysiol 24(abstr):575
20. Andersen HR, Kristensen L, Nielsen JC et al (2001) Atrial versus dual chamber pacing in patients with sick sinus syndrome. Atrial fibrillation, congestive heart failure and mortality during follow-up in a randomized trial of 177 consecutive patients. Pacing Clin Electrophysiol 24(abstr):575

Brady-Tachy Syndrome: What Is the Best Pacing Technique To Reduce the Burden of Atrial Fibrillation?

P. Azzolini*, G. Altamura, F. Bacca, F. Capestro, P. Dini, G.B. Del Giudice, S. Favale, L. Pavia, G. Pettinati and A. Puglisi*

Introduction

Atrial fibrillation (AF) is the most common sustained cardiac arrhythmia with an incidence of 0.4%-1% in the total adult population, 3%-4% in people aged 55-65 years and up to 9%-13% in those older than 70 years [1, 2]. Patients with AF have about two-fold higher risk of death than patients without AF. Above all, AF increases the risk of stroke and thromboembolism: AF is responsible of 20% of strokes, with 5-7-fold higher risk than in patients in sinus rhythm, and the risk ratio is 12-17 when hypertension, heart failure, diabetes and mitral stenosis coexist with AF [3, 4]. Moreover, AF results in electrical remodeling of the heart, which favors the induction and maintenance of the arrhythmia [5].

In patients with brady-tachy syndrome, atrial and dual-chamber pacing have been associated with a lower incidence of recurrent paroxysmal AF, mainly when compared with ventricular pacing [6-8]. Several possible mechanisms have been proposed to explain these antiarrhythmic benefits: prevention of bradycardia-triggered tachycardias, reduced frequency of premature atrial complexes, short-long atrial cycle prevention, reduced dispersion of conduction and refractoriness, and maintenance of a high degree of exit block from all natural subsidiary atrial pacemakers [9]. Recently clinical studies have suggested an increased beneficial effect of biatrial synchronous pacing [10], dual-site atrial pacing [11], interatrial septum pacing [12], and overdrive pacing [13-16] to prevent recurrent AF.

The present study was designed to evaluate the effect of different overdrive pacing modalities in AF.

*Division of Cardiology, S. Giovanni Calibita Fatebenefratelli Hospital, Isola Tiberina, Rome, Italy

State-of-the-art of Overdrive Algorithms to Prevent Atrial Fibrillation

Up to now there have been several overdrive algorithms available that have the aim of increasing the percentage of atrial-paced events and decreasing spontaneous atrial events. All these algorithms can be grouped into two different approaches:

1. *Heart rate modulation.* This group includes all the electromechanical sensor-based rate-responsive pacing modes, in which atrial overdrive is achieved by heart rate modulation induced by sensor-detected activity.
2. *Overall heart rate overdrive.* This group includes all those algorithms designed to reduce the escape interval following each sensed event and increase it after a programmable number of paced events. Thus, these algorithms do not modulate heart rate, they simply allow the atrium to be paced close above the sinus rate. The atrial pacing percentage associated with this class of algorithms is about 95%.

Both these approaches lead to a significantly reduced number of AF recurrences in patients with brady-tachy syndrome. However, even if the second class of overdrive algorithms is associated with a higher pacing percentage, a significant difference of atrial tachycardia (AT)/AF episodes between these two groups has detected only in a subgroup of patients with low values of atrial pacing percentage with DDDR pacing [17]. This consideration may suggest that pacing percentage is not the only parameter to keep under control and that heart rate modulation probably plays an important role in the prevention of AF.

There is another kind of prevention algorithm that should be included in the first class and that is based on the changes in the autonomic nervous system. *Closed loop stimulation* (CLS) is available with the pacemaker Biotronik Inos^{2+}, which, detecting the contractility force variation through the relative change in endocardial impedance, may produce a more effective pacing overdrive directly related to sympathetic activity [18, 19].

Materials and Methods

Devices Description

Two different Biotronik pacemaker models are used in this study: Inos^{2+} and Philos DR. With the Inos^{2+}, the heart rate modulation is achieved by an automatic indirect analysis of cardiac contractility. The contractility force variation is detected by a relative slope changes of endocardial impedance curve, collected during the systolic phase of the cardiac cycle. Thus, heart rate modulation is related to autonomic nervous system activity. Biotronik Philos DR is a last generation pacemaker with atrial prevention therapies (DDD+ mode) and full diagnostic features for evaluation of atrial tachyarrhythmia episodes, including the *atrial detection recording* (ADR) feature, overall AT/AF duration, prematurity-based atrial extra systole (AES) classification, and AES distribution vs atrial rate. All these features can be used to study the mechanism of AT/AF onset and the effect of overdrive pacing. Moreover, the ADR feature, stores the atrial and ventricular 2EGM signals prior to mode switch activation, providing a tool for the discrimination of false-positive AT/AF episodes. In Fig. 1 we report an example of a false-positive episode, printed during 1 month follow-up of a patient enrolled in the study.

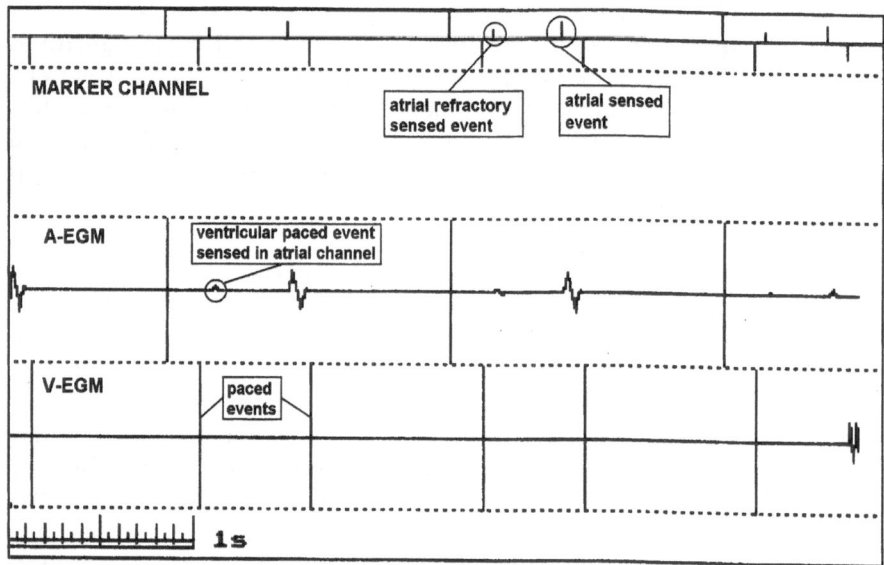

Fig. 1. A false-positive episode where atrial channel senses the ventricular paced event. This problem can be solved programming a longer *Far Field Blanking Period*

Study Design

This study is a randomized single-blind trial without crossover. Patients must meet the following requirements:

1. Patients must be indicated for the implant of a dual-chamber rate-responsive pacemaker system.
2. Patients with sick sinus syndrome (SSS) and brady-tachy syndrome (BTS) must have experienced at least one AT/AF episode during the last 3 months before implantation, which was not due to transient or reversible causes.

The *primary endpoint of the study* was to estimate the atrial pacing percentage and the AT/AF burden in patients with BTS, treated with conventional DDDR stimulation (accelerometer sensor), CLS stimulation and DDD+ mode, within 7 months after implant.

The *secondary study endpoint* is to verify any correlation between atrial pacing percentage and AT/AF burden with any of the following parameters: number of AESs; AES prematurity; AES distribution vs the mean atrial rate and the coupling interval between the first arrhythmic event and the last nonarrhythmic event.

Patients meeting the inclusion criteria were randomized into one of the following three arms: conventional DDDR stimulation group (control group); CLS stimulation; and DDD+ mode stimulation. Patients in the first and the third groups are implanted with the Biotronik Philos DR pacemaker system; patients in the second group are implanted with the Biotronik Inos^{2+} pacemaker system.

The standard procedure for any dual-chamber pacemaker implantation is followed. Moreover, three requirements have to be met: the atrial lead has to be bipolar to increase sensing performance; the atrial lead has to be positioned in the right atrial appendage; and the unfiltered bipolar sensing amplitude in atrium has to be ≥ 2 mV.

All patients are followed up 1, 4 and 7 months after implant. During the first month (system stabilization period), all pacemakers are programmed in DDD mode, with lower rate at 70 beats/min. At 1 month follow-up the programming requested by randomization is activated. Regular testing at follow-up visits are performed to evaluate the chronic performance of the Philos DR/ Inos^{2+} system, including pace/sense testing, pacing impedance, battery status, collection of the diagnostic data from the devices, and appropriateness of detection of spontaneous episodes logged by the systems.

Statistical Analysis and Study Dimension

Statistical comparisons among the atrial pacing percentages that will be obtained in the treatment arms of this ongoing study (DDDR, CLS, DDD+) will be performed through an F test. Due to the high atrial pacing percentage expected in the DDD+ arm, 150 patients are needed to observe a significant difference ($\alpha < 0.05$) among the mean atrial percentages observed in the three arms. A variance analysis between the atrial pacing percentage of the DDDR and CLS groups can be carried out using a t-test. A wide difference between these two groups is not expected. An absence of significance between DDDR and CLS will be considered to be a positive result of this trial.

Preliminary Results

Between February 2000 and April 2000 we enrolled 18 patients [4 male (22%) and 14 female (78%), mean age 70 ± 8 years]. Six patients were enrolled in the DDDR Group, seven in the DDD+ Group and five in the CLS Group. Six patients have been examined at 1 month follow-up. AF episodes were presented in 16 patients (84%), atrial flutter episodes in three patients (16%) and atrial tachycardia in four patients (21%). At implant the measured sensing was 3.2 ± 0.9 mV in the atrium and 13.9 ± 5.3 mV in the ventricle. The threshold and impedance values were, respectively, 0.7 ± 0.3 V and 642 ± 149 ohms (Ω) in the atrium and 0.4 ± 0.3 V and 794 ± 223 Ω in the ventricle. At predischarge follow-up the sensing, impedance and threshold values were similar to those obtained at implant.

Conclusions

Up to now the number of enrolled patients and the data collected have been too sparse to obtain any relevant results. One of the problems generally met in previous studies of AT/AF pacing prevention was the great number of false-positive episodes detected, due to oversensing and/or far-field detection in the atrial sensing channel of the pacemaker. This was due to the use of a detection algorithm with a low specificity (e.g. mode switch), without diagnostic features discriminating true AT/AF episodes from false ones. From this study we will be able to recognize false-positive episodes and calculate their incidence factor that we can use during data analysis. Moreover, using the Philos DR diagnostic function we will obtain further information about paroxysmal atrial episode onset and particularly about induction during spontaneous or paced rhythm, or during slow or fast atrial rhythm, and about the number and the behavior of premature atrial complexes before paroxysmal atrial fibrillation onset.

Centers participating in the study: Dr. G. Pettinati, Dr. D. Melissano - Ospedale F. Ferrari, Casarano (LE); Prof. F. Bacca, Dr. V. De Giorgi - Ospedale V. Fazzi, Lecce; Dr. A. Puglisi, Dr. P. Azzolini - Ospedale S. Giovanni Calibita Fatebenefratelli, Isola Tiberina, Roma; Dr. F. Capestro, Dr. P. Scipioni - Ospedale Cardiologico Lancisi, Ancona; Dr. G.B. Del Giudice - Ospedale S. Giovanni Addolorata, Roma; Dr. L. Pavia - Ospedale Piemonte, Messina; Dr. R. Quaglione - Policlinico Umberto I, Roma; Prof. G. Altamura, Dr. F. Biscione - Ospedale S. Giacomo, Roma; Prof. B. Castaldi - Ospedale F. Veneziale, Isernia; Dr. A. Mori - Ospedale E. Profili, Fabriano (AN); Prof. S. Favale – Policlinico Consorziale di Bari; Dr. P. Capone, Dr. P. Paoloni - Ospedale Civile di Fermo (AP); Dr. S. Rapino - Aurelia Hospital, Roma; Dr. P. Santarelli – Clinica Columbus, Roma.

References

1. Murgatroyd FD, Camm AJ (1995) Atrial fibrillation for the clinician. Futura, Mount Kisco, NY, pp 67-82, 97-98
2. Lang V, Bieberle T, Danilovic D (1999) Prevention of atrial tachyarrhythmias by cardiac pacing. Progr Biomed Res 5:504-512
3. Waktare JEP, Camm AJ (1997) Atrial fibrillation begets trouble. Heart 77:393-394
4. Wolf PA, Dawber TR, Thomas HE el al (1978) Epidemiologic assessment of chronic atrial fibrillation and risk of stroke: the Framinghan Study. Neurology 28:973-977

5. Franz MR, Karasik PL, Li C, et al (1997) Electrical remodeling of the human atrium: similar effects in patients with chronic atrial fibrillation and atrial flutter. J Am Coll Cardiol 30:1785-1792

6. Barold SS, Santini M (1993) Natural history of sick sinus syndrome after pacemaker implantation. In: Barold SS, Mugica J (eds) New perspectives in cardiac pacing, 3. Futura, Mount Kisco, NY, pp 169-211

7. Santini M, Ricci R, Puglisi A et al (1997) Long-term haemodynamic and antiarrhythmic benefits of DDIR versus DDI pacing mode in sick sinus syndrome and chronotropic incompetence. G Ital Cardiol 27:892-900

8. Andersen HR, Nielsen JC, Thomsen PEB et al (1997) Long-term follow-up of patients from a randomised trial of atrial versus ventricular pacing for sick-sinus syndrome. Lancet 350:1210-1216

9. Schoels W, Becker R (1998) Mechanisms of pacing interventions in atrial fibrillation. J Cardiovasc Electrophysiol 9[Suppl 8]:S13-S17

10. Daubert C, Mabo B, Berder V (1990) Arrhythmia prevention by permanent atrial resynchronization in advanced interatrial block. Eur Heart J 11:233-242

11. Saksena S, Prakash A, Hill M (1996) Prevention of recurrent atrial fibrillation with chronic dual site right atrial pacing. J Am Coll Cardiol 28:687-694

12. Padeletti L, Porciani MC, Michelucci A et al (1999) Interatrial septum pacing: a new approach to prevent recurrent atrial fibrillation. J Intervent Cardiac Electrophysiol 3:35-43

13. Garrigue S, Barold S, Cazeau S et al (1998) Prevention of atrial arrhythmias during DDD pacing by atrial overdrive. Pacing Clin Electrophysiol 21:1751-1759

14. Levy T, Walker S, Rochelle J, Paul V (1999) Evaluation of biatrial pacing, right atrial pacing, and no pacing in patients with drug refractory atrial fibrillation. Am J Cardiol 84:426-429

15. Ricci R, Azzolini P, Puglisi A et al (1998) Consistent atrial pacing: can this new algorithm suppress recurrent paroxysmal atrial fibrillation? G Ital Cardiol 28[Suppl 1]:115-118

16. Bellocci F, Spampinato A, Ricci R et al (1999) Antiarrhythmic benefits of dual chamber stimulation with rate-response in patients with paroxysmal atrial fibrillation and chronotropic incompetence. A prospective multicentre study. Europace 1:220-225

17. Ricci R, Santini M, Puglisi A et al (2001) Impact of consistent atrial pacing algorithm on premature atrial complexe number and paroxysmal atrial fibrillation recurrences in brady-tachy syndrome: a randomized prospective crossover study. J Intervent Cardiac Electrophysiol 5:35-46

18. Schaldach M, Hutten H (1992) Intracardiac impedance to determine sympathetic activity in rate-responsive pacing. Pacing Clin Electrophysiol 15(II):1778-1786

19. Attuel P, Pellerin D, Mugica J et al (1988) DDD pacing: an effective treatment modality for recurrent atrial arrhythmias. Pacing Clin Electrophysiol 11:237-242

Patients with Paroxysmal Atrial Fibrillation Undergoing "Ablate and Pace" Therapy: Is Prevention of Arrhythmic Recurrences Possible by Combined Overdrive and Biatrial Pacing?

D. IGIDBASHIAN

Paroxysmal atrial fibrillation (PAF) is one of the most common forms of arrhythmia and represents an important management problem [1] because of the usually alarming onset of symptoms, the disability these produce, the possibility of thromboembolic complications, and the often unsatisfactory results, or even undesirable effects [2], of drug therapy. The symptoms, especially in the setting of an underlying heart disease, significantly reduce the quality of life (QOL) of a large number of patients.

It has been estimated that 1.6%-2% of the general population has atrial fibrillation (AF), and that 40% of these have PAF. Approximately 12% of the latter group, corresponding to about 396 000 patients (216 000 > 65) of the European population, have severely symptomatic PAF that is refractory to multiple antiarrhythmic drug therapy [3]. This last group is the patient population toward which particular attention is directed to find ways and means to prevent or reduce the burden of this debilitating arrhythmia.

The onset of the arrhythmia implies the presence of triggers that induce AF, besides a substrate that sustains it, since triggers alone, without contributing factors, do not cause AF. Triggers may include atrial premature beats (APB) or tachycardia, bradycardia, sympathetic or parasympathetic stimulation, accessory atrioventricular pathways, and acute atrial stretch [4]. Ectopic activity originating from the pulmonary veins has been identified as a trigger at the origin of a very large percentage of PAF manifestations [5, 6]. The ectopic activities seem to originate from "sleeves" of atrial tissue extending into these veins.

Triggers propagating into the atria may initiate reentering wavelets, if the wavelength is sufficiently short. This can occur even in normal atria if the effective refractory period (ERP) or conduction velocity is decreased. Persistence of AF may result from structural and electrical remodelling, which is characterized by atrial dilatation and its shortening of ERP [4].

PAF has a tendency to evolve to progressively longer periods of generally non-self-terminating AF. While it initially responds to pharmacological or electrical cardioversion, with time, it usually tends to become resistant to these.

Electrophysiology Section, Cardiovascular Department, AULSS 21, Legnago Hospital, Italy

Otherwise, prompt cardioversion reduces the time patients remain in AF and increases the interval between recurrences. Rapid restoration of sinus rhythm could thus forestall progressive remodelling and the increase in frequency and duration of the AF episodes [4]. For this reason, prevention of PAF and/or its prompt resolution is of particular clinical importance.

Measures directed at the prevention, control, and "cure" of AF or PAF should where possible take into careful account the reason(s) underlying this extremely frequent arrhythmia, which is often an expression of different disease processes. Nevertheless, in approximately half of the patients presenting with PAF, no obvious clinical cause is found (lone or idiopathic PAF).

Aside from pharmacological treatment, several options have been proposed and put into practice, starting with atrioventricular (AV) junction ablation combined with implantation of a pacemaker, a treatment introduced almost 20 years ago [7]. These options can essentially be summarized as measures to prevent PAF, measures to control ventricular rate, measures to modify the substrate maintaining AF, and measures to eliminate the initiating trigger. The first two include the use of a pacemaker, while the last are currently performed by radio frequency (RF) ablation. Among the preceding, atrial pacing (AP), atrial overdrive pacing, and biatrial (BiA) pacing (single or dual site) have been proposed and used to prevent the recurrence of AF, suppressing triggers and modifying the electrophysiologic substrate.

The idea of a completely nonpharmacological therapy has been, at least in part, demonstrated to be insufficient to abolish or reduce AF recurrences alone [8]. The curative therapies, such as the Maze surgical procedure and RF atrial ablation, are nevertheless performed with this primary objective, but despite the promising results obtained by these techniques, they have to be combined with antiarrhythmic drug therapy, in a substantial number of patients undergoing these procedures if preventive/curative effects on PAF are to be obtained [9-11].

Based on the observation by Haïsaguerre et al. that "virtually 100% of PAF – with or without ectopy, with or without structural heart disease – have focal origins that can be targeted for ablation" and that "these foci have a characteristically predominant anatomic location in the pulmonary veins" [11], RF ablation of the pulmonary veins is being gradually accepted as the method of choice for the treatment of drug-refractory PAF [9-11]. However, in spite of the enthusiasm generated by this curative treatment, the current technical difficulties related to the technique, the length of the procedure, and the possible complications, besides the recurrence of the arrhythmia in a small percentage of cases [12], have limited the use of these methods to a few specialized and well-equipped centres.

Despite the accurate statement by Haïsaguerre et al. that "this curative approach is clearly superior to AV junction ablation" [5], the latter procedure, currently called "ablate and pace", has demonstrated great clinical efficacy in the past few years. It is essentially a palliative treatment, unable to eliminate the electrophysiologic substrate of the disease, that acts indirectly through control of the irregular and fast ventricular rate. In doing, it virtually abolishes palpitations, the most specific and troublesome symptom of PAF, in over 80% of the patients [3]. It also noticeably reduces other symptoms associated with PAF, such as effort dyspnea, exercise intolerance, and easy physical exhaustion, besides significantly improving the QOL scores [3]. These findings, documented by several uncontrolled studies and by two randomized controlled trials [8, 13], explain why this technique has been widely adopted. Thus, the typical candidate for "ablate and pace" appears to be an elderly patient with frequently recurring, highly symptomatic, multiple-drug-resistant PAF, experiencing a significative limitation of QOL and in whom the "curative" therapies are not feasible or desirable or have not succeeded.

Further clinical benefit can be obtained from this method by combining it with currently available pacing techniques and/or algorithms aimed at prevention of AF or the reduction of the AF burden. Pacing-based treatments, with the objective of preserving or restoring sinus rhythm, include atrial supported pacing modes (AAI/DDD), AP with an elevated basic rate, dynamic overdrive pacing, interatrial septum pacing, and dual right AP and BiA or multisite pacing. The role of these measures in AF control is, however, still under investigation.

Several studies have suggested a decreased frequency of AF recurrences during long-term AP in patients with sick sinus syndrome (SSS) compared with ventricular-based therapy [14]. Likewise, right AP at relatively rapid rates (80-90 bpm) in patients with AF and SSS prolonged the time to the first AF recurrence [15].

Except for bradycardia-dependent AF, there is uncertainty regarding the mechanism(s) of the possible preventive effects of antibradycardia pacing. Bradycardia may favor the emergence of ectopic activity, which can trigger intra-atrial reentry. Longer refractory periods associated with slow heart rates may additionally contribute to the occurrence of regional conduction block and conduction delay in response to a premature beat. Furthermore, there appears to be an inverse relation between heart rate and atrial refractoriness.

Although overdrive pacing, either permanent or dynamic, with minimum increments of atrial overdrive after premature atrial complexes (PACs), reduces the incidence of APBs [16], there is no clear evidence that this contributes significantly to preventing AF. A recent study comparing DDDR stimulation with and without a consistent atrial pacing (CAP) algorithm showed a significant reduction in PACs and a significant increase in atrial paced beats, without an undue increase in atrial rate, but also without any difference in mode switch (MS) activation [17]. This latter observation is confirmed by a previous paper and a similar personal experience.

Conversely, the preliminary results of an ongoing prospective study (PROVE) on the effectiveness of atrial overdrive pacing combined with an automatic rest rate function algorithm showed a 34% reduction of MS episodes and a 48% shortening of overall duration of the episodes by overdrive pacing [18]. Likewise, dynamic overdrive pacing after coronary bypass surgery significantly reduced AF [19]. Nevertheless, other studies [20, 21] and prospective investigations by Gillis et al. to evaluate the possible beneficial effects of atrial rate-adaptive pacing (ensuring AP most of the time) on the time of first AF recurrence, on the reduction of the recurrence, and on the AF burden did not meet expectations [22, 23].

Lastly, a recent prospective evaluation using three simultaneously active algorithms for prevention of atrial tachyarrhythmia (AT) reduced the number of arrhythmia episodes per patient per day but without reducing the time during which the patients remained in AT [24]. Therefore, the overall impact of overdrive pacing on AF prevention appears at least disputed.

The notion that spatial dispersion of atrial refractoriness and/or conduction, and that the presence of APBs favors the initiation of atrial arrhythmias, led to the development of synchronous BiA pacing by Daubert et al. [25] in 1989, with the intent of reducing these. This consisted in fixing a right atrial lead in the high right atrium (HRA) and a second lead positioned in the coronary sinus (CS), either proximal, mid or distal, in order to detect and pace the left atrium (LA). With a similar intent, Saksena et al. adopted a dual-site right AP technique some years later [26], which consisted in screwing the second lead near the ostium of the CS, in the posterior part of the triangle of Koch, a zone crucial to the genesis of arrhythmias. Simultaneous activation of both atria was also obtained by pacing through a right atrial lead screwed to the anterior interatrial septum [27].

Moreover, pacing at the distal CS level appeared to suppress the propensity of right atrial extrasystoles to induce AF, by limiting their precocity at the posterior part of Koch's triangle and by probably blocking microreentries [28].

It therefore appears that BiA or multisite atrial pacing probably contributes to preventing arrhythmia by correcting asynchrony and nonuniform activation (resulting from organic or functional conduction blocks), and by the possibility of preventing macroreentry occurrence. Compared with spontaneous sinus rhythm and single-site right atrial pacing, this technique reduces the P wave duration and the activation delay of the crista terminalis region and of the CS ostium.

Daubert et al. reported that 64% of their patients with drug-refractory AT and intra-atrial conduction delay who were treated with BiA synchronous pacing remained in sinus rhythm at the end of the follow-up, taking a significantly reduced number of antiarrhythmic drugs [29]. Likewise, dual-site right atrial pacing combined with pharmacological therapy in unselected patients with previously drug-refractory atrial flutter and fibrillation also significantly increased the proportion of patients free of AF recurrence to 89% [15]. Furthermore, Leclercq et al. demonstrated the superior efficacy of dual- versus single-site AP in modifying the natural history of patients with prolonged P wave and sinus node dysfunction [30].

Finally, preliminary results of the ongoing DRAPPAF study, comparing recurrences of AF during dual- and single-site right AP, showed a similar arrhythmia-free interval in both groups, but a significantly lower incidence of electrical cardioversions in those crossing over to from single- to dual-site pacing [31].

Despite some reports not in accord with this [32], the results obtained with BiA or multisite atrial pacing have been generally favorable in both selected and unselected patients. The possibility of testing the additive beneficial electrophysiologic effects of this pacing technique combined with an overdrive algorithm on a well-defined group of patients, is particularly challenging and might offer new insights. A recently proposed European multicentre, prospective, randomized, single-blinded, crossover study offers this opportunity in a selected group of patients. The study, to be started soon, called MISSION (an acronym for multisite stimulation for prevention of atrial arrhythmias [33]), will evaluate the effects of a combination of BiA and overdrive pacing in patients with an interatrial conduction defect (P > 120 ms), recurrent drug-refractory atrial tachyarrhythmias and a cardiac pacing indication. This study explicitly requires drug refractoriness, even to amiodarone. Conversely, exclusion criteria include conditions such as hyperthyroidism, severe valvular insufficiency, presence of a high number of PABs, and indications for other elective therapies, such as focal ablation, holiday heart syndrome, etc.

The possibility of testing this pacing-based therapy in patients presenting with highly symptomatic, drug-refractory, frequently recurrent PAF, with an indication for AV junction ablation, as an arm of MISSION, appears quite rational and stimulating. In these patients, in whom pharmacological antiarrhythmic treatment will be maintained, BiA stimulation with and without the overdrive algorithm and standard DDDR pacing will be compared. This aggregate should permit the maximum clinical benefit possible in this group of highly selected PAF patients while still keeping them free of palpitations and therefore virtually asymptomatic.

Utilising the diagnostic features of the dedicated pulse generator (PG), additional information regarding the arrhythmia and its onset may be obtained and may permit, where possible, optimization of the pacing functions available. BiA stimulation, to obtain synchronized pacing of both atrial chambers, will use a new trichamber PG (model Triplos LA) developed by Biotronik. This will be connected to a standard right atrial lead, located in the HRA or atrial appendage, in combination with a specially designed CS lead (Biotronik, model Corox LA) for pacing the LA. BiA sensing will use dipoles between the distal ring electrode of the CS and the tip electrode of the HRA versus the proximal RA ring electrode or the distal HRA and CS electrodes versus the PM case. BiA stimulation will be obtained with a circuit closed, between the distal CS and RA tip electrodes and the RA ring electrode. The DDT_A mode will be used to facilitate the prevention of AF through permanent synchronization of both atria. The DDT_A+ mode, in this PG, combines atrial synchronization with an overdrive algorithm that follows the spontaneous rhythm, slightly increasing the basic rate and following it. The standard DDD_AR will shall act as a control for the above two modes. The features of synchronous BiA pacing will include BiA stimulation after BiA sensing besides synchronization after RA and LA PACs. The PG has special statistical storing capabilities which will help to keep track of the arrhythmia detection recordings (ADR), the date and time of episodes, event markers and intracardiac electrogram (IEGM) (up to 40 cycles before onset), the number and duration of MS activation, PAC counter, etc. This type of diagnostics will make it possible to quantify the AF burden on the basis of the number and cumulative duration of AF episodes, calculated from all MS episodes.

A preliminary clinical evaluation will be performed to confirm the inclusion criteria and the collection of the following data: history and number of AF episodes, surface ECG P wave duration, Holter ECG, echocardiogram (diameter of LA and LV, LVEF), presence and severity of heart disease and any previous thromboembolic events, NYHA class, QOL questionnaire (SF 36 + specific symptoms) [34], and laboratory test results (TSH/T3/T4).

Stable antiarrhythmic medication will be favored. If changes are made in the drug regimen, exact documentation of the rationale will be required. Failure, contraindication or refusal of amiodarone must be reported. In the case that this drug is withdrawn, a 100-day washout period should pass before randomization.

Implantation of the above-mentioned system and AV junction ablation will be performed at this point. The lead locations in the HRA and CS will depend on the adequacy of the electrical parameters. Furthermore, at implantation, a study of the spread of atrial excitation will be performed. Conduction time at sinus rate and higher stimulated rates – up to 10 bpm less than the Wenkebach rate – between RA and LA and vice versa will be recorded. P wave duration during sinus rhythm, RA and BiA pacing on the surface ECG will also be recorded. Finally, the electrical characteristics will be registered and the lead positions documented in a biplanar fashion.

After a run-in period of 1 month, with the PG programmed in the standard DDDR mode in all the patients, during the first follow-up, patients will be randomized to:
-   A group with the PG programmed in the BiA-DDT$_A$ mode,
-   A group with the PG programmed in the BiA-DDT$_A$+ mode, or
-   A control group remaining with the PG programmed in BiA-DDDR mode.

The PG rate setting will be base rate 60 bpm with repetitive hysteresis at 40 bpm. Later, at the second and third follow-ups (respectively at the third and fifth months after implantation), the above PG programs will be crossed over (Fig.1, left).

Follow-ups will be performed at 1, 3, 5 and 7 months, according to the study flow chart (Fig.1, right). At each follow-up the following will be checked: PG interrogation; electrical characteristics; current medication; surface ECG P wave duration during sinus rhythm, RA, and BiA pacing respectively; interatrial conduction time RA - LA (CS); RA and LA signal amplitudes and amplitudes of the "cross-sensed" R-wave; echocardiogram (diameter LA and LV, LVEF); NYHA functional class; thromboembolic events; QOL questionnaire.

The primary endpoint of the study will be the cumulative duration of AF, on the basis of the MS function. The study hypothesis is that the cumulative duration of AF under BiA overdrive stimulation will be shorter intra-individually than with the BiA pacing alone or with the control pacing mode. Secondary endpoints will be the number of AF episodes, QOL, NYHA functional class, progress of heart failure, and changes in the pharmacological therapy.

Because of the rather stringent inclusion criteria, the number of patients expected to be enrolled is low.

On the basis of previous studies the hypothesis is that BiA stimulation may reduce the AF burden by up to 50% in the patient population considered eligi-

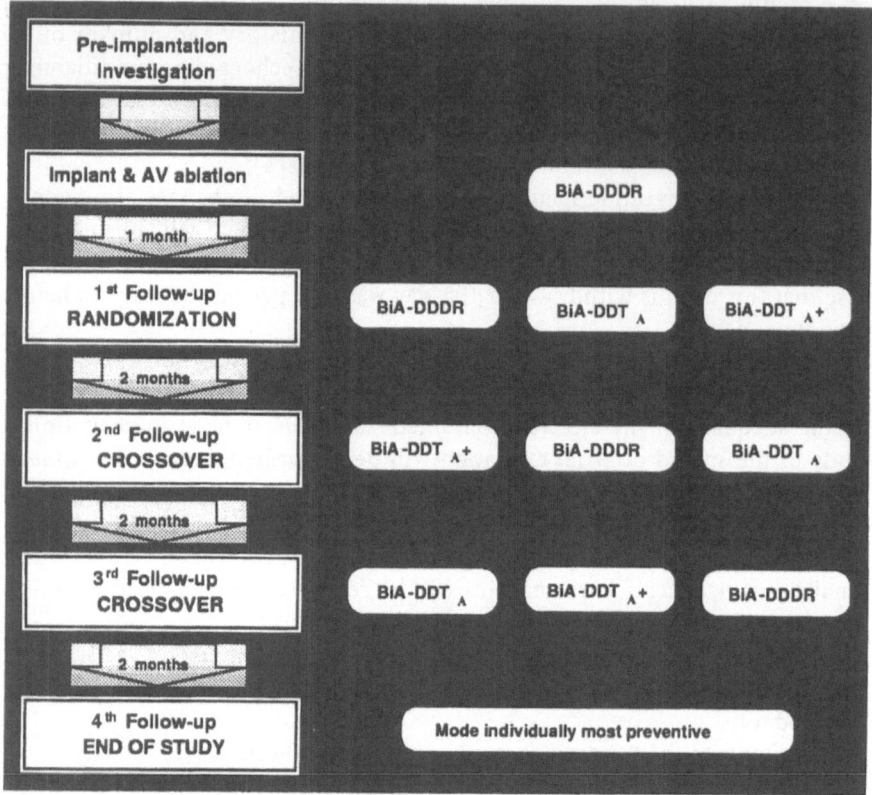

Fig. 1. Follow-up sequence (*left*) and crossover PG mode programming (*right*) in the three groups of patients participating the "ablate and pace" arm of the European MISSION trial. For explanation of programmed modes, see text

ble for the study. The expectation is also to be able to specify more clearly the additional potential benefits of synchronised BiA plus overdrive pacing in this well-defined and observed patient cohort.

In conclusion, the search for a reasonably safe cure for AF as a whole is still out of reach and may remain so indefinitely. The nearest to this goal the scientific community has reached, with promising results in a large percentage of patients, is anatomical ablation and/or modification of the triggering mechanism at its site of origin and/or of the substrate sustaining the arrhythmia. However attractive all that may seem, these procedures do not resolve all problems and in some cases can create new ones.

Nonpharmacological, pacing-based therapies have been and are being implemented with some success, especially in selected groups of patients and/or selected electrophysiologic situations. Among these pacing-based therapies, "ablate and pace", a palliative treatment, has demonstrated its efficacy in significantly reducing symptoms and improving QOL.

In patients with highly symptomatic drug-refractory PAF, in whom "curative" therapies are not feasible, or desirable or have not succeeded, the possibility of combining AV junction ablation and innovative pacing techniques may become particularly useful clinically. The possibility of combining this further with atrial and/or ventricular multisite cardiac stimulation and pacing algorithms to prevent or reduce PAF can maximize the clinical benefits which may be obtained by preserving sinus rhythm or reducing the burden of the arrhythmic bouts.

A prospective, randomized, European multicenter study called MISSION [33], to be started soon, offers the possibility of an arm of the trial dedicated to evaluating the AF burden reduction in this particular subset of patients, in whom "ablate and pace" will be combined with BiA and overdrive pacing.

References

1. Wolf PA, Abbott RD, Kannel WB (1991) Atrial fibrillation as an independent risk factor for stroke: the Framingham study. Stroke 22:983-988
2. Flaker GC, Blackshear JL, McBride R (1992) Antiarrhythmic drug therapy and cardiac mortality in atrial fibrillation. J Am Coll Cardiol 20:527-532
3. Brignole M (2000) Ablate and pace. Am J Cardiol 86[Suppl]:4K-8K
4. Alessie MA, Boyden PA, Camm J et al (2001) Pathophysiology and prevention of atrial fibrillation. Circulation 103:769-777
5. Haïsaguerre M, Jaïs P, Shah DC et al (1998) Spontaneous initiation of atrial fibrillation by ectopic beats originating in the pulmonary veins. N Engl J Med 339:659-666
6. Chen SA, Hsieh MH, Tai CT et al (1999) Initiation of atrial fibrillation by ectopic beats originating from the pulmonary veins. Circulation 100:1879-1886
7. Scheinmann MM, Morady F, Hess DS, Gonzalez R (1982) Catheter induced ablation of the atrioventricular junction to control refractory supraventricular arrhythmias. JAMA 248:851-855
8. Brignole M, Gianfranchi L, Menozzi C et al (1997) Assessment of atrioventricular junction ablation and DDDR mode-switching pacemaker versus pharmacological treatment in patients with severely symptomatic paroxysmal atrial fibrillation: a randomized controlled study. Circulation 96:2617-2624
9. Pappone C, Rosanio S, Oreto G et al (2000) Circumferential radiofrequency ablation of pulmonary vein ostia: a new anatomical approach for curing atrial fibrillation. Circulation 102:2619-2628
10. Haïsaguerre M, Shah DC, Jaïs P et al (2000) Mapping-guided ablation of pulmonary veins to cure atrial fibrillation. Am J Cardiol 86[Suppl]:9K-19K
11. Haïsaguerre M, Jaïs P, Shah DC et al (2000) Electrophysiologic end point for catheter ablation of atrial fibrillation initiated from multiple pulmonary venous foci. Circulation 101:1409-1417
12. Wellens HJJ (2000) Pulmonary vein ablation in atrial fibrillation. Hype or hope. Circulation 102:2562-2564
13. Marshall H, Harris Z, Griffith M et al (1999) Prospective randomized study of ablation and pacing versus medical therapy for paroxysmal atrial fibrillation: effects of pacing mode and mode-switch algorithm. Circulation 99:1587-1592
14. Andersen HR, Nielsen JC, Thomsen PE et al (1997) Long-term follow-up of patients from a randomised trial of atrial versus ventricular pacing therapy for sick sinus syndrome. Lancet 305:1210-1216

15. Delfaut P, Saksena S, Prakash A, Krol RB (1998) Long-term outcome of patients with drug refractory atrial flutter and fibrillation after single- and dual-site right atrial pacing for arrhythmia prevention. J Am Coll Cardiol 32:1900-1908

16. Garrigue S, Barold SS, Cazeau S et al (1998) Prevention of atrial fibrillation during DDD pacing by atrial overdrive. Pacing Clin Electrophysiol 21:1751-1759

17. Lam CT, Lau CP, Leung SK et al (2000) Efficacy and tolerability of continuous overdrive atrial pacing in atrial fibrillation. Europace 2:286-289

18. Funck RC, Adamaec R, Lurje L et al (1998) Atrial overdriving is beneficial in patients with atrial arrhythmias: first results of the PROVE study. Pacing Clin Electrophysiol 21:1751-1759

19. Blommaert D, Gonzalez M, Mucumbitsi J et al (2000) Effective prevention of atrial fibrillation by continuous atrial overdrive pacing after coronary artery bypass surgery. J Am Coll Cardiol 35:1411-1415

20. Igidbashian D, Mazzone P, Rillo M et al (1998) Dual chamber pacemaker in patients with atrial fibrillation submitted for ablation of the atrio-ventricular junction. G Ital Cardiol 28[Suppl 1]:322-325

21. Levy T, Walker S, Rex S, Paul V (2000) Does atrial overdrive prevent paroxysmal atrial fibrillation in paced patients? Int J Cardiol 75:91-97

22. Gillis AM, Wyse DG, Connolly SJ et al (1999) Atrial pacing periablation for prevention of paroxysmal atrial fibrillation. Circulation 99:2553-2558

23. Gillis AM, Connolly SJ, Lacombe P et al for PA3 Study Investigators (2000) Randomized crossover comparison of DDDR versus VDD pacing after atrioventricular junction ablation for prevention of atrial fibrillation. Circulation 102:736-741

24. Israel CW, Lawo T, Lemke B et al (2000) Atrial pacing in the prevention of paroxysmal atrial fibrillation: first results of a new combined algorithm. Pacing Clin Electrophysiol 23:1888-1890

25. Daubert JC, Mabo P, Berder V, Paillard P (1990) Arrhythmia prevention by permanent atrial resynchronization in patients with advanced interatrial block. Eur Heart J 11:237

26. Saksena S, Prakash A, Hill M et al (1996) Prevention of recurrent atrial fibrillation with chronic dual-site right atrial pacing. J Am Coll Cardiol 28:687-694

27. Spencer WH, Zhu D, Markowitz T et al (1997) Atrial septal pacing: a method for pacing both atria simultaneously. Pacing Clin Electrophysiol 20:2739-2745

28. Papageorgiu P, Anselme F, Kirchhof CJ et al (1997) Coronary sinus pacing prevents induction of atrial fibrillation. Circulation 96:1893-1898

29. D'Allonnes GR, Pavin D, Leclercq C et al (2000) Long-term effects of synchronous pacing to prevent drug-refractory atrial tachyarrhythmia: a nine year experience. J Cardiovasc Electrophysiol 11:1081-1091

30. Leclercq JF, De Sisti A, Fiorello P et al (2000) Is dual site better than single site atrial pacing in the prevention of atrial fibrillation? Pacing Clin Electrophysiol 23:2101-2107

31. Ramdat Misier AR, Beukema WP, Oude Luttikhuis HA, Willems R (2000) Multisite atrial pacing: an option for atrial fibrillation prevention? Preliminary results of the Dutch dual site right atrial pacing for prevention of atrial fibrillation study. Am J Cardiol 80[Suppl]:20K-24K

32. Mabo P, Paul V, Clémenty J et al (1999) Biatrial synchronous pacing for atrial arrhythmia prevention: The SYMBIAPACE Study. Eur Heart J 20:4

33. Igidbashian D on behalf of the MISSION steering committee (2000) Multisite stimulation for prevention of atrial arrhythmias. Europace 2[Suppl A]:A71

34. Linde C (1996) How to evaluate quality-of-life in pacemaker patients: problems and pitfalls. Pacing Clin Electrophysiol 19:391-397

ICD Patients: What Is the Efficacy of Early Activation of Atrial ATP Therapies in Atrial Fibrillation Termination?

M. Santini*, G. Altamura, S. Favale, P.L. Padeletti, P.A. Ravazzi and G. Biancalana

Background

Atrial fibrillation (AF)/atrial tachycardia (AT) is one of the most common arrhythmias. It has been reported that a relevant percentage of patients implanted with implantable cardioverter defibrillators (ICDs) have atrial tachyarrhythmias at the time of implant [1]. One of the most interesting results of the recently available atrial-ventricular dual-chamber ICD clinical investigations is the significantly high success rate of automatic atrial anti-tachy-pacing (ATP) therapies in AF/AT termination: atrial bursts, ramps and high frequency bursts (50 Hz bursts) successfully terminated 68% of the device-detected atrial episodes [2-4] in patients with an indication for ventricular ICD. In spite of the considerably high AF/AT termination rate, no significant reduction was observed in terms of AF/AT burden or mean duration of AF/AT episodes. A possible explanation of these surprising data may relate to no limit being imposed on the ATP intervention delay from the episode onset.

Currently, it is not known whether early delivery of atrial ATP therapies can reduce the overall duration of atrial episodes and/or increase the success rate of episode termination. A specific trial is therefore needed to measure the mean duration reduction of atrial tachyarrhythmic episodes and the successful termination rate of atrial ATP therapies, when ATP therapies are delivered with no delay from the atrial episode onset. Such an investigation should clarify the clinical meaning of the encouraging results obtained about the ATP success rate during the first clinical experiences. The Biotronik Tachos DR active housing is the only implantable, automatic tachyarrhythmia control device that makes it possible to choose the intervention delay from the atrial episode onset, through an atrial beat-to-beat control counter, thus providing very early atrial therapies activation (see Fig. 1). This device can therefore usefully represent an optimal tool to investigate whether early atrial therapies can reduce the mean duration of the AF/AT episodes. The objectives, methods and design of a starting multicenter trial on the clinical efficacy of early activation of atrial ATP therapies are summarized below.

* S. Filippo Neri Hospital, Division of Cardiology, Rome, Italy

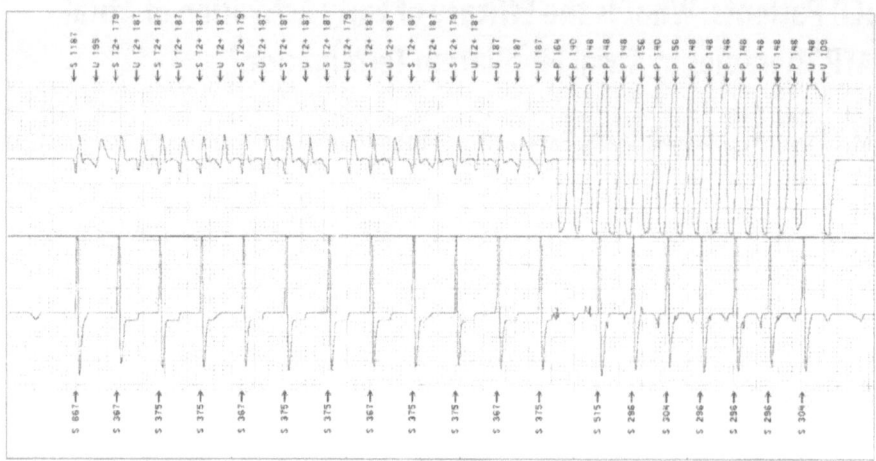

Fig. 1. Atrial flutter episode. Example of atrial flutter episode detected by the Biotronik Tachos DR ICD in less than 4 s (18 intervals). The first trace is the atrial EGM signal and the second is the ventricular EGM signal stored in the ICD memory. After detection, the mean atrial rate is updated (4 PP intervals) and anti-tachy pacing therapy then delivered

Study description

Study Endpoints

The primary objective of the study is to observe a reduction (if any) of the mean AF/AT episode duration when atrial ATPs are delivered within no more than 30 atrial beats if compared with no atrial therapy condition. In most cases, 30 AF/AT beats should correspond to about 7 s delay, thus providing very early activation of atrial ATP therapies. The parameter of interest will be the mean duration of device-detected atrial episodes, defined as the average of the time interval between device-detected onset and termination.

Further secondary objectives are: to measure the success rate of atrial ATP therapies delivered no more than 30 atrial beats after AF/AT episode onset; to study and classify the spontaneous onset and termination mechanisms of the AF/AT episodes; to estimate the AF/AT episode incidence rate in the patient population selected for this study; and to verify the specificity and sensitivity of the dual-chamber discrimination algorithm provided by the ICD under investigation in the AF/AT selected patient population.

Inclusion and Exclusion Criteria

The following criteria define the patient population selected for the study.

Patients included in this study must be indicated for the implant of a ventricular ICD and have experienced at least one documented AF/AT episode during 1 year prior to implant which was not due to transient or reversible causes. They also must be able to receive a pectoral implant.

Patients not indicated for ventricular ICD implantation, and/or with recurrent AF/AT episodes due to transient or reversible causes, and/or needing prolonged antiarrhythmic drug treatment are excluded from the study. Also, patients being in medical conditions that would preclude the testing required by the protocol or limit study participation, or inaccessible for follow-up at the study centre, as well as pregnant patients or patients aged over 80 cannot be enrolled in the study.

Study Design

This study is a comparison single-blinded randomized prospective study, without crossover.

The mean AF/AT episode duration collected during the study will be measured and compared between a patient group with atrial ATPs programmed on and a patient group with atrial ATPs programmed off. Thus, patients will be randomized in the atrial ATP ON group or in the atrial ATP OFF group at implant. They will be followed-up at 1 month and every 3 months afterwards, until 1 year follow-up is reached. This relatively long observation period should provide sufficient time to collect data on a significant number of AF/AT episodes and to study atrial arrhythmia evolution in the selected population along a significant time scale.

Antiarrhythmic Drug Treatment

As a general guideline, any ongoing antiarrhythmic drug treatment should be withheld after implant and without any recurrences of ventricular and/or atrial tachyarrhythmic episodes. Nevertheless, ventricular tachycardia (VT)/ventricular fibrillation (VF) episodes have the highest treatment priority. Therefore, any antiarrhythmic drug therapy is allowed at any scheduled or unscheduled follow-up visit, whenever at least one documented VT/VF episode has occurred. Any antiarrhythmic drug treatment of AF/AT episode recurrences should be avoided during the whole study. Whenever three unscheduled follow-up visits occur within less than 3 months, at which unsuccessfully treated AF/AT episodes are documented in the device memory, an antiarrhythmic drug therapy can be started at the discretion of the physician, using Amiodarone (free dosage). Other antiarrhythmic drug therapies are allowed exclusively when Amiodarone is clinically contraindicated, or when inefficacy of Amiodarone is documented. β-blockers are allowed.

Study Dimensions and Statistical Analysis

Previous data from the atrial-ventricular dual-chamber ICDs worldwide clinical investigations report an atrial ATP success rate of 68%. Within a 95% confidence interval (CI) of 10%, data collection of about 100 atrial episodes in each randomization period is needed. With 100 episodes in each arm, a significant variation of the mean atrial episode duration in the treatment group will be detected as long as the standard error of the variation is equal to or less than about four times the variation. With the hypothesis that each patient experiences at least two atrial episodes during the first 12 months, 100 patients should be required to reach the objectives of the study.

Discussion

The significantly high atrial ATP therapy success rate (68%) in terminating AF/AT episodes was one of the most interesting and somewhat surprising results of the first clinical experience of the atrial-ventricular dual-chamber ICD. But the clinical impact of this data still needs to be evaluated, addressing the possible correlation between the success rate of the atrial ATP therapies and the reduction of the AF/AT burden, which was never pointed out. The clinical trial presented here could put in evidence such a correlation (if any), as well as establish whether the immediate electrical treatment of atrial tachyarrhythmias at the onset could result in a more successful therapy strategy than delaying the atrial ATP intervention to wait for spontaneous termination. Further clinical insights into atrial fibrillation in ventricular ICD indicated patients are expected regarding AF spontaneous onset and termination mechanisms, and their incidence in the ICD patient population as well.

References

1. Schmitt C, Montero M, Melichercik J (1994) Significance of supraventricular tachyarrhythmias in patients with implanted pacing cardioverter defibrillators. Pacing Clin Electrophysiol 17:295-302
2. Bailin JS et al (1999) Clinical experience with a dual chamber implantable cardioverter defibrillator in patients with atrial fibrillation and flutter. NASPE, Pacing Clin Electrophysiol (II)22:685 (abstr)
3. Santini M (1998) Clinical experience with a dual defibrillator. Eur Heart J 19 [Suppl P585]:77(abstr)
4. Wharton M, Santini M (1998) Treatment of spontaneous atrial tachyarrhythmias with the Medtronic 7250 Jewel AF: Worldwide clinical experience. Circulation 98:984

Might a Better Understanding of Atrial Electrophysiology Help Atrial Fibrillation Treatment?

H. HEIDBÜCHEL

The "Electrical Rationale" of Atrial Fibrillation

The conceptual framework for understanding atrial fibrillation (AF) dates back to the early twentieth century, when it was realized that the electrocardiographic appearance of the arrhythmia is due to a multitude of activation wavefronts in the atria. Different mechanisms responsible for the initiation and maintenance of the arrhythmia were presented. Some authors postulated that multiple reentrant wavelets were propagating independently and perpetuously throughout the atria. Others argued that a dominant reentrant circuit or focal mechanism was "driving" the atria: since the entire atria are not capable of sustaining one-to-one conduction of the driver throughout the muscle mass, fragmentation of the wave into a multitude of wavelets is a secondary result. Moe further refined those early concepts by stressing that "multiple wavelets" around functionally refractory tissue could perpetuate the arrhythmia [1]. Therefore, maintenance of AF is dependent on the number of wavelets and the mass of tissue available.

Two new electrical concepts have brought added insight during the last 10 years. The first, introduced by Wijffels and Allessie, is that rapid atrial rates predispose the atria to ensuing atrial arrhythmias due to a shortening and maladaptation to rate of the atrial refractory period (ERP) [2]. Shortening of the refractory period leads to smaller wavelengths, so that the probability of persistence for multiple wavelets is increased. The leitmotif of their work is now known as "AF begets AF". Similar changes occur in humans prone to AF and can be demonstrated after short episodes of induced AF.

The second concept is the recognition that some forms of AF are indeed focal in nature or - more often - focally induced. A majority of foci reside in the orifices of the pulmonary veins. The group around Haïssaguerre has shown that targeting these foci by ablation can result in cure of the arrhythmia [3]. However, the long-term outcome of this approach is currently unknown.

Department of Cardiology, University Hospital Gasthuisberg, University of Leuven, Belgium

Issues Unresolved by Electrical Answers

Some important clinical observations remain unexplained. It is unclear why patients develop their first episode of AF, often after many decades of life. There clearly was no previously elevated heart rate to shorten ERP. Even if ectopic beats were present, it is questionable how far these sporadic runs are sufficient to start the "AF begets AF" spiral. In fact, it is not known what AF burden is required to induce the "AF begets AF" cascade. The role of other electrophysiological and hemodynamic factors in the induction and maintenance of AF is largely undefined.

Nonelectrical Observations

Many observations point to important structural changes underlying AF development. AF is in essence a disease of the elderly [4], and atrial dilatation or congestive heart failure (even asymptomatic) are its strongest clinical predictors [5]. This suggests that not only electrical but probably also structural alterations [6] have occurred over the years to make the atria prone to AF. Experimental work in our sheep laboratory showed that rapid atrial pacing led to much slower development of AF than the rapid early decrease in ERP (Fig. 1A, B). However, the slow induction of AF was paralleled by a slow increase in atrial pressure and size [7]. Moreover, burst-pacing the atria, resulting in high atrial rates for only 33% of the total time, led to much slower AF development than continuous high rate pacing, although the time course and degree of ERP shortening (i.e., electrical remodeling) were similar. The increases in atrial pressure and size were clearly larger in the continuously paced group [7]. An association between AF and progressive atrial enlargement is also obvious in patients [8]. Atrial ischemia during AF as manifested by typical subcellular changes [9] and depressed atrial contractility will contribute to further dilatation. Another important observation comes from randomized trials showing that atrial-based pacing results in a significant reduction of AF compared with ventricular pacing (VVI or DDD), but divergence of the curves only becomes apparent after 2-3 years [10, 11]. If a purely electrical phenomenon were to explain the lower propensity for AF with atrial pacing, one would expect a much earlier therapeutic effect. The delayed separation suggests a biological effect, which could be lower atrial loading due to the enhanced atrioventricular synchrony during atrial-based pacing.

Interestingly, heart failure in a dog model is as effective in inducing AF as is the classical model of rapid atrial pacing [12]. However, AF development in the heart failure model is not accompanied by ERP shortening. The main finding in the heart failure dogs was progressive atrial fibrosis, not seen in the rapidly paced dogs. Angiotensin 2 is elevated in heart failure, and was observed in the heart failure dog model. Interestingly, our sheep model of AF revealed an early

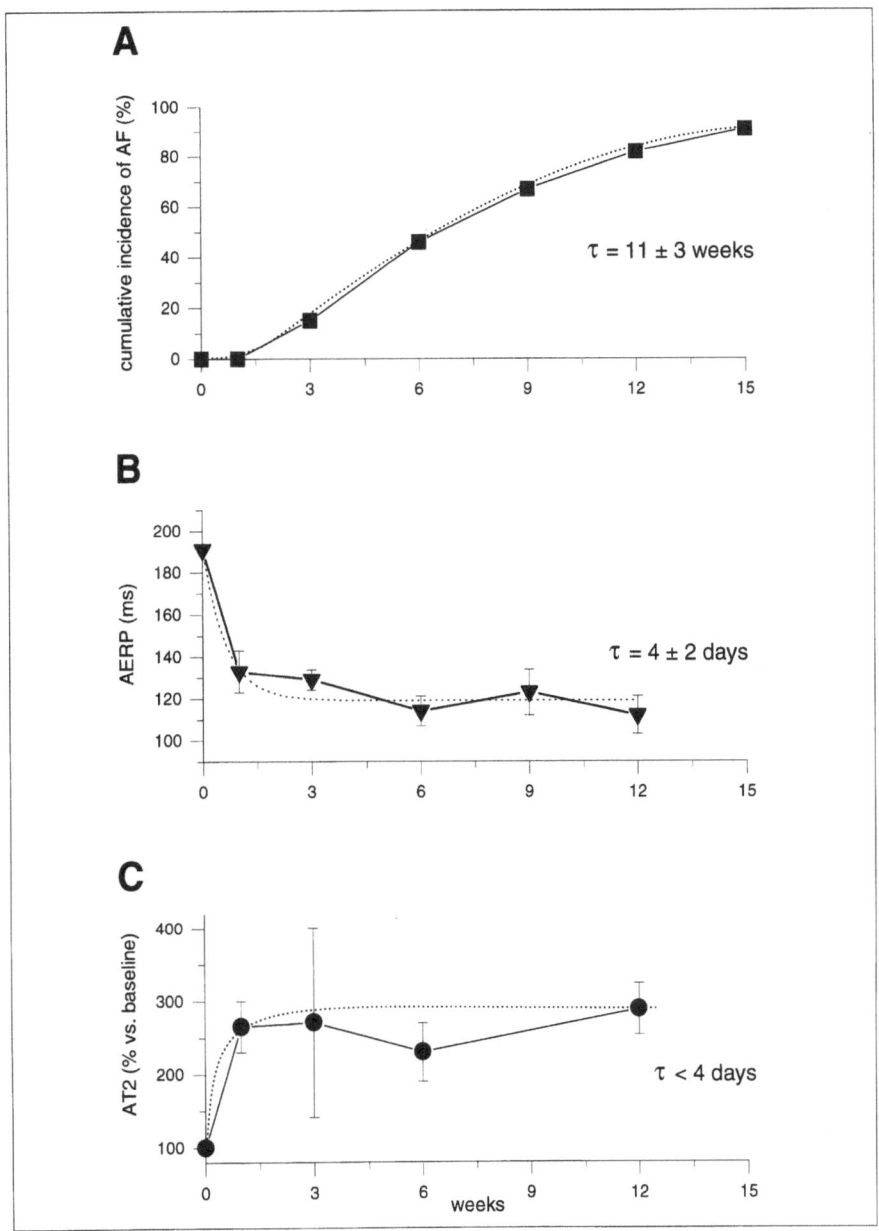

Fig. 1. A Development of sustained AF (i.e., lasting longer than 5 min) in a high rate atrial pacing model in sheep is slow. The time constant fitted for the curve was 11 weeks. **B** Refractory period (AERP) shortening was much faster, with a time constant of a few days. Therefore, AERP shortening by itself is not sufficient to induce AF, pointing to the presence of a "second factor" of electrical and/or structural remodeling. **C** Angiotensin 2 (AT2) levels increase rapidly after the start of pacing, suggesting a possible pathophysiological role in the development of the substrate for AF. It is known that angiotensin 2 induces both intercellular fibrosis and gap junction conductance decrease, each of which can promote AF

and steady activation of the renin-angiotensin system, indicating that it could play a pathophysiological role and not just be a bystander effect of atrial dilatation and AF induction (Fig. 1C) [13]. Angiotensin 2 has been shown to induce both intercellular fibrosis and a decrease in gap junction conductance [14, 15]. Both may result in decreased conduction overall (leading to smaller AF wavelengths) and increased heterogeneity of conduction and wavelength (predisposing to induction and maintenance of reentry). Together with the observation that ACE inhibition after myocardial infarction resulted in a decreased incidence of AF [16], all these observations point to important hemodynamic factors in the development of AF, and to the possible pivotal role of the renin-angiotensin system. Moreover, insight into other pathways such as apoptotic cell death during AF [17], altered connexin expression [18], and mechano-electrical feedback [19] is only just emerging. Finally, it has been shown that atrial pressure elevation acutely shortens ERP and increases the propensity for AF [20].

Many diseases that predispose to AF have in common the fact that they are associated with an increase in left heart pressures and interstitial fibrosis: heart failure, hypertension, old myocardial infarction, mitral disease, etc. The mean left atrial pressure in patients ablated for focal but lone AF in our institution is significantly higher than that in age- and sex-matched patients undergoing (transseptal) ablation for left-sided accessory pathways (17.3 ± 2.4 mmHg vs 14.3 ± 3.3 mmHg; p = 0.01; unpublished observations) although arterial pressures and left ventricular ejection fractions were similar. Therefore, our working hypothesis is that longer-lasting atrial pressure overload may lead to atrial structural changes that predispose to and maintain AF (Fig. 2). Other authors

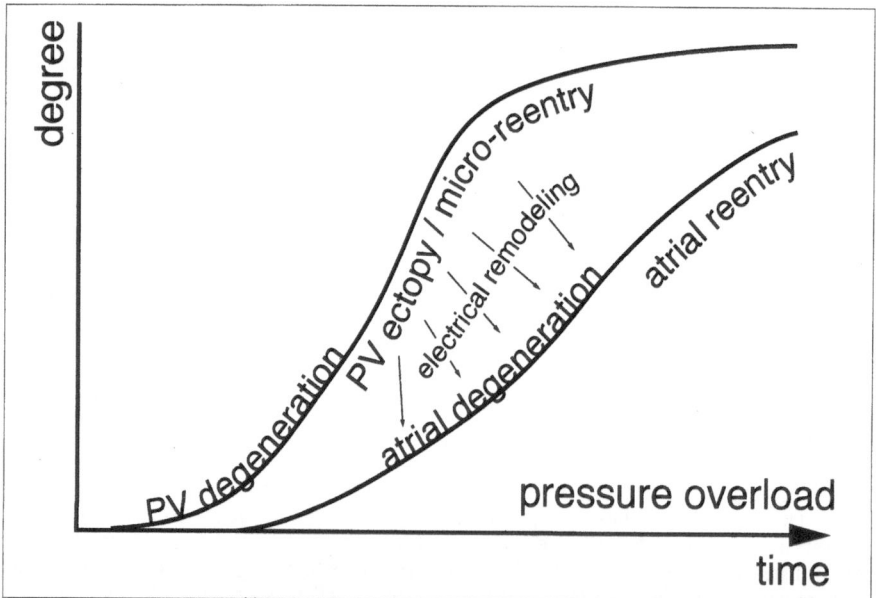

Fig. 2. Chronic atrial pressure overload may be one of the key factors in the cascade of events leading to AF. See text for discussion

have pointed to larger diameters of the pulmonary veins in patients with focally induced AF [21]. It is tempting to speculate that the atrial pressure increase leads to dilatation of the thin-walled (i.e., most compliant) pulmonary veins first, and to degeneration of the global atrial wall at a later stage. Pulmonary vein dilatation and degeneration may lead to focal activity. There are indications that the basic mechanism of this "focal activity" may not be enhanced automaticity but micro-reentry [22]. These bursts of ectopic discharges will be a trigger for AF but will also accelerate its development by electrical and structural remodeling. It is not known to what extent the focal firing contributes to atrial substrate changes. If pressure-related degeneration forms the basis of both focal (pulmonary vein) activity and multiple wavelet reentry in the atrial wall, ablation of the foci may be only a temporary cure when not accompanied by other measures to halt the degeneration of the atrial wall.

Electrical Tools for a Structural Classification?

Long-term monitoring in patients with paroxysmal AF (e.g., via the elaborate diagnostic capabilities of modern pacemakers) has revealed a wide variety of underlying rhythms and onset triggers preceding paroxysms. Moreover, "atrial fibrillation" on the surface ECG can have a very heterogeneous presentation during invasive electrophysiological evaluation, from purely focal arrhythmias ("drivers") via partially organized intraatrial reentrant tachycardias to completely chaotic reentry ("multiple wavelets"), with frequent conversions between those forms during a single episode. Some authors have presented classification schemes of these chaotic rhythms into different subgroups of (dis)organization based on bipolar intracardiac recordings. Clearly, AF is not simply AF, but forms a whole electrical spectrum. Most likely, AF also comprises a whole structural spectrum. Unfortunately, not much is known about how far these electrical presentations provide insight into the (degree of) underlying structural degeneration. Further research in this field could certainly help in defining which patients have passed a "point of no return" versus those who might benefit from therapeutical interventions.

Therapeutic Considerations

Treatment for AF may need to be tailored on the basis of the hemodynamic and electrical findings in a given patient. In highly damaged atria with degenerative reentry (i.e., multiple wavelets), medication will remain the mainstay to palliate AF, since full reversibility and cure is unlikely. Linear ablation may be an option in the future for this group of patients. In less damaged atria, elimination of the focal triggers and/or isthmus ablation if drugs can achieve organization of AF into flutter (or another form of organized intraatrial reentrant tachycardia) are valuable options today. Atrioventricular synchronous pacing certainly has a role in preventing further hemodynamic load to and structural degeneration of the atria. Research is ongoing to define how far and by what modalities it may also electrically prevent recurrences. If angiotensin 2 proves to be an important mediator in the cascade of electrical and structural remodeling, ACE inhibitors and/or angiotensin 2 receptor antagonists may in the future be part of the standard anti-AF armamentarium. They may be the precursors of a whole new approach to AF, targeting it less as an electrical disease and more as a structural problem.

References

1. Moe GK (1962) On the multiple wavelet hypothesis of atrial fibrillation. Arch Int Pharmacodyn 140:183-188
2. Wijffels MC, Kirchhof CJ, Dorland R, Allessie MA (1995) Atrial fibrillation begets atrial fibrillation. A study in awake chronically instrumented goats. Circulation 92:1954-1968
3. Haïssaguerre M, Jais P, Shah DC et al (1998) Spontaneous initiation of atrial fibrillation by ectopic beats originating in the pulmonary veins. N Engl J Med 339:659-666
4. The National Heart, Lung, and Blood Institute Working Group on Atrial Fibrillation (1993) Atrial fibrillation: current understandings and research imperatives. J Am Coll Cardiol 22:1830-1834
5. Vaziri SM, Larson MG, Benjamin EJ, Levy D (1994) Echocardiographic predictors of nonrheumatic atrial fibrillation. The Framingham Heart Study. Circulation 89:724-730
6. Frustaci A, Caldarulo M, Buffon A et al (1991) Cardiac biopsy in patients with "primary" atrial fibrillation. Histologic evidence of occult myocardial diseases. Chest 100:303-306
7. Willems R, Holemans P, Ector H et al (2001) Effect of different pacing protocols on the induction of atrial fibrillation in a transvenously paced sheep model. Pacing Clin Electrophysiol 24:925-932
8. Sanfilippo AJ, Abascal VM, Sheehan M et al (1990) Atrial enlargement as a consequence of atrial fibrillation. A prospective echocardiographic study. Circulation 82:792-797
9. Ausma J, Wijffels M, Thone F et al (1997) Structural changes of atrial myocardium due to sustained atrial fibrillation in the goat. Circulation 96:3157-3163
10. Andersen HR, Nielsen JC, Thomsen PE et al (1997) Long-term follow-up of patients from a randomised trial of atrial versus ventricular pacing for sick-sinus syndrome. Lancet 350:1210-1216
11. Connolly SJ, Kerr CR, Gent M et al (2000) Effects of physiologic pacing versus ventricular pacing on the risk of stroke and death due to cardiovascular causes. Canadian Trial of Physiologic Pacing Investigators. N Engl J Med 342:1385-1391
12. Li D, Fareh S, Leung TK, Nattel S (1999) Promotion of atrial fibrillation by heart failure in dogs: atrial remodeling of a different sort. Circulation 100:87-95
13. Willems R, Holemans P, Ector H et al (2000) Neurohumoral changes in atrial remodeling. Europace 1:B17 (abstract)
14. McEwan PE, Gray GA, Sherry L et al (1998) Differential effects of angiotensin II on cardiac cell proliferation and intramyocardial perivascular fibrosis in vivo. Circulation 98:2765-2773

15. De Mello WC (1996) Renin-angiotensin system and cell communication in the failing heart. Hypertension 27:1267-1272

16. Pedersen OD, Bagger H, Kober L, Torp-Pedersen C (1999) Trandolapril reduces the incidence of atrial fibrillation after acute myocardial infarction in patients with left ventricular dysfunction. Circulation 100:376-380

17. Aime-Sempe C, Folliguet T, Rucker-Martin C et al (1999) Myocardial cell death in fibrillating and dilated human right atria. J Am Coll Cardiol 34:1577-1586

18. Van der Velden HM, van Kempen MJ, Wijffels MC et al (1998) Altered pattern of connexin40 distribution in persistent atrial fibrillation in the goat. J Cardiovasc Electrophysiol 9:596-607

19. Sadoshima J, Izumo S (1997) The cellular and molecular response of cardiac myocytes to mechanical stress. Annu Rev Physiol 59:551-571

20. Tse HF, Pelosi F, Oral H et al (2001) Effects of simultaneous atrioventricular pacing on atrial refractoriness and atrial fibrillation inducibility: role of atrial mechanoelectrical feedback. J Cardiovasc Electrophysiol 12:43-50

21. Lin WS, Prakash VS, Tai CT et al (2000) Pulmonary vein morphology in patients with paroxysmal atrial fibrillation initiated by ectopic beats originating from the pulmonary veins: implications for catheter ablation. Circulation 101:1274-1281

22. Mandapati R, Skanes A, Chen J et al (2000) Stable microreentrant sources as a mechanism of atrial fibrillation in the isolated sheep heart. Circulation 101:194-199

Circadian Patterns of Atrial Fibrillation Onset Mechanism: Can Pacing Be Influential?

A. Capucci, G.Q. Villani, N. Marrazzo, D. Pozzetti and M. Piepoli

*Do androids dream
of electric sheep?*
P.K. Dick, 1968

Introduction

Circadian variation in the incidence of acute cardiovascular events is well known. However, this pattern has not been extensively investigated in paroxysmal atrial fibrillation (AF), although with the increasing number of aged people the significance of this arrhythmia is growing in our society. In the last few years, several authors have suggested the presence of a circadian pattern of AF onset and termination in different patient populations [1-4]. This observation, if further confirmed, could have implications for the timing of antiarrhythmic therapy. Recently, an influence of atrial pacing on the circadian pattern of AF has been proposed and investigated [5, 6].

Does a Circadian Pattern in AF Really Exist?

There are only limited data regarding the diurnal distribution of paroxysmal AF, and not all investigators have observed a distinct circadian pattern of AF initiation.

Kupari et al. [1] studied 251 patients aged 65 years or less and admitted for treatment of symptomatic supraventricular tachyarrhythmia (152 AF episodes), to assess whether these arrhythmias do or do not manifest a circadian variation in occurrence. They concluded that the frequency of onset of sustained supraventricular tachyarrhythmias varies through the day, showing nearly equal peaks in the morning and in the evening and a trough at night.

Yamashita et al. [2] evaluated 150 patients with paroxysmal AF in a drug-free state from among 25 500 consecutive Holter recordings. To determine whether the onset, maintenance, and termination of paroxysmal AF were random events, they analyzed the total recorded duration of arrhythmia, the incidence of AF and number of AF patients with onset, maintenance, and termination of this arrhythmia as hourly data and as hourly probabilities. A prominent

Divisione di Cardiologia, Ospedale Civile, Piacenza, Italy

circadian rhythm of the total duration of AF, approximately 90% of which was well explained by a single cosinusoidal function, was detected with a nadir around 11 A.M. Because the onset of the arrhythmia had little or no circadian rhythm, this finding was due to a diurnal pattern of maintenance and termination, both of which were well expressed by a double-harmonic density function. Maintenance showed a trough at 11 A.M., and termination showed a peak at the same time, leading to the nonuniform duration of single episodes of AF throughout the 24-h day.

Viskin et al. [3] reviewed all emergency telephone calls received in Shahal (a medical service covering 44 000 subscribers) from 1987 to 1997. Patients were included if new-onset AF was recorded. During this study period, 9989 episodes of paroxysmal AF were recorded. The time of onset was not uniformly distributed throughout the 24-h period. Instead, the distribution of arrhythmic episodes showed a double peak, with a significant increase in the number of episodes in the morning and a second rise in the evening ($p < 0.001$).

Recently, Yamashita et al. [4] suggested that aging significantly influences the circadian variation of paroxysmal AF, with the most prominent effect on its onset, leading to a more random time distribution of AF with increasing age. They evaluated the Holter recordings of 212 patients who had paroxysmal AF in a drug-free state. These patients were divided into two groups according to their age: 60 years old or less (94 patients) and over 60 years old (118 patients). In each group, the sum of the duration of each AF episode and the probability of onset, maintenance, and termination of AF were determined as hourly data and compared between the 2 groups. The time distribution of AF showed remarkable age dependence, with a well-modulated and monophasic circadian rhythm in the younger group in contrast to a toneless triphasic rhythm in the older group. Among the onset, maintenance, and termination of the arrhythmia, the most obvious age dependence was observed in the circadian variation of onset. In the younger group there were triple peaks, with the highest one in the night, whereas the older group exhibited a single peak in the daytime. In contrast, the probabilities of maintenance and termination showed similar circadian patterns between the groups, although their amplitudes were significantly reduced in the older group.

In conclusion, it seems that a circadian pattern of occurrence and termination of AF has been described by most researchers, although there is no concordance as to the exact time distribution.

Atrial Pacing in Prevention of AF

In the last few years several trials have been designed to evaluate the possibility that intelligently controlled pacemakers with new pacing algorithms may increase maintenance of sinus rhythm in patients with paroxysmal or persistent AF. If the atrium is predominantly or exclusively pacemaker-controlled, electrophysiological imbalances depending on variable cycle length, compensatory pauses following supraventricular extrasystoles and temporal dispersion of refractory periods can no longer induce AF. Preliminary results on new pacing systems are available.

Lam et al. [7] tested the effects of a consistent atrial pacing algorithm that automatically paced the atrium at 30 ms shorter than the sinus P-P interval for AF prevention. Fifteen patients with sick sinus syndrome implanted with a Thera DR (model 7940 or 7960, Medtronic Inc.) were randomly programmed to either rate-adaptive dual-chamber pacing (DDDR) only or DDDR plus consistent atrial pacing mode, each for an 8-week study period. The efficacy of consistent atrial pacing was assessed by the number of automatic mode switching episodes and the number of premature atrial complexes. Symptoms and quality of life were assessed by the SF-36 quality of life questionnaire and an AF symptom checklist. The percentage of atrial pacing increased from 57 ± 32% to 86 ± 28%; there was no significant difference in the number of automatic mode switching episodes between DDDR and DDDR plus consistent atrial pacing (47 ± 90 vs 42 ± 87, $p > 0.05$), but the addition of consistent atrial placing resulted in a significant reduction in premature atrial complexes by 74.7% ($p < 0.001$).

Recently, Funck et al. [8] reported the preliminary results of the AF Prevention by Overdriving (PROVE) trial, an ongoing prospective study of the effectiveness of atrial overdrive pacing combined with an "automatic rest rate function" in the prevention of atrial arrhythmias. In this study all patients receive a Talent DR 213 pacemaker and after a 1-month monitoring period are divided into two groups. Group I is made up of patients with two or more appropriate mode switch (MS) episodes, or 1 MS episode of 10 min or longer, and/or more than 300 atrial runs of more than 5 beats/month. Group II contains all the other patients. The number and duration of atrial arrhythmias are measured by the pacemaker's Automatic Interpretation and Data Analysis software (AIDA). Patients' quality of life is measured by a validated functional status questionnaire. After having been grouped, the patients are randomly assigned, in a crossover design, to standard DDDR or overdrive pacing plus rest rate, each programmed for a 3-month period. Preliminary results in 78 patients show a 34% reduction in the mean number of MS episodes and a mean 48% shortening of the overall duration of the episodes by overdrive pacing plus rest rate, achieved by a mean 84% prevalence of atrial pacing. Furthermore, overdrive pacing plus rest rate is well tolerated and associated with a slight improvement in quality of life.

Circadian Patterns of Onset Mechanism: Can Pacing Be Influential?

Recently, Gillis et al. [5] in the Canadian Atrial Pacing Peri-Ablation for Paroxysmal Atrial Fibrillation trial tested the hypotheses that atrial pacing may prevent paroxysmal AF in patients without symptomatic bradycardia and that

DDDR pacing is more likely to prevent paroxysmal AF following total atrioventricular (AV) node ablation than is VDD pacing. They studied the circadian variation of paroxysmal AF in the first 67 patients who received a dual-chamber pacemaker 3 months before a planned AV node ablation and the possible role of atrial pacing in the modulation of a circadian pattern of AF.

They observed [6] a distinct circadian variation of AF, with two time peaks of initiation, one in the early morning and one in the early evening. A clear bimodal distribution of AF initiation persisted for episodes of 2 h duration or less, whereas the late afternoon peak was diminished for episodes of more than 2 h duration. (Fig. 1) In the paced patients a bimodal pattern of AF initiation was also observed, with an early morning (4-7 A.M.) and an early evening (4-7 P.M.) peak. A reduction of AF episodes was observed in the morning and early afternoon. By contrast, in non-paced patients only an early morning (4-6 A.M.) AF peak was observed (Fig. 2).

On the basis of these observations it could be suggested that atrial rate-adaptative pacing may play a role in altering the diurnal pattern of AF by increasing the heart rate during atrial activity. The nocturnal pacing (at 70

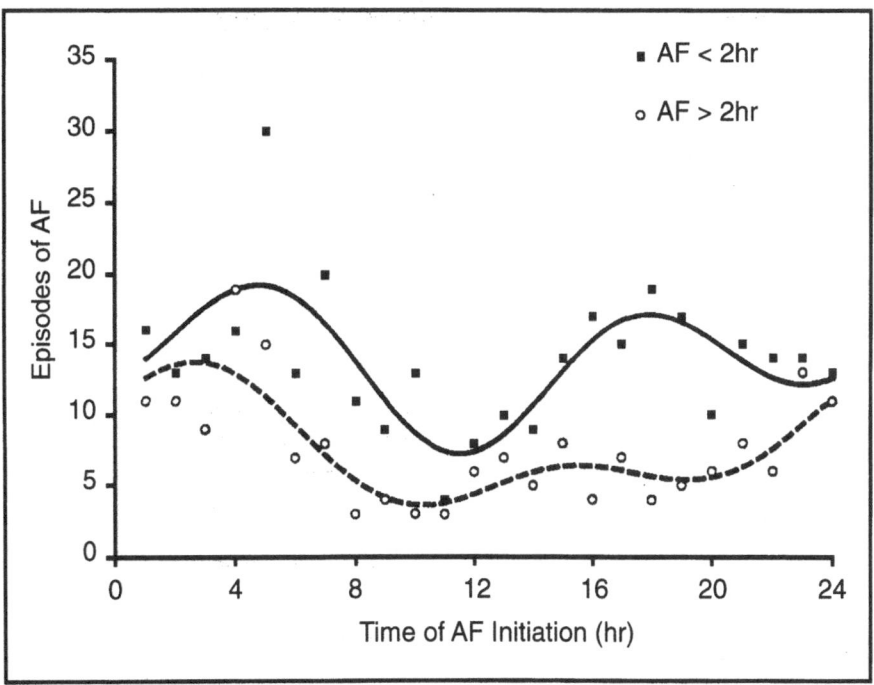

Fig. 1. Circadian variation of AF initiation based on duration of AF: AF ≤ 2 h (*solid squares*); AF < 2 h (*open circles*). The curves represent the best fits of the data to double harmonic functions. *Solid line:* AF ≤ 2 hours, $R^2 = 0.51$, $p = 0.006$ compared with fit of the data to single harmonic function; *dashed line:* AF > 2 h, $R^2 = 0.65$, $p = 0.02$ compared with fit of the data to single harmonic function. AF was dichotomized at 2 h because the median duration of AF was just greater than 1 h

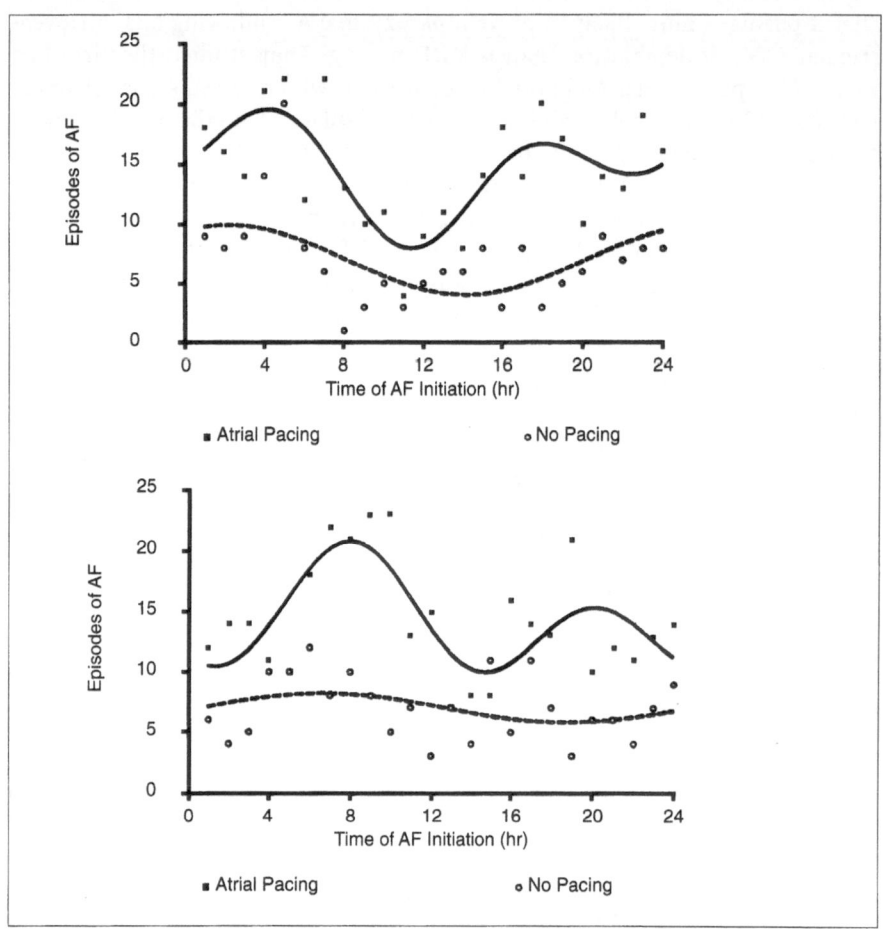

Fig. 2. *Upper panel:* effect of atrial pacing on the circadian variation of AF initiation. The AF episodes per hour are plotted versus time of initiation. The curves represent the best fits of the data to single or double harmonic functions. AF initiation in the atrial pacing group (*solid squares*) was best described by the double harmonic function ($R^2 = 0.54$, $p = 0.01$) reflecting 2 time peaks in AF initiation and the circadian variation of AF initiation in this group was best described by a single harmonic function ($R^2 = 0.30$). *Lower panel:* effect of atrial pacing on circadian variation of AF termination. The curves represent the best fits of the data to single or double harmonic functions. AF termination in the atrial pacing group is best described by a double harmonic function ($R^2 = 0.50$, $p = 0.008$ vs fit to single harmonic function). AF termination in the no pacing group does not manifest a distinct circadian variation

bpm) does not seem to influence the nocturnal pattern of AF, suggesting that AF onset is not related to vagally mediated bradycardia.

Recent data show that bradycardia is related to AF onset in only 19% of episodes [9]. It should be possible for a new pacing algorithm improving the rate of paced beats in these patients to reduce the electrophysiogical imbalance (variable cycle length, compensatory pauses following supraventricular extrasystoles, frequent ectopic atrial activity) and consequently the occurrence of AF.

References

1. Kupari M, Koskinen P, Leinonen H (1990) Double-peaking circadian variation in the occurrence of sustained supraventricular tachyarrhythmias. Am Heart J 120:1364-1369
2. Yamashita T, Murakawa Y, Sezaki K, Inoue M, Hayami N, Shuzui Y, Omata M (1997) Circadian variation of paroxysmal atrial fibrillation. Circulation 96:1537-1541
3. Viskin S, Golovner M, Malov N et al (1999) Circadian variation of symptomatic paroxysmal atrial fibrillation. Data from almost 10 000 episodes. Eur Heart J 20:1369-1370
4. Yamashita T, Murakawa Y, Hayami N et al (1998) Relation between aging and circadian variation of paroxysmal atrial fibrillation. Am J Cardiol 82:1364-1367
5. Gillis AM (1999) The Atrial Pacing Peri-ablation for Paroxysmal Atrial Fibrillation (PA3) Study: rationale and study design. Europace 1:40-42
6. Gillis AM, Connolly SJ, Dubuc M et al (2001) Circadian variation of paroxysmal atrial fibrillation. PA3 Investigators. Am J Cardiol 87:794-798, A8
7. Lam CT, Lau CP, Leung SK et al (2000) Efficacy and tolerability of continuous overdrive atrial pacing in atrial fibrillation. Europace 2:286-291
8. Funck RC, Adamec R, Lurje L, Capucci A on behalf of PROVE Study Group (2000) Prevention by overdriving: atrial overdriving is beneficial in patients with atrial arrhythmias: first results of the PROVE Study. Pacing Clin Electrophysiol 23:1891-1893
9. Kanko S, Dorwarth U, Gert C et al (1999) Analysis of onset scenarios in patients with drug refractory paroxysmal AF: implications for preventive pacing strategies. Pacing Clin Electrophysiol 22:307 (abstract)

Can Ventricular Rate Stabilisation Reduce Symptoms of Atrial Fibrillation?

P. Dini and F. Laurenzi

Introduction

Many haemodynamic studies showed that irregularity of the ventricular rhythm can affect the cardiac function [1]. This suggests that a significant additional mechanism for reducing cardiac output in patients with chronic atrial fibrillation is the irregularity of the ventricular rhythm. Additional experiences showed that pacing can possibly avoid not only ventricular pauses, but also short ventricular cycles as a consequence of concealed retrograde conduction after paced events [2, 3]. Patients with conducted chronic atrial fibrillation as a result of high and/or irregular ventricular rhythm are often symptomatic and present haemodynamic deterioration. Patients with chronic atrial fibrillation and indication for VVI pacing could benefit from simple algorithms for rate stabilisation during the spontaneous rhythm phases.

Results of Rate Stabilisation at Rest

The pacing percentage is an indirect indicator of the stabilising effect of the pacing algorithm. The Flywheel (FW) pacing mode (Vitatron) is designed to prevent sudden drops in heart rate: any rate drop exceeding 15 beats/min will result in pacing followed by a slow decrease of the pacing rate towards the lower rate limit. First of all we analysed the immediate effect of Flywheel in a group of ten patients at rest: in particular, we evaluated the difference between the ventricular rate histograms for 10 min with Flywheel on and for 10 min with Flywheel off (standard VVI pacing) in a randomised sequence. The stabilising effect of an algorithm can be assessed by the rate histogram evaluating the different distribution of the rates with respect to the standard VVI pacing. The obvious effect is the reduction of the lowest rates, as the rates lower than the dominant rate bin of the histogram. In addition, as reported in previous experiences [2, 3], we can also

Cardiology Department, S. Camillo Hospital, Rome, Italy

expect a reduction of the highest rates thanks to the hypothesised effect of the concealed retrograde conduction of paced events. For the ten patients studied at rest for 10 min with Flywheel on and 10 min with Flywheel off, the mean normalised difference of the rate histograms is shown in Fig. 1. This is done by computing the difference histogram, normalised with respect to the dominant rate component of each. This normalisation process allows consideration of a single rate axis for all patients, and thus permits evaluation of the mean effect of Flywheel function in the patient group studied. As can be seen in Fig. 1, this stabilisation algorithm increases the rate bin corresponding to the dominant rate bin of the patient (71-88 beats/min in Fig. 1) and reduces the incidence of both lowest and highest rates. In particular, the global reduction of highest (all rates over the dominant positive bin) and lowest rates is respectively 12.63% ($p = 0.01$) and 4.6% (p = n.s.). The global result of these effects means an enhancement of the rate bin corresponding to the dominant rate of the patient in that storing period, and consequently it represents a rate stabilisation effect.

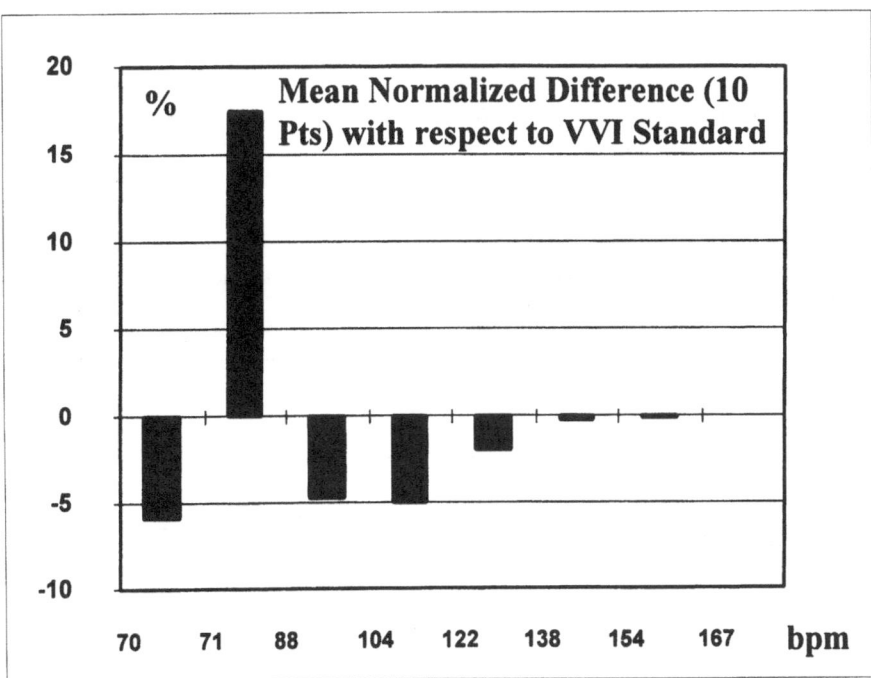

Fig. 1. Difference between the rate histogram of 10 min with Flywheel on and the histogram of 10 min with Flywheel off

Results of Rate Stabilisation during 1 Month of Normal Life

Next, a group of 19 patients was studied at the end of 1 month programming with Flywheel on and off by a crossover intrapatient analysis. As can be seen from Fig. 2, the stabilisation algorithm can significantly increase the pacing percentage only in patients who have a pacing percentage above 50% in VVI standard. This obviously means that the stabilisation algorithm can be applied in patients with prevalent spontaneous rhythm. In this case the pacing percentage significantly increases ($p = 0.02$) (Fig. 2). For the same reason there is little difference in the rate histograms for Flywheel on and Flywheel off when the pacing percentage is above 50% in VVI standard.

By contrast, we can evaluate the difference between these two histograms when the pacing percentage is lower than 50% in VVI standard. For this last group of patients the analysis of 1 month of follow-up with Flywheel on and

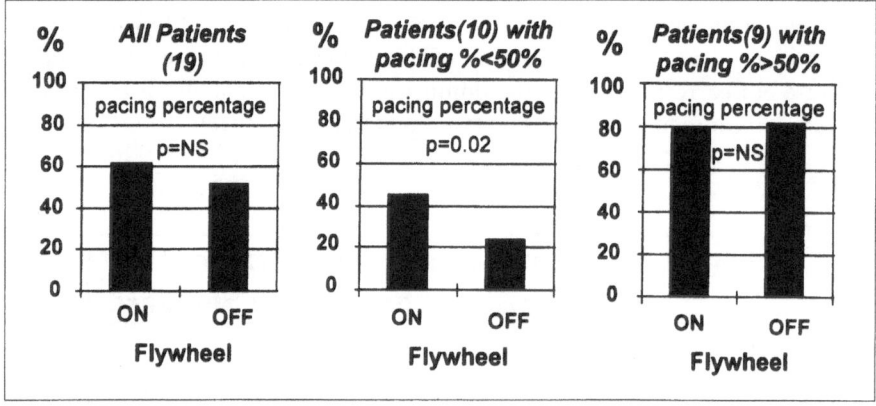

Fig. 2. Pacing percentage with Flywheel on and Flywheel off as shown by the rate histograms at 1-month follow-up in the two modalities

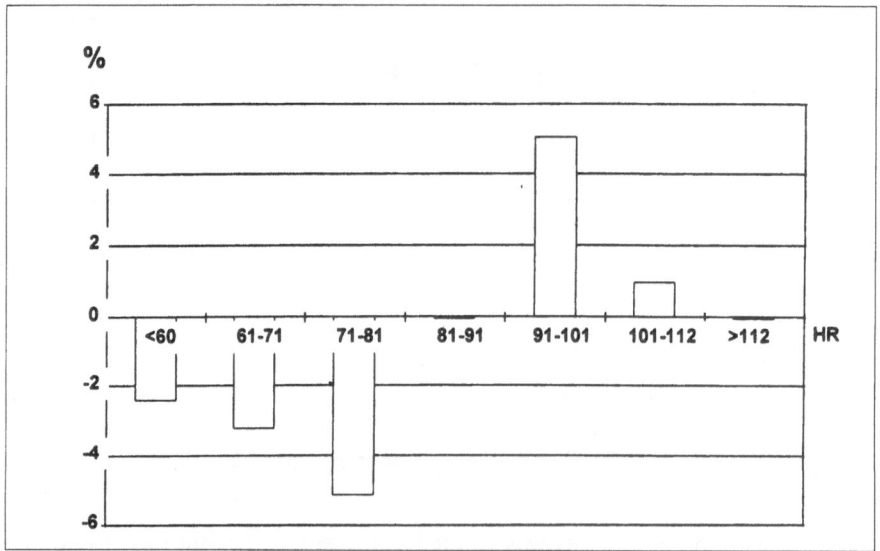

Fig. 3. Mean normalized histogram of the difference between the histograms with Flywheel on and Flywheel off at 1-month follow-up

Flywheel off is shown in Fig. 3, which summarises the mean normalised difference histogram. Like Fig. 1, this histogram shows a significant reduction of the lowest rates (10.81% in the range 60-91 beats/min, $p = 0.05$) and a consequent increase of the dominant positive bin (in the range 81-101 beats/min), which corresponds to the dominant rate component. Therefore, the result shown in Fig. 3 is different from the result in Fig. 1 as far as the highest rates are concerned: in this case, representing the normal life of patients, the total reduction of rates above 112 beats/min is only 0.08% (p = n.s.). Patients with conducted chronic atrial fibrillation can benefit from a stabilisation algorithm if characterised by a relatively low pacing percentage (< 50%) in standard VVI mode, which means they are patients with a prevalent spontaneous rhythm.

Patients

Ninety-three patients were enrolled in the RASTAF study: a single blind randomisation of Flywheel on or off with 1 month follow-up periods. The pacemaker's rate histogram and percentage of pacing were used to evaluate heart rate stabilisation. In addition, ECG recordings were used to analyse beat-to-beat variations in both pacing modes and for a baseline assessment (lowest rate 40 beats/min).

Results

Patients with more than 50% pacing during the ECG recording while in the Flywheel off mode were excluded since the Flywheel mode will only be sporadically activated. R-R instability was defined as the mean absolute difference of successive R-R intervals per the average R-R interval. Table 1 summarises the results [4].

Although pacing with the Flywheel mode on was only activated after significant drops in heart rate, we found that the higher percentage of pacing resulted in an improved stability of the heart rate in patients with conducted chronic atrial fibrillation. Another important fact is that the Flywheel pacing mode did not increase the average ventricular rate. Any statistically significant effect was seen on patients' symptoms. The same study also evaluated the quality of life of patients treated with this regularisation function [5], by means of Short-Form Health Survey (SF-36) questionnaire, symptom score and visual analogue scale. Patients with more than 50% pacing in VVI were excluded from the analysis because their rhythm can be considered already stabilised. Fifty-five patients were then analysed and the results are summarised in Table 2.

Table 1. Effects of pacing on heart rate stability

	Baseline	Flywheel off	Flywheel on
MAD (ms)	182 ± 150	137 ± 113	123 ± 109
R-R instability (%)	23.5	18.3	16.2
Average R-R (ms)	782 ± 169	756 ± 134	764 ± 125
Percentage pacing (%)	2.3	14.0	29.0

Table 2. Effects of pacing on quality of life and symptom frequency

	N	Flywheel on	Flywheel off	p value
SF 36 scale				
General health	55	62 ± 23	58 ± 18	< 0.05
Mental health	55	76 ± 14	73 ± 16	< 0.03
Physical component	55	41 ± 11	40 ± 11	0.07
Percentage pacing	55	36 ± 12	23 ± 13	< 0.01
Frequency of symptoms	29	11 ± 6	12 ± 7	0.06

Conclusions

Rate stabilisation by pacing is an interesting possibility to investigate with the aim of reducing R-R variability, which is considered to be an important cause of cardiac output impairment in patients with conducted chronic atrial fibrillation. The use of simple pacing algorithms can contribute to achieving this goal, even though it must be remembered that pacing the right ventricle is not haemodynamically so effective as the spontaneous beats.

Patients with conducted chronic atrial fibrillation can benefit from a stabilisation algorithm if characterised by a relatively low pacing percentage (< 50%) in standard VVI mode, which means they are patients with a prevalent spontaneous rhythm.

The analysis of symptom frequency does not show significant effects: the positive effect of rate regularisation was counterbalanced by the negative effect of right ventricular pacing. The recent technology of left ventricular stimulation and biventricular stimulation should be tested in this patient population in conjunction with rate stabilisation algorithms.

The RASTAF Study

The RASTAF Study was a multicenter clinical evaluation of rate stabilisation by Flywheel on patients with chronic atrial fibrillation and an indication for SSI(R) pacing [4].

RASTAF study: Austria: Dr. Goldsteiner (Wiener-Neustadt) *Canada:* Dr. Bauer (Toronto); Dr. Brown (New Westminster); Dr. Burgess (Regina); Dr. Geddes (Winnipeg); Dr. Hughes (Peterborough); Dr. Jue (Vancouver); Dr. Labonté (Sudbury); Dr. Lai (Nanaimo); Dr. Leather (Victoria); Dr. McMeekin (Saskatoon); Dr. Singh (Scarborough) *Italy:* Dr. Dini (Rome-S. Camillo); Dr. Cervellati (Imola); Dr. Mariotti (Senigallia); Dr. Fasciolo (Novi Ligure); Dr. Freggiaro (Tortona); Prof. Giani (Seriate); Dr. Mambelli (Cesena); Dr. Saccomanno (Ancona); Dr. Scirè (Esine) *United Kingdom:* Dr. Holdwright (London)

References

1. Daoud EG, Weiss R, Bahu M et al (1996) Effect of an irregular ventricular rhythm on cardiac output. Am J Cardiol 78:1433-1436
2. Wittkampf F, De Jongste M, Lie H et at (1988) Effect of right ventricular pacing on ventricular rhythm during atrial fibrillation. J Am Coll Cardiol 11:539-545
3. Meijler F, Jalife J (1997) On the mechanism(s) of atrioventricular nodal transmission in atrial fibrillation. Cardiologia 42:375-384
4. Dini P, Brunekreeft W, on behalf of the RASTAF I Study Group (2000) Rate stabilization in patients with conducted atrial fibrillation – RASTAF I results. Europace 1 [Suppl D] (abstr 10/5)
5. Labonte RE, Burgess J, McMeekin JD, Brunekreeft W, on behalf of the RASTAF Study Group (2000) Symptom reduction through ventricular rate stabilization in patients with conducted chronic atrial fibrillation. Europace 1 [Suppl D] (abstr 10/4)

Novel Pacing Algorithms Applied in Hybrid Therapies of Atrial Fibrillation: The Ultimate Solution?

T. Lewalter[1], A. Yang[1], J. Schrickel[1], R. Schimpf[1], H. Bielik[1], S. Herwig[1], B. Esmailzadeh[2], A. Welz[2] and B. Lüderitz[1]

Introduction

The Latin word "hybrida" describes a "mixture" or "two origins". In the treatment of atrial fibrillation (AF), the term "hybrid therapies" is used for various "mixed" therapeutic approaches, as for example pharmacologic and ablative hybrid therapy [1] and linear lesions or preventive pacing in combination with drug therapy to maintain sinus rhythm. Apart from sophisticated pacing algorithms, pacemaker therapy to prevent AF also offers elaborate AF diagnostic capabilities. In the following, we describe a case which illustrates the use of these advanced pacemaker diagnostics to guide catheter ablation therapy of class IC drug-induced atrial flutter in a patient with initially paroxysmal AF. We also introduce the VIP registry, because it is expected that more than 50% of these patients with recurrent AF and preventive pacing receive concomitant antiarrhythmic drug therapy. The VIP registry intends to enroll 350-400 pacemaker patients and therefore might offer an opportunity to analyze the impact of specific drugs on the efficacy of different preventive pacing algorithms.

Relevance of Pacemaker Diagnostics to Guide Pharmacologic and Ablative Hybrid Therapy of AF

A 58-year-old woman had hypertensive heart disease and so far drug-refractory paroxysmal AF. Medical therapy had included sotalol, verapamil, flecainide and amiodarone. For further treatment of the patient's highly symptomatic and drug-refractory AF atrioventricular node ablation was considered, but it was decided to carry out pacemaker implantation and preventive pacing in the

[1]Deptartment of Medicine-Cardiology; [2]Department of Cardiovascular Surgery, University of Bonn, Germany

first instance and to keep atrioventricular node ablation as an additional, optional second line of therapy. The AF-related symptoms did not improve within 3 months after pacemaker implantation (AF burden was 28.1% of follow-up time), and therefore 600 mg propafenone per day was additionally administered. The patient returned after 6 weeks complaining of increased palpitations and tachycardia. The pacemaker diagnostics revealed a burden of 47% atrial tachyarrhythmia during follow-up. The detailed onset reports exclusively demonstrated atrial flutter at a rate of 240/min. With the suspected diagnosis of a class IC drug-induced typical atrial flutter, an electrophysiological study was performed. Atypical atrial flutter and AF was mechanically induced which reorganized to counterclockwise isthmus-dependent atrial flutter after intravenous administration of 70 mg propafenone (Fig. 1). After successful isthmus ablation and continuing of the propafenone medication, atrial flutter did not return; the burden of paroxysmal AF was significantly reduced to less than 1% of follow-up time.

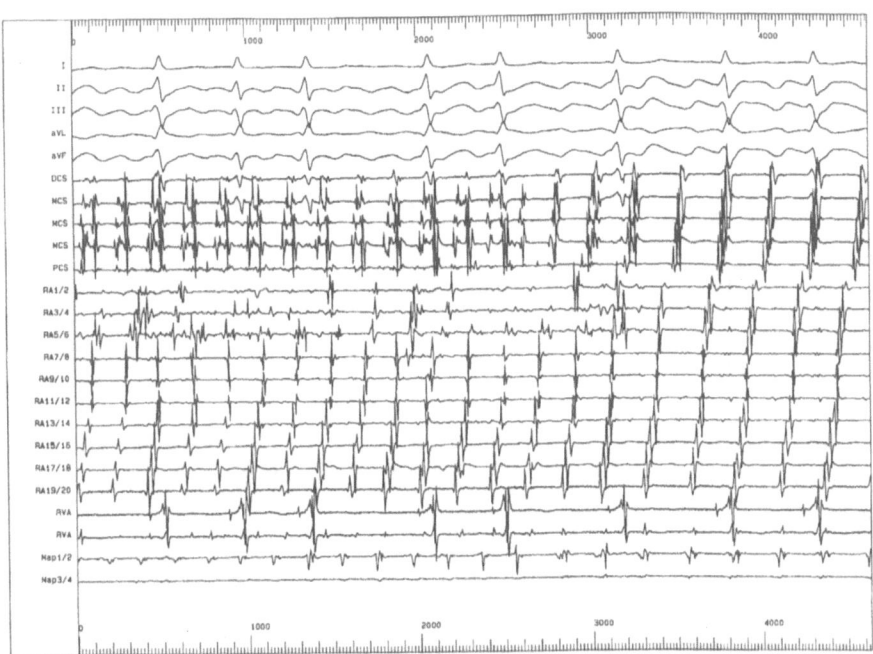

Fig. 1. Conversion of atrial fibrillation/atypical atrial flutter into typical counterclockwise atrial flutter. On the *left side* of this ECG one can observe fragmented electrograms in the cavotricuspid isthmus (RA1/2 to RA5/6) and rapid epicardial left atrial signals (DCS, MCS, and PCS). After intravenous administration of 70 mg propafenone, the atrial activation reorganized to typical atrial flutter with a counterclockwise activation of the right atrium, which allows radiofrequency catheter ablation therapy

VIP Registry

The VIP (AF prevention by individualised pacemaker programming) Registry will include patients with a conventional indication for antibradycardia pacing and known paroxysmal AF. After pacemaker implantation (Selection series, Vitatron) and a maturation phase of 6 weeks, the pacemaker is programmed to standard antibradycardia therapy for 3 months. The "premature atrial contractions (PACs) before atrial fibrillation onset" histogram is then used to guide the activation of different preventive pacing algorithms (Fig. 2). If more than 70% of episodes have less than two PACs, a continous overdrive algorithm ("pace conditioning") is activated. The rationale for this approach is that in cases of rare PAC activity before AF onset, PAC-triggered algorithms may miss the majority of induction scenarios for intervention (Fig. 3). However, if 70% or less of episodes have less than two PACs, PAC-triggered algorithms such as "post PAC response" or "PAC suppression" should have an opportunity to intervene and prevent AF from starting [2].

I. Recommended Decision Tree

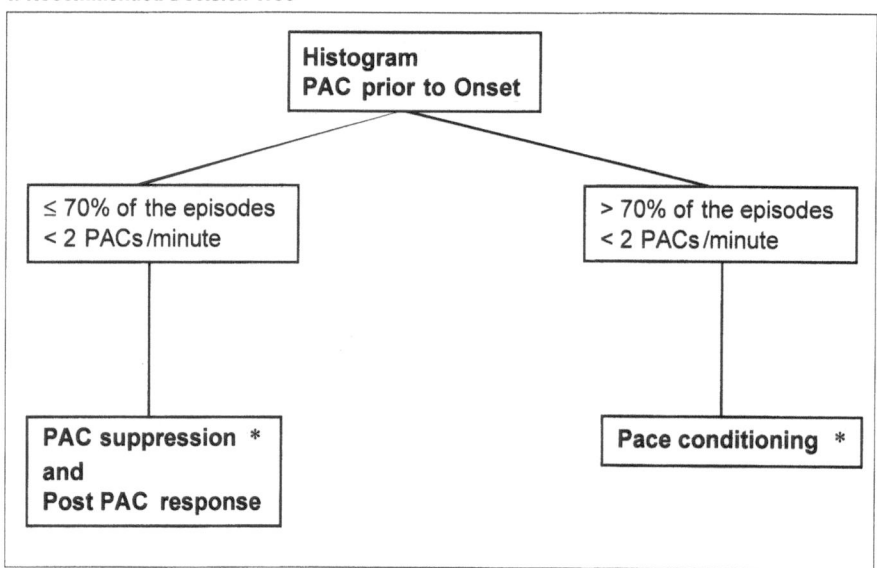

II. Additional criteria

| Post-exercise rate control |

It is to additionally activate "Post-Exercise rate control" if the patient indicates the start of "AF after emotion or exercise", or if AF after exercise has been documented in a detailed onset report

Fig. 2. Programming recommendations for the VIP Registry. *It is recommended to program the maximum therapy rate to a maximum of 90-100/min

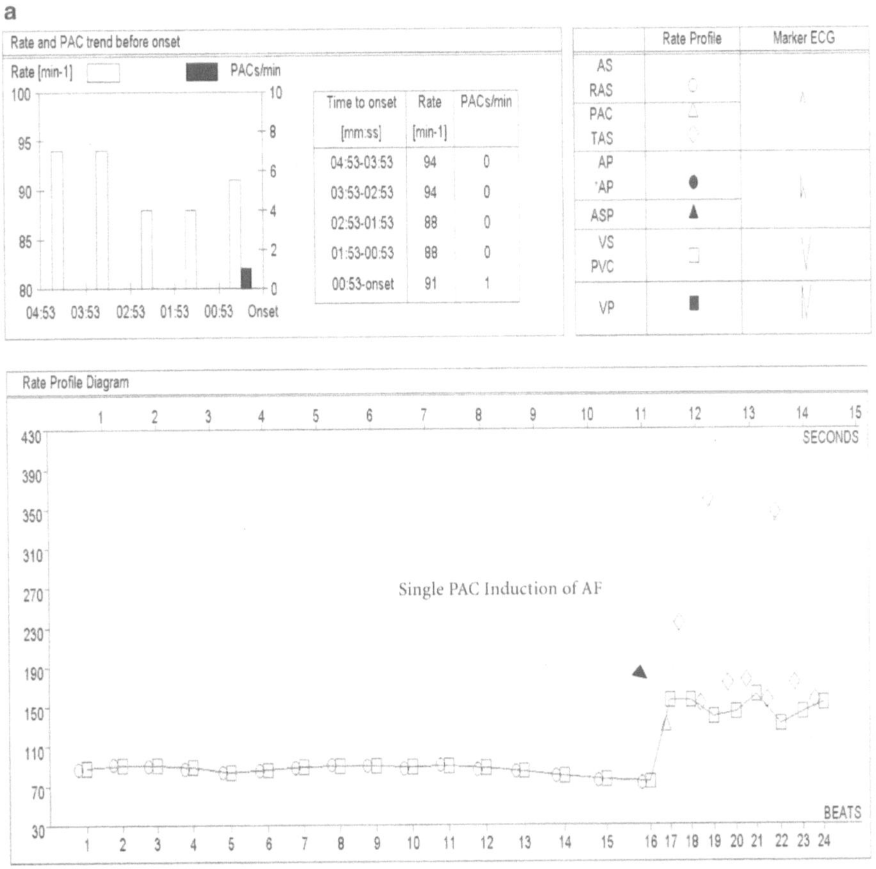

a

Rate and PAC trend before onset

Rate [min-1] ☐   ■ PACs/min

Time to onset	Rate	PACs/min
[mm:ss]	[min-1]	
04:53-03:53	94	0
03:53-02:53	94	0
02:53-01:53	88	0
01:53-00:53	88	0
00:53-onset	91	1

	Rate Profile	Marker ECG
AS		
RAS		
PAC		
TAS		
AP		
'AP	●	
ASP	▲	
VS		
PVC		
VP	■	

Rate Profile Diagram

Single PAC Induction of AF

Fig. 3. a The "Rate and PAC trend before onset" did demonstrate only a single PAC prior to this AF episode. The "Rate profile diagram" indicates that this single PAC did directly induce AF

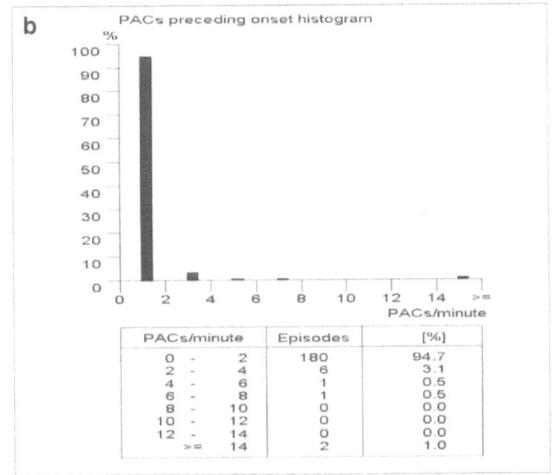

b PACs preceding onset histogram

PACs/minute		Episodes	[%]
0	- 2	180	94.7
2	- 4	6	3.1
4	- 6	1	0.5
6	- 8	1	0.5
8	- 10	0	0.0
10	- 12	0	0.0
12	- 14	0	0.0
	>= 14	2	1.0

Fig. 3. b This patient demonstrated in 94.7% of all AF episodes detected less or equal than 2 PAC s/minute in the five minutes prior to AF onset

References

1. Huang DT, Monohan KM, Zimetbaum P et al (1998) Hybrid pharmacologic and ablative therapy: a novel and effective approach for the management of atrial fibrillation. J Cardiovasc Electrophysiol 9:462-469
2. Lewalter T, Jung W, Lickfett L et al (2000) Pace prevention of atrial fibrillation: what can we expect from new algorithms? Herzschr Elektrophys 11/II:58-62

PACEMAKER THERAPY:
TECHNOLOGICAL AND PRACTICAL ASPECTS

Advanced Patient Management Using Knowledge-Based Systems

M. Schaldach[†1], B. Diem[2], P. Hanrath[2], M. Mlynski[3], V. Lang[1] and W. Ameling[3]

Introduction

Modern implantable devices such as the cardioverter-defibrillator (ICD) and pacemaker offer a wide variety of therapeutic and diagnostic options to adapt the devices to the specific needs of each patient [1, 2]. Unfortunately this flexibility of adjustment requires a large number of parameters, which makes programming complex and time consuming. As a result, some modern features of ICDs are not used because time constraints during the follow-up procedures do not allow the time-consuming tweaking of the parameters. This article describes new technologies which support the physician in the handling of modern implantable devices during implantation and follow-up. The first piece of technology described in this paper is an automatic database with an information manager to improve efficiency during follow-up and provide the physician with information whenever it is needed [3]. A knowledge-based follow-up system analyzes the Holter data of implantable pacemakers and supports the physician during the decision process. The second piece of technology is a knowledge-based programming system. The complete programming procedure is done using the physician's own language, so the learning effort required is considerably reduced [4].

Automatic Follow-Up Database with Automatic Holter Analysis

As the number of available pacemakers continues to grow, new added features are increasing their functionality and complexity. The greater number of statistical functions and stored data require ever increasing more attention and detailed assessment. However, the time and resources available for pacemaker follow-up and appropriate use of the stored information are relatively limited

[1]Department of Biomedical Engineering, University of Erlangen-Nuremberg; [2]Department of Cardiology, University Clinics, University of Aachen; [3]Department of Electrical Engineering and Computer Science, University of Aachen, Germany

(Fig. 1). Without a doubt, the possibility of an automatic analysis of the raw interrogated data, based on knowledge-based diagnosis (Fig. 2), could be of great help in supporting the physician's decisions [5, 6]. A Computer Data Manager system (CDM 3000, Biotronik, Germany), integrated with a special software module including the knowledge-based system, has been developed to meet this challenge. The knowledge-based system is intended to support physicians with the analysis of diagnostic data (Holter data) that have been stored in the pacemaker memory and are made accessible during the follow-up of pacemaker patients. The system uses a set of rules (rule base) to evaluate the avail-

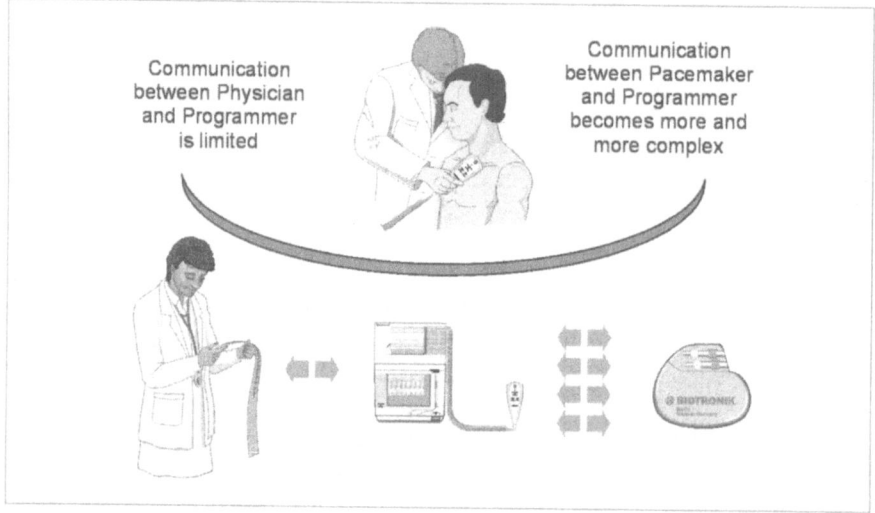

Fig. 1. The follow-up situation today

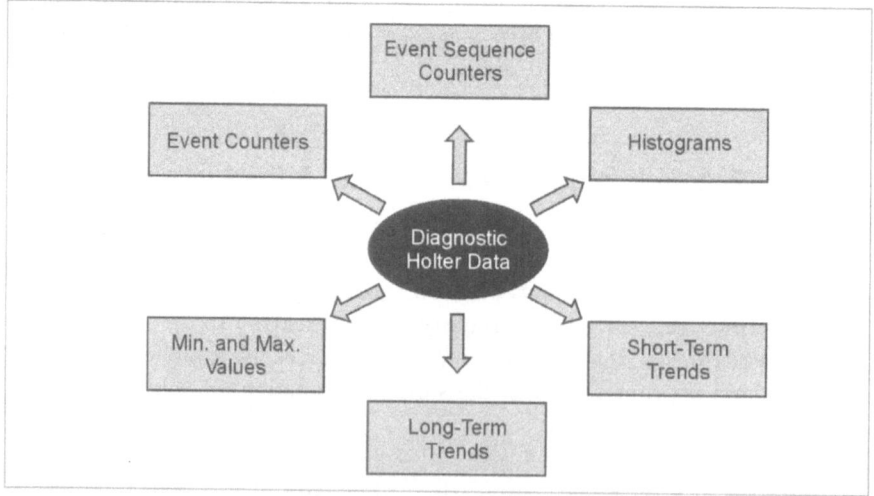

Fig. 2. Major contents of diagnostic Holter data

able diagnostic information, compare these with the limiting values or reference distributions, and actively support the decision process of the physician. The physician can judge the accuracy of both the conclusion and its underlying reasons (rationale), and can also contribute further comments and rules.

In the first phase of a clinical evaluation the following steps were considered:
- Verification (examination of the consistency, completeness, and accuracy of the system of rules, as well as of further qualitative attributes such as its differentiation, expressiveness, efficiency, and its avoidance of cycles and redundancy)
- Validation (quality and efficiency of the system as a whole, comprising all the components with respect to the clinical problem)
- Estimation of the system's functionality and ease of use.

Innovative Follow-up Procedure

The interrogated data are downloaded to the CDM 3000 database and then processed by the knowledge-based system. After the automatic analysis the data are displayed on the computer screen. The follow-up information, stored according to the respective patients (rendered anonymous), will appear in a tree-like structure. Simultaneously, the results of the analysis will be displayed on the working screen in two further windows (Fig. 3):
- Analysis window. This window contains the results of the analysis, with hypertext links to further background information.
- Graphics window. This window displays all Holter data compiled in graphic form, together with a list of all pacemaker programming parameters distributed on several register cards.

The software provides multiuser capability, with the possibility of granting specified individuals different levels of access to pacemaker and patient data.

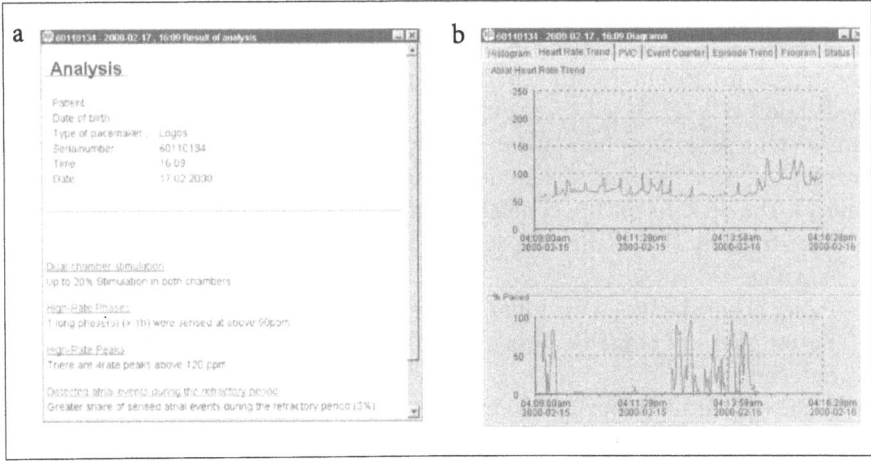

Fig. 3a,b. Examples of data obtained during follow-up assisted by the knowledge-based system. **a** Analysis window with a summary of the most important findings regarding the patient's status. **b** Graph window showing heart rate trend and percentage of paced events

Results

Thirty patients were included in this preliminary evaluation. Both the CDM 3000 and the knowledge-based system turned out to facilitate both access and use. The results of the data analysis were clearly arranged in different windows on the screen, with data, comments, and graphics, allowing rapid and comprehensive evaluation of the status of both the patient and the pacemaker. The evaluation of the statistical information obtained permitted optimization of the pacemaker's functional parameters according to the real individual needs of the patient. Wherever possible, the patient's spontaneous activity was promoted. The results demonstrated that in the patient population being studied, it was possible to improve nonoptimal pacemaker settings, especially those relating to the atrioventricular delay, the hysteresis option, and the rate-responsive sensor functions.

Automatic ICD Programming Assistant

The increasing complexity of implantable devices requires a continuous learning effort to maintain a complete picture of the interactions and functionality of the devices. Because of this, some therapeutic options may not always be activated even if the device provides them and even if they would be clinically useful. Since future implantable devices will offer even more therapeutic options by including enhanced multisite support or preventive pacing with rate stabilization algorithms, the gap between the functionality offered by the device and the functionality made use of by the clinician may widen. This gap can only be closed with the help of knowledge-based systems which support the user during the programming process by automatically generating an appropriate parameter set from the clinical data [4]. This patient-oriented programming assistant prompts the clinician to specify the patient's arrhythmias and symptoms, together with general disease and functional states and relevant medication (Fig. 4). Based on the clinical information, the programming assistant system generates the appropriate parameter set and explains the results (see Fig. 5). This provides a completely new way of programming implantable devices. The benefits for the clinical user are:
- User-friendly: The "language" of the device programming is the clinician's language
- Faster programming: Less input is necessary and it is easier
- Better therapy control: Appropriateness of the parameter set is cross-checked
- Reduced learning effort: New devices with new algorithms or features have the same user interface.

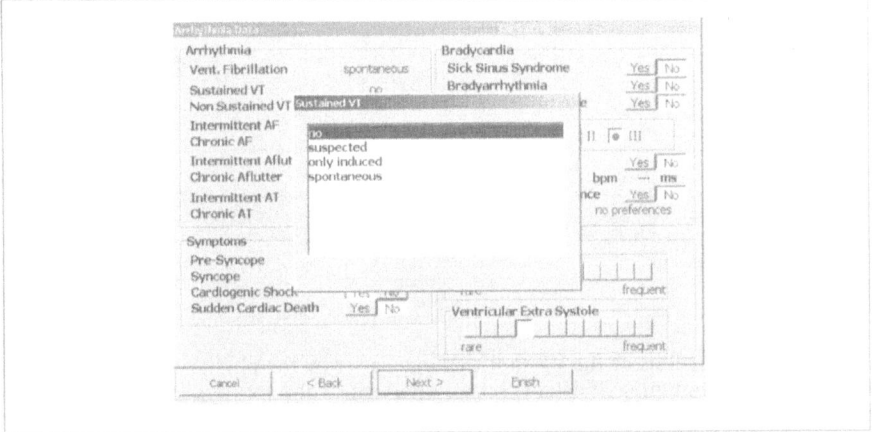

Fig. 4. The user enters the patient-specific arrhythmias into the programming assistant. On the basis of this information, a complete parameter set is calculated

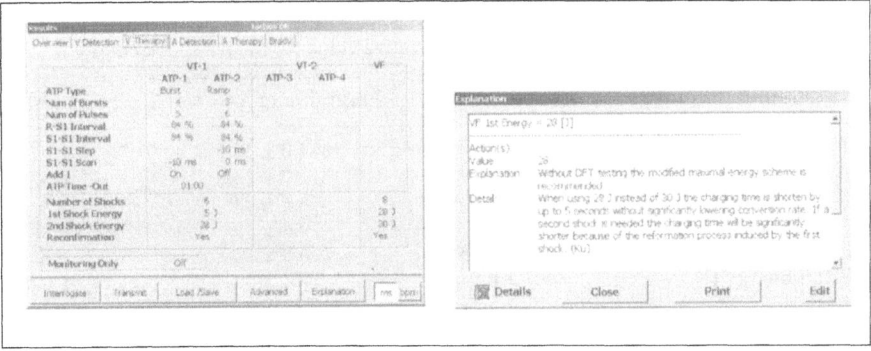

Fig. 5. Results of the automatic calculation are presented in a way known from commercial ICD programmers (*left*). The underlying reasons for the calculation steps for each value are shown on physician's request (*right*)

Results

The knowledge-based system was tested on the clinical data of 40 patients (9 female, 31 male, age 68 ± 10 years) who received the dual-chamber ICD Tachos DR. The calculation of the automatic programming system was compared to the physician's setting for each parameter. Figure 6 shows the difference in programming of the first and second VF shock energy, showing in more than 75% of the cases a difference of only 2 J, which is one programming step. The analysis using the Student's *t*-test demonstrates that only a few parameters show a statistical difference between the setting of the physician and that of the programming assistant (Table 1). This indicates that the programming assistant sets the values of most of the parameters within the acceptable range. Currently a clinical study is investigating the efficiency of this new tool in supporting the physician.

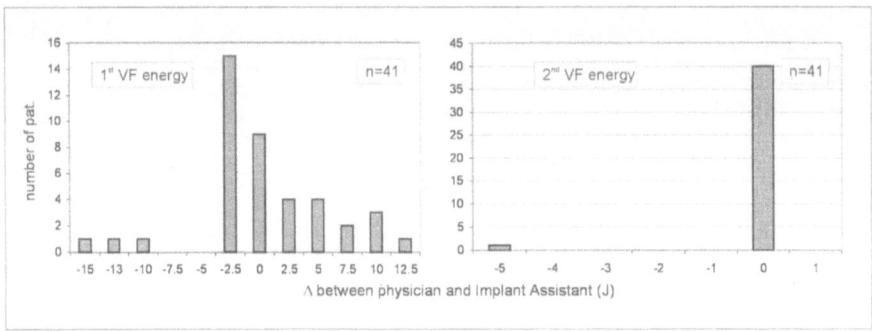

Fig. 6. Statistical analysis of the VF shock energy as set by the physician as the reference and by the programming assistant. Seventy percent of the settings for the first shock energy are within 2 J. No statistical difference was seen for the two parameters on the basis of Student's t-test ($p > 0.05$), demonstrating that the programming assistant calculates the parameter within an acceptable range

Table 1. Statistical analysis of the important parameters. Most of the parameters show no statistical difference between the settings of the physician and those of the programming assistant. However, the VT zone limit was set to higher rates by the physician, whereas the programming assistant chooses a more conservative value for the AF shock energy

	Physician	Programmer Assistant	t-test
VT1 Zone Limit (ms)	360.2 ± 30.0	384.0 ± 28.1	$p < 0.05$
VF Zone Limit (ms)	303.3 ± 26.7	312.0 ± 22.3	n.s.
VF 1st Energy (J)	25.9 ± 4.8	26.4 ± 4.0	n.s.
VF 2nd Energy (J)	30.0 ± 0.0	29.9 ± 0.6	n.s.
AF Zone Limit (ms)	270.5 ± 39.8	276.8 ± 12.7	n.s.
AF 2nd Energy (J)	9.7 ± 8.9	17.1 ± 8.6	$p < 0.05$

Conclusions

Integrating knowledge-based systems into the implantation and follow-up procedures reveals new possibilities for improving electrotherapy of the heart. Information management becomes more reliable and most routine processes can be automated. This increases not only the effectiveness of the follow-up but also contributes to improved quality of management in medical care. Knowledge-based systems integrated into programming systems for cardioelectric implant devices offer interesting possibilities and clinical benefits through:
- The full diagnostic capabilities provided by modern pacemakers and ICDs, which can be utilized without additional effort
- The detailed technical and medical expertise provided by a knowledge-based support for the physician
- The possibility of early and precise detection of the progression of diseases and of other risk factors
- Long-term optimization of the therapy
- Overall improvement in the quality of follow-up

References

1. Schaldach M (2000) Expert pacing system. Prog Biomed Res 5:336-348
2. Revishvili AS (1998) Dual-chamber automatic implantable cardioverter-defibrillator. Prog Biomed Res 3:9-13
3. Igidbashian D, Lonardi G, Gemelli M et al (2000) Clinical evaluation of a new computer based expert management system of pacemaker diagnostic functions. Prog Biomed Res 5:471-477
4. Diem BH, Lang V, Mlynski M et al (2001) Computer aided, patient-oriented programming of implantable cardioverter defibrillators. Prog Biomed Res 6:1-5
5. Sack S, Malinowski K, Appl U et al (1996) Analyse von Arrhythmien und Schrittmacherfunktionen durch die automa-tische Interpretation von Schrittmacher-Diagnosefunktionen. Herzschrittmacher 16[Suppl 11]:103-114
6. Limousin M, Geroux L, Nitzsché R et al (1997) Value of automatic processing and reliability of stored data in an implanted pacemaker: initial results in 59 patients. Pacing Clin Electrophysiol 20:2893-2898

Single-Lead Dual Chamber Pacing: How Reliable and Effective Is It?

I.E. Ovsyshcher and E. Crystal

In 1979, a single-lead (SL) dual chamber system with a non-contact unipolar electrode floating in the atrial blood pool and standard ventricular part was first tested in humans by Antonioli [1]. However, unipolar atrial sensing was suboptimal, encouraging the development of SL systems, incorporating bipolar atrial sensing [2-11]. SL systems became commercially available in Europe and USA about 10 years ago. The aim of this review is to analyze the present status of pacing by SL in both pacing modes: VDD and DDD.

Physical and Technical Aspects of Atrial Signal Detection in Bipolar SL-VDD Systems

Besides physiological maneuvers that have an effect on the atrial signal detected by floating electrodes, there are two groups of factors which influence the atrial signal. The first group consists of factors beyond the control of the operator device, such as aging, shape, size, the anatomy of the atrium, sequence of impulse propagation, and atrial arrhythmia. The second group depends on the design of the atrial lead, sensing amplifier, and technique of implantation, and includes such factors as the distance between the atrial wall and electrodes, electrode size, interelectrode spacing, dipole orientation, and sensing mode. Since the first group cannot be controlled, only the second will be addressed here.
- *Distance between atrial wall and electrode.* The greater the distance, the smaller the amplitude of the atrial signal.
- *Electrode size.* Small electrodes deliver high-quality signals recorded only from nearby myocardium; larger sensing electrodes ("antennas") can record more distant signals, but at the expense of recording lower-amplitude signals adjacent to the atrial wall, and increasing the detection of far-field signals. The optimal electrode size will, of necessity, be a compromise between the opposing factors.

Cardiology Department, Cardiac Research Center, Soroka University Medical Center and Faculty of Health Sciences, Ben Gurion University of the Negev, Beer-Sheva, Israel

- *Interelectrode spacing.* The effects of varying interelectrode spacing are analogous to those of varying electrode size: the larger the interelectrode space, the bigger the sensing antenna, but at the cost of decreased specificity. The larger the interelectrode separation, the more the bipolar lead system behaves as a unipolar system.
- *Dipole orientation.* Two types of electrode dipole orientation in bipolar SL designs have been developed:
    1. Diagonal atrial bipolar (DAB) leads consist of two small split rings separated by 5 mm, available in leads manufactured by Guidant Co. (previously by CCS, Inc., and Intermedics).
    2. The total ring pair electrode model exists in two configurations: with a short interelectrode distance of about 10 mm (Biotronik, Guidant, Medtronic, and Vitatron) or a long interelectrode distance of 12-30 mm (St. Jude Medical Company, 12 mm; Sorin, 13 mm; Medico, 30 mm).

Additional details on the SL systems and differential amplifiers may be found in recent reviews [7-10].

Atrial Sensing Performance and Long-Term Results

The clinical significance of intermittent atrial undersensing is as yet unclear. Probably, inappropriate atrial sensing in patients with SL devices is only relevant in the absence of >10% of atrioventricular (AV) synchrony [11]. The sensing in both SL configurations in clinical use (total and split ring systems) has been compared and shown to be equally efficacious in each [12]. Some degree of atrial undersensing was demonstrated by ambulatory ECG monitoring or during physiological maneuvers and exercise testing. No evidence of atrial oversensing, even at the most sensitive settings, was found with either device. At 6 months after implantation, the mean atrial signal for both systems was 0.8-1.2 mV. As both devices contain amplifiers capable of detecting atrial signals as low as 0.10-0.18 mV, these amplitudes still allow a substantial margin before undersensing occurs. Single-center analysis of the Medtronic SL device [5], the results of a multicenter investigation of the same pacing system [13], and direct comparison of the two SL systems (Intermedics and Medtronic) showed, despite the different sensing strategies of these two devices [14], that they were essentially equivalent [13-15]. Most importantly, adequate atrial sensing was obtained in 98% of patients with total ring atrial electrodes and was maintained throughout the 2-year follow-up [13]. Among 101 consecutive patients with an DAB-SL pacing system, the VDD mode survived in 84% for 36 months [16]. For three SL systems, Intermedics, Medtronic, and Vitatron, Holter recordings were performed at 1 and 12 months after implantation. AV synchrony with a 2:1 programmed safety margin of atrial sensitivity was 98.6 ± 2.6%, compared to 99.8 ± 0.4% at highest atrial sensitivity ($p = 0.002$), with no difference between the three systems [17]. Similar data were demonstrated with four VDD pacing systems (Biotronik, Intermedics, Medtronic, and Medico) implanted in 150 patients [18].

Others studies have also demonstrated the similar long-term reliability of bipolar atrial sensing in various SL systems [19-28]. The rate of reprogramming to the VVI/R mode because atrial fibrillation (AF) was 2%-5% (follow-up 3-63 months), was similar to that for DDD patients with heart block and predominantly atrial sensing [29]. In another study [30], the incidence of paroxysmal AF was significantly lower in patients with SL systems than in those treated with DDD pacemakers: 4.5% and 8.9% ($p < 0.05$), respectively (10 years' experience, 178 patients). The reliability of diagnosis of intermittent atrial undersensing by various diagnostic features of pacing devices was recently examined [31]. Only the "P-wave" (atrial signal) amplitude histogram was comparable with Holter monitoring in the detection of atrial undersensing. Atrial sensing reliability in SL systems (180 patients) has been compared with DDD pacing (180 patients): the incidence of atrial undersensing episodes was similar during a mean follow-up of 29 months [32]. The incidence of AF did not differ significantly, and only a trend to a higher reintervention rate in the DDD group was found. The complications related to atrial undersensing (3%) in the VDD group, were counterbalanced by complications in the DDD group: atrial lead dislodgment (4%), atrial far-field oversensing (1.4%), and pneumothorax (3%).

Sensing during activity and body posture. Atrial signal attenuation during exercise compared to resting upright was found with SL-VDD pacing [5, 33-35]. Although the values for each individual varied considerably according to maneuver, in all postures and during hyperventilation and maximal *exercise,* atrial undersensing was rare. When the atrial signal was evaluated by the "P-wave" amplitude histograms for posture changes, respiration, and during exercise, significant variation was shown, with a difference in amplitude of up to 200% in 20% of the patients. During daily activities, 23% of recorded "P-wave" amplitudes were below 0.5 mV [35].

The cost-effectiveness of SL pacing was evaluated and showed a significant estimated cost reduction with SL pacing versus traditional two-lead systems: a cost reduction of $112 million per year [36].

Patient Selection for SL-VDD Pacing

According to the American College of Cardiology/American Heart Association guidelines of 1998, SL-VDD pacing is indicated for patients with intact sinus node function and various degrees of heart block. Such simple criteria as atrial rest rate ≥ 70 bpm, before implantation, identified patients at low risk (0.6%-0.8%) of sinus node disease [37]. For diagnosis of sinus node disease, Antonioli [7] used criteria of 60 bpm at rest and 85 bpm during exercise. On the basis of a retrospective analysis of about 400 VDD implants, we have been employing the following rules of thumb in evaluating patients with complete heart block (before or after temporary VVI pacemaker): the sinus rate should be at least 90 bpm at rest; sinus rate below 90 bpm raises the suspicion of sinus node dysfunction; in sinus rhythm at rest between 71 and 89 bpm the likelihood of mild-to-moderate chronotropic incompetence is about 10%; and in sinus rhythm of 70 bpm or less the probability of significant chronotropic incompetence is very high (about 30%). In using these criteria, nocturnal and at rest sinus bradycardia below 50 bpm was observed in less than 5% of our patients 3 years after implantation. ECG monitoring may be useful at rest and, when possible, during walking at maximum rate. The preimplant right atrium volume as determined by echocardiography was found to be an accurate predictor of atrial undersensing [38]. It may be expected that in patients with significantly dilated right atrium, the probability of sinus node disease and atrial arrhythmias is higher than usual. All these criteria of sinus node disease for selected patients for VDD pacing should be evaluated in prospective studies.

According to recent publications, paroxysmal AF is not a contraindication for devices with mode switch [7, 39, 40]. However, it should be mentioned that patients with paroxysmal AF, prior to implantation, had poorer results for VDD pacing survival in a follow-up period of 14 ± 7 months [41]. We do not use any SL systems in patients with paroxysmal AF, or any frequent premature beats, since we believe that better results may be obtained with DDD/R pacing. SL-VDD pacing should also be avoided in patients who may require antiarrhythmic or any other medication which could lead to drug-induced chronotropic incompetence.

Single Leads for Sensing and Pacing: SL-DDD Systems

The major limitation of SL systems is that they cannot provide atrial pacing with the same success as they provide atrial sensing. Currently, there are two approaches to clinically managing atrial pacing by SL systems. The first is to use available SLs; the second is to change the lead shape and thus position the stimulation electrode closer to the atrial wall. A multicenter study using the Medico Phymos 830-S SL-VDD reported successful atrial stimulation on implantation in 76% of 315 patients with a mean threshold 3.2 ± 1.5 V at 0.5 ms [42]. At 6 months' follow-up, only 51% of the patients were responsive to atrial pacing without side effects, with a threshold of up to 5 V at 0.5 ms. An interesting approach using a floating atrial dipole for pacing has been proposed by Biotronik [42-45], an overlapping biphasic impulse (OLBI) mode of atrial stimulation. During this mode of pacing, two unipolar rectangular impulses of opposite polarity are delivered simultaneously to the floating atrial electrodes. A reduction of atrial stimulation threshold was achieved as compared to conventional biphasic stimulation (2.5 V ± 1.9 V vs 5.8 V ± 4.2 V). Atrial capture was reported in 84% of patients at 3 months after implantation [45]. However, in 21% of the patients, phrenic stimulation was observed. Similar results were reported in 125 patients in a multicenter study from 34 centers [45]. The pacing stability was investigated after reprogramming a lower rate of 20% above the resting sinus rate during sitting and left and right decubital positions by Holter

ECG monitoring in 32 patients with stable atrial capture in supine. In 83% of patients, loss of atrial capture was observed about 15% of the time. Of note is that the initial price of the SL-DDD system, even without OLBI stimulation, is more than that of the SL-VDD unit and at least equal to that of the two-lead DDD device [36]. Endeavoring to improve the results of atrial pacing, Biotronik proposed SL with three floating atrial rings: VECATS (vena cava atrial stimulation SL) [46]. The proximal ring is located in the superior vena cava, while the medial and distal rings float in the high and mid part of the right atrium. The pacing stimulus is derived between the proximal and medial rings, while sensing is assigned between the medial and distal rings. In the multicenter European and Canadian clinical study, the results of atrial stimulation in 78 patients 3 months after implantation were comparable with those achieved with standard SL and OLBI stimulation.

Thus, the results of floating SL pacing support the assumption that for clinically appropriate atrial pacing, the atrial dipole should be positioned as close as possible to the atrial wall, since only the contact lead is able to provide clinically appropriate pacing [8]. Of note was that the best results were achieved in the mid or lower atrium position [8, 15, 27, 43, 45, 47, 48].

The second approach to SL-DDD pacing is to change the shapes of the lead that provides contact between the atrial part of the SL and the atrial wall. Numerous SL-DDD designs are now being studied. Medtronic is currently conducting clinical trials of several DDD single pacing leads [8, 49, 50] and implantable cardioverter-defibrillator leads for DDD pacing [51] which have a preshaped L-curve with a protruding, electrically active side tip designed to lodge in the lower part of the right atrium. Although sensing in all these leads was appropriate, the mean chronic atrial threshold was 3.4 V ± 0.4 V at 0.5 ms [50] and 5 V at 0.57 ms, and diaphragmatic stimulation was noted in many patients [49].

Pacesetter of St. Jude has designed an atrial J-lead with ventricular limb that offshoots 1 cm proximal to the atrial precurved J and can be positioned in the apex of the right ventricle [52]. This lead was easily placed in dogs and achieved long-term atrial pacing thresholds of less than 1 V. Hirschberg et al. [53], also from Pacesetter, have designed a SL for DDD pacing in which the distal tip is an atrial electrode, which has an active fixation and is hooked in the right atrium, with the body of the lead passing via the tricuspid valve to the ventricle after fixation of the atrial tip. As the authors have reported in animals, implantation of this lead is quite simple.

Another type of SL for DDD pacing has been designed by CCS Inc. and has two preformed S-shaped curves: one at the level of the superior vena cava and the other at the level of the mid-to-lower right atrium [54]. The acute and chronic performance of this version of a SL-DDD has been recently evaluated [55, 56]. The mean acute atrial signal was 2.5 mV ± 1 mV and the mean atrial stimulation threshold was 1.6 V ± 0.5 V. In a follow-up for 6 months, there was a high rate of atrial part dislocation (3/14) and a relatively high threshold, despite OLBI stimulation, in the remaining patients (mean 3.1V ± 1.5 V).

Practical Aspects of SL Positioning

SLs are available in several different lengths of atrial to ventricular apex separations. The decision to choose any AV separation may be made empirically: large or tall vs child or short/small patient. A simple fluoroscopic technique may also be used to predict the best lead size, by laying a test electrode over the chest of a supine patient and positioning it under fluoroscopy to approximate the expected intracardiac course of the lead [57].

Regarding placement of atrial electrodes there is significant controversy. There are implanters who recommend placing the atrial lead in close proximity to the sinus node, but not far from the mid part of the right atrium [6, 7, 21, 22, 32]. Others, before selecting the optimum place for the atrial lead, strongly recommend right atrial mapping by the atrial part of the SL [5, 8, 13]. In several reports (about 500 implantations of SL devices) the optimum atrial signal was most frequently found in the mid-lower and lower parts of the right atrium [5, 8, 13, 15, 27, 48]. A comparison study regarding the best placement for the two types of leads (total and split rings) was conducted and no significant differences in optimum positioning or achievable atrial signal amplitude were found [58]. Nonuniformity of the anatomy in normal and diseased atria led to multiform atrial depolarization, making individual propagation and sensing of the atrial signal via the pacemaker's amplifier unpredictable. This complexity in the anatomo-electrophysiological substrate could explain the unpredictability of the optimum location of the atrial lead. It should be noted that usually the optimum cardiac signal is provided by contact or at least a very close position of the electrodes to the atrial or ventricular wall. If this is important for atrial sensing by floating electrodes, it is more important if the same leads are to provide atrial pacing. More details regarding the position of the atrial part of the SL and the technique of placing it were discussed in a recently published review [8].

Another important issue during implantation of SL is the minimum acceptable amplitude of the atrial signal. As was demonstrated for the first time with Medtronic's VDD system [5], and later with the Intermedics device [14-16, 20] as well as in the multicenter study using the Biotronik SL-VDD system [59], there is an approximately 50% diminution in atrial signal amplitude between the values obtained at implant with a PSA (usually measurements done via a ventricular channel) and the actual atrial sensing threshold detected by the pacemaker immediately after implantation. There are several reasons for this diminution of atrial signal [8, 13]. As mentioned above, the atrial signal may decrease by up to 200% during exercise or other physiological maneuvers [31-35]. This would suggest that it is necessary to employ a large margin of safety: at least more than twofold according to the above-mentioned data. Therefore, the minimum acceptable atrial signal amplitude during implantation should be at least twice the desired long-term atrial signal, and the desired long-term atrial signal should be at least 0.5-1.0 mV (if one assumes amplifiers are capable of detecting atrial signals as low as 0.10-0.18 mV, these amplitudes still allow for a substantial margin before undersensing occurs). Accordingly, during implantation of SL, for appropriate long-term survival of VDD pacing, minimum acceptable atrial signal amplitude measured by the ventricular channel of the PSA should be at least 1-2 mV [8, 13]. In follow-up such diagnostic features as atrial signal amplitude histograms (Saphir II, Vitatron; KAPPA 700, Medtronic) can provide further help in adequately programming atrial sensitivity.

Conclusions

1. Floating SL-VDD pacing is a reliable, convenient, and cost-effective pacing alternative for patients with various degrees of AV block and normal sinus node function. To obtain appropriate long-term results with SL systems, it is important to place the atrial lead at a site within the right atrium, where it exhibits the optimal atrial signal.
2. The performance of various models of floating SL with various stimuli configurations does not provide clinically adequate results and cannot currently be used as an alternative to DDD pacing.
3. Proposed models of SL dual chamber pacing, with the atrial part in contact with the right atrial wall, are very attractive, but they are still in their early stages of development.
4. There is good reason to hope that in the near future SL systems capable of both appropriate atrial sensing and pacing will be available. These systems are particularly suited to electrical therapy of arrhythmia and for heart resynchronization by future universal anti-brady-tachyarrhytmias devices.

References

1. Antonioli GE, Baggioni GF, Grassi G et al (1979) A simple P-sensing ventricle stimulating lead driving a VAT generator. In: Meere C (ed) Cardiac pacing. PaceSymp, Montreal, Canada
2. Goldreyer BN, Olive AL, Leslie J et al (1981) A new orthogonal lead for P synchronous pacing. Pacing Clin Electrophysiol 4:638-644
3. Brownlee RR (1989) Toward optimizing the detection of atrial depolarization with floating bipolar electrodes. Pacing Clin Electrophysiol 12:431-442
4. Furman S, Gross J, Andrews C (1991) Single lead VDD pacing. In: Antonioli GE, Aubert AE, Ector H (eds) Pacemaker leads. Elsevier, Amsterdam, pp 183-197
5. Ovsyshcher IE, Katz A, Bondy C (1994) Clinical evaluation of a new single pass lead VDD pacing system. Pacing Clin Electrophysiol 17:1859-1864
6. Antonioli GE (1994) Single lead atrial synchronous ventricular pacing: A dream comes true. Pacing Clin Electrophysiol 17:1531-1547
7. Antonioli GE (1999) Single A-V lead cardiac pacing. Arianna, Casalecchio, Italy
8. Ovsyshcher IE, Wagshal AB (1998) Single-lead VDD/DDD pacing. In: Vardas PE (ed) Cardiac arrhythmias, pacing and electrophysiology. The expert view. Kluwer Academic, Dordrecht, pp 389-398

9. Tse HF, Lau CP (1998) The current status of single lead dual chamber sensing and pacing. J Interv Card Electrophysiol 2:255-267

10. Furman S (1993) Sensing and timing on cardiac electrorogram. In: Furman S, Hayes DL, Holmes DR (eds) A practice of cardiac pacing. Futura, Mount Kisco, pp 104-108

11. de Cock CC, Huygens J, Visser CA (1997) Inappropriate atrial sensing in single lead VDD pacing: how much is clinically relevant? Eur Heart J 8 (Suppl):A662

12. Lau CP, Leung SK, Lee ISF (1996) Comparative evaluation of acute and long term clinical performance of two single lead atrial synchronous ventricular (VDD) pacemakers: diagonally arranged bipolar versus closely spaced bipolar ring electrodes. Pacing Clin Electrophysiol 19:1574-1581

13. Ovsyshcher IE, Katz A, Rosenheck S et al (1996) Single lead VDD pacing: multicenter study. Pacing Clin Electrophysiol 19:1768-1771

14. Wagshal AB, Ovsyshcher IE (1997) Letter to the Editor. Pacing Clin Electrophysiol 20:1888-1889

15. Tse HF, Lau CP, Leung SK et al (1996) Single lead DDD system: a comparative evaluation of unipolar, bipolar, and overlapping biphasic stimulation and the effects of right atrial floating electrode location on atrial pacing and sensing thresholds. Pacing Clin Electrophysiol 19:1758-1763

16. Palma EC, Andrews CA, Hanson S et al (1997) Atrial arrhythmia and mode survival in single pass VDD pacemakers. Pacing Clin Electrophysiol 20:A1538

17. Nowak B, Middeldorf T, Voigtlander T et al (1998) How reliable is atrial sensing in single-lead VDD pacing: comparison of three systems. Pacing Clin Electrophysiol 21:2226-2231

18. Rey JL, Tribouilloy C, Elghelbazouri F et al (1998) A single-lead VDD pacing: long-term experience with four different systems. Am Heart J 135:1036-1039

19. Crick JCP (1991) European multicenter prospective follow-up study of 1002 implants of a single lead VDD pacing system. Pacing Clin Electrophysiol 14:1742-1744

20. Naegeli B, Osswald S, Pfisterer M et al (1996) VDDI pacing: short and long-term stability of atrial sensing with a single lead system. Pacing Clin Electrophysiol 19:455-464

21. Longo E, Catrini V (1990) Experience and implantation techniques with a new single-pass lead VDD system. Pacing Clin Electrophysiol 13:927-936

22. Ansani L, Percoco GF, Guardigli G et al (1994) Long-term reliability of single lead atrial synchronous pacing systems using closely spaced dipoles: five year experience. Pacing Clin Electrophysiol 17:1865-1869

23. Curzio G and the Multicenter study Group (1991) A multicenter evaluation of a single-pass lead VDD pacing system. Pacing Clin Electrophysiol 14:434-442

24. Lau C-P, Tai Y-T, Li J P-S et al (1992) Initial clinical experience with a single pass VDDR pacing system. Pacing Clin Electrophysiol 15:1894-1900

25. Takei Y, Ishibashi H, Tanaka K et al (1997) The long term outcome after VDD pacemaker implantation. Pacing Clin Electrophysiol 20:A1454

26. Clinical Study Report (1995) VDD stimulation with fractally coated single pass leads. Biotronik, Berlin

27. Gessman L, White M, Ghaly N et al (1996) US experience with the AddVent VDDI pacing system. Pacing Clin Electrophysiol 19:1764-1767

28. Chamberlain-Webber R, Barnes E, Papouchado M et al (1998) Long-term survival of VDD pacing. Pacing Clin Electrophysiol 21:2246-2248

29. Chamberlain-Webber R, Petersen MEV, Ingram A et al (1994) Reasons for reprogramming dual chamber pacemakers to VVI mode. A retrospective review using a *computer* database. Pacing Clin Electrophysiol 17:1730-1736

30. Moracchini P, Tesorieri MC, Juliani M et al (1997) Atrial fibrillation incidence in

patients with VDD single lead and DDD pacing system. Pacing Clin Electrophysiol 20:A1549

31. Wiegand UK, Bode F, Schneider R et al (1999) Diagnosis of atrial undersensing in dual chamber pacemakers: impact of autodiagnostic features. Pacing Clin Electrophysiol 22:894-902

32. Wiegand UK, Bode F, Schneider R et al (1999) Atrial sensing and AV synchrony in single lead VDD pacemakers: a prospective comparison to DDD devices with bipolar atrial leads. J Cardiovasc Electrophysiol 10:513-520

33. Varriale P, Chryssos BE (1993) Atrial sensing performance of the single-lead VDD pacemaker during exercise. J Am Coll Cardiol 22:1854-1857

34. Toivonen L, Lommi J (1996) Dependence of atrial sensing function on posture in a single-lead atrial triggered ventricular (VDD) pacemaker. Pacing Clin Electrophysiol 19:309-313

35. Langford EJ, Smith REA, McCrea WA et al (1997) Determining optimal atrial sensitivity settings for single lead VDD pacing: the importance of the P wave histogram. Pacing Clin Electrophysiol 20: 619-623

36. Lee JK, Krahn AD, Yee R et al (1998) Long term reliability and cost effectiveness of VDD pacing. Circulation 98 (17 Suppl: I):A427

37. Wiegand UK, Bode F, Schneider R et al (1999) Development of sinus node disease in patients with AV block: implications for single lead VDD pacing. Heart 81:580-585

38. de Cock CC, Van Campen LC, Huygens J et al (1999) Usefulness of echocardiography to predict inappropriate atrial sensing in single-lead VDD pacing. Pacing Clin Electrophysiol 22:1344-1347

39. Nowak B, Voigtlander T, Rosocha S et al (1998) Paroxysmal atrial fibrillation and high degree AV block: use of single-lead VDDR pacing with mode switching. Pacing Clin Electrophysiol 21:1927-1933

40. Buys EM, van Hemel NM, Jessurun ER et al (1998) VDDR pacing after His-bundle ablation for paroxysmal atrial fibrillation: a pilot study. Pacing Clin Electrophysiol 21:1869-1872

41. Ben Ameur Y, Martin E, Jarwe M et al (1997) VDD mode single electrode cardiac stimulation: indications, results and limitations of the method. Ann Cardiol Angiol (Paris) 46:585-591

42. DiGregorio F, Morra A, Bongiorni MG et al (1997) A multicenter experience in DDD pacing with single-pass lead. Pacing Clin Electrophysiol 20:A1210

43. Del Giudici G, Frabeti L, Cioffi L et al (1997) DDD pacing using a single A-V lead with atrial floating dipole and biphasic overlapping stimulation. Pacing Clin Electrophysiol 20:A1516

44. Tse HF, Lau CP, Leung SK et al (1996) Single lead DDD system: a comparative evaluation of unipolar, bipolar, and overlapping biphasic stimulation and the effects of right atrial floating electrode location on atrial pacing and sensing thresholds. Pacing Clin Electrophysiol 19:1758-1763

45. Frabetti L, Sassara M, Melissano A et al (1997) OLBI pacing–the Italian experience. Prog Biomed Res 2:88-94

46. Res JCJ, Lau C (2000) First results of the Canadian and European single lead DDD studies. A report of two multicenter studies on vena cava atrial stimulation (VECATS). Pacing Clin Electrophysiol 23:1804-1808

47. Bongiorni MG, Moracchini PV, Nava A et al (1998) Radiographic assessment of atrial dipole position in single pass lead VDD and DDD pacing. Pacing Clin Electrophysiol 21:2240-2245

48. Calosso E, Verzoni A, Manzo R et al (1997) DDD pacing by the floating electrode of a VDD single lead pacemaker. Pacing Clin Electrophysiol 20:A1516

49. Israel CW, Kruse IM, Van Mechelen R et al (1999) Results from the use of a preshaped lead for single-pass VDD/DDD stimulation. Pacing Clin Electrophysiol 22:1314-1320

50. Naegeli B, Straumann E, Gerber A et al (1999) Dual chamber pacing with a single-lead DDD pacing system. Pacing Clin Electrophysiol 22:1013-1019

51. Gradaus R, Dorszewski A, Kleeman A et al (1999) Acute results with a new single pass, right ventricular defibrillation lead capable for pacing and sensing in right atrium and ventricle. J Am Coll Cardiol 33:134A

52. Morgan K, Bornzin GA, Florio J et al (1997) A new single pass lead. Pacing Clin Electrophysiol 20:A1211

53. Hirschberg J, Ekwall C, Bowald S (1996) DDD pacemaker system with single lead (SLDDD) reduces intravascular hardware. Long-term experimental study. Pacing Clin Electrophysiol 19:A601

54. Brownlee RR, Swindle MM, Bertolet R et al (1997) Toward optimizing a preshaped catheter and system parameters to achieve single lead DDD pacing. Pacing Clin Electrophysiol 20:1354-1358

55. Hazday MS, Mendelson D, Brownlee RR (1998) Acute evaluation of a preformed single-pass VDD/DDD pacing lead. J Interv Cardiovasc Electrophysiol 2:171-173

56. Antonioli GE, Sassara M, Guerra R et al (1999) First clinical experience with a new preshaped single AV lead for permanent DDD pacing. Pacing Clin Electrophysiol 22:A177

57. Nowak B, Voigtlander T, Liebrich A et al (1996) A simple method for preoperative assessment of the best fitting electrode length in single lead VDD pacing. Pacing Clin Electrophysiol 19:1346-1350

58. Karagouz R, Guldal M, Ertas F et al (1997) Comparison of the optimal position of the atrial electrodes in two different single lead VDD pacing systems. Pacing Clin Electrophysiol 20:A1444

59. Anonymous (1995) Clinical experience with VDD pacing systems. Review, 6:1, Biotronik, Berlin

Hemodynamic Sensors: Are They All the Same?

R. Chirife, M.C. Tentori, H. Mazzetti and D. Dasso

Introduction

The need for rate adaptation in cardiac pacing triggered interest in hemodynamic sensors. Although several different methods have been proposed, the simplicity of operation of the piezoelectric sensor (or accelerometer) placed within the pacemaker prevailed over the physiological value of other, more complex methods. More recently, however, the advent of electrical treatment of heart failure renewed the interest in hemodynamic sensors which could be used for follow-up, for rate control in patients with limited physical activity, and for DDD pacing optimization. The purpose of this paper is to describe in general terms those sensors applicable to implantable devices, in particular the impedance-derived hemodynamic sensor.

Background

The assessment of cardiac function has long been a matter of interest and controversy. In 1740 Stephen Hales [1] published his observations on the blood pressure behavior of the mare's heart when subjected to challenge: "*the violent straining to get loose, did by acting of most of her muscles, especially the abdominal, impel the blood from all parts of the vena cava and consequently there was the greater supply for the heart which must therefore throw out more in each pulsation*". Perhaps this was Starling's inspiration for what is now believed to be one of the fundamental principles of cardiac performance: Starling's Law of the heart [2]. On the preload-output curve one can observe the effect of contractility changes by shifts of the curve to the right or to the left. Based on this principle, the calculation of ejection fraction is a simplified expression of Starling's principle. Contractility can be assessed by various methods <[3-10] that remove the effect of preload and afterload. Although

Cardiology Division, Hospital Fernández, Buenos Aires, Argentina ventricular dP/dt is also used as a marker of contractility [4, 11], it is known to be strongly load-dependent. Preload assessment on the other hand can be made by wedge and pulmonary artery pressure measurements, and by right ventricular end-diastolic volume (EDV) using the conductance (impedance) catheter [12, 13].

Implantable Sensors in the Right Side of the Heart

Since chronic implantation of any hardware within the left heart or in the arterial system is generally disapproved of by most cardiologists due to the risk of systemic embolization, the right ventricle has been looked upon as an alternative. Based on the law of conservation of mass, and in the absence of intracardiac shunts, it is expected that whatever changes in pump function take place on the right side will eventually take place on the left heart and viceversa. Thus, the use of right ventricular sensors to assess overall cardiac performance is appealing. While neurohormonally mediated contractility changes will simultaneously affect both sides of the heart, preload changes modulating pump function (following the Starling principle) will be apparent first in the right heart [12]. Table 1 attempts to classify some of the available sensors on the basis of their type, physiological signal, hardware used, etc.

Table 1. Classification of implantable intracardiac sensors

Method Hemodynamics	Physiologic signal	Lead hardware	Measurement	
Pressure	RV dP/dt	Piezoelectric transducer	Peak amplitude	Contractility
Motion/sound	Peak intracardiac acceleration, "PEA"	Piezoelectric transducer	Peak amplitude	Contractility ?
	Z slope, area, "VIP"	None (standard leads)	Peak amplitude	Contractility ?
Impedance	RV end-diastolic Volume	None (standard leads)	Amplitude @ End diastole	Preload
	Pre-ejection period (PEP)	None (standard leads)	Timing	Contractility
	RV end-systolic Volume	None (standard leads)	Amplitude @ End systole	Contractility
	RV ejection Fraction	None (standard leads)	Amplitude ratio	Contractility
	Stroke volume Cardiac output	None (standard leads)	Amplitude X HR	Pump Function

Applications of Implantable Hemodynamic Sensors

Implantable hemodynamic sensors have been traditionally associated with rate-adaptive pacemakers. The first pacemaker to use an impedance-derived intracardiac hemodynamic signal was the pre-ejection period (PEP)-controlled rate-adaptive pacemaker [14]. Since the right ventricular impedance value is reciprocally related to right ventricular volume (the larger the volume, the smaller the impedance), volume-derived preload and contractility indices obtained from the absolute right ventricular impedance changes were also proposed for implantable devices [15, 16]. The slope of impedance change within a predetermined window ("ventricular inotropic parameter", VIP) may also give contractility information applicable to rate control [17, 18]. Another sensor, the intracardiac accelerometer (peak endocardial acceleration, PEA) was proposed as a marker of cardiac contractility changes and thus used for rate control [19, 20] and atrioventricular optimization [21]. Hemodynamic sensors have several applications (Table 2), depending on the type of sensor and the hemodynamic parameter that is being measured.

Table 2. Applications of intracardiac sensors

Contractility sensor	For rate response, arrhythmia discrimination and heart failure management
Preload sensor	For heart failure management
Cardiac output	For heart failure management and arrhythmia discrimination

Impedance Method

To record intracardiac impedance, a low-level (well below capture threshold) carrier signal (generally a constant-current square wave, with a pulse width of 0.005-0.1 ms) is driven to a pair of intracardiac electrodes at a rate of 40-1000 Hz. The resulting voltage from the same or from a different pair of electrodes is detected with an amplifier. The value of the sensed voltage will be inversely proportional to the volume where the electrodes are contained.

Electrode Configurations

Impedance can be measured using unipolar, bipolar, tripolar or quadripolar configurations. These terms refer to the number of electrodes used for delivery of the impedance carrier signal and for the detection of the resulting voltage. Unipolar VVI systems allow only the unipolar configuration, while bipolar DDD systems offer all choices. In addition, signal detection may have different physiological

Table 3. Different modes for intracardiac impedance detection. The driving current (carrier) and the detection of the resulting voltage can be applied to any electrode combination using from VVI unipolar leads to bipolar atrial and ventricular leads

Impedance configuration			
Driving	Detecting	Configuration	Type
Can-RVTip	Can-RVTip	Unipolar	Transthoracic
RVRing-RVTip	RVRing-RVTip	Bipolar	Intraventricular
RARing-RVTip	RVRing-RVTip	Tripolar	Intraventricular
RARing-RVTip	RARing-RVTip	Bipolar	Transvalvular
RARing-RVTip	RARing-RVRing	Tripolar	Transvalvular
RARing-RVTip	RARing-RVRing	Quadripolar	Transvalvular

implications depending whether it is done within the ventricle or across the tricuspid valve (transvalvular impedance, TVI)[22]. This classification is depicted in Table 3.

The Intracardiac Impedance Waveform

Figure 1 shows a multichannel recording of a canine experiment. The timing of the impedance-derived volume waveform (channel 2) is seen to correspond closely with the proper timing of invasive pressure and flow parameters.

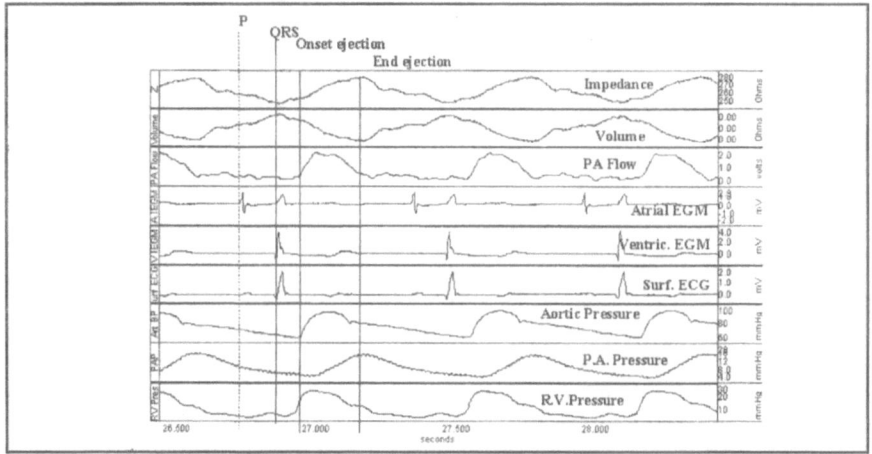

Fig. 1. Tracing obtained from a dog under general anesthesia. Pulmonary artery (PA) flow was determined with a catheter-tip electromagnetic flow meter. Aortic and right ventricular pressures were obtained with Millar catheter-tip manometers, PA pressure with a fluid-filled catheter. Of note is that the onset of ejection of the PA flow is aligned with the onset of ejection of the Z and volume waveforms. Prior to ejection, an increase in end-diastolic volume is noted, due to the atrial contraction. The end of ejection of the PA flow coincides with the minimum RV volume (maximum impedance). These findings indicate that the timing of the impedance-derived volume corresponds to the hemodynamic counterparts

Hemodynamic Validation of Impedance

Since there is no gold standard for beat-by-beat intraventricular volume measurement, indirect methods have been used. One of them is the construction of Starling regressions using impedance-derived cardiac volumes under preload challenges. Successful reproduction of the preload-stroke volume relationship is considered evidence for the validation of the method for volume assessment. Contractility challenges (such as isoproterenol or dobutamine infusion) are expected to increase the ejection fraction as measured from impedance [16]. Assuming that the patient's increase in heart rate is due to adrenergic stimulation, the measured percentual change in ejection fraction should match closely with the patient's intrinsic rate change. Also, any significant degree of positive feedback during incremental rate pacing at rest, an undesirable sensor response, should be absent from the contractility measurement.

Observations on Impedance Validation

Figure 2 shows a canine experiment during which balloon occlusion of the inferior vena cava was performed to abruptly reduce venous return. Impedance was recorded using the TVI method [22], sampling impedance between the atrial and ventricular ring electrodes. It can be seen that the onset of occlusion causes an immediate reduction of EDV, and upon release of occlusion there is a rapid return to normal with a little previous overshoot. A Starling regression during inferior vena cava occlusion in the dog is depicted in Fig. 3. End-diastolic impedance (EDZ) and end-systolic impedance (ESZ) were normalized to 100 ml and 50 ml respectively, and stroke volume (SV) plotted against EDV. The reduction of EDV upon increasing pacing rate is seen in Fig. 4. Figure 5 is a Starling regression obtained in a typical patient using impedance-derived volume, normalized to 200 ml for end-diastole and 100 ml for end-systole. Table 4 shows the resulting regression slopes and R values for all Starling regressions obtained in 24 patients. Figure 6 shows the concordance between a patient's intrinsic rate and the ejection fraction calculated rate during isoproterenol challenge. Figure 7 demonstrates that the contractility measurement remains unaffected by increasing and decreasing pacing rate at rest, thus ruling out positive feedback.

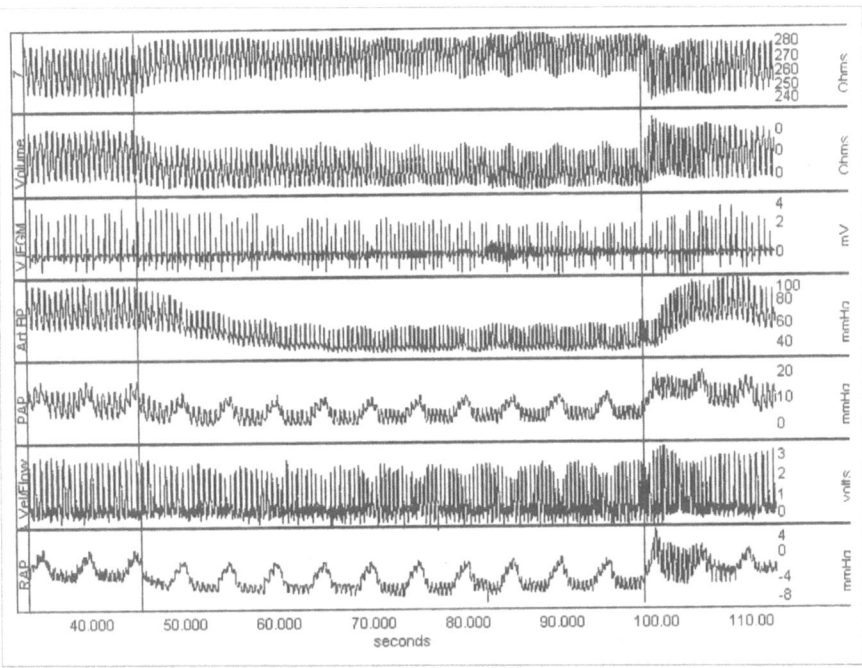

Fig. 2. Multichannel recording at slow speed of inferior vena cava occlusion in a dog. The vertical line to the *left* marks the onset of the occlusion and the one on the *right* the end. The abrupt reduction in preload causes a decrease in end-diastolic volume (the top envelope of the tracing in *channel 2*). At the end of the maneuver, EDV returns to normal, preceded by some overshoot, which has a similar counterpart in the arterial blood pressure waveform (*channel 4, Art BP*). The periodic modulation seen on most channels is due to the effect of the mechanical respirator

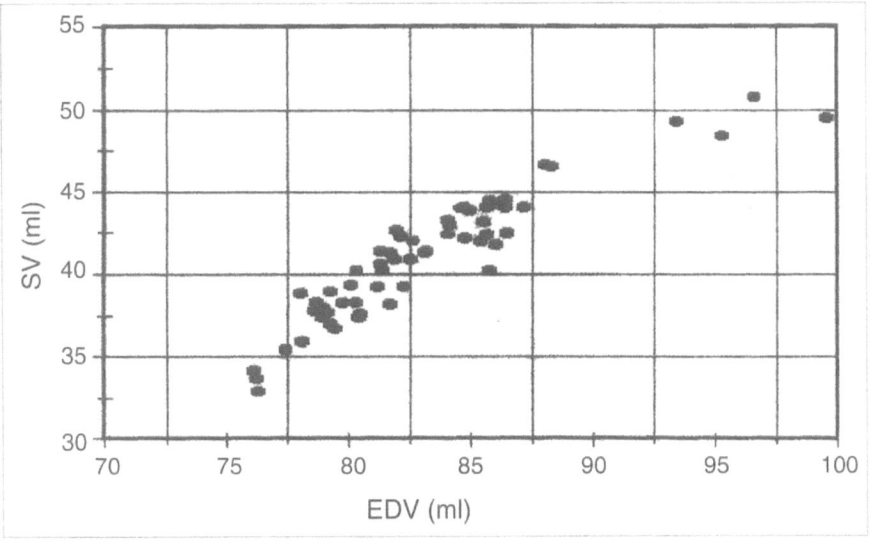

Fig. 3. Starling regression from the study in Fig. 2

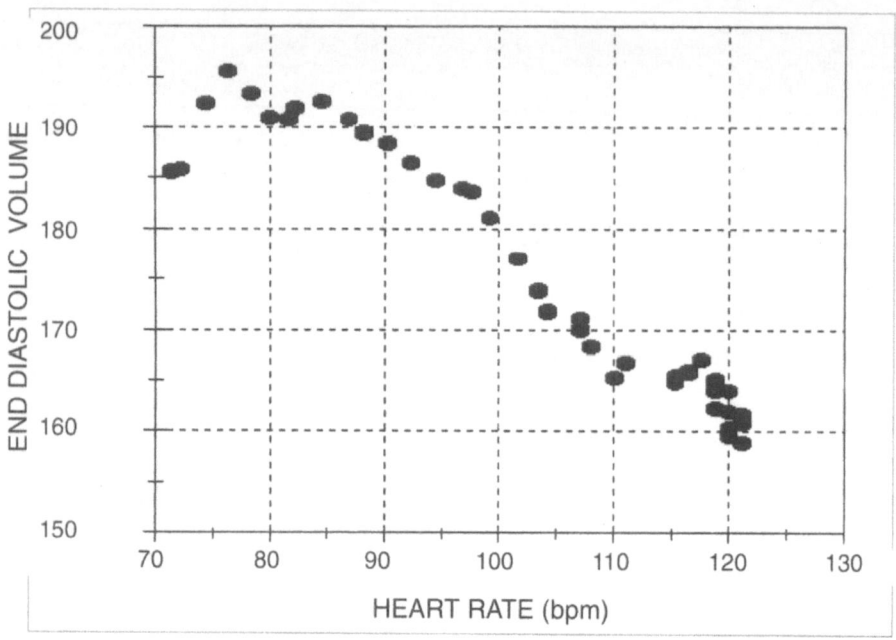

Fig. 4. The effect of increasing pacing rate on EDV is more noticeable between 85 and 110 bpm during VVI pacing in a patient

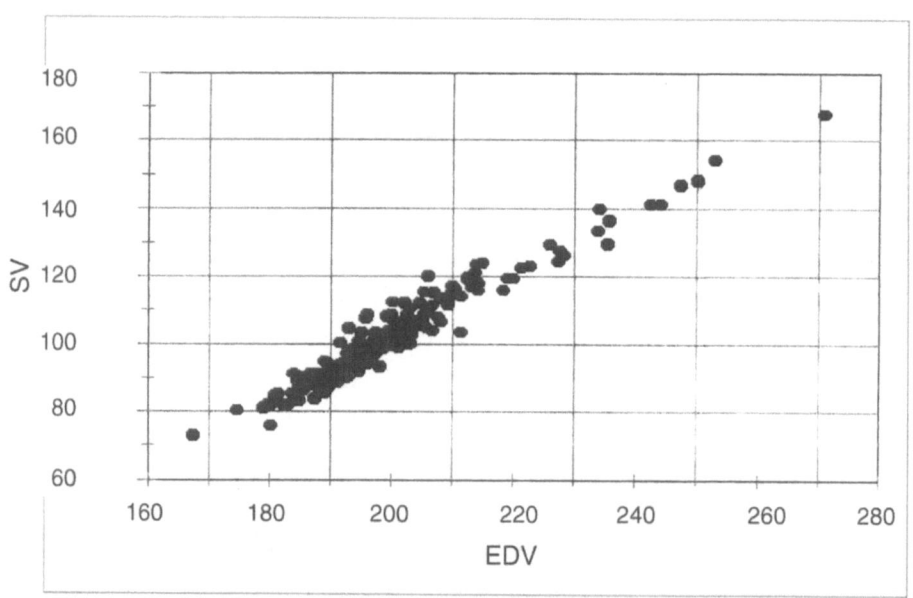

Fig. 5. Starling regression obtained in a typical patient using impedance-derived volume, normalized to 200 ml for end-diastole and 100 ml for end-systole

Table 4. Summary of results. The mean calculated Starling slope is very close to 1.0 with a range from 0.61 to 1.85. This variation is due to the non-linearity of the volume-impedance relationship, which varies from patient to patient. The R values observed were all statistically significant

	Results of preload challenge (Starling regressions)			
	Mean	SD	Minimum	Maximum
Starling slope	0.99	+/- 0.24	0.61	1.85
R value	0.87	+/- 0.11	0.61	0.98

P values, between 0.01 and 0.001

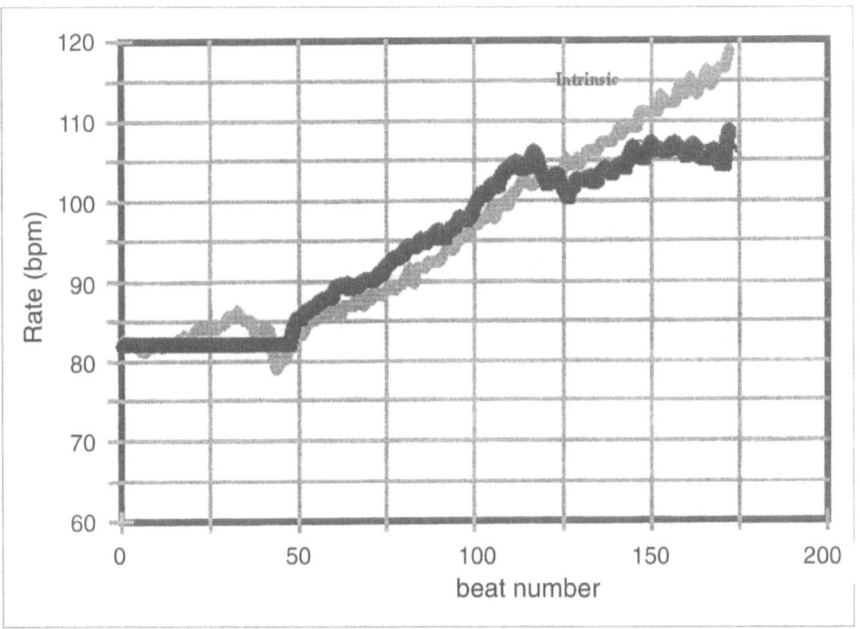

Fig. 6. Comparison between the patient's intrinsic rate and the contractility-calculated rate during isoproterenol study. The contractility rate was calculated from the percentage change in Z-derived ejection fraction

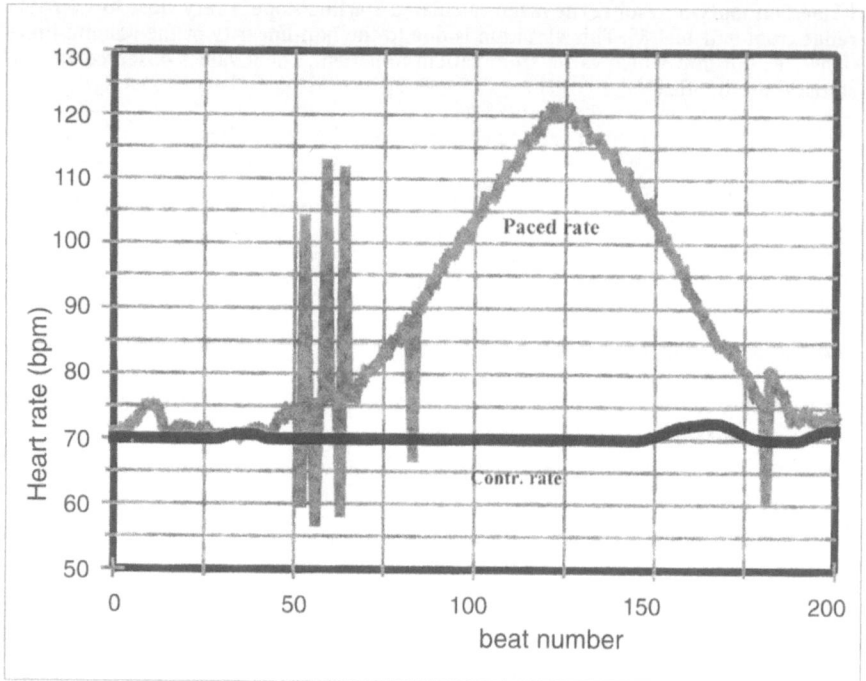

Fig. 7. An example of the independence between pacing rate changes at rest and Z-derived contractility rate. The slight rise of contractility observed during the declining rate of pacing is frequently observed, and interpreted as part of the baroreflex sensitivity reaction

Conclusions

1. Not all hemodynamic sensors are the same, for they measure different hemodynamic parameters with different techniques.
2. Intracardiac bipolar or multipolar impedance seems to be the most reasonable approach for hemodynamic assessment with implantable devices.
3. Unipolar ventricular impedance (VIP) and intracardiac accelerometer signals (PEA) may provide contractility information, but these sensors need further validation, for they may be preload-dependent.

References

1. Hales S (1740) Statistical essays: containing haemastaticks; or, an account of some hydraulic and hydrostatical experiments made on the blood and blood vessels of animals. Innys and others, London
2. Patterson SW, Starling EH (1914) On the mechanical factors which determine the output of the ventricles. J Physiol 48:357-379

3. Nicolosi AC, Hettrick DA, Warltier DC (1996) Assessment of right ventricular function in swine using sonomicrometry and conductance. Ann Thorac Surg 61:1381-1387

4. Strobeck JF, Sonnenblick EH (1981) Myocardial and ventricular function. Part II: Intact heart. Herz 6:275-287

5. Sharir T, Feldman MD, Haber H et al (1994) Ventricular systolic assessment in patients with dilated cardiomyopathy by preload-adjusted maximal power. Circulation 89:2045-2053

6. Ross J (1984) Applications and limitations of end-systolic measures of ventricular performance. Fed Proc 43:2418-2422

7. Sagawa K, Suga H, Shoukas AA, Bakalar KM (1977) End-systolic pressure/volume ratio: a new index of cardiac contractility. Am J Cardiol 40:748-753

8. Mahler F, Covell JW, Ross J Jr (1975) Systolic pressure-diameter relations in the normal conscious dog. Cardiovasc Res 9:447-455

9. Mehmel HC, Schwartz F, Manthey J et al (1984) Is the quotient: systolic peak pressure/end-systolic volume a useful parameter in the assessment of left ventricular function? Z Kardiol 73:242-247

10. Grossman W, Braunwald E, Mann T et al (1977) Contractile state of the left ventricle in man as evaluated from end-systolic pressure-volume relations. Circulation 56:845-852

11. Chirife R, Healy RW, Leland OS, Neff RK (1976) Computer analysis of left ventricular function in patients with ischemic heart disease. In: Saha S (ed) Proc Fourth New England Bioengineering Conference, Yale University. pp. 185-189

12. Lichtwark-Aschoff M, Beale R, Pfeiffer UJ (1996) Central venous pressure, pulmonary artery occlusion pressure, intrathoracic blood volume and right ventricular end-diastolic volume as indicators of cardiac preload. J Crit Care 11:180-188

13. Chen CH, Nevo E, Fetics B et al (1997) Comparison of continuous left ventricular volumes by transthoracic two-dimensional digital echo quantification with simultaneous conductance catheter measurements in patients with cardiac disease. Am J Cardiol 80:756-761

14. Chirife R (1988) Physiological principles of a new method for rate responsive pacing using the pre-ejection interval. Pacing Clin Electrophysiol 11:1545-1554

15. Chirife R (1991) Acquisition of hemodynamic data and sensor signals for rate control from standard pacing electrodes. Pacing Clin Electrophysiol 14:1563-1565

16. Chirife R, Ortega DF, Salazar AI (1993) Feasibility of measuring relative right-ventricular volumes and ejection fraction with implantable rhythm control devices. Pacing Clin Electrophysiol 16:1673-1683

17. Schaldach M, Hutten H (1992) Intracardiac impedance to determine sympathetic activity in rate responsive pacing. Pacing Clin Electrophysiol 15:1778-1786

18. Schaldach M (1990) Automatic adjustment of pacing parameters based on intracardiac impedance measurements. Pacing Clin Electrophysiol 13:1702-1710

19. Bongiorni MG, Soldati E, Arena G et al (1996) Is local myocardial contractility related to endocardial acceleration signals detected by a transvenous pacing lead? Pacing Clin Electrophysiol 19:1682-1688

20. Rickards AF, Bombardini T, Corbucci G, Plicchi G (1996) An implantable intracardiac accelerometer for monitoring myocardial contractility. The Multicenter PEA Study Group. Pacing Clin Electrophysiol 19:2066-2071

21. Padeletti L, Porciani MC, Ritter P et al (2000) Atrioventricular interval optimization in the right atrial appendage and interatrial septum pacing. Pacing Clin Electrophysiol 23(part I):1618-1622

22. Di Gregorio F, Morra A, Finesso M et al (1996) Transvalvular impedance (TVI) recordings under electrical and pharmacological cardiac stimulation. Pacing Clin Electrophysiol 19:1689-1693

Hemodynamic Sensors: What Clinical Value Do They Have in Heart Failure?

M. Gasparini[1], A. Curnis[2], M. Mantica[1], G. Mascioli[2], P. Galimberti[1], F. Bianchetti[2], F. Coltorti[1], L. Bontempi[2], A. Barbetta[3] and F. Di Gregorio[3]

Introduction

Up to recent years, electrical pacing has mainly been intended as a therapeutic tool in the treatment of cardiac rhythm disorders due to either atrial disorders or atrioventricular conduction defects. In order to synchronize the exogenous stimulation with the intrinsic activity, pacing devices are provided with electrical sensors and sensing circuits which reliably detect the depolarization spread in atrium and ventricle [1, 2]. Conventional pacemakers (PMs) and implantable defibrillators (ICDs), however, only regulate their function according to the timing of electrical cardiac activity, while information on the force developed by myocardial contraction and the related hemodynamic variables is lacking.

Nowadays, resynchronization of myocardial contraction by multisite or biventricular pacing is a widely accepted new application of cardiac stimulation, intended to improve the mechanical performance of the heart in patients with failing systolic function and slow interventricular conduction [3-5]. However, biventricular PMs and ICDs are generally not equipped with sensors suitable for monitoring the hemodynamic effects of the therapy and regulating the pacing parameters which can affect the functional results and the clinical benefit from the treatment.

Various hemodynamic sensors could be proposed for this task, but in the clinical setting it is essential that the sensor be small, simple to implant, and reliable in the long term, since the hardware required in dual-chamber biventricular pacing cannot be complicated any further. In view of this, hemodynamic sensors based upon cardiac impedance recordings may play a crucial role [6-9]. Impedance sensing can be performed by the same electrodes used for cardiac pacing, without the need for additional components [10].

[1]Electrophysiology Unit, Humanitas Clinical Institute, Rozzano, Milan; [2]Cardiology Division and Chair, Spedali Civili, Brescia; [3]Clinical Research Unit, Medico SpA, Rubano, Padua, Italy

The present study has been designed to check whether cardiac impedance recorded in a transvalvular configuration (TVI) along the cardiac cycle [11-13] can provide insight into the ongoing variations in stroke volume (SV), ejection fraction (EF), and ventricular contractility, and whether TVI-derived information might be applied in the self-regulation of a biventricular pacing system in heart failure patients.

Materials and Methods

TVI was recorded on implantation of right-sided or biventricular dual-chamber pacing systems, by deriving the signal between the ring electrode in the right atrium and either the tip or the ring electrode in the right ventricle. The TVI waveform was stored in memory by a dedicated nonimplantable device, together with the atrial electrogram (AEGM), the ventricular electrogram (VEGM), one surface standard ECG lead, and the systemic blood pressure, measured by a transducer from either the radial or the femoral artery. The time derivative of arterial pressure was then obtained by off-line data processing, in order to determine the maximum systolic rate of rise (dP/dt_{max}) in each cardiac cycle.

The patients undergoing right-sided dual-chamber implantation were affected by sick sinus syndrome. Recordings were performed under sinus rhythm and AAI pacing at various rates, during baseline conditions, during intravenous administration of isoproterenol (IPN), and in the subsequent recovery phase. The arterial pressure and the cardiac rate were monitored throughout the drug infusion, which was stopped as soon as the intrinsic rate increased by 30 beats/min above the starting value.

Patients undergoing biventricular dual-chamber implantation presented with dilated cardiomyopathy with atrioventricular (AV) and interventricular conduction disturbances. The right ventricular (RV) lead was positioned in the ventricular apex and the left ventricular (LV) lead in the lateral or posterolateral cardiac vein. Recordings were performed under sinus rhythm and VDD or DDD pacing with AV delay ranging from 80 to 150 ms, by stimulating in sequence the right ventricle, the left ventricle, and both ventricles connected in parallel.

TVI data were analyzed according to Chirife et al. [7], on the assumption that cardiac impedance is a linear function of the ventricular volume. End-diastolic volume (EDV) and end-systolic volume (ESV) at rest were scaled to 200 and 100, respectively, to determine the negative slope coefficient for TVI - volume conversion in each patient and allowing EDV, ESV, SV, and EF calculation under different experimental conditions. In addition, a corrected ejection fraction (EF_c) was worked out by removing from the estimated SV the fraction due to preload changes, according to Starling's law, in order to obtain an estimate of cardiac contractility. Hemodynamic parameters derived from TVI measurements were compared with related changes in sinus rate, arterial pressure, and dP/dt.

Results were expressed as mean ± standard deviation in steady-state conditions, or as the moving average calculated over 30 consecutive cardiac beats as a function of time. The statistical significance of differences between groups was calculated by one-way ANOVA and the two-tailed Student's *t*-test.

Results

Right-Sided Dual-Chamber Pacing

TVI signals recorded with the tip and the ring ventricular electrode in sinus rhythm at rest are shown in Figs. 1 and 2, respectively. In both electrode configurations, the TVI waveform shows a first negative deflection during the P-R interval, followed by progressive increase during the ventricular systole. TVI recorded on the detection of the R wave was considered as the expression of the ventricular EDV, while the maximum TVI value in each cardiac cycle, which is generally recorded at the end of the T wave, represented the ventricular ESV. Figure 2 shows an example of a premature ventricular complex (PVC) breaking the sinus rhythm and starting a cycle with reduced systolic pressure and dP/dt_{max}. The same event is recorded on the TVI channel as an increased diastolic impedance, representing a reduced EDV, in the presence of unchanged end-systolic impedance and ESV. The corresponding SV is therefore reduced, in agreement with the observed reduction in systolic and pulse arterial pressure.

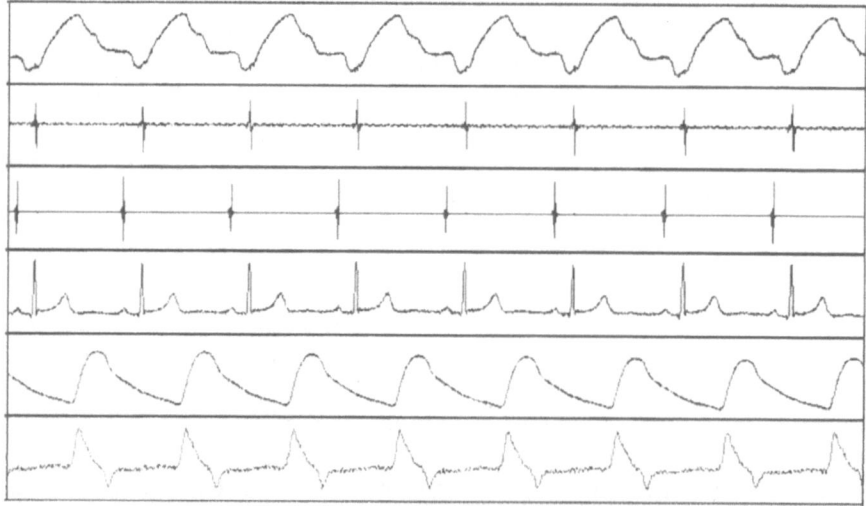

Fig. 1. *From top to bottom:* TVI recorded between the ring atrial electrode and the tip ventricular electrode in a standard dual-chamber implant, ventricular (VEGM) and atrial electrogram (AEGM), ECG lead I, radial arterial pressure, dP/dt. End-diastolic and end-systolic TVI averaged, respectively, 435 ± 7 and 559 ± 3 Ω

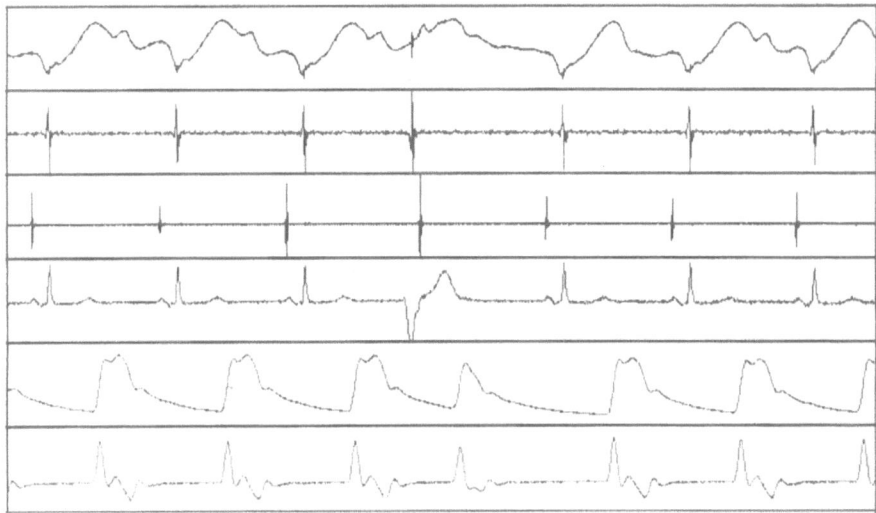

Fig. 2. *From top to bottom:* TVI recorded between ring atrial and ventricular electrodes in a standard dual-chamber implant, VEGM, AEGM, ECG lead II, radial arterial pressure, dP/dt. End-diastolic and end-systolic TVI averaged, respectively, 211 ± 6 and 263 ± 4 Ω

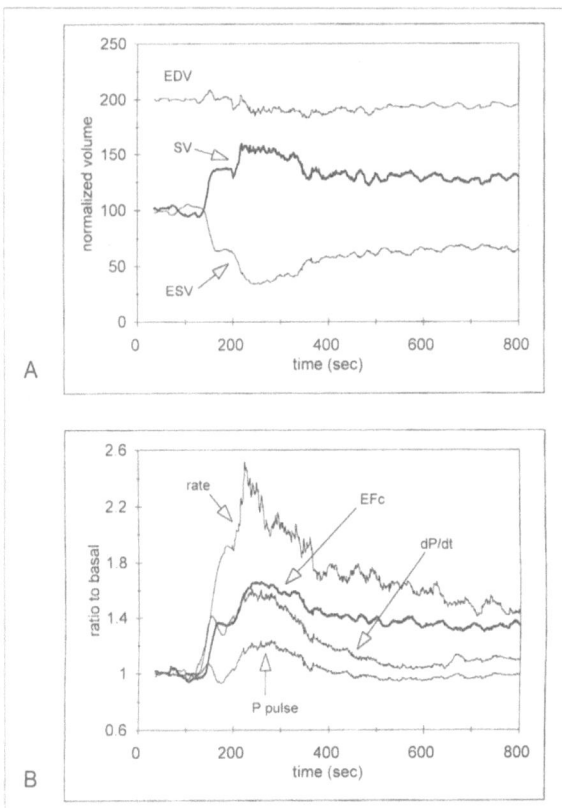

Fig. 3. A,B. Intravenous isoproterenol administration in the recording shown in Fig. 2. Data represent the moving average over 30 consecutive cardiac cycles. **A.** Effects on TVI-derived end-diastolic volume (EDV), end-systolic volume (ESV), and stroke volume (SV), which are scaled, respectively, to 200, 100 and 100 arbitrary units under resting conditions. **B.** Relative changes with respect to base values of heart rate, radial pulse pressure, radial dP/dt, and TVI-derived corrected ejection fraction (EF$_c$). See text for detailed explanation

The effects of IPN infusion in a representative recording are shown in Fig. 3. β-Adrenergic stimulation induced a fast increase in sinus rate, followed by a phase of junctional rhythm and then sinus rhythm again, frequently broken by premature atrial complexes (PACs) and PVCs. The diastolic arterial pressure was transiently decreased at the onset of the drug action, while the pulse pressure showed a delayed increase. The maximum dP/dt increased in two steps, and was mirrored by the corresponding reduction in TVI-derived ESV. Since EDV remained almost constant in spite of more than two-fold changes in cardiac rate, SV, EF, and EF_c were all increased with a similar time course. After the peak response to IPN, dP/dt_{max} returned to base level more quickly than the heart rate and all TVI-derived parameters, which remained elevated for several minutes after the IPN infusion was stopped.

Biventricular Dual-Chamber Pacing

Continuous monitoring of arterial pressure and dP/dt during the implantation of dual-chamber biventricular pacing systems demonstrated that the hemodynamic performance of the paced heart is markedly dependent on the individual AV delay regulation. Figure 4 illustrates the case of a patient affected by dilated cardiomyopathy undergoing biventricular pacing by a bipolar lead positioned in the RV apex and a coronary sinus lead advanced into the posterolateral cardiac vein. With VDD stimulation of the left ventricle, the dP/dt_{max} in the

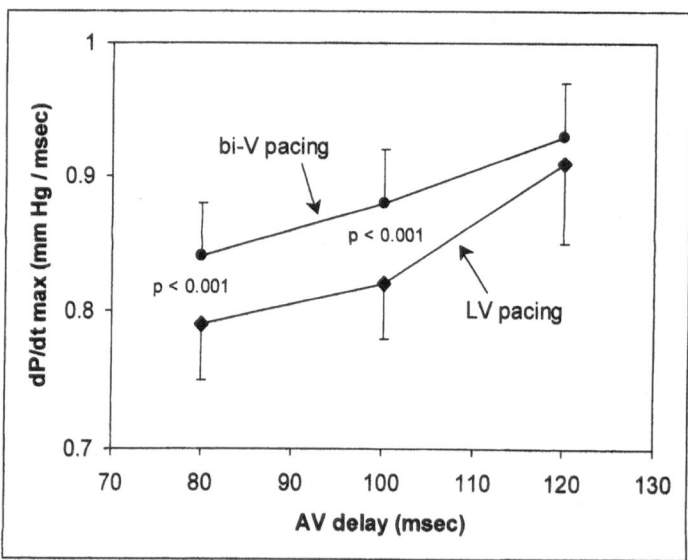

Fig. 4. Effects of different AV delays on dP/dt_{max} during LV or biventricular pacing. The variation of dP/dt_{max} as a function of the AV delay is significant in both stimulation modalities ($p < 0.001$, one-way ANOVA). The difference between LV and biventricular stimulation is significant with 80 and 100 ms AV delay ($p < 0.001$, two-tailed Student's t-test), but not with 120 ms AV delay

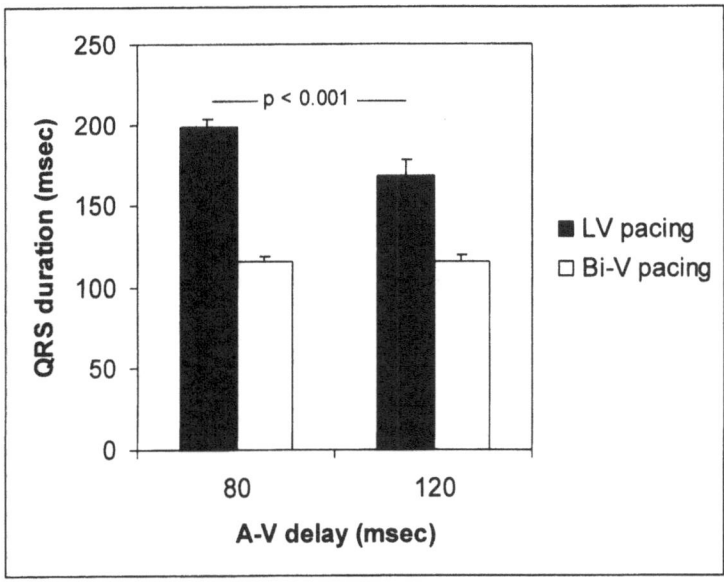

Fig. 5. Effect of different AV delays on QRS duration during LV or biventricular pacing. The difference is significant for LV pacing ($p < 0.001$, two-tailed Student's t-test), but not for biventricular pacing

femoral artery increased significantly when the AV delay was raised in the range of 80 to 120 ms. The effect was coupled with a substantial reduction in the duration of the paced QRS complex, which was further reduced and became independent of the AV delay setting during biventricular pacing (Fig. 5). Biventricular pacing also improved the pump function with respect to LV pacing, but did not abolish the influence of AV delay on dP/dt_{max} (Fig. 4).

To ascertain whether TVI can provide analogous indications, the impedance signal was recorded between the atrial ring electrode and the RV and LV tip electrodes, connected in parallel to allow biventricular stimulation. An example of the resulting waveform is shown in Fig. 6. Panel A shows spontaneous activity in sinus rhythm: two R waves are evident on the VEGM channel, the first (RV) with a P-R interval of 214 ± 6 ms and the second (LV) with a P-R of 283 ± 5 ms. The duration of the intrinsic QRS as measured on ECG lead III was 131 ± 6 ms. Panel B shows biventricular VDD pacing, with pacing energy reduction and transition from effective biventricular capture (first two cycles) to the capture of RV alone. The loss of LV capture is underlined by the appearance of a conducted R wave in the VEGM tracing and the simultaneous widening of QRS from 120 ± 7 to 163 ± 6 ms. At the same time, the TVI peak-to-peak excursion showed a nonsignificant increase from 45 ± 6 to 51 ± 8 Ω.

TVI recording between the right atrial and ventricular ring electrodes, by contrast, allowed endocardial impedance measurement with no influence from the epicardial LV electrode, even when RV and LV tip electrodes were connected in parallel to perform biventricular pacing. In an endocardial configuration, TVI showed higher sensitivity, changing in agreement with the trend of conventional hemodynamic parameters in the varying test conditions. Figure 7 clearly shows the effect of reducing the AV delay reduction from 150 to 120 msec, during biventricular pacing. In this patient, the longer AV delay resulted in fusion beats and impaired interventricular synchronization, while effective biventricular capture was obtained as a result of shortening the AV delay. This promptly induced a remarkable increase in systolic pressure, pulse pressure, and dP/dt_{max}, with a concurrent significant increase in TVI peak-to-peak amplitude (Table 1).

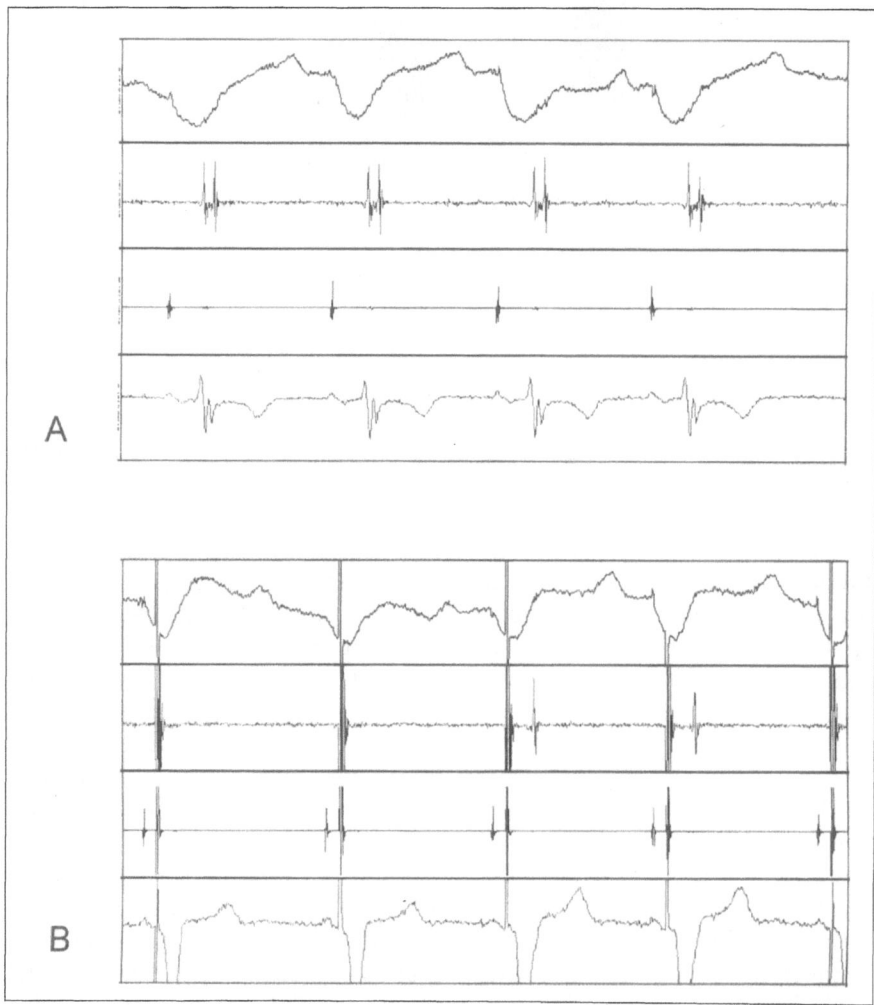

Fig. 6. A,B. *From top to bottom:* TVI recorded in biventricular configuration (between the ring atrial electrode and the tip RV and LV electrodes connected in parallel), VEGM, AEGM, and ECG lead III. Intrinsic activity under sinus rhythm. **B.** Traces as in **A.** Biventricular VDD pacing with effective capture on both sides (first two cycles) or in RV only (last two cycles)

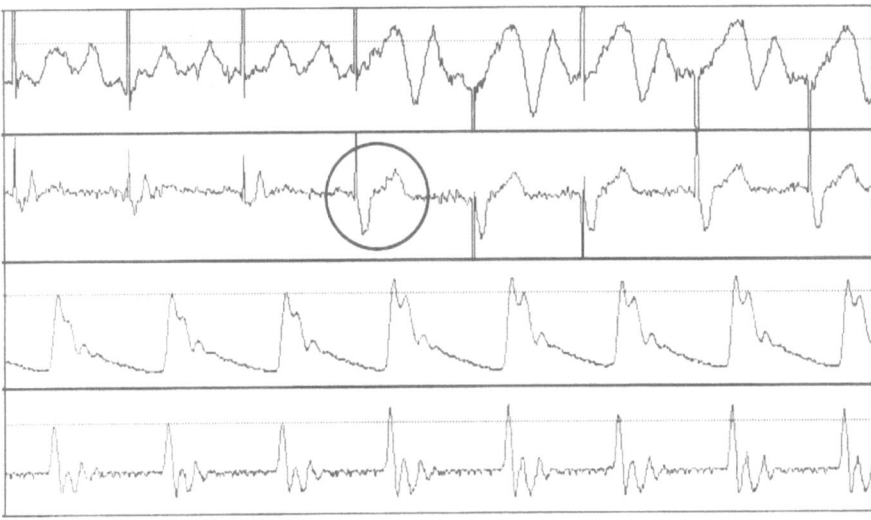

Fig. 7. *From top to bottom:* TVI recorded in endocardial configuration (between the ring atrial electrode and the ring RV electrode), ECG lead I, femoral arterial pressure, dP/dt_{max}. Biventricular VDD pacing. The *circle* on the ECG marks the transition from 150 ms AV delay, resulting in fusions, to 120 ms AV delay, resulting in effective biventricular capture. Biventricular stimulation promptly induced a clear-cut increase in systolic pressure, dP/dt_{max}, and TVI peak-to-peak amplitude (see the *dotted lines* for comparison)

Table 1. Effects of reduction of AV delay from 150 to 120 ms during biventricular VDD pacing on sinus rate, femoral pressure parameters, end-diastolic and end-systolic TVI, and TVI peak-to-peak excursion. TVI was recorded in endocardial mode, between the atrial ring electrode and the RV ring electrode

| | AV delay | | | |
	150 ms	120 ms	% Change	p^a
Rate (/min)	60.4 ± 1.4	59.6 ± 1.7	-1.3	n.s.
Diastolic pressure (mmHg)	70.6 ± 0.3	71.9 ± 0.8	1.8	< 0.001
Systolic pressure (mmHg)	138.3 ± 1.4	146.4 ± 1.5	5.9	< 0.001
Pulse pressure (mmHg)	67.6 ± 1.4	74.5 ± 1.9	10.2	< 0.001
dP/dt_{max} (mmHg / ms)	1.29 ± 0.04	1.55 ± 0.08	20.2	< 0.001
ED-TVI (Ω)	394.3 ± 2.2	394.7 ± 2.3	0.1	n.s.
ES-TVI (Ω)	411 ± 2.5	418.6 ± 2.2	1.8	< 0.001
Peak-to-peak TVI (Ω)	16.7 ± 2.3	23.8 ± 2.2	42.5	< 0.001

[a] Two-tailed Student's *t*-test
ED, end-diastolic; *ES*, end-systolic

Discussion

The general properties of the TVI signal derived from either the tip or the ring ventricular electrode strongly suggest a correlation between TVI and ventricular volume. According to this assumption, minimum and maximum TVI values can provide an estimate of EDV and ESV, respectively, while peak-to-peak TVI amplitude would reflect the SV [7, 10]. The evidence from IPN infusion shows that TVI-derived hemodynamic estimates change during the drug action in agreement with the observed variation in sinus rate, arterial blood pressure, and dP/dt_{max}. In all tests performed, the onset of IPN effects on the reference cardiovascular parameters was accompanied by a simultaneous increase in the EF_c, which is calculated by removing the preload influence from the actual SV. Therefore, EF_c can only be affected by changes in cardiac contractility or by deep modifications in the vascular tone, which are both expected to occur as a result of β-adrenergic stimulation. The time course of EF_c closely resembled that of sinus rate, suggesting this TVI-derived parameter as a potential physiological sensor in rate-responsive pacing.

Since the indications provided by impedance recording are consistent with cardiac hemodynamics [7], TVI might also be applied as a tool to evaluate functional performance in heart failure patients. This could be helpful in monitoring the clinical evolution of the disease, as well as in the assessment of the acute and chronic effects of pharmacological and electrical treatments. Moreover, TVI could be proposed as a suitable hemodynamic sensor in the control and self-regulation of an implanted biventricular pacemaker. In agreement with previous studies [14, 15], our data clearly indicate the essential role of AV delay optimization in biventricular pacing to obtain maximum enhancement of cardiac contractility. By stimulating only the ventricle showing delayed intrinsic activation, the hemodynamic improvement correlates with the reduction of QRS duration, indicating that better synchronization of intrinsic and paced AV conduction may underlie the observed effect. Under biventricular pacing, the influence of AV delay on cardiac contractility might better reflect the timing of passive and active transmitral flow, which would affect LV filling, as well as the timing of the LV contraction, which would affect mitral valve closure and functional regurgitation [14].

Preliminary experience of biventricular TVI recording with the RV endocardial electrode and the LV epicardial electrode connected in parallel resulted in reduced TVI sensitivity to changes in cardiac contractility. In contrast, when TVI was recorded by the RV ring electrode in an endocardial configuration, the sensor performance improved substantially, since the signal peak-to-peak amplitude changed in agreement with the direct measurement of arterial pressure and dP/dt. Even though biventricular pacing is mainly intended to improve LV hemodynamics [16], any change in cardiac output should involve LV and RV to the same extent, thus making right-sided TVI a valuable probe of overall systolic performance. Further studies are planned to fully check the sensitivity, specificity, and reliability of TVI-derived information in the assessment of cardiac function.

References

1. Furman S, Hayes DL, Holmes DR Jr (1989) A practice of cardiac pacing. Futura, Mount Kisco, NY
2. Sutton R, Bourgeois I (1991) The foundation of cardiac pacing. Part I. Futura, Mount Kisco, NY
3. Cazeau S, Ritter P, Lazarus A et al (1996) Multisite pacing for end-stage heart failure: early experience. Pacing Clin Electrophysiol 19:1748-1757
4. Daubert JC, Ritter P, Le Breton H et al (1998) Permanent left ventricular pacing with transvenous leads inserted into the coronary veins. Pacing Clin Electrophysiol 21:239-245
5. Gras D, Mabo P, Tang T et al (1998) Multisite pacing as a supplemental treatment of congestive heart failure: preliminary results of the Medtronic Inc InSync study. Pacing Clin Electrophysiol 21:2249-2255
6. Salo RW, Wallner TG, Pederson BD (1986) Measurement of ventricular volume by intracardiac impedance: theoretical and empirical approaches. IEEE Trans Biomed Eng 33:189-195
7. Chirife R, Ortega DF, Salazar A (1993) Feasibility of measuring relative right ventricular volumes and ejection fraction with implantable rhythm control devices. Pacing Clin Electrophysiol 16:1673-1683
8. Schaldach M, Hutten H (1992) Intracardiac impedance to determine sympathetic activity in rate responsive pacing. Pacing Clin Electrophysiol 15:1778-1786
9. Schaldach M (1994) The myocardium-electrode interface at the cellular level. In: Aubert AE, Ector H, Stroobandt R (eds) Cardiac pacing and electrophysiology. A bridge to the 21st century. Kluwer Academic, Dordrecht, The Netherlands, pp 169-188
10. Chirife R (1991) Acquisition of hemodynamic data and sensor signals for rate control from standard pacing electrodes. Pacing Clin Electrophysiol 14:1563-1565
11. Di Gregorio F, Morra A, Finesso M, Bongiorni MG (1996) Transvalvular impedance (TVI) recording under electrical and pharmacological cardiac stimulation. Pacing Clin Electrophysiol 19:1689-1693
12. Bongiorni MG, Soldati E, Arena G et al (1997) Transvalvular impedance as a marker of cardiac activity. In: Vardas PE (ed) Europace '97, free papers. Monduzzi, Bologna, pp 525-528
13. Morra A, Panarotto D, Santini P, Di Gregorio F (1997) Transvalvular impedance (TVI) sensing: a new way toward the hemodynamic control of cardiac pacing. In: Vardas PE (ed) Europace '97, free papers. Monduzzi, Bologna, pp 529-533
14. Auricchio A, Sommariva L, Salo RW et al (1993) Improvement of cardiac function in patients with severe congestive heart failure and coronary disease by dual-chamber pacing with shortened AV delay. Pacing Clin Electrophysiol 16:2034-2043
15. Auricchio A, Stellbrink C, Block M et al (1999) Effect of pacing chamber and atrioventricular delay on acute systolic function of paced patients with congestive heart failure. Circulation 99:2993-3001
16. Kass D, Chen CH, Curry C et al (1999) Improved left ventricular mechanics from acute VDD pacing in patients with dilated cardiomyopathy and ventricular conduction delay. Circulation 99:1567-1573

How Reliable and Effective Are Hemodynamic Sensors in Correcting Chronotropic Incompetence?

E. Occhetta, M. Bortnik, G. Francalacci, C. Pedrigi, B. Marenna and C. Vassanelli

Introduction

Conventional dual chamber rate-responsive pacing is the treatment of choice in patients with severely impaired of chronotropic competence. In currently available DDDR pacemakers, appropriate modulation of the heart rate depends on the degree to which the artificial rate-control algorithm approximates the physiological response, and therefore on the specificity of the signal detected by the sensor [1]. Activity sensors respond to body movements or muscle tremors and are specific for physical exercise only. Other sensors, such as those based on minute ventilation, detect signals more closely correlated to metabolic needs. The time response of activity sensors (rate vs signal variation) is quite fast but often not truly physiological; by contrast, the response of metabolic sensors is more "physiologic" but it is slow; however these latter are claimed to have a more appropriate response to metabolic demand [2]. A device combining activity and metabolic (minute ventilation) sensing could obviate the problems of the faster less, "physiologic" and the slower, more "physiologic" system; cross-checking between the two sensor systems could also eliminate false positive heart rate increases [3, 4].

The main limitation of all these rate-adaptive approaches remains in the control system. Since all of them operate in an open loop, the pacemaker is unable to verify whether the paced rate is appropriate both to the patient's metabolic needs and his overall pathophysiological status, or, on the contrary, if it is inducing side effects (e.g., an improper increase of arterial blood pressure, left ventricular failure, etc.) that cannot be well tolerated [5].

Hemodynamic sensors could revise the concept of physiologic pacing. By close, real monitoring of the ventricular hemodynamics they optimize the paced heart rate. Then the ideal heart rate has to correlate to the activity status (and quickly respond to the physical needs), to the metabolic demand and, especially in the presence of heart failure, to the myocardial contractility [6]. In the spectrum of presently available devices, the concept of closed loop stimula-

Division of Cardiology, University of Piemonte Orientale School of Medicine, Novara, Italy

tion (CLS) could be regulated by hemodynamic sensors [7]. To fully understand the CLS concept, a concise review of the basic mechanisms of cardiovascular regulation is necessary.

The mechanism of cardiovascular regulation is complex; its function is to provide constant and appropriate perfusion of all tissues in the body. It operates in a closed loop system with negative feedback which reacts to external influences with the aim of maintaining a constant and adequate mean arterial blood pressure. When signals sent to the central nervous system by biological transducers such as baroreceptors, mechanoreceptors, and chemoreceptors indicate a shift of the controlled variable from the current value, a reaction takes place that modulates a counter-effect designed to change the regulated parameter (e.g., cardiac output).

The main feature of an effective closed loop control is the negative feedback. This means that whenever a parameter deviation in one direction is detected, the control system induces changes in the opposite direction, to compensate for the deviation and restore the equilibrium.

The baroreceptors located in the aortic arch and the carotid sinus continuously monitor the mean arterial blood pressure, which is influenced by cardiac output and total peripheral vascular resistances. The signal generated by the baroreceptors is directed to the medullary circulatory control center, where it is integrated with other incoming signals from the cerebral cortex and eventually reaches the autonomic nervous system. The sympathetic and parasympathetic branches of the autonomic nervous system influence both cardiac function and peripheral vasoconstriction, continuously adjusting cardiac output and total peripheral resistances. The cardiac function is kept under control mainly through three parameters: chronotropism, which has the major influence on the cardiac output, inotropism (contractility), and dromotropism. Thus, under physiologic conditions, the cardiovascular system depends on the ability of the autonomous nervous system to react to physical and mental stress.

In general, the closed loop control of the circulatory system is active even in patients whose chronotropic mechanism is impaired. The circulatory centers attempt to compensate the chronotropic incompetence by increasing myocardial contractility at the expense of the patient's maximum exercise and stress tolerance, which are severely impaired. The contractile force of the myocardium can be adjusted only within certain limits, with increased stress on the myocardial fibers and higher energy consumption [8].

Closed Loop Stimulation

The role of CLS is to maintain appropriate cardiovascular regulation by integrating an implanted device into the natural system. Closed loop pacing can be accomplished, converting the changes of myocardial contractility into individual stimulation rates. With such a device, the pacing rate is linked to the circulatory centers, and adequate perfusion is provided under various conditions.

Hemodynamic sensors could be linked to the sympathetic nervous discharge (such as the QT dynamics) and they could work in the manner of a positive feedback: at high plasma levels of catecholamine, increase in heart rate follows the reduction of QTc duration. This system acts as an indirect hemodynamic rate-responsive sensor and needs to be integrated with a fast activity sensor (in a dual sensor system) to achieve good physiological sensitivity [9].

Better closed loop hemodynamic rate-responsive stimulation could be obtained by negative feedback driven by variations in cardiac contractility: a system may carry out rate-responsive pacing while adapting to the hemodynamic needs of the patient and, in consequence, improve his or her quality of life.

At present, myocardial contractility is monitored by two different systems: (1) peak endocardial acceleration (PEA) and (2) intracardiac impedance.

1. In the BEST Living pacemaker (from Sorin Biomedica, Italy) there is a special unipolar ventricular lead, which contains a micro-accelerometer sensor in its distal portion. This sensor measures PEA values on a cycle-by-cycle basis. The continuously updated average value measured over 24 h represents the reference signal (PEA REF) and a dual-slope linear algorithm utilizes the changes in PEA (ΔPEA) to modulate the pacing rate, closely related to the levels of myocardial contractility [10, 11].

2. The INOS^{2+} pacemaker (from Biotronik, Germany) uses an algorithm based on variations in right ventricular (RV) impedance, generated by changes of the myocardium-to-blood ratio in the volume around the tip of a conventional ventricular pacing lead, during systole. The measuring signal consists in a sequence of constant-current pulses of subthreshold amplitude. The signal is applied between the ventricular tip and the pacemaker can, in a temporal window of 245 ms that starts 47 ms after the ventricular pacing pulse. This system does not require dedicated leads to be effective, and can therefore be considered for replacement of previously implanted DDDR devices that have reached the end of their life or have failed for any other reason [12, 13].

These contractility-related sensors, directly correlated to the RV dP/dt_{max}, are processed through negative feedback and are converted in a closed-loop rate control [14, 15]. Therefore, if the pacing rate is set too high, the baroreceptors detect the excessive increase in the blood pressure. This leads to an immediate downregulation of contractility and, consequently, to a reduction in the pacing rate. Unlike other, non-closed-loop DDDR systems, the CLS mode has demonstrated its capability to modulate the heart rate not only in response to physical activity, but also to other nonvoluntary stress situations (mental stress, drug infusion, and circadian variations), besides re-establishing the baroreceptor response to the Valsalva maneuver. A better quality of life was also reported using the CLS system [16, 17].

Validation of CLS Approaches

Several studies have been performed in order to elucidate the advantages and reliability of these new approaches to rate control.

Peak Endocardial Acceleration

Validation of the PEA-based approach is based on multicenter experiences.

The European PEA clinical investigation group [18] evaluated 105 patients implanted with the Living-1 dual chamber pacemaker connected to a lead with a BEST (Biomechanical Endocardial Sorin Transducer) sensor. The performance of the PEA signal was tested under conditions of physical and mental stresses and during daily life activities by 24-h recordings of PEA (PEA Holter) 1-2 months and approximately 1 year after implantation. Implantation of the BEST lead was performed without complications in all patients. The sensor operated properly in the short and long term in 98% of patients. Although PEA values differed from patient to patient, the values closely reflected the variations in sympathetic nervous activity induced by physical and mental stress in each individual patient. During exercise and daily life activities, a close correlation between PEA and the heart rate was observed in patients with normal sinus rhythm, showing that PEA allows nearly physiological control of the pacing rate.

Clementy et al. [19] recently performed a validation of the PEA by serial standardized testing. This study compared the chronotropic performance of 14 patients with chronotropic incompetence treated with this device and that observed in 18 control subjects in normal sinus rhythm. Five daily life activities (hall walk, walking up and down stairs, squatting, and hyperventilation) and two types of exercise (Bruce treadmill protocol and bicycle ergometry) were performed in a random order after individual programming of each pacemaker. For each test, correlation coefficients were calculated between changes in PEA and variations in paced rate, between instantaneous variations in heart rate (by telemetry and continuous measurement by the pacemaker), and between sensor-driven rate in patients and normal sinus rhythm in controls. The variations in paced heart rate closely correlated with those observed in subjects with normal sinus rhythm, and proved to be sensitive, specific, rapid, and independent of the type of exercise. After optimal programming of this sensor, PEA modulated the heart rate as expected during normal sinus rhythm.

Intracardiac Impedance Approach

Several Italian studies have evaluated the INOS^{2+} CLS system.

The CONPRES Study

The CONPRES (Contractility index vs ventricular Pressure variation) study [20] was divided into two phases. The first aimed to verify whether the variations in the contractility index (CI) correlated with the variations in the dP/dt_{max} measured in the right ventricle (RV$dP/dt_{max}$) during a sequence of provocative tests. The second phase was addressed to test whether a correlation still existed between the variations in the CI and those in the dP/dt_{max} measured in the left ventricle (LV$dP/dt_{max}$).

Phase I. During implant procedures, direct catheter-derived measurements of RVdP/dt_{max} were correlated with the CI (telemetrically detected by the implanted device) in a group of 15 patients (12 male and 3 female, mean age 64.5 years) with chronotropic incompetence and second- or third-degree AV block. The CI was continuously monitored using a dedicated device (UNIL-YSER, Biotronik) connected to a laptop PC programmer. During the procedure, all patients underwent exercise testing (handgrip to the patient's limit), a mental stress test, and isoproterenol infusion (dose titration to obtain a heart rate increase of 20 bpm). RVdP/dt_{max} and CI were measured simultaneously and the trends compared. A good correlation was found between the two parameters ($r_{mean} = 0.91$).

Phase II. In order to verify whether the variations of CI measured in the right ventricle correlated to those of the left ventricular chamber, the LVdP/dt_{max} and the CI (telemetrically detected by an exteriorized device) were measured during diagnostic left heart catheterization in 15 consecutive patients (9 male and 6 female, mean age 62.8 years) without evidence of conduction disturbances. The CI was monitored while the patient was paced in VDD mode by means of an exteriorized INOS^2 CLS pulse generator interfaced to an UNILYSER device system. During the procedure, the two parameters were simultaneously measured before and after isometric exercise test (handgrip up to 80% of patient's tolerance) and left ventricular angiography and the trends of variation were compared. After handgrip the correlation between the variations of the CI and LVdP/dt_{max} was acceptable ($r = 0.79$). This type of stress increases the peripheral vascular resistances and left ventricular afterload. The sympathetic response to isometric stress influences the contractile level of both ventricles simultaneously, and, since the CI is measured in the right ventricle, this accounts for the better correlation between this index and variations of the RVdP/dt_{max}.

Left ventricular angiography affects the preload by increasing the ventricular diastolic filling during isovolumetric ventricular contraction. These changes are shared by the right ventricle, accounting for the good correlation ($r = 0.92$) between the CI and LVdP/dt_{max} during this procedure.

The results of the CONPRES study demonstrate that the device responds properly to the variation of contractility in the whole heart.

The VICRA Study

The VICRA (Validation of Inos Contractility Rate Modulation Algorithm) study [21] aimed to evaluate the appropriateness of response of CLS to both conscious and unconscious metabolic demands. Sixty-two patients underwent a treadmill exercise test (modified Bruce protocol, symptoms limited). In all patients the trend of the heart rate (HR) was appropriate, with rate acceleration and deceleration in accordance with the individual systolic (SABP) and diastolic (DABP) blood pressure changes. Forty-five of these patients were subjected to a mental stress test (color words-two steps). All patients showed prompt and appropriate

HR modulation, not only during the two steps of the test, but, for most of them, even during the test's preliminary phase in which the patient became emotionally involved by the physician's explanation of the procedure.

In all patients a 24-h Holter ECG recording was performed at 3-month follow-up. The analysis of the Holter recordings showed proper and typical dynamics of HR modulation throughout the whole monitoring time. A sixth-degree polynomial regression of the HR trend was performed for all records. This fitted trend matched well with the natural circadian variations of the HR, confirming that CLS operates under the control of the cardiovascular system. Only two patients reported an occasional sudden feeling of waking-up during the night associated with a high paced rate. The analysis of Holter recordings showed that the HR increases were caused by hyperactivity of the parasympathetic tone during REM sleep in one patient and by supine position in the second, both conditions inducing an increase in myocardial contractility.

The INPAR Study

The purpose of the INPAR (Inotropy controlled Pacing Replacing conventional DDDR pacing) study [22] is to evaluate whether patients previously implanted with a conventional DDDR pacemaker show significant hemodynamic improvement and experience a better quality of life (QOL) when the implanted device is replaced by a pulse generator operating in closed loop control. So far, seven patients with a DDDR pacemaker (56-87 years old) have undergone elective device replacement with an $INOS^2$ CLS pacemaker. In each patient, the basic and upper rates programmed in the $INOS^2$ CLS pacemaker were the same set as in the explanted RR device. The replaced RR device models were: 2 Thera DR (Medtronic), 2 Marathon DR (Intermedics), 1 Relay (Intermedics), 1 Dromos DR (Biotronik), and 1 Meta DDDR (Telectronics). One week before and 3-5 weeks after replacement, patients underwent a set of provocative tests, both physical (treadmill, 6 min walking, modified Bruce protocol) and mental (color words-two steps) stresses and, whenever possible, administration of positive inotropic drugs (isoproterenol). HR, SABP, and DABP were monitored during all tests but mental. After the tests, patients were asked to fill a QOL questionnaire (Karolinska Institute modified).

During exercise, HR modulation was satisfactory for all DDDR devices, independent of the sensor used, but the rate reached by RR devices during the last 4 min of exercise was on average 15%-20% higher than that reached with CLS pacing. In contrast, during the recovery phase, RR devices reduced HR more rapidly than CLS pacemakers. In RR conventional pacemakers, HR was artificially brought back to the baseline value in about 5 min after the end of the exercise, while with $INOS^2$ CLS, the HR decreased more gently and was, on average, still higher than the basic rate 7 min after the end of the stress.

Some conclusions can be drawn from the data obtained during the exercise test. During the last 4 min of the exercise, the increase of the HR in RR pacing was nonphysiologic (too fast and disproportionate), causing hemodynamic imbalance and possibly sympathetic hyperactivity. This might lead to increased cardiac contractility and to a disproportionate increase in blood pressure. Similarly, the rapid decrease of the HR in the recovery phase during RR pacing might leave the organs with a unbalanced supply/demand ratio while energy requirements are raised due to the increased afterload. This forced the SABP up to high levels during the first stage of recovery time, an effect which might be particularly harmful in hypertensive patients at higher risk of acute myocardial ischemia and stroke. The CLS pacing shows a more physiologic trend [23]. Following the baroreceptor signals that influence contractility, the CLS pacing properly balances the HR-blood pressure ratio, maintaining a proper hemodynamic balance during both the exercise and recovery phases. This exerts a preventive action against excessive peaks of blood pressure and/or HR that may lead to adverse events in patients with cardiac disease.

The CLS pacing responded appropriately to unconscious metabolic demand, modulating HR not only during the test, but also in the preliminary phase in which the physician explained the test procedure to the patient.

In the context of this study, the significance of QOL evaluation is of particular value, as the two conditions of the patient were comparable. The QOL questionnaire analysis showed that the patients experienced a better quality of daily life after pacemaker replacement, with a mean QOL score that increased from 41.8 ± 13.8 during RR pacing to 59.5 ± 12.0 with CLS pacing.

The response to inotropic agents (isoproterenol) was investigated in only two normotensive control patients (the first with a Marathon DR and the second with a Thera DR pacemaker). No HR adaptation was achieved by the DDDR pacemaker, with an excessive increase of both SABP and DABP at the time of maximal contractile response to the drug. By contrast, the CLS device modulated HR appropriately, in accordance with the blood pressure trend, smoothing and considerably limiting the pressure increase.

Conclusions

It has now become evident that even DDDR pacemakers, whether with simple or sophisticated artificial sensors (including dual-sensor devices), are unable to fully restore a complex function impaired by the cardiovascular system. The hemodynamic sensors driving closed loop stimulation are a significant advance in preserving intrinsic circulatory regulation. They integrate the pacemaker into the physiological control system, enabling the heart rate to be controlled by the autonomic nervous system and not by an artificial pacing algorithm.

The first clinical experiences confirm the overall beneficial effects of a pacing approach kept under the control of the autonomic nervous system and show that DDD-CLS is superior to conventional DDDR pacing systems because it:

•   Reacts proportionally to conscious and unconscious metabolic needs in every patient, taking into account individual circulatory conditions;

- Does not induce excessively high heart rates, which may be beneficial to patients with ischemic heart disease;
- Improves the quality of life of patients through appropriate physiological control;
- Can be used with dedicated leads (for PEA), but also in any patient with previously implanted leads, since the CLS system does not require a specific sensor to detect variations in contractility.

Clinical experience with CLS is so far limited to the treatment of chronotropic incompetence, although the possible indications include the prevention of malignant vasovagal syncope [24, 25] and the monitoring of sympathetic activity with the aim of tailoring antiarrhythmic therapy.

References

1. Lau CP (1993) Rate adaptive cardiac pacing: single and dual chamber. Futura, New York
2. Rossi P (1987) Rate responsive pacing: biosensor reliability and physiological sensitivity. Pacing Clin Electrophysiol 10:454-466
3. Connelly DT (1993) Initial experience with a new single chamber dual sensor rate responsive pacemaker. Pacing Clin Electrophysiol 16:1833-1841
4. Conell R, Morris-Thrugood J, Paul V et al (1993) Are we being driven to two sensors? Clinical benefits of sensor cross-checking. Pacing Clin Electrophytsiol 16:1441-1444
5. Malinowski K (1998) Interindividual comparison of different sensor principles for rate adaptive pacing. Pacing Clin Electrophysiol 21:2209-2213
6. Occhetta E, Vassanelli C, Ravazzi AP et al (2000) Myocardial contractility guided dual chamber rate-responsive pacing: towards a closed-loop stimulation. In: Santini M (ed) Progress in clinical pacing 2000. CEPI-AIM Group Rome, pp 268-277
7. Schaldach M (1998) What is closed loop stimulation? Prog Biomed Res 3:235-241
8. Pichelmaier AM, Ebner E, Greco OT et al (1993) A multicenter study of a closed-loop ANS-controlled pacemaker system (abstract). Pacing Clin Electrophysiol 16:1930
9. Occhetta E, Francalacci G, Perucca A et al (1996) Improving exercise tolerance efficiently: how much sensor driven pacing is required? In: Santini M (ed) Progress in clinical pacing 1996. Futura Media Service, Armonk, New York, pp 197-203
10. Rickards AF, Bombardini T, Corbucci G et al (Multicenter PEA Study Group) (1996) An implantable intracardiac accelerometer for monitoring myocardial contractility. Pacing Clin Electrophysiol 19:2066-2071
11. Menozzi C, Tomasi C, Brignole M et al (1996) Cardiac contractility: concepts and advances in implantable system applications. In: Adornato E (ed) Therapies for cardiac arrhythmias in 1996. Where are we going? Pozzi, Rome, pp 383-396
12. Schaldach M, Hutten H (1992) Intracardiac impedance to determine sympathetic activity in rate responsive pacing. Pacing Clin Electrophysiol 15:1778-1786
13. Pichelmaier AM, Braile D, Ebner E et al (1992) Autonomie nervous system controlled closed loop cardiac pacing. Pacing Clin Electrophytsiol 15:1787-1791
14. Osswald S, Hilti P, Crohn TH et al (1999) Correlation of intracardiac impedance and right ventricular contractility during dobutamine stress test. Prog Biomed Res 4:166-170
15. Occhetta E, Perucca A, Rognoni G et al (1995) Experience with a new myocardial

acceleration sensor during dobutamine infusion and exercise test. Eur J Cardiac Pacing Electrophysiol 5:204-209

16. Andrade JCS (1998) Cardiac contractility sensor evaluation in a DDDR system. A multicenter study. Prog Biomed Res 3:137-142

17. Novak M, Hoffmann G, Schaldach M (1998) Multi-center investigations with automatically initialised closed loop stimulation-rate response during daily life and exercise tests. Prog Biomed Res 3:147-151

18. Langenfeld H, Krein A, Kirstein M et al (European PEA Clinical Investigation Group) (1998) Peak endocardial acceleration based clinical testing of the "BEST" DDDR pacemaker. Pacing Clin Electrophysiol 21:2187-2191

19. Clementy J, Kobeissi A, Garrigue S et al (2000) Validation by serial standardized testing of a new rate-responsive pacemaker sensor based on variations in myocardial contractility. Europace 3:124-131

20. Ravazzi AP, Diotallevi P, Zecchi P (2000) Influence of rate modulation on hemodynamics. In: Adornato E (ed) Cardiac arrhythmias: how to improve the reality in the third millenium? Pozzi, Rome, pp 511-520

21. Zecchi P, Bellocci F, Sanna T et al (1999) Clinical benefit of closed loop stimulation. Preliminary results of an intensive validation study. Prog Biomed Res 4:185-189

22. Sanna T, Di Martino G, Bellocci F, Zecchi P (2000) Rate modulation algorithms. Have all the same influence on hemodynamics? In: Adornato E (ed) Cardiac arrhythmias: how to improve the reality in the third millenium? Pozzi, Rome, pp 521-531

23. Zecchi P, Bellocci F, Ravazzi AP et al (2000) Closed loop stimulation. A new philosophy of pacing. Prog Biom Res 5:126-131

24. Deharo JC, Peyre JP, Ritter PH et at (1998) Treatment of malignant primary vasodepressive neurocardiogenic syncope with a rate responsive pacemaker driven by heart contractility. Pacing Clin Electrophysiol 21:2688-2690

25. Occhetta E, Bortnik M, Pedrigi C et al (2000) Pacing rate automatic reaction to neuromediated hemodynamic changes. In: Santini M (ed) Progress in clinical pacing 2000. Rome, pp 542-547

Hemodynamic Sensors: What Clinical Value Do They Have in Chronotropic Incompetence?

M.G. Bongiorni[1], E. Soldati[1], G. Arena[1], F. Di Gregorio[2], A. Barbetta[2] and M. Mariani[1]

Introduction

The physiological capacity to regulate heart rate according to changing metabolic needs is impaired to a various degree in all clinical forms of sick sinus syndrome (SSS), as well as in the presence of pathologies affecting the autonomic nervous system or the brainstem centers which control cardiovascular function (e.g., carotid sinus syndrome, malignant vasovagal syndrome, and various autonomic neuropathies). In such conditions, rate-responsive cardiac pacing has proved a valuable therapeutic solution, provided that the artificial sensors used to assess the metabolic demand give reliable information [1]. To this purpose, an interesting approach is pacing rate regulation according to changes in cardiac hemodynamic parameters such as stroke volume (SV), ejection fraction (EF), and the maximum rate of rise of systolic blood pressure (dP/dt), with the aim of restoring the physiological correlation between inotropic and chronotropic cardiac function [2-6].

Hemodynamic information can be inferred from electric impedance measurements by means of standard pacing leads, on the assumption that cardiac impedance depends on the blood volume present in the cardiac chambers [7, 8]. Different electrode configurations have been used for cardiac impedance recording in pacemaker implants, including unipolar, bipolar and tripolar ventricular systems [9]. In addition, an alternative approach has been proposed, based on recording of transvalvular impedance (TVI) between right atrial and ventricular electrodes [10-12]. The TVI signal can be detected by means of either the tip ventricular electrode (in contact with the ventricular wall), or the ring ventricular electrode, thus recording impedance variation along the cardiac cycle in the absence of direct myocardial influence. The present study has been designed to analyze TVI signal properties in patients free to move and during the performance of a physical stress test, in order to assess TVI reliability as a potential new sensor in rate-responsive pacing.

[1]Cardiothoracic Department, University of Pisa; [2]Clinical Research Unit, Medico SpA, Rubano, Padua, Italy

Materials and Methods

At present, TVI can only be recorded by an external nonimplantable device, which is connected with the intracardiac pacing leads during pacemaker implantation or replacement. The main limitation of this approach is that during surgery the patients cannot move or perform any significant physical activity. Therefore, any influence of posture on TVI cannot be investigated, and the effects of adrenergic stimulation on the signal properties can only be studied by acute drug administration.

To overcome these constraints, TVI was recorded in patients with abandoned infected pacing leads, where the lead connectors were exposed to allow exudate draining before lead extraction. Meanwhile, the patients were free to move and carry on normal physical activity. TVI, atrial electrogram (AEGM), ventricular electrogram (VEGM), and surface ECG were recorded simultaneously with the patients lying supine, sitting upright, standing and walking for few steps. Patients were then seated on the ergometric bicycle and an exercise protocol was performed, increasing the power in 20 W steps every 3 min. The arterial blood pressure was measured under basal conditions and after each power increase.

TVI data were analyzed off-line according to the method of Chirife et al. [3]. In brief, TVI recorded on the detection of the R wave or after the emission of a ventricular spike was assumed to be proportional to the ventricular end-diastolic volume (EDV), and the maximum TVI value during the Q-T interval was related to the end-systolic volume (ESV). The negative linear slope relating the two variables was calculated under resting conditions by assigning an arbitrary volume of 200 to the average end-diastolic TVI and a volume of 100 to the average end-systolic TVI. Any TVI change with respect to the resting values thus allowed calculation of the corresponding relative variation in EDV, ESV, stroke volume (SV), and ejection fraction (EF). In addition, a cardiac contractility index (EF_c) was derived as the corrected EF obtained by removing the preload effect from the calculated SV, according to Starling's law.

Results

The evidence obtained in a typical experiment is illustrated in the following example. The patient, affected by third-degree atrioventricular block, had had an implanted-dual-chamber device for 5 years. The pacemaker was explanted due to lead infection and replaced with a new, contralateral implant. Before extraction of the chronic leads, TVI was recorded through the exposed lead connectors, between the atrial ring and the ventricular tip electrodes, during atrium-driven ventricular pacing.

The signals derived with the patient resting supine are shown in Fig. 1. TVI minimum and maximum values were detected at the end of ventricular diastole and systole, averaging $418 \pm 3 \, \Omega$ (mean $\pm$ SD) and $482 \pm 1 \, \alpha$, respectively. The

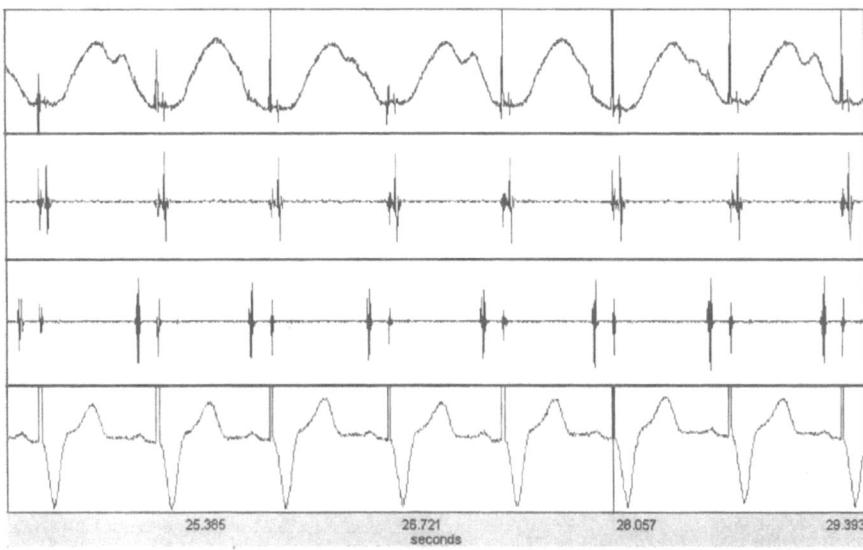

Fig.1. From *top* to *bottom*: transvalvular impendance (TVI), ventricular electrogram (VEGM), atrial electrogram (AEGM), ECG lead II. The intracardiac signals are recorded from the exposed connectors of abandoned chronic pacing leads prior to their extraction. VDD pacing is performed by a contralateral new implant. TVI is derived between the ring electrode of the atrial lead and the tip electrode of the ventricular lead, with the patient resting supine. Peak-to-peak TVI fluctuation averages 63 ± 3 Ω

peak-to-peak TVI excursion in the cardiac cycle was 63 ± 3 α, corresponding to an increment of $15 \pm 1\%$ with respect to the end-diastolic value.

The TVI waveform maintained the same morphology and signal-to-noise ratio, despite changes in the patient's posture. However, body movements resulted in quantitative changes in TVI-derived parameters, which are reported in Fig. 2. Raising the chest from supine to sitting up caused a small decrease in EDV, accompanied by a transient rate increase and ESV reduction. Consequently, SV showed little change and EF_c was transiently increased. Moving to the standing up position promptly induced a further EDV reduction and rate increase, followed by a delayed rate decrease and ESV increase, suggesting a weakening of the pump function. This was also indicated by a reduction in SV and contractility. All changes were reversed when the patient started some activity: first, slow walk, and then climbing onto the bed again. Finally, returning to the resting supine position restored all parameters to the starting values.

TVI, AEGM, VEGM, and surface ECG were then recorded in the same patient during a stress test on the ergometric bicycle. With the patient sitting on the bike before starting the exercise, the sinus rate and EF_c were already increased, while the SV was remarkably decreased, with respect to the values recorded at rest in the supine position. During the test, the sinus rate increased further, reaching the maximum at the end of the exercise and slowly declining thereafter (Fig. 3). TVI-derived SV quickly rose at the onset of exercise and fell

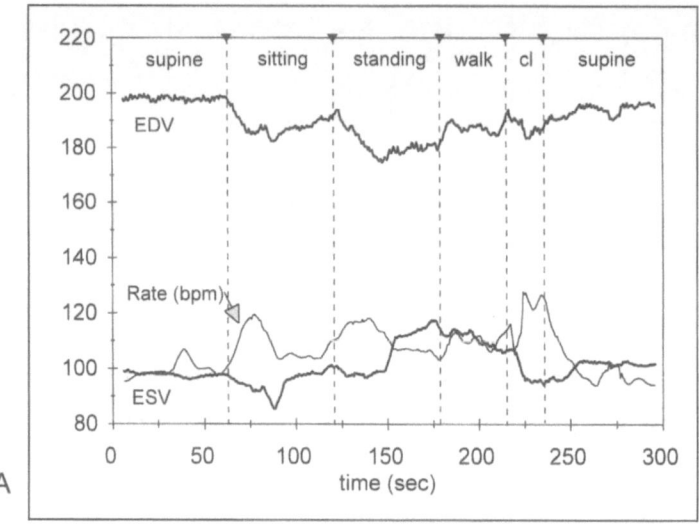

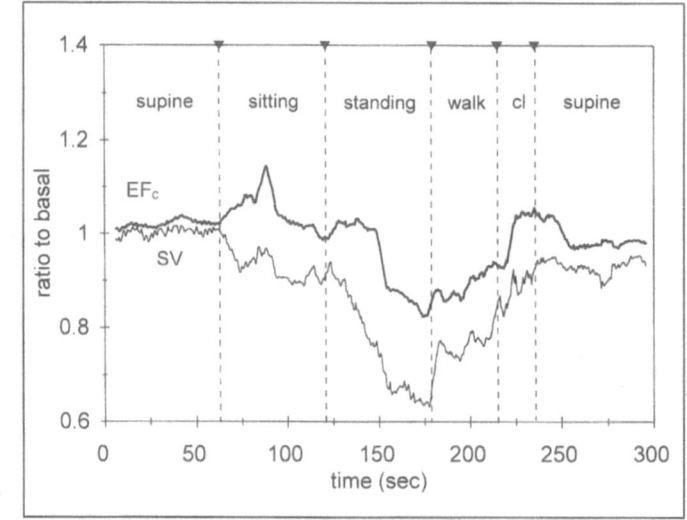

Fig. 2A,B. A Effects of postural changes on sinus rate, end-diastolic volume (EDV) and end-systolic volume (ESV), as derived from TVI data. Each value is the moving average calculated over ten consecutive cycles. The sinus rate (*light curve*) is expressed in beats per minute. EDV and ESV (*heavy curves*) are expressed in arbitrary units assuming a linear relationship between TVI and the ventricular volume, which is scaled at 200 in end-diastole and 100 in end-systole with the patient resting supine. The stroke volume is determined as the difference between EDV and ESV. Recordings were performed continuously while the patient moved from the supine position to sitting upright, standing up, slow walking, climbing onto the bed (*cl*) and resting supine again. **B** Relative changes in stroke volume (SV) and contractility index (EF$_c$) with respect to resting values, as derived from the data reported in **A**. While SV is directly affected by posture, EF$_c$ shows a compensatory reaction on sitting (i.e., increases when EDV decreases) and a delayed reduction on standing up, which might reflect a transient failure in inotropic regulation. Both SV and EF$_c$ rose again when the patient started to walk

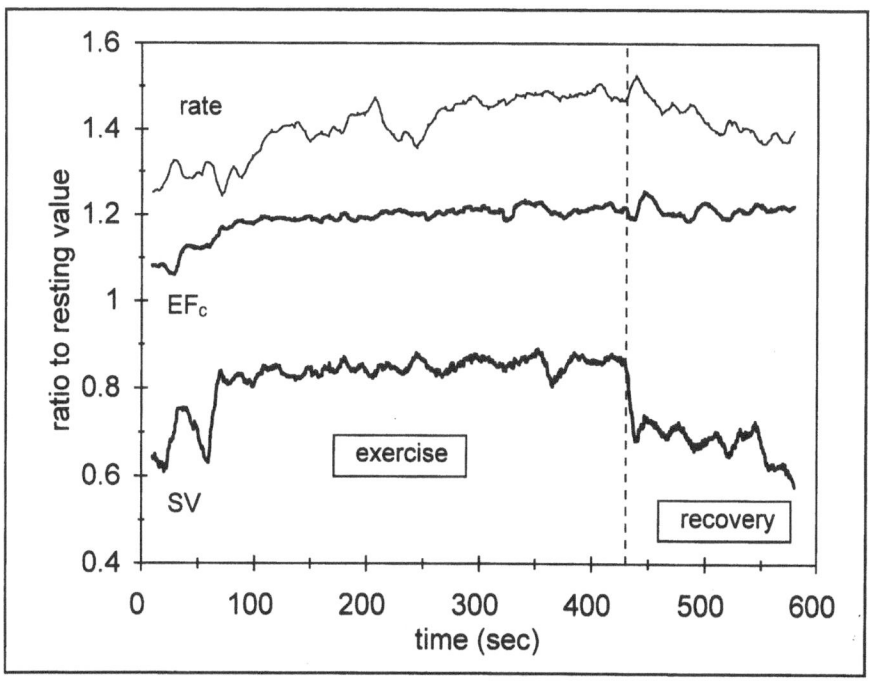

Fig. 3. Relative changes in sinus rate (*lighter curve*), stroke volume (SV) and contractility index (EF$_c$) with respect to base values (resting supine) during a stress test on the ergometric bicycle and in the following recovery phase. Each point represents a moving average calculated over 20 consecutive beats

back to the base value when the exercise was stopped. EF$_c$ increased following a similar time course, then maintained the elevated values into the first minutes of the recovery phase.

Discussion

Despite the need for physiological monitoring to ensure the ideal feedback control of cardiac output, the most common rate-responsive systems are still represented by accelerometric sensors providing information on body movements. With these, the pacing rate must be empirically linked to the level of acceleration detected by individual adjustment of the sensor gain. As physical sensors, currently available accelerometric rate-responsive systems generally ensure good sensitivity and a quick response to motion, but may lack specificity, being incapable of distinguishing between active and passive body movements [9].

This limitation should not affect physiological sensors, including systems designed for assessing minute ventilation (relating the pacing rate to the rate and depth of breathing), the Q-T interval (which is partially dependent on the activity of the autonomic nervous system), and the cardiac inotropic state. These correspond to the so-called hemodynamic sensors, which are intended to drive rate-responsive pacing following changes in cardiac contractility [4-6]. Hemodynamic sensing systems may require the use of pacing leads equipped with specific electromechanical devices, as is the case for the detection of right ventricular pressure and dP/dt or for recording the vibrations produced during the isometric systole (peak endocardial acceleration). Sensors of this kind have provided good results in clinical studies [4, 13], but their use in routine practice is limited by the need for special leads and by the unavoidable deterioration of mechanical sensor components with the progress of time.

On the other hand, valuable information on cardiac mechanical activity can be derived by conventional pacing electrodes, from electrical impedance measurements along the cardiac cycle. Changes in cardiac impedance can reflect both local events in the close proximity of the electrode and in the myocardial wall [14, 15], as well as changes in the amount of blood present in the cardiac chambers at any time [2, 3]. In the latter hypothesis, the instantaneous electric impedance (Z) is dependent on the conducting volume (V) according to the relationship:

$$Z = K \times L / V$$

where L is the distance between the measuring electrodes and K is a constant coefficient.

In the present study, we processed impedance data recorded in TVI configuration (i.e, between one atrial and one ventricular electrode) by approximating the above function as a line with negative slope [3]. This allowed quick calculation of relative variations in EDV, ESV, SV, EF, and EF_c (a contractility index), with respect to the resting values. Moving from lying to upright position induced EDV reduction, which is probably the expression of the decrease in venous return and diastolic ventricular filling, and affected SV according to Starling's law. Even if SV was decreased, the contractility index EF_c was not directly affected by posture, showing only small variations which paralleled the changes in sinus rate. In contrast, both SV and EF_c promptly increased during physical exercise. The good sensitivity to conditions of increased cardiac output demand, in the absence of postural influence and of any positive feedback due to cardiac rate changes [10-12], makes TVI a promising hemodynamic sensor in pacing treatment of chronotropic incompetence.

References

1. Malinowski K (1998) Interindividual comparison of different sensor principles for rate adaptive pacing. Pacing Clin Electrophysiol 21:2209-2213
2. Chirife R (1991) Acquisition of hemodynamic data and sensor signals for rate control from standard pacing electrodes. Pacing Clin Electrophysiol 14:1563-1565

3. Chirife R, Ortega DF, Salazar A (1993) Feasibility of measuring relative right ventricular volumes and ejection fraction with implantable rhythm control devices. Pacing Clin Electrophysiol 16:1673-1683

4. Heynen H, Sharma A, Sutton R et al (1991) Clinical experience with VVIR pacing based on right ventricular dP/dt. Eur J Cardiac Pacing Electrophysiol 1:138-146

5. Bennett T, Sharma A, Sutton R et al (1992) Development of a rate adaptive pacemaker based on the maximum rate-of-rise of right ventricular pressure (RV dP/dtmax). Pacing Clin Electrophysiol 15:219-234

6. Kay GN, Philippon F, Bubien RS et al (1994) Rate modulated pacing based on right ventricular dP/dt: quantitative analysis of chronotropic response. Pacing Clin Electrophysiol 17:1344-1354

7. Salo RW, Wallner TG, Pederson BD (1986) Measurement of ventricular volume by intracardiac impedance: theoretical and empirical approaches. IEEE Trans Biomed Eng 33:189-195

8. Woodard JC, Bertram CD, Gow BS (1987) Right ventricular volumetry by catheter measurement of conductance. Pacing Clin Electrophysiol 10:862-870

9. Lau CP (1993) Rate adaptive cardiac pacing: single and dual chamber. Futura, Mount Kisco, NY, pp 161-180

10. Di Gregorio F, Morra A, Finesso M, Bongiorni MG (1996) Transvalvular impedance (TVI) recording under electrical and pharmacological cardiac stimulation. Pacing Clin Electrophysiol 19:1689-1693

11. Bongiorni MG, Soldati E, Arena G et al (1997) Transvalvular impedance as a marker of cardiac activity. In: Vardas PE (ed) Europace '97, free papers. Monduzzi, Bologna, pp 525-528

12. Morra A, Panarotto D, Santini P, Di Gregorio F (1997) Transvalvular impedance (TVI) sensing: a new way toward the hemodynamic control of cardiac pacing. In: Vardas PE (ed) Europace '97, free papers. Monduzzi, Bologna, pp 529-533

13. Rickards AF, Bombardini T, Corbucci G, Plicchi G, on behalf of the Multicenter PEA Study Group (1996) An implantable intracardiac accelerometer for monitoring myocardial contractility. Pacing Clin Electrophysiol 19:2066-2071

14. Schaldach M, Hutten H (1992) Intracardiac impedance to determine sympathetic activity in rate responsive pacing. Pacing Clin Electrophysiol 15:1778-1786

15. Schaldach M (1994) The myocardium-electrode interface at the cellular level. In: Aubert AE, Ector H, Stroobandt R (eds) Cardiac pacing and electrophysiology. A bridge to the 21st century. Kluwer Academic, Dordrecht, pp 169-188

Hemodynamic Sensors: Clinical Value in Vasovagal Syncope

Introduction

Devising hemodynamic sensors capable of recognizing an imminent vasovagal faint in the absence of abrupt bradycardia remains a challenge. The ultimate goal is to enable implantable treatment devices, whether pacemakers, drug infusion systems, neural stimulators, or combined systems, to react promptly and reliably interrupt an impending event, whether the hypotension be the result of cardioinhibition, vasodilation, or a combination of both. A more limited goal is to enhance operation of diagnostic instrumentation (e.g., implanted or external loop recorders) in order to facilitate the initial evaluation of syncope patients.

At the present time, cardiac pacemakers are the only implantable devices for which sensors targeted at identifying an imminent vasovagal faint are beginning to see application. However, to date, there is insufficient evidence to demonstrate whether such sensors are either able to detect vasovagal syncope reliably, especially in the absence of abrupt heart rate slowing (i.e., a pure hemodynamic or neurological sensor), or whether indeed sensor operation is critical to treatment efficacy.

Potential Sensor Targets

Most neurally mediated faints are the result of transient cerebral hypoperfusion due to a combined circulatory disturbance in which both peripheral vasodilatation (vasodepressor component) and marked or relative bradycardia (cardioinhibitory component) result in inadequate cerebrovascular perfusion pressure [1-4]. In the case of the vasovagal faint, the routes of afferent neural traffic which trigger these hemodynamic responses are not well established. In certain instances, such as syncope associated with fear or emotional upset, the cerebral cortex clearly plays an important role in initiating and/or "interpret-

Cardiac Arrhythmia Center, University of Minnesota Medical School, Minneapolis, Minnesota, USA

ing" the afferent signals. In others, such as dehydration or prolonged upright posture, the role of central cardiopulmonary receptors sensitive to changes in vascular volume and stretch is strongly suspected. However, in most cases, the origin of the afferent signals is obscure.

Ultimately, afferent neural impulses, whether from cortical or peripheral sites, converge in the medulla (nucleus tractus solitarius) near the nuclei of the vagus nerve, the vasomotor centers, and the hypothalamus. Thereafter, the efferent limb of the reflex incorporates both neural and humoral aspects. In regard to the neural contribution, vasodilatation is thought to be primarily the result of diminished sympathetic vasoconstrictor activity, whereas the cardioinhibitory response in humans is principally due to enhanced efferent vagal tone.

A final element in the "vasovagal reflex" is the arterial baroreceptor system. This system should act to prevent syncope by countering the evolving vasodilatation and bradycardia. In this regard, the often large fluctuations in heart rate, blood pressure, tidal volume, respiratory rate, and other circulatory markers (e.g., subcutaneous blood flow) observed during tilt-table induction of vasovagal faints are probably indicative of attempts at baroreceptor compensation [5, 6]. In some cases circulatory stability is achieved and the faint is aborted.

Each limb of the vasovagal reflex provides opportunities for developing indicators of an imminent faint [7]. However, in reality, only certain aspects of the efferent and feedback loops are addressable with current implantable technology.

Nonhemodynamic Sensors

Several reports, including two multinational randomized clinical trials, have confirmed the treatment effectiveness of cardiac pacing when vasovagal syncope has been recurrent, long-standing, difficult to control, and appears to have a cardioinhibitory component [8-11]. In several of these studies, pacemakers had one or other form of automatic vasovagal syncope detection algorithm; recognition of a vasovagal event by the algorithm resulted in a period of high rate pacing designed to compensate for both the bradycardia and the inevitable concomitant vascular dilatation. In each of these cases, the detection technique was limited to ongoing monitoring of cardiac rate, with intervention based on recognition of abrupt heart rate slowing (i.e., the anticipated accompaniment of cardioinhibitory vasovagal syncope). However, none of the available studies was designed to address directly the actual importance of having a diagnostic sensor system, as opposed to simply having a conventional pacemaker implanted. The on-going VPS2 (Vasovagal Pacemakers Study 2) trial may in part address this issue.

The possibility exists that recognition of altered parasympathetic nervous system activity could be employed as a means of suggesting an imminent faint in susceptible individuals. In theory, direct vagus nerve recording is possible. However, implementation of such a system has yet to be accomplished. In fact, if recognition of changes of vagal nerve traffic have any utility in the identification of imminent vasovagal events, it is more likely that such changes will be detected through surrogate measures of vagal activity such as changes in respiratory pattern or sinus arrhythmia (heart rate variability). In regard to the former, changes in respiration are well recognized to accompany vasovagal faints, beginning with increased tidal volume followed by increased respiratory rate [12, 13].

Microneurographic recordings from muscle sympathetic nerves have advanced our understanding of the vasovagal faint. Such recordings could, in theory, be useful for identifying an imminent vasodepressor response. However, from a practical perspective there are important barriers to be overcome before this approach could become a reality. Most importantly, the methodology for obtaining these recordings is cumbersome, and their long-term stability in "free living" patients is doubtful. Furthermore, it is unknown whether all sympathetic nerve activity is affected simultaneously during a vasovagal faint, and at an appropriately early time. Indeed, in several published examples of microneurographic recordings obtained during spontaneous or induced vasovagal faints [14, 15], muscle sympathetic nerve activity appears to diminish only after a considerable preceding period of hypotension.

Given the low likelihood that direct sympathetic neural recordings will prove feasible in clinical practice, an altered sympathetic neurohumoral environment may be more readily detectable through changes in certain cardiac electrophysiological measures. In this regard, recognition of altered relationships between certain conduction intervals (AV interval, QT interval) and concomitant heart rate (RR interval) are readily accomplished by current implantable systems. However, whether these methods can provide adequate warning of imminent faints is as yet unknown.

Hemodynamic Sensors

Several types of "hemodynamic" sensors have been developed with the potential for application in vasovagal syncope detection. These include systems designed to detect changes in myocardial contractile state (a surrogate for sympathetic neural traffic), and sensors designed to monitor central circulatory pressures.

Cardiac Sympathetic Neurohumoral and Neural Influences

Marked increase of circulating epinephrine levels is a characteristic premonitory feature of the vasovagal faint, especially in younger patients [1-4]. Thereafter, a fall in neural sympathetic outflow to the peripheral vasculature seems to play a role in triggering peripheral vasodilation and hypotension. Therefore, monitoring evolving changes in sympathetic neural and neurohumoral status may provide a means for detecting an imminent vasovagal faint. However, in the absence of practicable techniques for direct in vivo measurement of circulating catecholamines or sympathetic neural activity (see above), indirect methods may prove useful. To this end, both changes in myocardial contractile performance as well as catecholamine-induced changes in cardiac conduction intervals may be useful measures.

A vigorous myocardial contraction, presumably resulting from increased circulating catecholamines and diminished central volume (e.g., upright posture, dehydration, fright, etc.), has been closely associated with vasovagal faints. Consequently, recognition of an abrupt increment in contractile activity (especially in the absence of increased physical activity) may be indicative of an imminent faint [16-22]. Efforts have been made to make use of these effects by measuring changes in right ventricular pressure, pre-ejection index (PEI) and dP/dt [16], and measurements of peak endocardial acceleration (PEA) [18, 19].

Preliminary studies suggest that right ventricular pressure alone is an unsuitable sensor due to the small magnitude of the pressure changes in a chamber as compliant as the right ventricle. PEI, although reported to be useful to trigger rapid pacing in one patient with severe orthostatic hypotension [20], also appeared to exhibit only small and highly variable changes. On the other hand, right ventricular dP/dt_{max} fell about 30% (median) from peak value beginning about 2 min before syncope; thus, changes in right ventricular dP/dt_{max} may merit further evaluation.

In regard to PEA, recordings have been obtained from an endocardial microaccelerometer located in a pacing electrode during induced vasovagal faints [17]. In this configuration, although the lead is in the right ventricular cavity, this recording has been reported to track left ventricular dP/dt closely. Nevertheless, syncope occurred with both low and high PEA values [18, 19]. Consequently, this approach requires further assessment before it can be recommended.

Finally, an impedance plethysmographic technique has been proposed to provide a method for detecting changes in myocardial contractile state [21, 22]. This technique offers a measurement which parallels dP/dt, and thereby may be applicable as a vasovagal syncope sensor. However, clinical studies to date are limited and uncontrolled.

Cerebral Blood Flow

The early recognition of diminishing cerebral blood flow could be among the most specific indicators of an imminent faint. Perivascular flow probes, using ultrasonic or perhaps laser Doppler techniques, might be capable of providing such information. However, miniaturizing such systems to limit power consumption and facilitate implantation is as yet an unmet challenge. Further, the invasiveness of such an approach would clearly limit its applicability in other than extreme cases of recurrent vasovagal syncope.

Heart Rate, Blood Pressure, and Blood Flow Variability

Heart rate, blood pressure, and blood flow variability are recognized accompaniments of evolving vasovagal faints. It is likely that the observed oscillations at least in part reflect attempts by the arterial baroreceptor system to fend off the evolving faint. Whether the early recognition of such oscillations can be used to predict an imminent faint is as yet uncertain.

Heart rate oscillations (i.e., heart rate variability, HRV) during induced vasovagal faints have been studied primarily to provide insight into neurophysiologic changes associated with tilt-induced syncope. Specifically, HRV findings support the concept that susceptible individuals manifest a relative failure of parasympathetic withdrawal immediately following assumption of the upright posture [5]. Conceivably, this observation could form part of a detection algorithm, but the time required to make HRV measurements remains a critical limitation. Some form of "rolling" method could be useful, but it is uncertain whether such an approach could respond promptly enough to recognize a rapidly evolving syncopal event. Subcutaneous blood flow oscillations may be used in a similar manner, but the measurement technique may not be readily adaptable to an implanted device [6].

Conclusions

Early reliable detection of an impending vasovagal faint provides the opportunity for automatic delivery of preventive therapies ranging from cardiac pacing and parenteral drug delivery to neural stimulation. Findings to date, although very preliminary, suggest that no single sensor system will be sufficient. Further, although the potential utility of sensors capable of recognizing vasovagal syncope at an early stage is appealing, there are as yet no conclusive studies documenting their utility.

Acknowledgements. The author thanks Barry L.S. Detloff and Wendy Markuson for assistance in preparation of the manuscript.

References

1. Van Lieshout JJ, Wieling W, Karemaker JM, Eckberg DL (1991) The vasovagal response. Clin Sci 81:575-586
2. Benditt DG, Goldstein MA, Adler S et al (1995) Neurally mediated syncopal syndromes: pathophysiology and clinical evaluation. In: Mandel WJ (ed) Cardiac arrhythmias, 3rd edn. Lippincott, Philadelphia, pp 879-906
3. Quan KJ, Carlson MD, Thames MD (1997) Mechanisms of heart rate and arterial blood pressure control: implications for the pathophysiology of neurocardiogenic syncope. Pacing Clin Electrophysiol 20 (pt II):764-774
4. Lurie KG, Benditt DG (1996) Syncope and the autonomic nervous system. J Cardiovasc Electrophysiol 7:760-776
5. Lippman N, Stein KM, Lerman BB (1995) Failure to decrease parasympathetic tone during upright tilt predicts a positive tilt-table test. Am J Cardiol 75:591-595

6. Benditt DG, Chen M-Y, Hansen R et al (1995) Characterization of subcutaneous microvascular blood flow during tilt-table-induced neurally-mediated syncope. J Am Coll Cardiol 25:70-75

7. Benditt DG, Lurie KG (1997) Sensors for early recognition of imminent vasovagal syncope. In: Raviele A (ed) Cardiac arrhythmias. Springer-Verlag Italia, Milan, pp 428-434

8. Benditt DG, Sutton R, Gammage M, Markowitz T, Gorski JA, Nygaard GA, Fetter J, and International Rate Drop Investigators Group (1997) Clinical experience with Thera DR rate-drop response pacing algorithm in carotid sinus syndrome and vasovagal syncope. Pacing Clin Electrophysiol 20 (Suppl II):832-839

9. Sra J, Jazayeri MR, Avitall B et al (1993) Comparison of cardiac pacing with drug therapy in the treatment of neurocardiogenic (vasovagal) syncope with bradycardia or asystole. N Engl J Med 328:1085-1090

10. Connolly SJ, Sheldon R, Roberts RS, Gent M (1999) The North American Vasovagal Pacemaker Study (VPS). A randomized trial of permanent cardiac pacing for the prevention of vasovagal syncope. J Am Coll Cardiol 33:16-20

11. Sutton R, Brignole M, Menozzi C, Raviele A, Alboni P, Giani P, Moya A for the VASIS Investigators (2000) Dual-chamber pacing is efficacious in treatment of neurally-mediated tilt-positive cardioinhibitory syncope. Pacemaker versus no therapy: a multicentre randomized study. Circulation 102:294-299

12. Kurban AS, Erickson M, Petersen MEV et al (2000) Respiratory changes in vasovagal syncope. J Cardiovasc Electrophysiol 11:607-611

13. Benditt DG, Samniah N (2000) Respiratory changes during the evolving vasovagal faint: physiologic and clinical implications. J Cardiovasc Electrophysiol 11:612-615

14. Wallin BG, Sundlof, G (1982) Sympathetic outflow in muscles during vasovagal syncope. J Autonom Nerv Syst 6:287-291

15. Ellenbogen KA, Morillo CA, Wood MA et al (1997) Neural monitoring of vasovagal syncope. Pacing Clin Electrophysiol 20 (Suppl II):788-794

16. Petersen MEV, Williams TR, Erickson M, Sutton R (1997) Right ventricular pressure, dP/dt and PEI, during tilt-induced vasovagal syncope. Pacing Clin Electrophysiol 20 (Suppl II):806-809

17. Brignole M, Menozzi C, Corbucci G et al (1997) Detecting incipient vasovagal syncope: atrioventricular acceleration. Pacing Clin Electrophysiol (Suppl II):801-805

18. Deharo JC, Peyre JP, Ritter PHet al (1998) A sensor-based evaluation of heart contractility in patients with head-up tilt-induced syncope. Pacing Clin Electrophysiol 21:223-226

19. Deharo JC, Peyre J-P, Chalvidan T et al (2000) Continuous monitoring of an endocardial index of myocardial contractility during head-up tilt test. Am Heart J 139:1022-1030

20. Grubb BP, Wolfe DA, Samoil D et al (1993) Adaptive rate pacing controlled by right ventricular pre-ejection interval for severe refractory orthostatic hypotension. Pacing Clin Electrophysiol 16:801-805

21. Osswald E (1997) Correlation of intracardiac impedance and right ventricular contractility during dobutamine stress test. In: Raviele A (ed) Cardiac arrhythmias. Centro Scientifico Editore, Venice, p 89

22. Occhetta E, Bortnik M, Pedrigi C et al (2000) Pacing rate automatic reaction to neuromediated hemodynamic changes. In: Santini M (ed) Progress in clinical pacing. CEPI, Rome, pp 542-547

Sophisticated Pacemaker Diagnostics: Are They Really Useful in Clinical Practice?

E.M.F. ADORNATO, P. MONEA AND E. ADORNATO

Introduction

With the progress of the electrophysiological and hemodynamic understanding of the heart and further improvements of hardware and software technology, significant progress has been made in cardiac pacemakers (PM) that have made pacing therapy safe and effective, allowing improvement of the patient's hemodynamic status and quality of life as well as his/her survival. However, after PM implantation, a series of problems, sometimes very serious, can arise that can compromise regular PM operation or necessitate its removal.

Diagnostic Functions of Pacemakers

Documentation of clinical events occurring during the follow-up of PM patients and evaluation of the integrity of implanted devices are of great importance. The patient's clinical history is not always diagnostic because of the lack of relationship between symptoms and clinical events in the majority of cases; the usefulness of 24 h Holter monitoring is limited in paroxysmal cardiac arrhythmias and in intermittent clinical events because it reflects a relatively short recording period. On the other hand, the need for diagnostic functions in the implantable PM derives from the newer and nonconventional clinical indications for PM implantation, such as prevention and treatment of supraventricular tachyarrhythmias, vaso-vagal syncope, congestive heart failure, and from complexity of the PM with an increasing number of functions that may reduce the effectiveness of pacing therapy in case of uncritical use of multiple algorithms in inappropriate combinations. However, the complex functions facilitate non-invasive electrophysiologic study, allow the treatment of supraventricular and ventricular tachyarrhythmias by programmed stimulation and allow measurement of the pacing and sensing threshold.

Dipartimento di Cardioscienze, Azienda Ospedaliera "BMM", Reggio Calabria, Italy

Diagnostic functions recently implemented in the newer models of permanent PM are:

- Counters providing quantitative data on atrial and ventricular events, without giving any information on their chronology
- Histograms that collect atrial and ventricular events, place them in rate bins, reporting, over a defined time period, the percentage of sensed and paced cardiac beats, the percentage of atrial and ventricular ectopic beats, the specific types of AV sequence, the trend of daily cardiac rate and the correct operation of the automatic switching of pacing modality, if this function has been activated
- Curves for specific data that are continuously analyzed by the PM (daily heart rate, sensor-modulated rate, response of the sensor activity, etc.)
- Events markers that have different morphology and amplitude in respect to the sensed or paced cardiac beats; registration of events markers, in conjunction with atrial and ventricular intervals, may be particularly helpful when displayed simultaneously with an ECG
- Stored intracardiac electrograms (EGMs) during clinical events, analogous to conventional Holter monitoring. This function, which can be automatically activated in coincidence with a programmable trigger or externally activated by the patient at the onset of any predetermined symptom, is the most important technological innovation in the permanent PM because it provides a storage of numerous data, no longer restricted to statistics concerning PM functioning [1].

The diagnostic functions of permanent PMs help physicians to:

- Obtain information concerning the integrity of the implanted device (battery status and longevity, lead impedance, current drain, etc.) and the value of the programmed parameters
- Assess the operation of the PM and the cause of possible troubleshooting (inefficacy of pacing therapy, sensing problems, detection of false signals, etc.)
- Establish the relationship between symptoms and disorders of cardiac rhythm or other clinical events
- Diagnose type, incidence, rate and duration of symptomatic or asymptomatic cardiac arrhythmias
- Identify the mechanisms associated with the onset of cardiac arrhythmias

Pacemaker Troubleshooting

Troubleshooting of potential device malfunctions and their management in the implanted patients has become a challenge for physicians, considering the rapid escalation of PM therapy and the increased complexity of the new devices [2].

The cardiac pacing threshold is affected by several factors and a loss of atrial or ventricular capture may occur immediately after the implantation procedure or during long-term follow-up.

Accurate and reliable sensing of intracardiac signals is of clinical importance for the effectiveness and safety of antibradycardia pacing therapy. A fixed value of PM sensitivity may lead to detection problems, because atrial and ventricular endocardial signal amplitudes are influenced by several physiologic and pathologic factors, lead design and lead maturation. Atrial undersensing is a frequent phenomenon in DDD and VDD PM because of the low amplitude of atrial signals, and during atrial tachyarrhythmias, especially atrial fibrillation (AF), because of large variations in signal amplitude and signal slew-rates of consecutive tachycardia depolarizations. On the other hand, the programming of high amplifier sensitivity may lead to oversensing of cardiac (T wave, late potentials) and extracardiac signals, leading to pacing output inhibition, high-rate atrial tracked ventricular pacing or antitachycardia pacing programs delivery in cases where an antitachycardia PM has been implanted.

VA cross talk is a relatively common complication of modern DDD or VDD pacing; the atrial circuit senses the R wave and the algorithm diagnoses an existent atrial tachycardia resulting in inadequate mode switching. AV crosstalk (the ventricular circuit senses the atrial stimulus), causing inhibition of the ventricular output, is also frequent in DDD PM.

Diagnostic data from marker events in combination with EGM are extremely useful tools in understanding the clinical patterns and obtaining a normal pacing operation.

Cardiac Arrhythmias in Pacemaker Patients

Patients with permanent PM often have cardiac arrhythmias, different from those requiring the PM implantation, that may be related to the PM activity (asynchronous pacing), the presence of retrograde atrioventricular (AV) conduction or the deterioration of cardiopathy [3, 4].

Endless-loop tachycardias are an arrhythmic complication of DDD pacing, due to retrograde VA conduction detected by the atrial circuit. Modern PM automatically recognize and terminate these arrhythmias by an extension of the post-ventricular atrial refractory period (retrograde P' wave falling in the refractory period is not detected) or commutation of the pacing modality in the DVI mode in cases of a ventricular extrasystole or detection of any tachycardia at a rate equal to the value of the programmed upper rate.

Several clinical studies have documented, during a relatively short follow-up period, a high incidence of AF in patients with both VVI/VVIR or DDD/DDDR pacemakers, especially when implanted for the treatment of sick sinus syndrome; in a large proportion of these patients, no arrhythmias had been detected before the PM implantation. Immediate diagnosis and treatment of AF are important to avoid symptoms and hemodynamic consequences, to reduce the risk of thromboembolism without anticoagulation, and to restore sinus rhythm.

Episodes of sustained or nonsustained ventricular tachycardia (VT) may be present in patients with permanent PM, especially in those with organic cardiopathy and low left ventricular ejection fraction (LVEF), even if the true incidence of these arrhythmias is unknown because of the lack of information from epidemiologic studies. There are many reasons to recognize the presence of VTs in PM-dependent patients. Sustained VT, even when hemodynamically well tolerated, may require electrophysiologically-guided antiarrhythmic therapy, including implantable cardioverter defibrillators (ICDs). Two recent prospective randomized trials have documented that patients with coronary artery disease, LVEF < 35%, nonsustained VT at Holter monitoring and inducibile sustained VT at the electrophysiologic study are at high arrhythmic risk and may benefit from an ICD [5, 6]. Automatic detection of nonsustained VT may be of great importance also in PM patients because it identifies a subgroup of patients at high arrhythmic risk.

Mechanisms of Cardiac Arrhythmia Onset

The diagnostic functions of the sophisticated PM may contribute to the knowledge of the pathophysiologic mechanisms responsible for the onset of cardiac arrhythmias, and are important not only for theoretical considerations but also for therapeutic implications. Analysis of the stored EGMs has detected that frequent atrial premature beats with a "short-long-short" sequence (31% of cases), relative sinus tachycardia (30% of cases), sinus bradycardia (14% of cases) or supraventricular tachycardias (type II atrial flutter, atrial tachycardia) were the main triggering factors of the recurrent AF episodes. It is important to note that retrograde AV conduction or an asynchronous atrial pacing stimulus, falling during the vulnerable atrial period, may be the cause of recurrent AF episodes. Modern models of permanent PM are capable of recognizing the electrophysiologic mechanisms triggering the onset of AF and to correct them by using special algorithms; the same permanent device may also be utilized for the treatment of atrial tachycardias (ATs) which often degenerate into AF by delivering several antitachycardia pacing programs.

Some investigators reviewing stored EGMs have reported different patterns of initiation of VTs that may be particularly useful for the interpretation of the pathophysiological mechanisms of sudden cardiac death in men; "short-long-short" coupling intervals before the initiation of VT were documented in almost of 25% of the analyzed stored events, indicating an increased dispersion of refractoriness as possible trigger. Supraventricular tachyarrhythmias with a rapid ventricular response before the onset of ventricular tachyarrhythmias were documented in approximately 20% of the analyzed stored events, while ventricular premature beats or R-on-T phenomena occurred in a limited number of patients. Moreover, implantable PM could help to clarify the role of the autonomic nervous system in determining sudden cardiac death by the analysis of RR intervals before, during and after the occurring arrhythmias; in fact, several studies have shown that a reduced heart rate variability, indicating an imbalance of autonomic tone, is associated with a high incidence of total mortality in patients surviving acute myocardial infarctions.

Conclusions

The answer to the question raised should be, "The diagnostic functions of sophisticated PM are really useful in clinical practice". However, limitations of the most current PM derive from the limited memory of the device, which do not allow the recording of ECG waveform for several hours, and from difficulties in interpreting the stored intracardiac EGMs in some particular cases.

Diagnostic features and stored EGM recording may be considered the most important technological advances in the last generation of PM; they allow monitoring of the activity of the implanted device, evaluation of the appropriateness of pacing therapy, diagnosis of PM troubleshooting and elucidation of the onset and maintenance of spontaneous cardiac arrhythmias. An increased memory to obtain a wider range of capabilities is required.

References

1. Huikuri H (2000) Effect of stored electrograms on management in the paced patient. Am J Cardiol 86[Suppl]:101K-103K
2. Dodinot B, Houruez P, Sadoul N (1999) Pacemaker troubleshootings. Mediterr J Pacing Electrophysiol 1:268-274
3. Cazeau S, Ritter P, Nitzsche R et al (1994) Diagnosis of atrial arrhythmias using the Holter function of a new DDD pacemaker. Pacing Clin Electrophysiol 17 (Part II):2106-2113
4. Kamalvand K, Tan K, Willems R et al (1996) Use of pacemaker diagnostic functions for recognition and management of cardiac arrhythmias. Pacing Clin Electrophysiol 19 (Part I):514-515
5. Moss AJ, Hall WJ, Cannom DS et al for the Multicenter Automatic Defibrillator Implantation Trial (1996) Improved survival with an implanted defibrillator in patients with coronary artery disease at high risk for ventricular arrhythmia. N Engl J Med 335:1933-1940
6. Buxton AE, Lee KL, Fisher JD et al (1999) A randomized study of the prevention of sudden death in patients with coronary artery disease: Multicenter Unsustained Tachycardia Trial Investivator. N Engl J Med 341:1882-1890

Pacemaker Automaticity: Real Progress or Increased Complexity and Costs?

M.H. Schoenfeld[1] and H.T. Markowitz[2]

Pacemaker automaticity may be defined as the "algorithmic regulation of pacer function based on patient conditions and pacemaker system conditions without the need for clinician input" [1]. Indeed, it does not represent a new concept. More than twenty years ago the "autodiagnostic pacemaker" was described as a device capable of detecting failure to capture and failure to sense, allowing for automatic adjustment of output voltage [2]. Demand pacing automatically adjusts and resets pacemaker timing based on endogenous rhythm. Pulse width stretching was an old concept whereby the pacemaker attempted to maintain constant energy: as battery voltage depleted, the pulse generator would increase pulse width so as to maintain a margin of safety relative to stimulation thresholds. "Regulated outputs" use regulator circuitry for the output voltage of pacing pulses to compensate for gradually decreasing battery voltage. Unipolar systems automatically reverted to asynchronous pacing when myopotentials were sensed so as to prevent undue inhibition of pacer output. "Power on reset" and related approaches allowed for the automatic detection of electromagnetic interference such as electrocautery and set the pacemaker to predetermined settings to prevent unintended setting of parameters by severe interference. With the advent of dual chamber systems, current drains became higher than previous traditional VVI systems; an early elective replacement indicator (ERI) was the automatic change of mode from DDD to VVI so as to conserve battery energy and signal to the patient and physician that ERI had been reached (in effect, an early form of "automatic mode switch").

With time, additional forms of automaticity were incorporated into pacing systems. Rate-responsive systems allowed for pacing rate to be determined automatically as a function of a measured parameter such as activity or minute ventilation. Previously, "hysteresis" allowed for automatic changes in pacing rate depending on the utilization by the patient. Programmers incorporated automaticity by providing default parameters and parameter warnings, i.e.,

[1] Cardiac Electrophysiology and Pacer Laboratory, Hospital of Saint Raphael, Yale University School of Medicine, New Haven, Connecticut; [2]Medtronic Inc., Minneapolis, Minnesota, USA

suggestions to the clinician as to what values were considered safe or "nominal" by the manufacturer, and specific parameter combinations felt to result in potentially inappropriate pacer function were locked out. Potential problems uniquely associated with dual chamber systems were addressed by automatic extension of post-ventricular atrial refractory period (PVARP) following a premature ventricular contraction (PVC) and automatic triggering of ventricular pacing to prevent ventricular inhibition from sensing of atrial pacing ("nonphysiologic atrioventricular delay" or "ventricular safety pacing"). "Automatic" steroid elution at the tip of pacing leads has allowed a lowering of chronic stimulation thresholds.

Current enhancements of automatic function include simple tests for guiding rate-response setup, calculation of strength-duration curves, and the ability to temporarily suspend atrial synchronized ventricular pacing when atrial dysrhythmias are encountered (so-called "automatic mode switching" [3]). Atrioventricular intervals may be programmed to change automatically based on whether the atrial complex is paced or spontaneous or adapted to shorten as a function of increasing atrial rate, or to vary automatically based on the patient's intrinsic atrioventricular conduction. Special features now allow prevention of atrial competitive pacing and the implementation of special algorithms to interrupt pacemaker-mediated tachycardias. In addition, certain devices allow for an automatic switch in polarity to unipolar configuration when failure of a bipolar lead is detected. Perhaps most exciting has been the advent of some pacer systems that automatically confirm capture and adjust pacer output parameters on the basis of the patient's stimulation threshold [4, 5]. Automatic detection of endogenous signals and corresponding self-adjustment of sensitivity to allow adequate sensing margins has also been developed. Automatic antitachycardia pacing algorithms and enhanced defibrillating capabilities have been increasingly refined in the current generation of automatic implantable cardioverter-defibrillators.

To reiterate, then, automaticity has been a concept integral to pacing systems for quite some time, and has been progressively advanced in its application to pacing systems. It has become technologically facilitated with the introduction of microprocessors into implanted pacemakers and rapidly advancing semiconductor technology. Large amounts of memory, fast processors, and sophisticated software have enabled the use of complex algorithms, allowing adaptations in pacing therapy to address changes in the condition of the patient or pacemaker system.

The potential impact of automaticity must be considered as it affects four sectors: patient, physician, industry, and government/third party payors. We have witnessed increasing complexity of generators and programmers in an age when ironically time and/or reimbursement are less commensurate with the task of monitoring patients and their pacing systems. Thus, the incorporation of automaticity into patient follow-up may allow a reduction in frequency and duration of patient visits – certainly more convenient for the patient who lives remote from a follow-up facility or is constantly "on the move." It may also ameliorate some of the problems encountered by the pacer physician, namely increasing patient loads, less time, and demands for increased productivity and improved documentation of enhanced patient outcomes. It may also allow for the timely and appropriate delivery of pacer intervention, e.g., in the case of automatic mode switching for paroxysmal atrial fibrillation, independent of the physician's ability to actually see the patient. On the other hand, there is the concern that automaticity may place pacer follow-up in the hands of inexperienced physicians, inadequately compensating for their lack of expertise in monitoring these devices.

Automaticity may benefit the industrial sector by facilitating pacemaker utilization in developing markets. It may also reduce the reliance upon field engineers and sales representatives for assisting in pacer follow-up, particularly in areas remote from pacemaker centers. Government and third party payors may also appreciate cost savings by the incorporation of automaticity into pacer follow-up. To this day, remarkably, up to one-third of devices may be left programmed to nominal outputs, particularly by implanters who always rely upon a manufacturer's representative [6]. The marked advancement of automaticity may be especially valuable to this cohort of patients. The widespread application of automatic output adjustment may result in fewer generator replacements over time and fewer routine office visits, thereby reducing the economic burden; current guidelines for follow-up and transtelephonic monitoring schedules [7] may warrant revision.

Clearly there are multiple caveats that must be raised in the universal adoption of automaticity to supplant or replace pacer follow-up. Automaticity cannot substitute for important information obtained from a careful history obtained by the physician, such as the presence or absence of symptoms ameliorated or possibly worsened by the pacing system. Physical examination remains paramount to follow-up, particularly in assessing the wound early after implantation [8]. Radiographic assessment provides important information about lead integrity [9] and lead position (early after implantation) that may be otherwise unobtainable.

Furthermore, automatic features may *detect a problem* but may not necessarily *identify the source* of that problem. If an increase in capture threshold is identified, for example, does this reflect a problem with lead position, lead integrity, a change in the electrophysiologic or anatomic milieu, or an alteration in concomitant medication? Timely input from the physician remains critical, so that appropriate interventions may be undertaken before a high-output situation results in premature battery depletion. Automatic features may temporarily remedy a situation, but more definitive action may often be required. Therefore, there must be a mechanism by which to alert the patient and/or physician when more prompt/urgent evaluation is necessary. Device "beeping" (audible alert) has been employed as one alert mechanism, particularly to signal battery depletion or system malfunction in the case of certain defibrillator models, though this has limited application in the case of the hearing-impaired *patient.*

Frequent and automatic determinations of threshold and lead impedance are useful in monitoring device survival and, as previously stated, may enhance longevity. Nonetheless, battery depletion may at times rapidly and unexpectedly occur, despite projected trends based on device utilization and battery capacity. The pacer may not always predict its untimely demise: device failures and recalls remain "a way of life" for the pacer physician [10-12]. Large databases assessing device performance may dictate the need for more frequent visits in the case of a particular pacer model [13, 14]. Thus, the alternative approach to exclusive reliance upon automaticity for device follow-up is a regular follow-up schedule with the pacer physician… but with what frequency?

A variety of follow-up scenarios may be envisioned: (1) total dependence on automaticity (including complete elimination of scheduled clinic follow-ups) possibly aided by future remote monitoring systems; (2) absolute reliance upon regularly arranged patient visits; or (3) something in between (fewer patient visits and/or less time per visit, facilitated by automaticity). It would appear that automaticity will have different impacts on follow-up at different phases in the life of a device [1]. While wound healing, lead positioning, stimulation thresholds, and electrogram sensing are important early following implantation, these issues are of less concern once lead stabilization has occurred; similarly, rate response and timing adjustments are typically of greatest concern early in follow-up and less likely to be an issue unless there is a change in a patient's comorbid clinical conditions. Conversely, projection of remaining device longevity is less of a concern early following implantation but assumes greatest importance as the device approaches elective replacement. While concern about the pacemaker and patient are greatest early after implantation and just prior to generator replacement, automaticity may have its greatest impact during the normal service life of the pacemaker by monitoring, providing adjustments where necessary, and alerting the physician to more intensified follow-up when needed unexpectedly. Advances in telemetry and the availability of world-wide networked computing may lead to further enhancements of automaticity including patient/physician alerting.

Thus, automaticity will undoubtedly enhance, at times complicate, but not eliminate pacer follow-up. It may reduce the frequency of patient visits, especially during the device's middle-of-life. Most likely it will shorten the required time for device evaluation per visit: triaging may take place based on interrogated data, with more extensive assessments required for pacemaker-identified problems. It is conceivable that, with time, enhanced gathering of diagnostic data about both the patient and the pacer system will allow automatic identification and correction of problems and timely/convenient reporting to the following physician; if the pacing system identifies a problem that cannot be readily remedied, it will signal both to the patient and physician that prompt medical attention with corrective action is required. Indeed, the potential utility of automaticity in problem recognition and correction appears infinite, easing the follow-up of increasingly complex devices. Nonetheless, we must apply automaticity to pacemaker follow-up with some degree of caution, lest we place undue reliance upon the technology and insufficient reliance upon ourselves.

References

1. Schoenfeld MH, Markowitz HT (2000) Device follow-up in the age of automaticity. Pacing Clin Electrophysiol 23:803-806
2. Auerbach AA, Furman S (1979) The autodiagnostic pacemaker. Pacing Clin Electrophysiol 2:58-68
3. Lau CP, Tai YT, Fong PC et al (1991) Atrial arrhythmia management with sensor controlled atrial refractory period and automatic mode switching in patients with minute ventilation sensing dual chamber rate adaptive pacemakers. Pacing Clin Electrophysiol 15:1504-1514
4. Jacquemart JF (1995) Autocapture: principe et interêt du concept. Stimucoeur 23:259-262
5. Feld GK, Love CJ, Camerlo J et al (1992) A new pacemaker algorithm for continuous capture verification and automatic threshold determination: elimination of pacemaker afterpotential utilizing a triphasic charge balancing system. Pacing Clin Electrophysiol 15:171-178
6. Bernstein AD, Parsonnet V (1996) Survey of cardiac pacing and defibrillation in the United States in 1993. Am J Cardiol 78:187-196
7. Schoenfeld MH (1996) Follow-up of the pacemaker patient. In: Ellenbogen KA (ed) Cardiac pacing, 2nd edn. Blackwell Science, Cambridge, pp 456-500
8. Byrd CL, Schwartz SJ, Gonzales M et al (1986) Pacemaker clinic evaluations: key to early identification of surgical problems. Pacing Clin Electrophysiol 9:1259-1264
9. Saliba BC, Ardesia RJ, John RM et al (1997) Predictors of fracture in the Accufix atrial "J" lead. Am J Cardiol 80:229-231
10. Goldman BS, Newman D, Fraser J et al (1996) Management of intracardiac device recalls: a consensus conference. Pacing Clin Electrophysiol 19:7-17
11. Kawanishi DT, Song S, Furman S et al (1996) Failure rate of leads, pulse generators, and programmers have not diminished over the last 20 years: formal monitoring of performance is still needed. BILITCH Registry and STIMAREC. Pacing Clin Electrophysiol 19:1819-1823
12. Blitzer ML, Marieb MA, Schoenfeld MH (2001) Inability to communicate with ICDs: an underreported failure mode. Pacing Clin Electrophysiol 24:13-15
13. Schoenfeld MH (1992) Recommendations for implementation of a North American multicenter arrhythmia device/lead database. Pacing Clin Electrophysiol 15:1632-1636
14. Moller M, Arnsbo P (1996) Appraisal of pacing lead performance from the Danish Pacemaker Register. Pacing Clin Electrophysiol 19:1327-1336

Pacemaker/ICD Lead Infection: What Are the Main Intracardiac Echocardiographic Features?

M.G. Bongiorni, G. Arena, E. Soldati, M. Ratti, C. Nardi and M. Mariani

The techniques of transvenous lead extraction have developed over the last ten years, allowing an high success rate [1-8]. Recently, recommendations, indications, facilities and training for extraction of chronically implanted transvenous pacing and defibrillator leads have been published from the North American Society of Pacing and Electrophysiology Lead Extraction Conference Faculty [9]. However, the researches in this field are continuously growing to make it as safe as possible.

The imaging methods currently used in the extraction procedures are fluoroscopy and, sometimes, transesophageal echocardiography (TEE). However, fluoroscopy allows visualization only of radio-opaque structures; thus, important findings such as the presence of vegetations or the relation between the leads and endothelial/endocardial surfaces cannot be appreciated. TEE is very useful for studing the intracardiac portion of leads but it is very difficult to visualize the superior and inferior venous system; moreover, its use during the procedure should require heavy sedation or general anesthesia.

The use of intracardiac echocardiography (ICE) has been demonstrated to be useful in many fields of invasive hemodynamics and electrophysiology [10-13]. ICE allows imaging of cardiac structures from a different perspective than from conventional ultrasound, in which the transducer is external to the structure of interest. Since ICE imaging typically originates from within the structure of interest, an entirely new perspective for the evaluation of vascular and cardiac structure, as well as pathology, has developed.

To date, the use of ICE in the field of pacemaker and ICD lead extraction procedures has not been described. The use of ICE should be helpful in obtaining morphological information visualizing the relationship between the leads and the anatomical structures. It could allow real-time continuous radiation-free monitoring during extraction procedures and an early detection of the possible complications.

Interventional Arrhythmology Unit, Cardiothoracic Department, Cisanello Hospital, University of Pisa, Italy

Materials and Methods

Since the beginning of 1999 we have applied ICE in selected cases of extraction procedures to verify whether this new imaging method could be useful in this field of invasive cardiology. We used a commercially available 9-French/9 MHz catheter (Ultra ICE™, Boston Scientific Corp., San Josè, CA, USA); this is a "direct view" mechanical ultrasound catheter with a rotating transducer mounted at the tip, connected to the motor unit via a flexible drive shaft. The piezo-electric transducer is constructed with a special angle that allows an optimal scanning of the surrounding structures. At the tip of the catheter is a filling port, used to fill the space around the piezo-electric transducer with distilled water, because the ultrasound waves are not well transmitted in the air. It provides a 360°, 4 cm depth penetrating two-dimensional image, perpendicular to the transducer and, therefore, to the shaft of the catheter. The images are viewed in real time and recorded on S-VHS videotape, connecting the catheter to the Clearview Ultra™ console (Boston Scientific Corp.).

The ICE catheter was introduced in the right femoral vein using the 10-French braided soft tip sheath and dilator kit (Boston Scientific Corp.), designed to provide support for positioning the catheter at specific locations in the heart and the vascular system. The catheter was advanced along the sheath to study most of the course of the lead from the superior venous system to the right ventricle.

We used ICE in 17 selected patients submitted to removal of their pacing or defibrillating system. There were 27 leads to remove, 24 pacing and three defibrillating leads. Among the pacing leads 15 were ventricular and nine atrial, while two defibrillating leads were ventricular and one in the superior vena cava. The indications to lead removal were septicaemia (18/27, 66.6%), local infection (6/27, 22.2%), coil fracture (2/27, 0.8%) and severe tricuspid valve incompetence (1/27, 0.4%).

Results

In this particular population, 26/27 (96.3%) of the leads were removed without any significant complication.

The use of ICE was demonstrated to be quite easy and safe; moreover, it provided many items of morphological information. Adherences of leads to vascular and endocardial wall were clearly visualized; as previously described from indirect signs during dilation by sheaths [5], the adherences were frequent at the level of the junction between the innominate vein and the superior vena cava, at the tricuspid valve and at the ventricular portion of the leads. An unexpected observation, exploring the course of leads along the venous system, was that they often appeared outside the lumen of the vein (Fig. 1). The presence and tissue characteristics of the adherences could be visualized, as well as the contacts of leads with the tricuspid valve.

With proper tools it was possible to advance the ICE catheter into the ventricle and study in which way the lead tip was encapsulated. The vegetations along the leads (Fig. 2) and the anatomical structures could be easily visualised and measured. Vegetations were present in five patients; in two of these cases, the TEE was negative, suggesting that ICE is more sensitive than TEE for the detection of vegetations.

The ICE findings also gave information about the integrity of the leads, allowing, for example, to visualize the loss of lead insulation.

In the case of free-floating leads, the proximal end could also be found when the coil was shorter than the insulation, which was not visible with fluoroscopy; this made it easier to capture the leads with particular tools like lassos.

Moreover, the use of ICE allowed us to visualize the progression of the dilating sheaths, often causing a clearly visible mechanical stress of the venous wall during dilatation. No complications related to the use of ICE were observed.

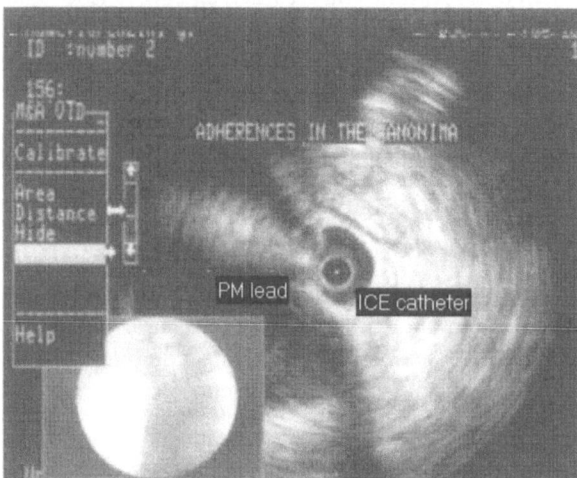

Fig. 1. Cross-section at the level of innominate vein. The ICE catheter is placed inside the vein, while the PM lead is surrounded by an adherence seeming outside of the vein

Fig. 2. Cross-section at the level of junction between superior vena cava and right atrium. The vegetation is clearly visible in close contact with the pacemaker lead

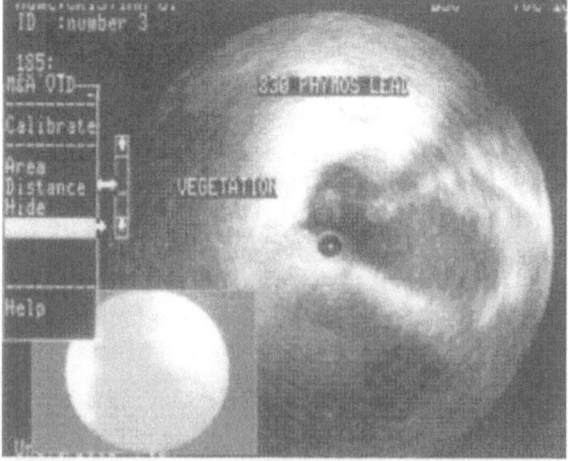

Discussion

The transvenous permanent lead removal procedures are another possible field of application of ICE. Our results showed that ICE gives clear views of the relationship between leads and most anatomical structures as well as pathological findings; therefore it is a very useful radiation-free technique for monitoring extraction procedures.

Catheter-based ultrasound systems, however, have several well-recognized limitations. By necessity, use of these systems is invasive and requires a dedicated with operator expertise; a full array of braided sheaths shapes must also be available. The sheaths and transducers are generally not reusable and can amount to a significant cost. Imaging artifacts, such as nonuniform rotational distortion with mechanical systems, can also limit the accurate use of these systems.

After our initial experience, we suggest that the use of ICE in extraction procedures is mandatory in cases of septicemia or any suspicion of possible vegetations. Moreover, we also recommend its use in the presence of multiple, long-lasting and free-floating leads.

References

1. Bongiorni MG et al (1998) The transvenous removal of definitive electrocatheters for stimulation and defibrillation: the indications, methods and results. Cardiologia 43:1105-1109
2. Byrd CL, Schwartz SJ, Hedin NB et al (1990) Intravascular lead extraction using locking stylets and sheaths. Pacing Clin Electrophysiol 13(part 2):1871-1875
3. Fearnot NE, Smith HJ, Goode LB et al (1990) Intravascular lead extraction using locking stylets, sheaths, and other techniques. Pacing Clin Electrophysiol 13(part 2):1864-1870
4. Byrd CL, Schwartz SJ, Hedin N (1992) Lead extraction. Indications and techniques. Cardiol Clin 10:735-748
5. Smith HJ, Fearnot NE, Byrd CL et al (1994) Five-years experience with intravascular lead extraction. U.S. Lead Extraction Database. Pacing Clin Electrophysiol 17(part 2):2016-2020
6. Manolis AS, Maounis TN, Chilaclakis J et al (1998) Successful percutaneous extraction of pacemaker leads with a novel (VascoExtor) pacing lead removal system. Am J Cardiol 81:935-938
7. Epstein LM, Smith TW (1999) Initial experience with larger laser sheaths for the removal of transvenous pacemaker and implantable defibrillator leads. Circulation 100:516-525
8. Wilkoff BL, Byrd CL, Love CJ et al (1999) Pacemaker lead extraction with the laser sheath: results of the pacing lead extraction with the excimer sheath (PLEXES) trial. J Am Coll Cardiol 33: 1671-1676
9. Love CJ, Wilkoff BL, Byrd CL et al (2000) Recommendations for extraction of chronically implanted transvenous pacing and defibrillator leads: indications, facilities, training. North American Society of Pacing and Electrophysiology Lead Extraction Conference Faculty. Pacing Clin Electrophysiol 23(part 1):544-551

10. Epstein LM (2000) The utility of intracardiac echocardiography in interventional electrophysiology. Curr Cardiol Rep 2:329-334
11. Bruce CJ, Packer DL, Belohlavek M, Seward JB (2000) Intracardiac echocardiography: newest technology. J Am Soc Echocardiogr 13:788-795
12. Ren JF, Schwartzman D, Callans DJ et al (1999) Intracardiac echocardiography (9 MHz) in humans: methods, imaging views and clinical utility. Ultrasound Med Biol 25:1077-1086
13. Daoud EG, Kalbfleisch SJ, Hummel JD (1999) Intracardiac echocardiography to guide transseptal left heart catheterization for radiofrequency catheter ablation. J Cardiovasc Electrophysiol 10:358-363

Percutaneous Extraction of Infected Pacemaker/ICD Leads: What Are the Current Technological Advances and Results?

M.G. Bongiorni, E. Soldati, G. Arena, G. Gherarducci, M. Ratti and M. Mariani

Background

Transvenous removal of permanent pacing and implantable cardioverter-defibrillator (ICD) leads is today an effective and relatively safe technique; its use will probably spread in the future because of the increasing number of pacemaker- or ICD-related complications. Abandonment of functionless pacing leads is becoming relatively common because the performance of the leads decreases with the implant duration [1, 2]. Infection is another complication of implanted devices; it is reported to occur in from 0% up to 19% of the patients [3, 4]. Endocardial ICD leads seem to give rise to the same complications as pacing leads; in ICD patients lead malfunction may result in dangerously inappropriate therapy or none. Infections occurring after implantation of an ICD are reported at an incidence of 2%-7%. All these complications can be treated by percutaneous lead removal. The indications for the procedure have been codified [5, 6] and today's techniques are effective. The success rate of transvenous removal in most reports is now more than 90%, with a low rate of serious, life-threatening complications. Despite these excellent results, however, efforts are still being made to improve both the techniques and the outcome of the procedures, in order to achieve better success rates and a lower incidence of complications.

Transvenous Techniques for Lead Removal

To date, the most extensive experience has been gained with the use of mechanical sheath dissection / contertraction and powered sheath extraction.

Mechanical sheath dissection was introduced into clinical practice by Byrd in the late 1980 and is still the most used technique worldwide. The most widely used extraction system is provided by Cook Vascular Inc. This system is provided with

Interventional Arrhythmology Unit, Cardiothoracic Department, Cisanello Hospital, University of Pisa, Italy

locking stylets and dilator sheaths [7-10]; they are used as first choice when the proximal end of the lead is exposed (superior approach). New stylets developed by Cook allow withdrawal if the attempt is unsuccessful, thus enhancing the flexibility and the safety of the system [11]. The technique in the case of the superior approach consists of a combination of traction by the locking stylet, mechanical dilation of adherences by the dilating sheaths, and countertraction at the tip of the lead by the outer telescopic sheaths. A transvenous workstation with a tip-deflecting wire, Dormier basket, and loop retriever is the tool of choice in cases of totally intravascular leads (inferior approach). The wide experience gained with this system, as reported by the USA registry [12], showed its effectiveness and safety. The removal of ICD leads by using this system has achieved the same results as the removal of pacing leads [13].

A similar system has been developed by VascoMed [14] and has been used in the European registry. The VascoExtor system consists of a locking stylet provided with a remote-control anchoring mechanism at the tip. A rotating motor can be applied to the stylet in order to facilitate the advancement or the withdrawal of the stylet; the system can be used on a wide range of coil lumen dimensions. A dilator sheath and a transfemoral workstation provided with a snare-loop catheter for intravascular lead extraction are also available. Although this system does not provide many tools for dilation of binding sites, the reported results seem to be satisfactory. Table 1 shows the results of two great multicenter registries on mechanical sheath dissection, using the two different systems. As shown in the table, the results of the two systems were quite similar.

The most frequent and dangerous complications of the mechanical dilation techniques are related to tears in the venous wall during dilation or in the heart wall while freeing the tip, leading to hemopericardium or cardiac tamponade. The incidence of complications is anyway not high and seem to be related to the experience of the operators.

In order to improve the effectiveness of the dilation, *powered sheath techniques* were developed in the 1990s, using a source of energy to make dissection of binding sites easier and faster. The first technological advance consisted of laser-assisted sheaths. In these, laser energy is delivered at the edge of a special sheath; at binding sites "lasing" dissects the scar tissue, thus freeing the lead. Table 2 shows the results of two multicenter studies, PLEXES [15, 16] and

Table 1. Results of lead removal using mechanical sheath dissection

	USA registry	Europe registry
No. of leads	2195	150
No. of leads per center	11.4	21.4
System	Cook Vascular	Vascomed
Success rate		
Total	86.8%	81%
Partial	7.5%	12%
Failed	5.7%	7%
Major complications	2.5%	0
Deaths	0.9%	0

Table 2. Results of lead removal using excimer laser-assisted techniques

	Plexes	Plesse
No. of leads	1285	113
System	Spectranetics	Spectranetics
Success rate		
Total	90%	92%
Partial	3%	4%
Failed	7%	4%
Major complications	2.7%	1.1%
Deaths	0.4%	0
Median extraction time (min)	n.r.	12 (1-180)

n.r., not recorded

PLESSE [17], carried out in recent years using the excimer laser sheaths produced by Spectranetics. The final outcome of the removal was similar to that with the mechanical sheath technique, while the incidence of serious complications appeared in many reports to be higher, due to the aggressiveness of the powered dilation. Limitations of the laser technique are the impossibility of dissecting calcified scar tissue or of performing dilation near the tip of the lead, due to the risk of myocardial wall tear [18, 19].

Electrodissection using radiofrequency by Cook Vascular Inc. is another new technique for transvenous lead removal; it is based on the use of dilating sheaths connected to a radiofrequency generator able to induce a thermal effect at their distal end and allows adherences to be cut. This technique is at present under clinical evaluation in the USA; the early reports [20] show effectiveness and safety similar to those of mechanical and laser dilation.

Although the results of the mechanical and powered sheath techniques are similar, the duration of the procedures and consequently of radiation exposure are shorter using powered sheaths; on the other hand, laser techniques are more expensive. The cost/benefit ratio of the two techniques will require careful evaluation in the near future; probably most procedures could be performed by mechanical techniques, while powered sheath techniques could be reserved for selected difficult cases.

Finally, another recent technological improvement in the field of transvenous lead removal is the use of intracardiac echography (ICE), performed using catheters with an echo-transducer at the tip. The use of ICE during transvenous removal procedures can allow determination of the relationships between leads and most anatomical structures better than fluoroscopy; it can be very useful either to detect the presence of vegetation and what becomes of it during dilation, or to monitor the possible occurrence of complications. However, because for the costs, the need for an additional venous puncture and a dedicated operator, we anticipate that ICE will find its role in selected cases where it will be most useful, such as where there are difficult leads, multiple leads, suspicion of vegetation, old leads, or free-floating leads.

Internal Transjugular Approach

Technological advances in transvenous lead removal can be achieved by modi-fying the techniques and the approach as well as improving the materials.

In our personal experience [21] and that of many others [22, 23] it was observed that the success rate of removal was strongly affected by the presence of free-floating leads, calcified scar tissue, or the impossibility of advancing a stylet to the lead. In the presence of these factors, an approach through the right internal jugular vein has some advantages. Most free-floating leads can be exposed via the jugular approach and can thus be subjected to a standard procedure for exposed leads. In addition, the straight course of the lead from the jugular vein to the right atrium or ventricle allows dilation along the longi-tudinal axis of the lead, making both dilation and countertraction easier. These conditions appeared to increase the effectiveness of mechanical dilation and to reduce the risk of complications. On the basis of these observations we devel-oped an internal transjugular approach for free-floating and difficult exposed leads.

Indications

Free-Floating Leads

Since 1994 the internal transjugular approach has been used as the first-choice technique for all free-floating leads submitted for removal at our institution.

Exposed Leads

Since 1996 this approach has been considered in the case of exposed leads where dilation of the binding sites appears particularly difficult. Conversion to the internal transjugular approach was decided on when:
- Lack of progress in dilation of the scar tissue continued for more than 5 min, or
- The stylet did not advance into the coil or stopped proximally to the binding sites requiring dilation.

Technique

The transjugular approach was performed in the electrophysiology laboratory; availability of cardiosurgical intervention should major complications arise was always ensured.

Preconditions for this approach are the possibility of percutaneously cannu-lating the right (or left) internal jugular vein, in the absence of venous obstruc-tion of the innominate and subclavian veins of the same side or of the superior vena cava, and the possibility of grasping the lead proximally to the binding site to dilate it or slip the lead through the binding sites.

Free-Floating Leads

The first step of the procedure consists of investigation of the possibility of catching the lead. If the proximal end of the lead is free, a tip-deflecting wire is advanced through the right femoral vein in order to catch the lead and retrieve it in a position where the proximal end can be approached. A loop retriever is advanced through the internal jugular vein in order to catch the lead as near as possible to the proximal end. Once the lead is grasped, it is exposed through the jugular vein; a standard procedure for exposed leads can be then performed.

Exposed Leads

The technique consists of exposure of the lead through the internal jugular vein. Different approaches are performed in different conditions. If the lead cannot be slipped through the adherences, a deflecting wire is introduced by the femoral vein, the lead is grasped proximally to the binding site and it is made free-floating. If the lead can be slipped though the binding sites, it is grasped distally to these and then slipped and made free-floating by traction performed by the deflecting wire. Once the lead is free-floating, a loop retriever is advanced via the jugular vein, the proximal end of the lead is grasped, and it is exposed through the jugular vein. A standard procedure for exposed leads is then carried out.

Results

From December 1989 to April 2001 we managed 596 patients (405 men, 191 women; mean age 65.2 years, age range 5-93 years) with indications for removal of 936 leads (872 pacing and 64 ICD leads) that had been implanted for a mean of 56.5 months (range 1-276 months). The indications for extraction were class I for 53.8% of the leads and class II in 46.2%.

Since 1994 we have managed 33 consecutive free-floating leads (11 atrial and 20 ventricular pacing leads, and 2 ventricular ICD leads) implanted for a mean of 76.7 months (range 4-216 months) in 29 patients. All these leads were subjected to a transjugular approach. Thirty-two out of 33 leads were exposed and successfully removed by mechanical dilation. For the remaining lead, which was too short to be exposed, the loop retriever was used as an extenstion of the lead, thus allowing effective mechanical dilation. All 33 leads were removed without complications.

Since 1996 the internal transjugular approach has been used for difficult exposed leads, according to the indications listed above. During this period 645 leads (588 pacing and 57 ICD leads) were subjected to a superior approach. Conversion to the transjugular approach was performed for 70 leads (11 atrial and 50 ventricular pacing leads, and 9 ventricular ICD leads). For all leads the technique allowed exposure through the jugular vein; the subsequent mechanical dilation allowed removal of 69 out of 70 leads (98.6%). For one lead dilation of a very tight calcified binding site proved impossible and the patient, who was suffering from systemic infection, underwent surgical lead removal. No complication related to the approach occurred. In one patient cardiac tamponade occurred after the removal of a ventricular pacing lead with a very extensive and tight ventricular binding site; emergency pericardiocentesis and surgical repair were successfully performed.

Between November 1996 and April 2001 670 leads (645 exposed and 25 free-floating leads, 612 pacing and 58 ICD leads) underwent transvenous removal at our institution. The combined use of a standard mechanical dilation technique and the transjugular approach allowed removal of 664/670 leads (99.1%). Among the six unremoved leads, in one the transjugular approach was not effective, in two superior vena cava obstruction made the approach impossible, and in three it was not performed because of the absence of mandatory indications for removal.

Conclusions

Today transvenous removal of pacing and ICD leads is feasible with high success rates and few complications. The results reflect the importance of improvements in both materials and techniques. The presence of binding sites is a key reason for partial or failed removal of a lead; most complications are related to difficulties in freeing leads from binding sites.

Mechanical dilation has been proved in large series to be effective and acceptably safe; on the other hand it often causes chest pain and it is time consuming. The use of powered dilation can probably reduce the duration of most procedures, but so far it has not been proven to increase the overall success rate. On the contrary, the incidence of serious complications seems to have increased with the use of a more aggressive dilation energy source, and the costs of these techniques are higher. The removal of free-floating leads is another problem; using the standard femoral approach, dilation of endoventricular adherences and countertraction is often problematic and sometimes impossible. Powered dilation cannot be used with conventional approaches in the case of free-floating leads.

In our experience, the transjugular approach can be employed in both these difficult situations. It can enhance the effectiveness of mechanical dilation and, by making straight the course of the lead and avoiding narrow turns, can enhance the safety of powered dilation. In addition, it makes it possible to subject free-floating leads to dilation and countertraction techniques. Analyzing our experience, it is impossible to determine what the outcome of removal would have been without this approach, but the success rate achieved (99.1%), without using powered dilation, suggests its high effectiveness. For exposed leads subjected to the superior approach, without conversion to the internal transjugular approach, removal was successful for 570/645 leads (88.2%); the new approach allowed a success rate of 99% (639/645 leads). In our overall experience, excluding free-floating leads, the success rate for removal was 80% before the introduction of the internal transjugular approach and 98.9% after it was introduced. These results may have been influenced by the increasing experience of the operators, but the role of the new approach is surely of key importance.

According to these observations, the combined use of technological improvements and new techniques makes transvenous removal high effective and acceptably safe when performed by experienced operators, thus changing the management of infected or malfunctioning pacing and ICD leads.

References

1. Furman S, Behrens M, Andrews C et al (1987) Retained pacemaker leads. J Thorac Cardiovasc Surg 94:770-772
2. Zerbe P, Ponizynski A, Dyszkiewicz W et al (1985) Functionless retained pacing leads in the cardiovascular system. Br Heart J 54:76-79
3. Rettig G, Doenecke P, Sen S et al (1979) Complications with retained transvenous pacemaker electrodes. Am Heart J 98:587-594
4. Parry G, Goudevenos J, Jameson S et al (1991) Complications associated with retained pacemakers leads. Pacing Clin Electrophysiol 14:1251-1257
5. Byrd CL, Schwartz SJ, Hedin NB (1992) Lead extraction: indications and techniques. Cardiol Clin 10:735-748
6. Love CJ, Wilkoff BL, Byrd CL et al (2000) Recommendations for extraction of chronically implanted transvenous pacing and defibrillator leads: indications, facilities, training. North American Society of Pacing and Electrophysiology Lead Extraction Conference Faculty. Pacing Clin Electrophysiol 23:544-551
7. Byrd CL, Schwartz SJ, Hedin NB et al (1990) Intravascular lead extraction using locking stylets and sheaths. Pacing Clin Electrophysiol 13:1871-1875
8. Byrd CL, Schwartz SJ, Hedin NB (1991) Intravascular techniques for extraction of permanent pacemakers leads. J Thorac Cardiovasc Surg 101:989-997
9. Bongiorni MG, Petz E, Levorato D et al (1991) Removal of chronic leads for permanent pacing. Clinical experience with transvenous extractors. In: Antonioli GE (ed) Pacemaker leads 1991. Elsevier Science, Amsterdam, pp 289-294
10. Bongiorni MG, Arena G, Soldati E, De Simone L (1994) A "step by step" protocol for lead extraction procedures: relation with success rate and complications. Pacing Clin Electrophysiol (abstr)
11. Kennergren C, Schaerf RH, Sellers TD et al (2000) Cardiac lead extraction with a novel locking stylet. J Interv Card Electrophysiol 4:591-593
12. Byrd CL, Wilkoff BL, Love CJ et al (1999) Intravascular extraction of problematic or infected permanent pacemaker leads: 1994-1996. US Extraction Database, MED Institute. Pacing Clin Electrophysiol 22:1348-1357
13. Kantharia BK, Padder FA, Pennington JC et al (2000) Feasibility, safety and determinants of extraction time of percutaneous extraction of endocardial implantable cardioverter defibrillator leads by intravascular countertraction method. Am J Cardiol 85:593-597
14. Reinhardt J, Alt E, Neuzner J et al (1993) Clinic pacemaker lead removal using a new method in 38 patients with 61 implanted leads. Multicenter experience. Pacing Clin Electrophysiol 16:1175 (abstr)

15. Byrd C, Wilkoff B, Love C et al (1997) Clinical study of the laser sheath: results of the PLEXES trial. Pacing Clin Electrophysiol 20:1053 (abstr)
16. Wilkoff BL, Byrd CL, Love CJ et al (1999) Pacemaker lead extraction with the laser sheath: results of the pacing lead extraction with the excimer sheath (PLEXES) trial. J Am Coll Cardiol 33:1671-1676
17. Kennergren C (1997) Initial European experience with excimer laser assisted extraction of permanent pacemaker leads. Pacing Clin Electrophysiol 20:1111 (abstr)
18. Parsonet V, Roelke M, Trivedi A et al (2001) Laser extraction of entrapped leads. Pacing Clin Electrophysiol 24:329-332 (abstr)
19. Epstein LM, Byrd CL, Wilkoff BL et al (1999) Initial experience with larger laser sheaths for the removal of transvenous pacemaker and implantable defibrillator leads. Circulation 100:516-525
20. Wilkoff BL (2000) Transvenous leads extraction with electrosurgical dissection sheaths. Initial experience. Pacing Clin Electrophysiol 23:679-684
21. Bongiorni MG, Soldati E, Arena G et al (1998) The transvenous removal of permanent pacing and defibrillator leads: indications, methods and results. Cardiologia 43:1105-1109
22. Heidi JM, Neal EF, Byrd CL et al (1994) Five-years experience with intravascular lead extraction. Pacing Clin Electrophysiol 17:2016-2020
23. Robboy SJ, Harthorne JW, Leinbach RC et al (1969) Autopsy findings with permanent pervenous pacemakers. Circulation 39:495-501

Interference to Pacemaker/ICD Function by Commonly Encountered Electronic Devices: When and How Much to Worry About?

M. Santomauro, C. D'Ascia, A. Costanzo, L. Ottaviano, G. Donnici and M. Chiariello

Introduction

Electromagnetic interference (EMI) and electromagnetic compatibility (EMC) are problems that increasingly claim the attention of the biomedical industry all over the world. The potential risk of interaction between radiofrequencies of transmitters and medical devices is well documented and frequently reported in the scientific press [1-7]. In a technogically advanced world, radiating EMIs are omnipresent at home, work and other everyday environments (Table 1). They are spread by different modes (Table 2), such as electrical lines or cables, electrostatic induction, electromagnetic radiation, intentional transmitters (radar, radio, TV and satellite transmissions, mobile telecommunication systems, scientific equipment) and unintentional transmitters (induction heaters, electrical equipment, car ignition systems, diathermy generators), and they constitute the main source of disturbance to active medical devices equipped with an electrical circuit prone to detect them.

EMI is a phenomenon that alters the functions of a medical device when it is exposed to an electromagnetic field. EMC is the capability of a device, piece of equipment or system to operate satisfactorily in its own electromagnetic environment, without generating unacceptable electromagnetic disturbances for other equipment. Since 1 January 1996, in compliance with EEC Directive 89/336, Italian law requires that only those products for which the aforementioned capability has been verified can be sold. The EMC problem is created by the coexistence of high-power equipment that generates noise with lower-power devices performing vital functions.

The international organizations (ICNIRP, International Commission On Non-ionizing Radiation Protection; ANSI, American National Standards Institute; and, in Italy, the CENELEC, European Committee for Electrotechnical Standardization) established limits of exposition that, if observed, ensure individual's health protection (Table 3). When an electronic medical device is exposed to radiofrequency (RF) (Fig. 1) signals, RF energy (Table 4) is absorbed by the electronic circuitry and other components, and functioning may be altered.

Department of Cardiology and Cardiac Surgery, University Federico II, Naples, Italy

Table 1. Danger scale of electric household appliances

Household appliance	Microtesla
Ice-cream machine	12
Food grinder	11
Washing machine (during spin-drying)	11
Electric typewriter	11
Electric shaver connected to power line	10
Carpet cleaner	10
Vacuum cleaner	10
Personal computer (the monitor is the major source of magnetic field)	10
Air conditioner (single room, movable)	7-8
Hairdryer	5
Electric oven	4
Television set	4
Sewing machine	3
Portable radio-tape recorder	2
Printer	2
Deep-fryer	2
Video tape recorder	2
Washing machine (during washing)	2
Hi-fi stereo	2
Clock radio	1
Electric knife	1
Desk lamp (halogen lamp)	1
Electric grill	0.6
Toaster	0.5
Iron	0.3
Refrigerator	0.3

Table 2. Sources of electromagnetic interference

Sources of EMI	Frequency range
Monitor	3-30 kHz
Radio AM	30 kHz-3 MHz
Diathermy	3-30 MHz
Radio FM	30-300 MHz
Mobile communication	900-1800 MHz
TV, microwave ovens, radiotherapy	0.3-3 GHz
Radar, satellite transmission	3-30 GHz

Pacemakers (PMs) and implantable cardioverter defibrillators (ICDs) are made up of electronic circuits which can be affected by electromagnetic fields in a negative way even if, currently, these devices are protected from most of electromagnetic sources.

Table 3. Limits of exposition at electromagnetic fields

Corporation	Limits in power's density (W/mq)	
	900 Mhz	1800 Mhz
ICNIRP (Switzerland, Austria, France)	4.5	9
CENELEC	4.5	9
DIN VDE (Germany)	4.5	9
ANSI (USA)	6	12
NRPB (UK)	33	100
Italy	1	1
Places with permanence ≥ 4 h	0.1	0.1

Table 4. Electromagnetic band

Frequency	Denomination
0-10 kHz	Extremely low frequency (ELF)
30 kHz-300 MHz	Radio frequency (RF)
300 MHz-300GHz	Microwave (MW)

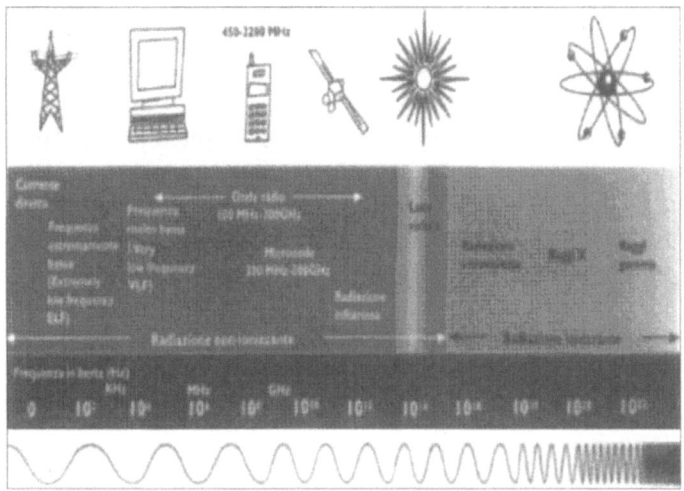

Fig. 1. Electromagnetic band

The effects of EMI on PMs and ICDs are based on several physical factors, such as the strength of the external signal, the distance between the signal and the PM and ICD, the frequency range, modulation type and immunity level of the PM and ICD. The outcome of the effect of EMI on PMs and ICDs can be a temporary or permanent malfunction, such as pacing inhibition by triggering of a ventricular pacing rhythm that is more rapid with VDD and DDD PMs, or asynchronous pacing, or other pacing modes [8-19] (Table 5, 6).

Table 5. Possible pacemaker responses to interferences

a	Single beat inhibition
b	Total inhibition
c	Asynchronous stimulation
d	Increase of stimulating frequency
e	Stimulation at improper frequency

Table 6. Possible defibrillator responses to interferences

a	Unsuitable delivery of shock
b	Unsuitable delivery of antitachycardia therapy
c	Inhibition of antitachycardia therapy
d	Cardioversion therapy inhibition
e	Defibrillation therapy inhibition

Cellular Mobile Phone

Cellular phones have become the most recent concern of sources of electro-magnetic fields [10-23]. Cellular mobile phone services operate within the frequency ranges 872-960 MHz and 1710-1875 MHz (Table 7). The first cellular system employed was the analogue Total Access Communication System (TACS) for which the phones have a nominal output of 0.63 W. This system is being phased out, so that the frequency channels it uses, around 900 MHz, may be allocated to more recent systems. It uses frequency modulation, which results in only very small and essentially random changes in the amplitude of the carrier wave.

Systems using the TACS standard have largely, although not entirely, been replaced by the European digital phone standard, GSM, the acronym for Global System for Mobile Communications, and mostly operate in either the 900 MHz or 1800 MHz bands. This standard is now widely used in many parts of the world. The digital processing uses phase modulation, which again results in only very small and essentially random changes in the amplitude of the carrier

Table 7. Frequency range and power level for mobile communication

Mobile communication	Frequency range	Higher power level (W)	Medium power level (W)
ETACS	872 - 950	0.6	0.006
GSM	890 - 915	2	0.25
DCS 1800	1710 - 1780	1	0.125
DECT	1880 - 1900	0.25	0.01
UMTS	1885 - 2200	n.d.	n.d.

n.d., not determined

wave. In the GSM system, each user requires a frequency channel of bandwidth 200 kHz, so there is a maximum of 174 channels (175, minus one needed for technical reasons) within the 35 MHz width of the 900 MHz band, and 374 within the 75 MHz width of the 1800 MHz band, available for allocation to network operators. The channels are distributed across the cells in a way that allows neighbouring cells to operate at different frequencies to avoid interference. Cells are very often divided into 120 sectors with different frequencies for each. These considerations limit the number of frequency channels available to users in a particular sector. Since the wavelengths at 900 MHz are twice as long as those at 1800 MHz, they are better at reaching the shielded regions behind buildings, etc., as a result of diffraction (bending). Therefore, to obtain the same coverage, fewer base stations and hence fewer channels are needed at 900 MHz than at 1800 MHz.

To increase the number of users that can communicate with a base station at the same time, a technique called time division multiple access (TDMA) is employed, which allows each channel to be used by eight phones. This is achieved by compressing each 4.6 ms chunk of information to be transmitted into a burst or pulse 0.58 ms long (1 ms or millisecond is a thousandth of a second). So the phones and base stations transmit for 0.58 ms, every 4.6 ms, which results in a 217 Hz pulse modulation or variation in their output (217 Hz = 1/4.6 ms). For technical reasons, there is, in fact, additional data compression which leads to the phones and base stations transmitting 25 pulses but omitting every 26th, and so on. This produces further pulse modulation of the power output at the lower frequency of 8.34 Hz (= 217 Hz/26). There is, however, no detectable amplitude modulation at the frequency of 271 kHz (every 4 µs), at which the individual digits (0 or 1) are transmitted, since this leads to a negligible change in amplitude.

The maximum powers that GSM mobile phones are permitted to transmit by the present standards are 2 W (900 Hz) and 1 W (1800 Hz). However, because TDMA is used, the average powers transmitted by a phone are never more than one-eighth of these maximum values (0.25 W and 0.125 W, respectively) and are usually further reduced by a significant amount due to the effects of adaptive power control and discontinuous transmission. Adaptive power control (APC) means that the phone continually adjusts the power it transmits to the minimum needed for the base station to receive a clear signal. This can be less than the peak power by a factor of up to a thousand if the phone is near a base station, although the power is likely to be appreciably more than this in most situations. Discontinuous transmission (DTX) refers to the fact that the power is switched off when a user stops speaking, either because he/she is listening or because neither user is speaking. So if each person in a conversation is speaking for about half the time, he/she is only exposed to fields from the phone for that half of the conversation. In summary, the largest output from a phone occurs if it is mainly used at large distances from the base station or shielded by buildings, etc. In this situation, the peak powers could approach the values of 2 W (900 Hz) and 1 W (1800 Hz) and the average powers could approach the values of 0.25 W (900 Hz) and 0.125 W (1800 Hz).

A third generation of mobile telecommunications technology has now been agreed and will be introduced in the next few years. In Europe this is called the universal mobile telecommunication system (UMTS) and worldwide it is known as international mobile telecommunications–2000 (IMT-2000). The frequency bands identified for this system are 1885-2010 MHz and 2110-2200 MHz. The specifications allow some choice in the modulation to be used but it is expected that the main choice will be code division multiple access (CDMA). The frequency channels will have 5 MHz bandwidths and, as in GSM, each can be used by a number of users at the same time. However, in CDMA, a transmission is "labelled" by a coding scheme that is different for each user. Since all the transmissions occur at the same time, the changes in amplitude of the carrier wave are essentially random (noise-like).

Two types of CDMA are likely to be implemented: frequency division duplex (FDD), where separate 5 MHz channels are used for the two directions (to and from the mobile phone), and time division duplex (TDD), where the same channel is used but in different time slots. Both types lead to pulse modulation because of the need to send regular commands from the base station to change the power level. In FDD the pulse frequency is 1600 Hz, while for TDD it can vary between 100 Hz and 800 Hz.

Digital enhanced cordless telecommunication (DECT) is now in widespread and increasing use and operates at similar frequencies, around 1850 (1800-1900) MHz, to cellular mobile phones. There are ten channels, with a spacing of 1.728 MHz. In each channel there are 24 time slots within a 10 ms frame and the transmission within a slot uses a form of frequency modulation. So a particular phone emits a pulse every 10 ms (100 Hz) during one of the time slots. Since the maximum power emitted is 250 mW, the average power emitted is about 10 mW. Possibly, DECT technology may form part of an overall UMTS system.

The expected demand for the use of UMTS for both speech and data and Internet services is such that systems may be expected to employ macrocells and microcells, and also short-range picocells, to meet the various requirements for mobility and wide bandwidth services, e.g. in the office environment.

Cordless phones are used at very short ranges between a base station located at the telephone socket outlet within the house or office and the cordless phone handset. Earlier cordless phones used analogue technology and are now being replaced by DECT, which has performance advantages in terms of privacy and protection against interference.

The RF power from a phone is mainly transmitted by the antenna together with circuit elements inside the handset. The antenna is usually a metal helix or a metal rod a few centimetres long, extending from the top of the phone. Neither type is strongly directional, although more power is radiated in some directions than others. At points 2.2 cm from an antenna (the distance at which calculations were made), the maximum values of the electric field are calculated to be about 400 V/m for a 2 W, 900 MHz phone, and about 200 V/m for a 1 W, 1800 MHz phone, and the maximum magnetic field is calculated to be about 1 υT for both phones. For both 2 W, 900 MHz phones and 1 W, 1800 MHz phones, the maximum intensity 2.2 cm from the antenna is very roughly about

200 W/m² (this is about one-quarter of the intensity of the sun's radiation on a clear summer day, although the frequency of the emission from a phone is a million or so times smaller). These are the fields and intensities when the antenna is a long way from the head or body. When the antenna is near the body, the radiation penetrates it but the fields inside are significantly less, for the same antenna, than the values outside. For example, the largest maximum fields inside the head when its surface is 1.4 cm from the antenna are calculated to be about three times smaller than the values given above. (The average field values are all appreciably less than these maximum values, for the reasons explained earlier.) As well as these RF fields, which are pulsed at 8.34 Hz and 217 Hz, there are magnetic fields near to the phone that oscillate at these same frequencies, and are a few υT in magnitude. These are generated by currents flowing from the battery, which are switched on and off at these frequencies as a result of TDMA.

An indication of the size of these fields (although not of course any effect they may have) may be obtained by noting that the maximum values of these low- and high-frequency oscillating magnetic fields are about one-tenth or less the size of the Earth's static magnetic field, 50 υT, while the maximum values of the oscillating electric fields outside the body are a few times greater than the electric field at the surface of the Earth due to its static charge. This is directed towards the ground and on a fine day has a constant value of about 100 V/m.

Personal Experience

Our study has evaluated the possible negative effects of environmental electromagnetic radiation on PM and ICD, in vitro and in vivo, which increase the possible health risk for patients due to PM and ICD malfunction.

In our in vitro study, in order to facilitate the study of electromagnetic compatibility problems and certify equipment manufactured, we have used an anechoic chamber in collaboration with Ansaldo Trasporti (Naples Research Center). The anechoic chamber comprises a screened chamber, control and computation system, antenna generation and amplification system, closed circuit television and intercom system.

This system has been used to generate electric fields up to a maximum intensity of 40 V/m in the 10 kHz-1 GHz frequency range. The radiofrequency power level needed to generate electric fields of the required intensity is ensured by two amplifiers, which deliver 1000 W in the 10 kHz-220 MHz range, and 100 W in the 100-1000 MHz range, respectively.

Pacemaker In Vitro Test

We evaluated the effects of a magnetic field with damped wave form motion in the anechoic chamber on four single-chamber PMs (VVI): Opus RM (test a) (Ela Medical); Reflex 8220 (test b); Meta MV (test c) (Medtronic) and Optima

MPT (test d) (Telectronics). The PMs were set on standard activity function by a remote control device that monitored PM before, during and after the test. The PMs were tested in an anechoic chamber at 1 m above the ground in horizontal and vertical positions in order to simulate patient posture. The PMs were connected to the monitor of a Biotronik PM 30 parameter controller by means of a 5.8 m long shielded cable.

The PMs were first immersed in a magnetic field with damped wave form motion at variable current amplitudes (400 impulses/s, from 10-15-20-30-40-50-60-80 voltage/control, current range 100 Å) and then, with electromagnetic fields ranging from 30-220 MHz and 220-1000 MHz. The susceptibility was demonstrated at 70-80 voltage/control.

PM parameters did not change between 200 MHz and 1000 MHz. However, from 30 MHz to 220 MHz we observed temporary malfunctions on all four PMs tested (particularly between 40.78 MHz and 87.85 MHz), with temporary VOO setting at the programmed rate. In two PMs we observed temporary pacing inhibition.

- *Test a*: horizontal PM, nonsusceptible; vertical PM, influenced at 44.03 MHz. Amplitude (A), ↑; pulse width (W), K; frequency (F), K.
- *Test b*: horizontal PM, nonsusceptible; vertical PM, influenced at 51.33 MHz (temporary inhibition) and 87.85 MHz. A, ↑; (W), ↑; (F), ↑.
- *Test c*: horizontal PM, nonsusceptible; vertical PM, influenced at 47.54, 51.33 and 87.85 MHz. A ↑; (W), K; (F), K.
- *Test d*: horizontal PM, nonsusceptible; vertical PM, influenced at 40.78, 81.36, 87.85, and 119.43 MHz (temporary inhibition at 51.33 MHz) (see Figs. 3, 4).

Our in vitro results show that operating ETACS cellular phones do not interfere with PMs. In fact, we did not observe any malfunction when irradiating PMs with frequencies in the 220-1000 MHz range.

Pacemaker In Vivo Test

In our study, we have analyzed 60 PMs and tested 30 different models of PM. The PMs were set on standard activity function. Tests have been practised on PM patients during a standard ambulatory follow-up. The patients were randomized and monitored using a remote control device (Biotronik PM3) and with ECG before, during and after the test. The test consisted of positioning cellular phones, ETACS, GSM and GSM dual-band, during the reception of a phone call, at a distance which from 30 cm was gradually reduced to 15-10-5 cm and finally placed in contact with the patient's pacemaker. The times for which the PMs were exposed to electromagnetic fields generated by cellular phones varied from 8 s to 10 s for each distance, and was for a total of 50 s. At the end of each test, we carried out a functional control and telemetric control of all the parameters programmed.

We observed few effects of interference caused by GSM and GSM dual-band cellular phone, except for the antenna, in 13 (21.6%) PMs of the older generation, constructed before 1997. In particular, there was asynchronous stimulation in eight (13.3%) patients, increase of stimulating frequency in five (8%) patients and inhibition in two (3.3%) patients (Fig. 2). In some cases, the interference was associated with variable symptoms. In no case were symptoms reported when the cellular phone was placed at the ear. Palpitations (3%) were the most commonly reported symptom, light-headedness (1%) or dizziness (1%) and pre-syncope (0.1%) occurred in very few cases, but syncope was never reported (Table 8). All symptoms stopped on removing the cellular phone from the PM.

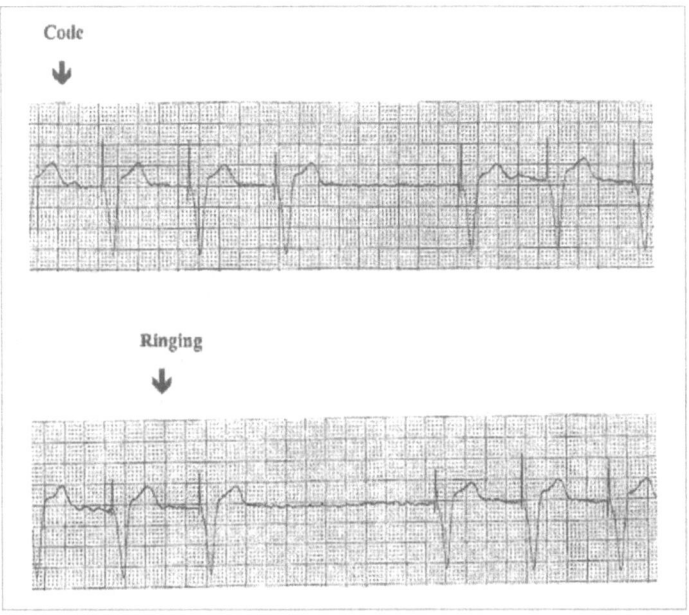

Fig. 2. GSM interference

Table 8. Symptoms caused by EMI

Symptoms	%
Palpitations	3
Light-headedness	1
Dizziness	1
Pre-syncope	0.1
Syncope	0

Defibrillators In Vitro Test

We evaluated the effects of a magnetic field with damped wave form motion in the anechoic chamber, on two ICDs Guardian ATP III (Telectronics) and PCD 7217B (Medtronic). The ICDs were set on standard activity function by a remote control device that monitored the ICD before, during and after the test. The ICDs were tested in an anechoic chamber at 1 m above the ground in horizontal and vertical positions in order to simulate patient posture. The ICDs were connected to the monitor of a Biotronik PM 30 parameter controller by means of a 5.8 m long shielded cable. The ICDs were first immersed in a magnetic field with damped wave form motion at variable current amplitudes (400 impulses/s, 10-15-20-30-40-50-60-80 voltage/control, current range 100 Å) and then with electromagnetic fields of 30-220 MHz and 220-1000 MHz. We did not observe interference on the ICDs.

Defibrillator In Vivo Test

In our study, we analyzed 19 ICDs and tested four different models of ICD. The ICDs were set on standard activity function. The tests were practised on ICD patients during a standard ambulatory follow-up. The patients were randomized and monitored with a remote control device (Biotronik PM3) and with ECG before, during and after the test. The test consisted of positioning cellular phones, ETACS, GSM and GSM dual-band, during the reception of a phone call, at a distance which from 30 cm was gradually reduced at 15-10-5 cm and finally placed in contact with the patient's ICD. The times for which the ICDs were exposed to electromagnetic fields generated by cellular phones varied from 8 s to 10 s for each distance, and was for a total of 50 s. At the end of each test, we carried out a functional control and telemetric control of all parameters programmed.

We observed no effects of interference caused by GSM and GSM dual-band cellular phone.

Our Results

Our results show that PM functioning can rarely be altered by electromagnetic fields generated by cellular phones. The risk of interference is like zero if the cellular phone is placed at 15 cm from the PM location. We have not observed anomalies in ICD functioning [24-26]. Other authors, such as Barbaro et al. [12, 19-21, 27] and Hayes et al. [15], have shown that the risks of interference with cellular phones during everyday utilization do exist, but at a very low risk.

Our recommendations are: keep a distance of at least 13 cm between the phone and the implantable device; do not carry a phone in the breast-pocket or attached to the belt if the device is implanted on the chest or on the abdomen, respectively – this because digital mobile phones keep emitting signals even though they are on stand-by or in receiving mode; use earphones to keep the phone away from the ear; utilize a mobile phone with a maximun power of 2 W (Table 9); if the phone is prevalently used in the car, the phone set must be connected to an external antenna (the strong electromagnetic field emitted by a built-in internal antenna is reflected by the car's metallic frame and reaches the user repeatedly); switch on the phone only when necessary; if symptoms occur, move away from the source or turn off the transceiver.

Table 9. Cellular phones' emission

Less dangerous cellular phones	Watts/ Kg	More dangerous cellular phones	Watts/ Kg
Motorola StarTAC 7860	0.24	Ericsson T28 World	1.49
Qualcomm PdQ-1900	0.26	Nokia Digital 5160	1.45
Mitsubishi Trium Galaxy G-130	0.35	Nokia 5170	1.45
Motorola TalkAbout 2297	0.35	Denso TP 2200	1.44
Motorola ST7797	0.39	Qualcomm QCP-1960	1.41
Motorola StarTAC 7797i	0.42	Sanyo SCP-4500	1.40
Motorola I1000blus	0.43	Sony CMB1200 2200 3200	1.39
Motorola G520	0.46	Nokia 8860	1.39
Motorola M3682	0.46	Motorola StarTAC 7867	1.38
Ericsson KF-688 e DF-688	0.48	Motorola ST7767D	1.38

Antitheft Electronic Article Surveillance Systems

With regard to antitheft electronic article surveillance systems, which are used particularly in supermarkets, shopping centres and bookstores (Figs. 3, 4) Barbaro et al. [29] have observed a sensing threshold variation due to the higher electromagnetic field of the continuous wave gate than the limit established by the standards prEN 45502-2-1 and prEN 45502-2-2 (1998) for the immunity of PMs and ICDs, respectively. McIvor [30] has observed in ICD patients an inappropriate firing in close proximity to a controlled access system. On some occasions, alarm systems and hand-held metal detectors have resulted in shifts in pacing rate and the alterations programmed the pacing, which caused patients with pacemakers to suffer chest pain and syncope. People with implantable defibrillators have received shocks when they got too close to these alarm systems.

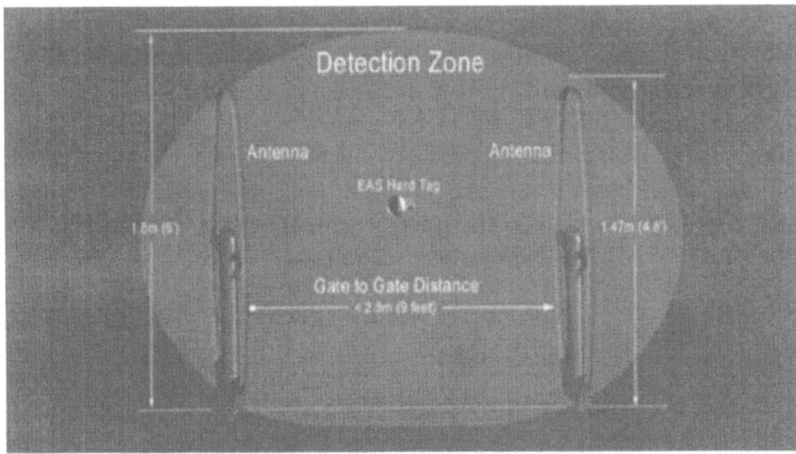

Fig. 3. Antitheft surveillance system

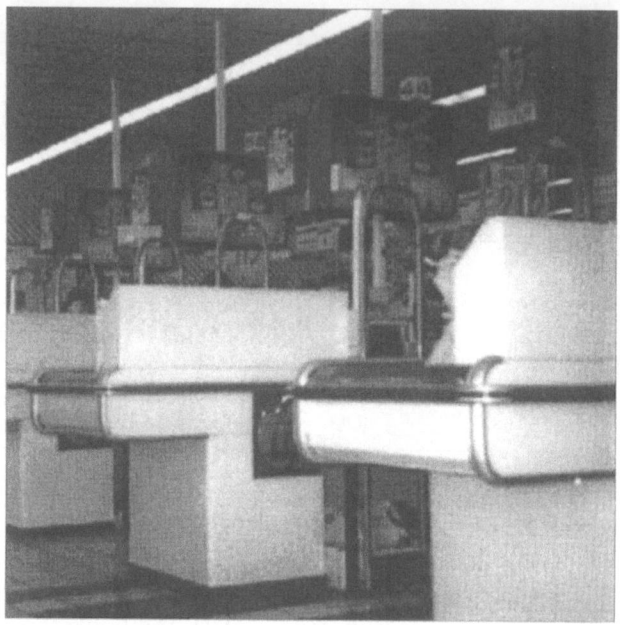

Fig. 4. Antitheft surveillance system in a supermarket

Mugica [36] has analysed data from a total of 408 patient exposures to an antitheft system. The study consisted of an "acoustomagnetic" system that emited an intermittent 58 kHz signal, and a magnetic audiofrequency system that emited a continuous 73 Hz signal. One or more interferences occurred in 17% of patients. Among pacemakers programmed in the DDD mode, a considerably greater prevalence of interference was observed at the atrial vs the ventricular level, despite the same programmed sensing polarity in both chambers. Sensing anomalies were the most commonly induced disturbance and typically lasted for the duration of exposure. No changes occurred in the programming of the pacemakers, and a single patient experienced palpitations during antitheft system-induced rapid pacing. The device interactions were transient and lasted as long as the patients remained in the electromagnetic field of the antitheft system. It is highly desirable that stores using security systems should display a sign stating "Antitheft System in Operation", particularly if they are hidden in walls or under the floor. Patients should identify the locations of the security systems and pass at an ordinary pace through these surveillance gates without standing near or leaning against them.

High-voltage Power Lines

A system that causes EMI is high-voltage power lines (Fig. 5), which switch the PM into asynchronous pacing when the subject is directly under the power line. Inhibition is a much more improbable event, as it depends on the coincidence of several simultaneous causes [4].

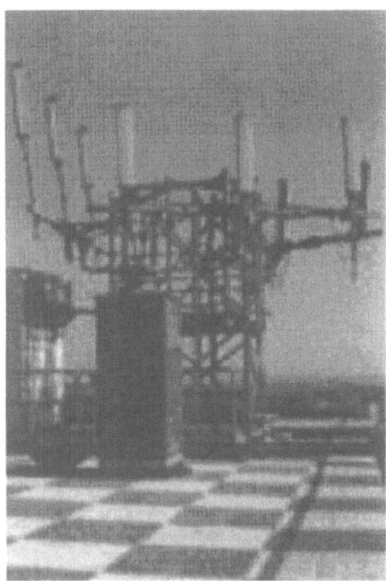 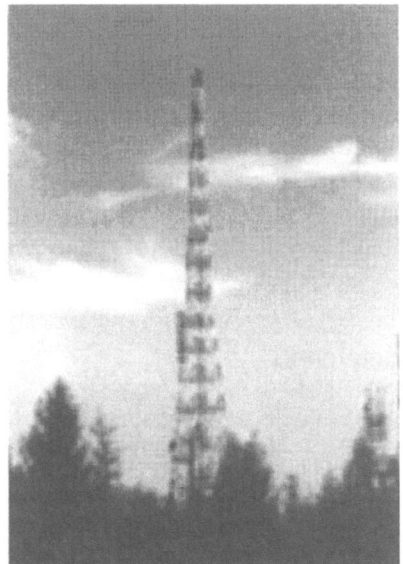

Fig. 5. High-voltage power lines

Nuclear Magnetic Resonance

In contrast, electromagnetic fields generated by nuclear magnetic resonance (NMR) equipment induce permanent or temporary malfunctioning. Consequently, in Italy there is a regulation (Ministerial Decree No. 51 of 1991), in line with the other European countries, that prevents PM and ICD patients from being subjected to NMR analysis. Actually, because in certain cases the risk-benefit relationship could justify this clinical test, Barbaro et al. have demonstrated that in some cases the patients with medical devices can be subjected to NMR. Where sensing was not inhibited, the PMs worked normally, could perfectly detect the variable fields, and were therefore open to interference [31, 32].

High-speed Train ETR 450

In the high-speed train ETR 450, no permanent or temporary malfunctioning of PMs was demonstrated [31].

TELEPASS System

The TELEPASS system causes no permanent or temporary malfunctioning of PMs during transit past the toll-station [28].

Conclusions

EMI is a well-known and long recognized problem that can interfere with implanted electronic medical devices. PM and ICD patients can have, with only some cautions, a low risk of interference by electromagnetic field. However, it is necessary to maintain continuous surveillance on the development of electronic and new technological systems that can generate electromagnetic fields that can interfere with the normal functioning of PMs and ICDs.

References

1. Walter WH, Mitchell JC, Rustan et al (1973) Cardiac pulse generators and electromagnetic interference. J Am Med Assoc 12:1628-1631
2. Imich W (1984) Interference in pacemakers. Pacing Clin Electrophysiol 7:1021-1048
3. Barbaro V, Bartolini P (1999) External electromagnetic interference with implantable cardiac pacemakers and defibrillators. MESPE 1:128-133
4. Barbaro V, Bartolini P, Tarricone L (1991) Evaluation of static magnetic field levels interfering with pacemakers. Physiol Med 7:73-76
5. Toivonen L, Valjus J, Hongisto M, Mesto R (1991) The influence of elevated 50 Hz electric and magnetic fields on implanted cardiac pacemakers: the role of the lead configuration and programming of sensitivity. Pacing Clin Electrophysiol 14:2114-2122
6. Belott P, Sands S et al (1984) Resetting of DDD pacemakers due to EMI. Pacing Clin Electrophysiol 7:169
7. Hayes D (1992) EMI update. 9th Annual National Symposium on Pacing and Arrhythmia control, February
8. Irnich W (1984) Interference in pacemakers. Pacing Clin Electrophysiol 7:1021
9. Telectronics Technical Note (1996) Electromagnetic interference and the pacemaker patients: an update
10. Barbaro V, Bartolini P, Andrea D et al (1995) Do European GSM mobile cellular phones pose a potential risk to pacemaker patients? Pacing Clin Electrophysiol 18:1218-1224
11. Naegeli B, Osswald S, Deola M, Burkart F (1996) Intermittent pacemaker disfunction caused by digital mobile phones. J Am Coll Cardiol 27:1471-1477
12. Barbaro V, Bartolini P, Bellocci F et al (1998) Elecromagnetic interference of digital and analog cellular telephones with implantable cardioverter defibrillators: in vitro and in vivo studies. Pacing Clin Electrophysiol 22:626-6234
13. Ehles C, Andresen D, Bruggemann T et al (1995) Functional pacemaker interference by mobile telephones. Circulation 92[Suppl 1]:1-738 (abstr)
14. Meisei E, Kopscek H, Klinghammer L, Daniel WG (1995) Interference of mobile phones with function of implanted pacemakers – how significant is the risk? Circulation 92[Suppl 1]:1-738 (abstr)
15. Hayes DL, VonFeldt LK, Neubauer SA et al (1995) Effect of digital cellular phones on permanent pacemaker. Pacing Clin Electrophysiol 18:863-871
16. Nowak B, Rosocha S, Zeuerhoff C et al (1996) Is there a risk for interactions between mobile phones and single lead VDD pacemakers? J Am Coll Cardiol 27[Suppl A]:236A (abstr)
17. Carillo R, Williams DB, Traad EA, Schor JS (1996) Electromagnetic filters impede

adverse interference of pacemakers by digital telephones. J Am Coll Cardiol 27[Suppl A]:15 (abstr)

18. Ellenbogen KH, Wood MH (1996) Chiamata urgente o numero sbagliato? J Am Coll Cardiol 27:1478-1479

19. Barbaro V, Bartolini P, Donato A, Militiello C (1996) Interferenze tra telefoni cellulari e pacemaker. Stato dell'arte al 1995. Cardiostimolazione 14:10-19

20. Barbaro V, Bartolini P, Donato A et al (1995) GSM and TACS cellular phones can alter pacemaker function. BEMS Abstract Book: Seventeenth Annual Meeting. Boston, MA, USA, June 18-22; pp 24-26

21. Barbaro V, Bartolini P, Donato A, Militello C (1996) Electromagnetic interference of analog cellular telephones with pacemakers. Pacing Clin Electrophysiol 19:1410-1418

22. Tofani S (1996) Stazioni radio base per la telefonia cellulare e sanità pubblica. AIRM - XIV Atti Congresso Nazionale Caserta, 1-3 Luglio

23. Carrillo R (1995) Preliminary observations on cellular telephones and pacemakers. Pacing Clin Electrophysiol 18:863

24. Santomauro M, Amendolara A, Costanzo A et al (1997) Cellular phones and pacemakers: how do they interact? Cardiac Arrhythmias. Springer-Verlag, Berlin, Heidelberg, New York, pp 514-521

25. Santomauro M, D'Ascia C, Costanzo A et al (2000) Interferenze elettromagnetiche nei portatori di device impiantabili: rischi potenziali o reali? Cardiologia 34th Convegno Internazionale pp 410-414

26. Santomauro M, D'Ascia C, Costanzo A et al (2000) How risk mobile telephones for patients with pacemaker or ICD? Cardiac Arrhythmias. Fifth International Symposium, Springer, Berlin, Heidelberg, New York, pp 58-63

27. Barbaro V, Bartolini P, Donato A et al (1981) GSM cellular phones interferences with implantable pacemakers: in vitro observations. Proceeding of the Vth International Symposium on Biomedical Engineering, Santiago de Compostela, Spain, September pp 275-276

28. Barbaro V, Bartolini P, Donato A, Militello C (1996) Sistema Telepass: analisi dei rischi di interferenza elettromagnetica con pacemaker. Istituto Superiore di Sanità (Rapporti ISTISAN 96/42). Rome, p 56

29. Barbaro V, Bartolini P, Donato A et al (1996) Sistemi automatizzati per il controllo degli accessi: analisi dei rischi sanitari. Istituto Superiore di Sanità (Rapporti ISTI-SAN 96/2). Rome, p 52

30. McIvor ME (1995) Environmental electromagnetic intereference from electronic article surveillance devices. Pacing Clin Electrophysiol 18:2229-2230

31. Barbaro V, Bartolini P, Battisti S et al (1991) Esposizione al campo elettromagnetico e corretto funzionamento dei pacemaker: il caso del treno ad alta velocità ETR450. 54 th Congresso Nazionale della Società Italiana di Medicina del Lavoro e Igiene Industriale, L'Aquila (Italy), October 9-12, pp 1147-1150

32. Bartolini P (1994) Interazione dei campi elettromagnetici prodotti da una risonanza magnetica con protesi e materiali ferromagnetici. Ann Ist Super Sanità 30:51-70

33. Gimbel JR, Johnson D, Levine PA, Wilkoff BL (1996) Safe performance of magnetic resonance imaging on five patients with permanent cardiac pacemakers. Pacing Clin Electrophysiol 19:913-919

34. Dodinot B, Godenir J, Costa AB (1993) Electronic article surveillance: a possible danger for pacemaker patients. Pacing Clin Electrophysiol 16:46-53

35. Lévy S (1999) FESC: ESC statement on possible interference between electronic article surveillance system and implanted pacemakers or defibrillators. Newsletter, May 8

36. Mugica J, Henry L, Podeur H (2000) Study of interactions between permanent pacemakers and electronic antitheft surveillance systems. Pacing Clin Electrophysiol 23:333-337

Biventricular Pacing: How to Predict the Clinical Response in the Single Patient?

M. Gulizia

Congestive heart failure (CHF) is one of the most widespread diseases of the Western world. Its prevalence is about 22.5 million people worldwide and 6.5 million in Europe (747 000 in Italy), with an incidence of 2 million patients/year in the world and 470 000/year in Europe (66 000 in Italy).

In addition to the clinical symptoms such as left ventricular dysfunction, reduced exercise tolerance, and impaired quality of life, these patients often have a markedly shortened life expectancy, with a further worsening in those with heart conduction defects [1-4]. The mortality is 50% in 5 years in all NYHA classes, and 50% in 1 year in NYHA class IV. From 1979 to 1996 mortality due to heart failure increased by 120%. The main causes of death are 40% "sudden cardiac death" and 50% "pump failure", with 10% other causes.

Pharmacological therapy with ACE inhibitors [5-7] and some β-blockers (carvedilol) [8-10] has been shown to reduce the mortality and improve the clinical status in CHF patients, but did not bring any improvement in the electrical conduction abnormalities often present in these patients.

Ten years ago cardiac pacing was proposed as an alternative therapy in patients with drug-refractory heart failure [11]. After initial controversial observations in which some authors described an improvement in cardiac function in patients with CHF treated with dual-chamber right-sided pacing [12-15], in 1995 the results of randomized studies [16, 17] with same pacing parameters as used by the first investigators failed to show any short-term or long-term benefit of right ventricular pacing.

At the end of this period when many authors were investigating the best pacing mode for CHF patients [18], finally, almost at the end of 1990s, some of them demonstrated a role for biventricular pacing compared to conventional pacing (right ventricular apex or right ventricular outflow tract) to increase hemodynamic and functional status in 26 CHF patients with left ventricular bundle branch block (LBBB) [19]. On the basis of this evidence, many other authors explored the role of biventricular pacing as an adjunctive therapy to drugs to treat symptoms in patients with advanced CHF (NYHA

Cardiology, S. Luigi-S. Currò Hospital, Catania, Italy

class III-IV), dilated cardiomyopathy (left ventricular ejection fraction, LVEF < 35%; left ventricular end-diastolic diameter, LVEDD ≤ 60 mm), and ventricular conduction disturbances (QRS ≥ 150 ms). Although the studies were in a small cohort of patients, they all demonstrated the enhancing effect of cardiac resynchronization therapy (CRT) on heart hemodynamic performance, working ability, and quality of life in patients with CHF and uncoordinated contraction [20-24].

These promising improvements in functional capacity with CRT have been recently confirmed by the results of two international studies: the Pacing Therapies for Congestive Heart Failure study (PATH-CHF) [25] and the Multisite Stimulation in Cardiomyopathies study (MUSTIC) [26]. From the results of these two studies and the data from the Italian InSync Registry (InSIR), it has been demonstrated that while the majority of patients "feel better" with CRT (and the benefit has an On-Off effect), approximately 20%-30% of them will experience no clinical improvement with multisite pacing.

Because, in the current cost-conscious health care environment, cost/effectiveness and cost/utility analysis of a new therapeutic strategy will be increasingly used in order to implement a new option only when it really works, and because so far we have no certain way of telling who will benefit most from this therapy, most investigators are looking for a way to predict the clinical response in the individual patient who is a candidate for CRT.

The results of the above-mentioned studies plus the InSIR [27] data will be used to speculate on this matter. Table 1 shows the proposed patient selection of the three studies.

All three studies demonstrated a statistical ($p < 0.001$) improvement in mean NYHA class (almost one class of the classification) in the biventricular (BiV) paced population, as well an increase ($p < 0.0001$ in MUSTIC and InSIR and $p < 0.001$ in PATH-CHF) in the mean distance walked in 6 min. All studies also showed an improvement in the quality of life of the patients by a reduction of more than 30% of the Minnesota Living with Heart Failure test score.

Table 1. Proposed patient selection in the MUSTIC study, PATH-CHF study, and the InSync Italian Registry

MUSTIC
   NYHA class III-IV
   Ejection fraction ≤ 35%
   QRS duration ≥ 150 ms

PATH-CHF
   NYHA Class III-IV
   Ejection fraction ≤ 35%
   QRS duration ≥ 120 ms

InSync Italian Registry
   NYHA Class III-IV
   Ejection fraction ≤ 35%
   QRS duration ≥ 120 ms

MUSTIC and PATH-CHF BiV-paced patients also increased peak oxygen consumption (VO_2) from baseline by more than 8% and than 23% respectively.

All three studies demonstrated a statistically significant reduction in the length of hospital stay, the overall number of hospitalizations, and the rate of hospitalizations per patient in the BiV-paced period [28, 29] (Fig. 1).

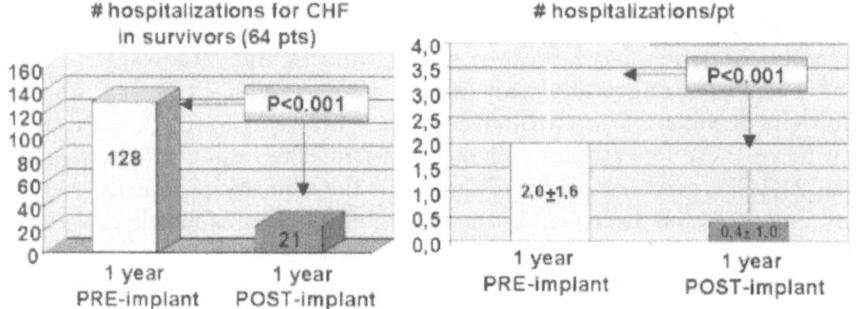

Fig. 1. Reduction in the overall number of hospitalizations and in the rate of hospitalizations per patient in the BiV-paced period in the InSync Italian Registry. Data presented by M Gulizia et al, EUROPACE 2001 [28]

However, although the two published studies and many abstracts on the InSIR data have shown that atriobiventricular pacing increases exercise capacity and quality of life in CHF patients with intraventricular conduction delay without a specific indication for a conventional pacing, no definite indication has been given towards finding any clinical routine-practice predictors able to identify patients who will respond to CRT.

In order to assess the potential acute benefit of multisite cardiac pacing with optimized atrioventricular synchrony and simultaneous BiV pacing in patients with drug-refractory CHF, Leclerq et al. [30] performed an acute hemodynamic study in 18 patients with severe CHF (NYHA class III and IV) and major intraventricular conduction block (QRS duration 170 ± 37 ms). They measured the pulmonary artery pressure, the pulmonary capillary wedge pressure (PCWP), and the cardiac index (CI) in different pacing configurations: atrial pacing (AAI) mode, used as reference, single-site right ventricular DDD pacing, and BiV pacing with the right ventricular lead placed either at the apex or at the outflow tract. Results of the study showed a significant increase in CI with BiV pacing compared to AAI or right ventricular DDD pacing (2.7 vs 2 and 2.4 l/min/m², $p < 0.001$). The PCWP also decreased significantly during BiV pacing compared to AAI (22 vs 27 mmHg; $p < 0.001$).

Although neither QRS duration nor PR interval nor left axis deviation proved to be predictors for distinguishing between responders and nonresponders to DDD BiV pacing, as shown in Table 2, the authors identified a *clinical* predictive parameter in the LVEF ($p < 0.036$) and an *acute* predictive one when they recorded an increase in cardiac output and decrease in PCWP by more than 10% during DDD BiV pacing compared to baseline (AAI mode).

Table 2. Responders and nonresponders patients in the acute studies. (Modified from [30])

	Responders ($n = 12$)	Nonresponders ($n = 6$)	p
QRS (ms)	175 ± 33	163 ± 44	0.5
PR (ms)	234 ± 44	220 ± 38	0.5
LVEF (%)	17 ± 2.7	21.6 ± 5.8	0.036

QRS, Electrocardiographic QRS duration in m/sec; *PR,* PR duration in m/sec; *LVEF,* left ventricular ejection fraction

In another acute study, Kass et al. [31] demonstrated the positive correlation existing between the baseline QRS duration and the %$\Delta dP/dt_{max}$ during left ventricle and BiV pacing. However, because of some discrepancies in the response to BiV pacing observed in some patients with wide QRS, authors postulate that finding the optimal pacing site can play a major role in CRT.

The same results were found by Auricchio et al. [32], who underlined the importance of baseline QRS duration > 150 ms, which was able to identify most of the acute responders to BiV pacing.

To determine whether some factors could predict the long-term clinical effectiveness of CRT, Alonso et al. [33] studied 26 patients with drug-refractory heart failure and wide QRS implanted with a BiV pacemaker. NYHA class, exercise tolerance, and LVEF were recorded at baseline and after pacemaker implantation. Patients were divided into two groups: group I, responders; group II, nonresponders. QRS duration and axis at baseline and during biventricular pacing, interventricular conduction time, and left and right ventricular lead positions were compared between the two groups.

Only QRS duration during BiV pacing differed between the two groups, with a significantly shorter value in group I than in group II (154 ± 17 vs 177 ± 26 ms; $p = 0.016$).

In a study on sensitivity and specificity of QRS duration to predict the acute benefit in CHF patients (PATH-CHF I and II) treated with CRT, Kadhiresan et al. [34] demonstrated that at smaller QRS duration thresholds the specificity tends to be lower, while accuracy was highest (80%) at a QRS duration of 155 ms, with positive and negative predictive values of 77% and 92% respectively.

Recently, Nelson et al. [35] performed cardiac catheterization in 22 CHF patients with a dual-sensor micromanometer to measure LV and aortic pressure during sinus rhythm and LV free wall pacing. Results demonstrated that, although mechanical dyssynchrony is a key predictor for pacing efficacy in CHF patients with conduction delay, combining information about QRS and basal dP/dt_{max} provides an excellent tool by which to identify maximal responders.

Other authors [36] speculating on the idea that pacing two sites with the longest conduction delay will result in the largest improvement in cardiac function *in CHF* demonstrated that applying CRT in these sites does not necessarily produce better hemodynamic improvement in CHF patients.

Some authors [37] have hypothesized that the percentage increase in QRS duration at short atrioventricular delays during BiV pacing can distinguish responder from nonresponder site, while others [38] have demonstrated, in a group of 18 CHF patients in atrial fibrillation treated with BiV pacing compared to a group of 56 in sinus rhythm, that CRT improved both patient groups, suggesting that inter- and intraventricular resynchronization had a more important effect that atrioventricular delay optimization.

In partial contrast with these just-mentioned results, in the analysis of 54/316 patients enrolled in the InSIR [39] who completed the 6-month Minnesota quality-of-life questionnaire or died of progressive heart failure during the first year after implantation, LVEDD was the only significant predictor of clinical outcome. The authors postulate that this could be due to the poor contractility reserve of a very dilated left ventricle, as shown by the LVEF % increasing only in the responders group (Table 3).

Table 3. InSync Italian Registry data: responders vs nonresponders. Responders ($n = 39$) were those who survived for more than 12 months or who at 6-month follow-up showed an increase of more than 30% in the Minnesota quality-of-life questionnaire. Nonresponders ($n = 12$) were those who died during the first 12 months of progressive heart failure or whose quality of life had not improved at 6-month follow-up. Responders had increased EF to 33 ± 3% at 6-month follow-up ($p < 0.001$), whereas nonresponders did not. (Adapted from [39])

	Responders	Nonresponders	p value
Basal NYHA class	3.1 ± 0.6	3.2 ± 0.7	0.62
Basal QRS (ms)	168 ± 37	171 ± 44	0.82
Paced QRS (ms)	144 ± 28	145 ± 32	0.88
LVEDD (mm)	69.7 ± 6.9	74.6 ± 5.3	< 0.05
Basal EF (%)	26 ± 8	24 ± 11	0.54

LVEDD, left ventricular end-diastolic diameter; *EF*, ejection fraction

In conclusion, many investigators are speculating to find reliable predictors of which CHF patients will benefit most from CRT and identify a marker that can predict the clinical response to it. So far, the only certainty is that either BiV or LV pacing alone can significantly improve LV function in the acute term and quality of life and exercise tolerance in the short-to-mid term in a large cohort of patients with intra- or interventricular conduction delay. The results of ongoing trials will perhaps clarify some aspects, such as: the best LV pacing sites, when it is important to perform an acute test before the definitive implantation, how to manage patients with incomplete conduction defects or those with right bundle branch block, when to treat patients with atrial fibrillation, and which patients are candidates for an ICD backup apart from those with conventional class I ACC/AHA indications.

References

1. Cohn JN, Johnson G, Ziesche S et al (1991) A comparison of enalapril with hydralazine-isosorbide dinitrate in the treatment of chronic congestive heart failure. N Engl J Med 325:303-310
2. Captopril Multicenter Research Group (1983) A placebo-controlled trial of captopril in refractory chronic congestive heart failure. J Am Coll Cardiol 2:755-763
3. Stevenson WG, Stevenson LW, Middlekauff HR et al (1996) Improving survival for patients with atrial fibrillation and advanced heart failure. J Am Coll Cardiol 28:1458-1463
4. Aaronson KD, Schwartz S, Chen T-M et al (1997) Development and prospective validation of a clinical index to predict survival in ambulatory patients referred for cardiac transplant evaluation. Circulation 95:2660-2667
5. Opie LH (1995) Fundamental role of angiotensin-converting enzyme inhibitors in the management of congestive heart failure. Am J Cardiol 75:3F-6F
6. Packer AC, Gheorghiade M, Young J et al (1993) Withdrawal of digoxin from patients with chronic heart failure treated with angiotensin-converting-enzyme inhibitors. N Engl J Med 329:1-7
7. The Acute Infarction Ramipril Efficacy (AIRE) Study Investigators (1993) Effect of ramipril on mortality and morbidity of survivors of acute myocardial infarction with clinical evidence of heart failure. Lancet 342:821-828
8. Packer M (1998) Do beta-blockers prolong survival in chronic heart failure? A review of the experimental and clinical evidence. Eur Heart J 19[Suppl B]:B40-46
9. Packer M, Bristow MR, Cohn JN et al (1996) The effect of carvedilol on morbidity and mortality in patients with chronic heart failure. N Engl J Med 334:1349-1355
10. Packer M (2001) Effect of carvedilol on survival in severe chronic heart failure. N Engl J Med 344:1651-1658
11. Hochleitner M, Hortnagl H, Ng CK et al (1990) Usefulness of physiologic dual-chamber pacing in drug-resistant idiopathic dilated cardiomyopathy. Am J Cardiol 66:198-202
12. Auricchio A, Sommariva L, Salo P et al (1993) Improvement of cardiac function in patients with severe congestive heart failure and coronary artery disease by dual chamber pacing with shortened AV delay. Pacing Clin Electrophysiol 16:2034-2043
13. Hochleitner M, Hortnagl H et al (1992) Long term efficacy of physiologic dual chamber pacing in the treatment of end stage idiopathic dilated cardiomyopathy. Am J Cardiol 70:1320-1325
14. Brecker SJ, Xiao HB, Sparrow J et al (1992) Effects of dual-chamber pacing with short atrioventricular delay in dilated cardiomyopathy. Lancet 340:1308-1312
15. Kataoka H (1991) Hemodynamic effect of physiological dual chamber pacing in a patient with end-stage dilated cardiomyopathy: a case report. Pacing Clin Electrophysiol 14:1330-1335
16. Gold MR, Feliciano Z, Gottlieb SS et al (1995) Dual-chamber pacing with a short atrioventricular delay in congestive heart failure: a randomized study. J Am Coll Cardiol 26:967-973
17. Linde C, Gadler F, Edner M et al (1995) Results of atrioventricular synchronous pacing with optimized delay in patients with severe congestive heart failure. Am J Cardiol 75:919-923
18. Brecker SJ, Xiao HB et al (1992) Effects of dual chamber pacing with short AV delay in dilated cardiomyopathy. Lancet 70:1320-1325

19. Blanc JJ, Etienne Y et al (1997) Evaluation of different ventricular pacing sites in patients with severe heart failure: results of an acute hemodynamic study. Circulation 96:3273-3277

20. Cazeau S, Ritter P et al (1994) Four chamber pacing in dilated cardiomyopathy. Pacing Clin Electrophysiol 17:1974-1979

21. Auricchio A, Stellbrink C et al (1999) Pacing therapies for congestive heart failure. (PATH-CHF study). Rational, design and endpoints of a prospective, randomized, multicentric study. Am J Cardiol 83:130-135

22. Saxon L, Boehemer J, Hummel J (1999) Biventricular pacing in patients with CHF: two prospective randomized trials (Vigor CHF). Am J Cardiol 83:120-123D

23. Saxon L, Kerwin WF, De Marco T et al (1998) The magnitude of sympathoneural activation in advanced heart failure is altered with chronic biventricular pacing. Arch Mal Coeur 91:153

24. Gras D, Mabo P, Tang T et al (1998) Multisite pacing as a supplemental treatment of CHF: preliminary results of the Medtronic InSync study (NASPE abstr). Pacing Clin Electrophysiol 21:2249-2255

25. Huth C, Friedl A, Klein H, Auricchio A (2001) Pacing therapies for congestive heart failure considering the results of the PATH-CHF study. Z Kardiol 90[Suppl 1]:10-15

26. Cazean S, Leclercq C, Lavergne T et al (2001) Effects of multisite biventricular pacing in patients with heart failure and interventricular conduction delay. N Engl J Med 344:873-880

27. Padeletti L, Porciani MC, Santini M et al (2001) InSync Italian Registry: long term clinical results of cardiac resynchronization. Europace Suppl 2:B58:787

28. Gulizia M, Ricci R, Lunati M et al (2001) InSync Italian Registry: does biventricular pacing impact on patients hospitalizations? Europace Suppl 2:B59:816

29. Auricchio A, Stellbrink C, Sack S et al (2001) PATH-CHF study: reduced hospitalization days due to heart failure. Europace Suppl 2:B49:471

30. Leclercq C, Cazeau S, Le Breton H et al (1998) Acute hemodynamic effects of biventricular DDD pacing in patients with end-stage heart failure. J Am Coll Cardiol 32:1825-1831

31. Kass DA, Chen CH, Curry C et al (1999) Improved ventricular mechanics from acute VDD pacing in patients with dilated cardiomyopathy and ventricular conduction delay. Circulation 30:1567-1573

32. Auricchio A, Stellbrink C, Block M et al (1999) Effect of pacing chamber and atrioventricular delay on acute systolic function of paced patients with congestive heart failure: the Pacing Therapies for Congestive Heart Failure Study Group: the Guidant Congestive Heart Failure Research Group. Circulation 99:2993-3001

33. Alonso C, Leclercq C, Victor F et al (1999) Electrocardiographic predictive factors of long-term clinical improvement with multisite biventricular pacing in advanced heart failure. Am J Cardiol 84:1417-1421

34. Kadhiresan V, Vogt J, Auricchio A et al (2000) Sensitivity and specificity of QRS duration to predict acute benefit in heart failure patients with cardiac resynchronization. NASPE 2000, part II:555

35. Nelson G, Curry CW, Wyman BT et al (2000) Predictors of systolic augmentation from left ventricular preexcitation in patients with dilated cardiomyopathy and intraventricular conduction delay. Circulation 101:2703-2709

36. Butter C, Auricchio A, Stellbrink C et al (2001) Longer LV-RV delay may not yield better BiVRT outcome in HF. Europace Suppl 2:B11:649

37. Yu Y, Auricchio A, Butter C et al (2001) Assess effectiveness of BiVRT using surface QRS duration. Europace [Suppl 2]B11:770

38. Achilli A, Bocchiardo M, Sassara M et al (2001) Biventricular stimulation: comparison of results of sinus rhythm and chronic atrial fibrillation patients. Europace Suppl 2:B11:612

39. Montenero AS, Santini M, Lunati M et al (2001) InSync Italian Registry: baseline predictive factors of the clinical outcome. Europace Suppl 2:B49:613

40. Lunati M et al (2001) NASPE 2001

Subject Index